Rev. Eugene P. Parisari

BIOETHICS

Third Edition

BIOETHICS

*basic writings on the
key ethical questions that surround
the major, modern biological
possibilities and problems*

edited by
THOMAS A. SHANNON

Cover Design: Tim McKeen

Library of Congress Cataloging-in-Publication Data

Bioethics : basic writings on the key ethical questions
    that surround the major, modern biological
    possibilities and problems.

    Includes bibliographies.
    1. Medical ethics. 2. Bioethics. I. Shannon,
Thomas Anthony, 1940–
R724.B47 1987   174'.2   86-25545
ISBN 0-8091-2805-5 (pbk.)

Published by Paulist Press
997 Macarthur Blvd.
Mahwah, New Jersey 07430

Printed and bound in the
United States of America

"Ethical Problems of Abortion" by Sissela Bok is reprinted from *Hastings Center Studies*,
Vol. 2, No. 1 (January 1974) by permission of the Institute of Society, Ethics and the
Life Sciences, Hastings-on-Hudson, N.Y. 10706. "Breaking Through the Stereotypes"
by Sidney and Daniel Callahan is reprinted by permission from *Commonweal*, Oct. 5,
1984, © 1984 by Commonweal Foundation. "Abortion: On Fetal Indications" by Susan
Nicholson is reprinted by permission of the *Journal of Religious Ethics*, Dept. of Religious
Studies, Knoxville, Tenn. "Abortion: A Review of Ethical Aspects of Public Policy" by
Thomas A. Shannon is reprinted with permission from the *Annual* of the Society of
Christian Ethics, 1982. "Abortion, Euthanasia, and Care of Defective Newborns" by
John Fletcher, Ph.D. is reprinted by permission from *The New England Journal of Med-
icine*, Vol. 292, No. 2 (January 1975). "Mongolism, Parental Desires, and the Right to
Life" by James M. Gustafson is reprinted from *Perspectives in Biology and Medicine*, Summer 1973, by permission of The University of Chicago Press. "Guidelines for Deciding
Care of Critically Ill or Dying Patients" by Raymond S. Duff is reprinted by permission
from *Pediatrics*, Vol. 64, 1979. "Brain Death" by Frank J. Veith and others is reprinted
by permission of the *Journal of the American Medical Association*, Vol. 238 (17 October
1977), © 1977, American Medical Association. "The Right To Die" by Hans Jonas is
reprinted by permission of the *Hastings Center Report*, August 1978, © by the Institute
of Society, Ethics and the Life Sciences, Hastings-on-Hudson, N.Y. 10706. "On Removing Food and Water: Against the Stream" by Gilbert Meilaender is reprinted by permission of the *Hastings Center Report*. "Keeping Dead Mothers Alive During Pregnancy"
by Thomas A. Shannon is reprinted from *The Human Fetus: Dilemmas and Decisions*,
McGraw-Hill 1987, by permission of the McGraw-Hill Book Company. "Philosophical
Reflections on Experimenting with Human Subjects" by Hans Jonas, Ph.D. is reprinted
by permission of *Daedalus*, Journal of the American Academy of Arts and Sciences, Boston, Mass., Spring 1969, *Ethical Aspects of Experimentation with Human Subjects*, 219–247.
"The Ethical Design of Human Experiments" by David R. Rutstein, M.D. is reprinted

*This third edition is rededicated
to my mother and to the memory of my father,
in gratitude for all they have given to me*

Contents

PART THREE
DEATH AND DYING

PART FOUR
RESEARCH AND HUMAN EXPERIMENTATION

PART FIVE
ETHICAL DILEMMAS IN OBTAINING INFORMED CONSENT

PART SIX
GENETIC ENGINEERING

PART SEVEN
THE ALLOCATION OF SCARCE RESOURCES

*   *   *

Preface

The study, evaluation, and resolution of problems in the field of bioethics are complicated by the basic fact of the interdisciplinary nature of such problems. In few other fields does such a wide range of disciplines converge on particular problems. This disciplinary problem is further complicated by continuing advances in medical-scientific technology. As a result, the questions and problems of bioethics come much easier and faster than resolutions—or even clear statements—of the problems. But the very urgency and significance of the problems demand an almost immediate resolution.

The rise of major institutes, the introduction of bioethical courses in colleges, universities, and medical schools, and a veritable flood of publications indicate the seriousness with which these issues are perceived. They also show a wide variety of interpretations and solutions to the problems. Consensus—a difficult task in any case—is more difficult in bioethics because of both the social and personal dimensions of the issues. In addition, there is the diversity of ethical, philosophical and religious frameworks that are brought to bear in an evaluation of the issues. But it also is causing certain issues to come to the fore and be perceived as thematically important for all problems in bioethics. Examples of these issues are the constitutive elements of personhood, the rights of a person, the rights of society, personal integrity, consent and distributive justice. As these are discussed from various perspectives and in differing contexts, the issues are becoming more sharply defined and the topography of the problems is becoming a little clearer.

This reader in bioethics is presented as a contribution to the ongoing discussion of issues such as these. Each article has a specific ethical argument or position, but the various arguments come from an interdisciplinary perspective which helps to broaden their impact. The articles are also very basic and important contributions to the discussions of a particular problem area in bioethics. In addition, each article frames its argument in such a way as to have a long-term interest and significance. The result is a set of articles that are both critical and informative and which also make an on-going contribution to the analysis of problems in bioethics. The topics selected are the standard problem areas of bioethics; they are also very significant human and ethical problems. The way in which these problems are resolved may very well set the tone for our future.

THE THIRD EDITION

I am very flattered to bring this Reader into a third edition. I hope that this version continues to be as helpful to faculty and students as the other editions have been.

When I published the first edition in 1976, bioethics was already a complex field. The complexity of the issues has continued, as well as a proliferation of articles. The selection task has become much more difficult.

The 1976 edition contained twenty-nine articles. The second edition retained seventeen of those articles and added sixteen new ones. The second edition also added a new chapter and included articles on new areas of discussion.

The third edition retains the same organization of sections in distinct topics, with one change. The section on behavior modification has been dropped. This is because not much new material has come out on this topic and because the topic is not as frequently discussed.

Seven articles are retained from the 1976 edition because I think they are classic articles that cogently define several issues. Ten of the new articles from the second edition remain. These, I think, continue to define and discuss thematic issues in bioethics. The third edition adds fifteen new articles for a total of thirty-one articles. These articles discuss a range of current topics, continue old—but unresolved—debates, and open new dilemmas.

The other major change is the deletion of the introductory chapter on Roman Catholic medical ethics. I have replaced this section with a chapter on thematic ethical concepts taken from my revised edition of my *Introduction to Bioethics,* also available from Paulist Press. This chapter will provide a quick overview to thematic concepts in the field of bioethics and can serve as a helpful frame of reference for those studying this topic for the first time.

I would like to thank in a special way my Department Chair, Professor JoAnn Manfra, and Worcester Polytechnic Institute for supporting my work for many years and for providing me with the resources to pursue my interests. While ultimately one works alone, the work is easier when supported by colleagues.

Thomas A. Shannon
Department of Humanities
Worcester Polytechnic Institute

introduction | *Thematic Ethical Concepts*

In treating topics within medical ethics, there are several concepts that recur frequently. It is impossible, for example, to discuss any problem within medical ethics without discussing informed consent. It is also impossible to escape discussions of justifications for our reasoning process.

To prepare you for some of the discussions that will emerge in the various topics and to help give you a basic framework for ethical analysis, this chapter will present, first, a discussion of ethical theories or methods and, second, definitions of basic ethical concepts.

1. ETHICAL THEORIES

In general, an ethical theory is the process by which we justify a particular ethical decision. It is a means by which we organize complex information and competing values and interests and formulate an answer to the question "What should I do?" The main purpose of a theory is to provide consistency and coherence in our decision making. That is, an ethical theory or framework gives us a common means to approach various problems. If we have a theory, we don't have to figure out where to begin each time we meet a new problem. A theory also allows us to develop some degree of consistency in our decision making. We will begin to see how different values relate to each other. If we are consistent and coherent in our decision making, we will have a greater degree of internal unity and integrity in our decision making. Given the complexity of problems to be addressed, these qualities are extremely worthwhile.

a. *Consequentialism*

The ethical theory of consequentialism answers the question "What should I do?" by considering the consequences of various answers. That is, what is ethical is that consequence which brings about the greatest number of advantages over disadvantages or which brings about the greatest good for the greatest number of people.

3

Basically, in this method, one looks to outcomes, to consequences, to the situation, and, from that perspective, one decides what is ethical. The ethical theories of situation ethics and utilitarianism are frequently used types of consequentialist ethical theories.

The major benefit of this theory is that it looks to the actual impact of a particular decision and asks how people will be affected by it. Consequentialism is attuned to the nuances of life and seeks to be responsive to them. The major problem of this theory is that the theory itself provides no standard by which one would measure one outcome against another. That is, while being sensitive to the circumstances, consequentialism has no basis for evaluating one outcome against another.

b. *Deontologism*

Deontological ethics, which derives its name from the Greek word for duty, *deon*, looks to one's obligations to determine what is ethical. This theory answers the question "What should I do?" by specifying my obligations or moral duties. That is, the ethical act is one in which I meet my obligations, my responsibilities, or fulfill my duties. For a deontologist, obligation and rules are primary, for only by attending to these dimensions of morality can one be sure that self-interest does not override moral obligations. The Ten Commandments and Kant's Categorical Imperative are probably the most common examples of deontological ethics.

The major benefit of deontological ethics is the clarity and certainty of its starting point. Once the rules are known or the duties determined, then what is ethical is evident. The major problem is the potential insensitivity to consequences. By looking only at duty, one may miss important aspects of a problem.

c. *Rights' Ethics*

This theory resolves ethical dilemmas by first determining what rights or moral claims are involved. Then dilemmas are resolved in terms of the hierarchy of rights. Paramount for a person of this orientation is that the moral claims of individuals—their rights—are taken seriously. The ethical theory of rights is a popular one in our American culture. Consider, for example, the central role this theory plays in the abortion debate.

The main advantage of a rights' theory is that it highlights the moral centrality of the person and his or her moral claims in a situation of ethical conflict. On the other hand, this theory does not tell us how to resolve conflicts of rights between individuals. The theory makes the claims of the individual central without telling us how to resolve potential conflicts of rights.

d. *Intuitionism*

Intuitionism resolves ethical dilemmas by appealing to one's intuition, a moral faculty of the person which directly apprehends what is right or wrong. Thus an intuitionist knows what is right or wrong, not by appeal to circumstances, duties, or rights, but by appeal to one's moral sense. While one's intuition may confer duties, the duty is not the point of departure; one's moral sense is.

We all know of situations in which all we can say is "I'm doing this because I know it's right," and that is the end of the moral argument. Experientially we know we frequently rely on this method, and the strength that comes from such a moral intuition is great. Nonetheless, if we cannot externalize or publicize in some fashion our process of decision making, we cannot be totally accountable to others. Thus while intuitionism may give us the necessary courage of our convictions, it does not provide us with a way of convincing others that our way is correct.

e. *Summary*

As you read this book and discuss the problems contained in it, you will find yourself using one or more of these methods in trying to convince yourself or others of the correctness of a particular position. You may also find it interesting to adopt one method to see how it works and where it will lead you. Discovering which method you are more comfortable with and being attentive to the methods others are using is a first step toward gaining clarity in one's discussions and debates about complex medical-ethical dilemmas.

2. ETHICAL TERMS

In the course of this book various terms will be frequently used. Philosophers, like physicians, nurses, lawyers, and other professionals, have their own language and jargon. This section will introduce you to some of the basic terms used in bioethical discussions so you can join in on the conversations.

a. *Autonomy*

Autonomy is a form of personal liberty of action in which the individual determines his or her course of action in accordance with a plan of his or her own choosing. Autonomy involves two elements. First is the capacity to deliberate about a plan of action. One must be capable of examining alternatives and distinguishing between them. Second, one must have the capacity to put one's plan into action. Autonomy includes the ability to actualize or carry out what one has decided.

In many ways, autonomy is the all-American value or virtue. It affirms that we ought to be the master of our own fate or the captain of our ship. Autonomy mandates a strong sense of personal responsibility for our own lives. Autonomy celebrates the hardy individualism for which our country is famous. It emphasizes creativity and productivity while being the enemy of conformity. Autonomy mandates that we choose who we wish to be and take responsibility for that.

In celebrating individuality and control of one's self, too heavy a reliance on autonomy can isolate one from the community, from one's family, from one's friends. While ultimately I am responsible for myself and my actions, the community can also be involved in my learning what my responsibilities are and can also set obligations that I need to respect as I make my decisions.

Thus, while autonomy is important, and plays a critical role in bioethics, it needs to be understood within the context of the community as well as other moral responsibilities that I may have.[1]

b. *Nonmaleficence*

Nonmaleficence is the technical way of stating that we have an obligation not to harm people, one of the most traditional principles of medical ethics. "First of all, do no harm." This is the basic principle derived from the Hippocratic tradition. If we can't benefit someone, then at least we should do that person no harm.

The harm we are to avoid is typically understood as physical or mental. But harm can also include injuries to one's interests. Thus I can be harmed by having my property unjustly taken or by having my access to it restricted. Or I can be harmed by having my liberty of speech or action unfairly restricted. Although there is no necessary physical impact on me from these latter harms, nonetheless I am harmed by having my interests constrained.

The duty of nonmaleficence clearly imposes an obligation not to harm someone intentionally or directly. However, it is also possible to expose others to a risk of harm. For example, if I am driving too fast, I may not actually harm someone, but I am clearly exposing individuals to the risk of harm. Thus the duty of nonmaleficence would prohibit speeding.[2]

But there are other situations in which individuals are exposed to the risk of harm and the duty of nonmaleficence is not necessarily violated. An individual receiving chemotherapy is exposed to various risks of harm from the therapy. Can such risks of harm be justified and, if so, how?

The traditional method for examining the legitimation of risks or harmful effects is the principle of double effect. This tradition has its origin in traditional Roman Catholic theology but has gained wide acceptance as a means of judging the moral acceptability of risks and harms.

The principle of double effect[3] has four conditions:

1. What we are going to do must not be evil or wrong. This is simply a restatement of the traditional moral axiom that we are never allowed to do wrong.

2. The harm we are considering must not be the means of producing the good effect. Our proposed action has a harmful dimension but the good end does not justify the means. We cannot do something wrong simply because a good consequence may also follow.

3. The evil or harmful effect may not be intended, but merely permitted or tolerated. For example, when someone has cardiac bypass surgery, one undergoes a risk of death and suffers the direct physical harm of having one's rib cage split open. However, the purpose of the operation is to repair blocked heart arteries, not to cut open one's chest. To repair the arteries, the chest must be cut open.

4. There must be a proportionate reason for performing the action in spite of the consequences the act has. This requires us to weigh a variety of benefits and costs, of values and disvalues. In doing this, one should ensure that the good outweighs the bad. Otherwise the second condition is violated.

In making this proportionalist judgment, Richard McCormick[4] has identified three factors to take into consideration. First, there is at stake a value at least equal in importance to the one sacrificed. Second, there is no less harmful way, here and now, of protecting the good we are seeking to attain. Third, the way the value is achieved should not undermine that value in the future.

McCormick's point is that establishing a proportionate reason is not like solving an arithmetic problem. Rather we need to exercise prudence and gauge the effect of our acts on other values. The duty of nonmaleficence stands as a strong reminder that we have an obligation not to harm, but that when some harm or risk of harm appears to be necessary, then we need to be accountable. The principle of double effect provides that process of justification.

c. *Beneficence*

Beneficence is the positive dimension of nonmaleficence. The duty of beneficence claims that we have a duty to help others further their interests when we can do this without risk to ourselves. Thus the duty of beneficence argues that we have a positive obligation to regard the welfare of others, to be of assistance to others as they attempt to fulfill their plans. The duty of beneficence is based on a sense of fair play. It basically suggests that because we have received benefits from others, because we have been helped along the way, we have an obligation to return that same favor to others. Beneficence is a way of ensuring reciprocity in our relations and of passing along to others the goods we have received in the past.[5]

But this duty is not without limit. The limit is harm to one's self. Beauchamp and Childress have identified a process which one can use to evaluate the risk of harm to determine our degree of obligation. First, the individual we are to help is at risk of significant loss or danger. Second, I can perform an act directly relevant to preventing this loss or damage. Third, my act is likely to prevent this damage or loss. Fourth, the benefits the individual receives as a consequence of my actions (a) outweigh harms to self and (b) present minimal risk to self.[6]

Again we have the necessity of making a prudential calculation about risks and benefits. Sometimes this calculation may be clear. If someone is drowning and I cannot swim, I am not obligated to go in the water to help the person, although I would be obligated to assist in other ways. But the calculation may be problematic. Does a health care professional have a duty to care for someone with AIDS? Here the moral calculus is complicated because of unclarity about the method of transmission, the time of incubation, and the effectiveness of traditional isolation techniques, as well as the as yet incurable nature of the disease.

d. *Justice*

On the one hand, the basic meaning or intent of justice is rather straightforward. Justice deals with the allocation of resources. It is the distribution of benefits and burdens, of goods and services according to a just standard. But determining that just standard has perplexed and puzzled people down through the ages.[7]

There are two basic types of justice. Comparative justice argues that what one person or group receives is determined by balancing the competing claims of other individuals or groups. In comparative justice, what one receives is determined by one's conditions or needs, and how those relate to similar needs of others in society. Thus one person may need a kidney transplant more than another because person A is dying of renal failure while person B has just been diagnosed as having kidney disease. The point of comparative justice is a balancing of the needs of individuals competing for the same resource.

Noncomparative justice determines distribution of goods or resources by a standard independent of the claims of others. Here we have a principle of distribution or treatment, not an evaluation of the specifics or the case of the needs of individuals. Good examples of noncomparative standards are the distribution according to strict numerical equality experience or the legal rule that all are innocent until proven guilty. In noncomparative justice, allocation, distribution and treatment are determined by principle, not need.

Similarly, there are two basic principles of justice: formal and material. The formal principle of justice specifies a procedure to be followed in allocating goods or distributing burdens. The traditional principle of justice is derivative from the Greek philosopher, Aristotle: equals are to be treated equally and unequals unequally. Or to restate it, to each, his or her own.

The formal principle of justice is noncomparative in that it states a rule by which distributions are to be measured. It proposes a standard independent of needs or individuals. However, the rule does not tell how we determine what qualifies for equality or inequality. That is, with respect to what standard is someone equal or unequal? What is morally relevant in our determining equality and inequality? The strength of the formal principle of justice is that it gives us a clear rule; its major deficit is that it does not specify how to apply it.

To cope with the problem of applications, material principles of justice have been devised. Generally speaking, a material principle of justice identifies some relevant property or criterion on the basis of which a distribution can be made. Thus material principles of justice are typically, though not always, comparative in that they examine needs or qualifications and on that basis determine what to do. Let me illustrate this by identifying several of these material principles of justice.

First is the noncomparative material principle of to each an equal share. The standard is strict numerical equality and one arrives at this by dividing what is to be allocated by the number of actual recipients. Second is distribution according to individual need. Here one looks at specific needs of individuals and judges them, one against the other. This, like the third principle of justice—social worth—is obviously comparative. Social worth criteria go beyond needs and evaluate the status of an individual or his or her actual or potential contributions to society. The final form of material justice, which is also comparative, is distribution according to individual effort. This criterion does not examine accomplishments but looks at what one attempted and the efforts to realize that. The higher the effort, the greater the reward.

Each of these principles has its benefits and problems and because of this a middle way has been suggested. This method of allocation emphasizes formal equality but shifts this by utilizing equality of opportunity rather than one of the comparative forms of justice. This method of distribution is randomization either through a lottery or by distribution to people as they show up.

The obvious benefit of this method is that it protects strongly our intuitive sense of respect for people. That is, randomization provides a formal rule of allocation that does not force us to make invidious and potentially harmful choices between people based on assumptions about social worth. Individuals maintain their dignity because they will be treated fairly by having an equality of opportunity. Finally, such a system will help maintain trust between members of the health care team and the patient. The patient is not at the mercy of biases of an institution or individuals, but rather knows he or she will be treated fairly.

On the other hand, this standard does not deal with some important questions. First, should there be some medical screen through which one should pass before entering the door? Second, should one's condition or likelihood of benefit be considered? That is, if a fifteen year old is more likely to benefit from a procedure than an eighty year old, should the eighty year old have an equal opportunity for treatment? Third, the mode of distribution assumes an endless supply of resources in that the only relevant criterion is equality of opportunity, not appropriateness of intervention or resource allocation.

From this discussion one can easily see why discussions of justice are important in bioethics, but also why they are among the most complex.

e. *Informed Consent*

Informed consent is, I think, the most critical problem in bioethics. This is the time when health care professionals and patients can discuss value implications of treatments or clarify what is important for each of them. Consent negotiations allow discussions of issues of importance for all involved parties.

Informed consent is the knowledge of and consent to a particular form of treatment before that treatment is administered. In this definition are four major elements.[8]

1. *Competence.* Competence generally refers to a person's capacity for decision making. A person may experience full competence, in that he or she is in control of his or her life. Or competence may be limited. A person may have decision making capacities in one area but not in another. An individual may not comprehend the value of money and may be restrained in its use but may be quite capable of making other decisions of daily living concerning nutrition, personal hygiene, or

appointment making. Age may also limit competence in that one may be competent for some activities but not others. Finally, and most difficult, one may be intermittently competent. Consider, for example, a person becoming senile. At times this individual may be competent, but at other times he or she may be unaware of the implications of his or her choices.

To help sort out the difficult issues of evaluating competence, three different standards have been proposed. I will present them in order of increasing complexity. The first standard states that a person is competent when he or she has made a decision. When presented with a choice, the individual chooses an alternative. The fact of a choice is evidence of competence. Second is the capacity to give reasons for one's choice. Competence here requires some process of justification, an articulation of why one made this choice. The third standard argues that not only should one be able to give reasons for one's choice, but also that this choice should be a reasonable one.

Each of these standards is different and raises a variety of value judgments. What is most critical is that individuals be aware of what standard of competence they are using and recognize that it may conflict with the judgments of others.

2. *Disclosure.* Disclosure refers to the content of what a patient is told during the consent negotiation. Two general standards for disclosure have been proposed. The first, and more traditional standard, is the professional standard. What a person is told is what professionals typically tell patients. The obligation to inform patients is fulfilled by telling a patient what one's colleagues would tell that same patient. The obvious problem with this standard is that one's colleagues may tell a patient little or nothing. That is, the professional standard may be simply to tell a patient as little as possible about his or her condition. In this situation, the standard is met, the obligation is fulfilled, but the patient remains ignorant.

Obvious problems with that standard led to the development of the more recent standard of the reasonable person. In this perspective, the health care provider is obligated to disclose what the reasonable person would want to know. One cannot fulfill the obligation by saying nothing; some information must be communicated. And the degree of specificity is centered outside the profession in the hypothetical reasonable person. Such a standard promotes autonomy and is protective of patients' rights. Nonetheless it remains on a general level.

This level of generality is why I think it important to go further and determine what *this particular* patient wants to know. Such a standard of disclosure recognizes a patient's right to be informed but, more importantly, it mediates that right with respect to the patient's desires. Some patients may want to know nothing; others may want additional reading they can do. Only by determining what this particular patient wants to know can his or her rights be respected and protected.

3. *Comprehension.* In addition to having information disclosed, one must also comprehend that information. If a patient doesn't understand what he or she has been told, there is no way that individual can use the information.

Comprehension presents many problems and may test the patience of health care professionals. Some may assume that patients simply cannot understand the complexity of the issues. Others may assume that one does not comprehend unless one receives a minicourse in medicine. Or one may assume that there is not sufficient time to fully inform an individual.

Several issues should be noted here. First, from the fact that someone is not *fully* informed, it does not follow that he or she is not *adequately* informed. Second, health care professionals have a professional language. While that language is appropriate for peer communication, it is inappropriate for communication with patients. Thus, professionals need to translate their terms and jargon so it will be intelligible to others. Third, comprehension typically requires time, especially when what needs to be told is not good news. Being informed does not necessitate being told everything at once. Fulfilling the condition of comprehension requires a sensitivity to what a patient can take in at one time.

4. *Voluntariness.* Voluntariness refers to one's ability to make a choice without being unduly pressured to make a particular choice by any specific person. Being free in making a decision means that we own the decision, that the decision is ours, that we have chosen the option.

It seems clear to me that no decision is ever made without some constraints or pressures. No one chooses in a vacuum, in the absence of values or experiences. The moral issue is to remove as much coercion or undue influence as possible so that the decision is the individual's, not someone else's.

Coercion refers to the use of an actual threat of harm or some type of forceful manipulation to influence the person to choose one alternative rather than another. Coercion may take physical, psychological or economic forms. The nature of coercion is perhaps best captured in the widely quoted phrase from the movie *The Godfather:* "I made him an offer he couldn't refuse." This connotes the illusion of choice (made an offer) but, in effect, forecloses all options but one (the one that can't be refused).

Undue influence refers to the use of excessive rewards or irrationally persuasive techniques to short-circuit a person's decision making process. Thus one may use behavior modification techniques to get someone to agree with your decision. One may offer large cash payments or the promise of benefits to induce people to participate in research that has a high risk.

But in either case, the appeal is not to a person's interests, rights, or values. The purpose of coercion or undue influence is to do an end run around choice or judgment so the patient will do what he or she might not ordinarily have done.

f. *Paternalism*

Generally speaking, paternalism involves some sort of interference with the individual's liberty of action. Typically this interference is justified with reference to the person's own good. Paternalism may be *active* in that one acts on behalf of a person but not at his or her request. One may provide a therapy for a person that he or she has not asked for. Or paternalism may be *passive* in that one refuses to help another achieve some goal he or she may have. For example, a physician may refuse to prescribe a tranquilizer because of his or her fears of its abuse by the patient.

James Childress, in his recent book on paternalism,[9] has identified several types that refine this general idea and indicate its different aspects.

1. *Pure and Impure.* Pure paternalism bases its intervention into a person's life on an appeal to the welfare of that person alone. This is the classic model in which parents tell children to eat spinach because it's good for them. Impure paternalism justifies interference with another person because of the welfare of that person *and* the welfare of another. Thus, some argue that a parent who is also a Jehovah's Witness should have a blood transfusion not only because of the good for that person, but also for the good of his or her children.

2. *Restricted and Extended.* A restricted paternalistic intervention is one which overrides an individual's act because of some defect in the person. Thus, one may prohibit a child from doing something because of chronological or psychological incompetence. In extended paternalism, an individual is restrained because what he or she wants to do is risky or dangerous. Thus there are laws that mandate wearing helmets while riding motorcycles or seatbelts while in front seats of cars or when under ten years of age.

3. *Positive and Negative.* A positive paternalistic act, such as forcing a patient into a rehabilitation program, seeks to promote his/her own good. A negative paternalistic intervention, such as taking cigarettes away from someone, seeks to prevent a harm.

4. *Soft and Hard.* In a soft paternalistic act, the values used to

justify the intervention are the patient's values. For example, unconscious or comatose patients are frequently removed from life support systems because they stated that preference in advance of being in that situation. In hard paternalism, the values used to justify an act are not the patient's. This is the classic case of someone else knowing what is good for you and then having you do it or having it done to you.

5. *Direct and Indirect.* In direct paternalism, the person who receives the alleged benefit is the one whose values are overridden. The motorcyclist forced to wear the helmet is the one who assumedly will benefit if there is an accident. In indirect paternalism, one person is restrained so that another individual can receive a benefit. A classic instance is child abuse in which parents are restrained in some fashion to benefit the child.

The desire to help someone or provide a benefit for someone runs deep within the human spirit. Also there are the specific obligations of nonmaleficence and beneficence that we discussed earlier in this chapter. Yet people are autonomous. They know their interests and what is important to them. Respect for persons mandates a presumption against paternalistic interventions. Yet we see harm being done that could be prevented. Can the issues be resolved?

One argument for a paternalistic intervention includes these four steps:

a. The recipient of the paternalistic act actually has some incapacity which prevents or inhibits him or her from making a decision. The person is under undue stress, is a minor, or his or her judgment is impaired in some way.

b. There is the probability of harm unless there is an intervention. Here one needs to determine if all harms are equal. Are physical, mental, or social harms interchangeable?

c. Proportionality. The probable benefit of intervention outweighs the probable risk of harm from nonintervention. Here one needs to be careful of uncritical interventions of extended paternalism.

d. The paternalistic intervention is the least restrictive, least humiliating and least insulting alternative. This criterion argues that one remain as respectful of the individual as possible during the intervention.

This method will not resolve all issues connected with paternalism, but it will force individuals to recognize and justify such paternalistic interventions.[10]

g. *Rights*

The term "rights" is one of the most frequently used in ethics and bioethics. Yet the term is problematic because of its varied meanings and different connotations. This problem is evident even in the origin of the term "rights." In the medieval ethical tradition, we do not find the term "rights"; rather, we find the term "duty." The term "duty" referred to the reciprocal obligation members of a community had to each other. Duties were specific ways in which each helped the other realize the common good of all. In the modern tradition, beginning with the Enlightenment, rights referred to claims of the individual against the state. Rights were a means of carving out a zone of privacy or protection against the ever increasing powers of the state. Thus the term "rights" has two major historical origins and two different connotations.

Current usages of rights language reject elements of this history. Some think of rights as privileges, as social goods that go beyond routine moral obligations. Other think of rights as a sort of social immunity, a protection from powers of the state. Rights are also seen as powers, capacities to act in society. Entitlements are another way of thinking of rights. These are social responses which are seen as deserved, as derivative from being a member of a society. Finally, rights are seen as claims, a moral demand made upon someone or on society.

Also there are different ways to think of rights. One way is to understand them as *moral*. Moral rights are based on an ethical argument and exist prior to and independent of the guarantees of any institution. Frequently these moral rights are rooted in the nature of the person and his or her dignity and are, therefore, understood to be universal and inalienable. A second type of right is *legal*: those rights spelled out by the laws, constitution or political institutions of a particular country or political unit. Legal rights are only those rights granted to citizens by the government. They are specific to particular cultures and are subject to social qualifications. A *positive* right is a claim to a positive action on the part of another person. A positive right entails a duty on the part of someone else to do something. For example, the right of informed consent confers an obligation on the part of a health care professional to tell me relevant information about my diagnosis and treatment options. A *negative* right establishes an obligation for someone to refrain from action. Negative rights establish obligations of noninterference. The legal right to abortion, for example, does not secure an obligation for someone to perform an abortion, rather only that a woman not be interfered with in seeking an abortion.

One of the most difficult problems in rights' theory is establishing who is the subject of a right and on what basis. Animal rights' activists argue, for example, that to have rights one need only be capable of feeling pain or be sentient. Others would suggest that consciousness is enough to secure rights. Still others argue that only self-consciousness can secure rights. Another suggestion is that one be able to use a language. This of course presents interesting issues with respect to the chimps who have been taught sign language as well as with other animals who appear to have some form of communication. Finally, the argument is made that only persons are bearers of rights. Persons are generally understood to be moral agents with an enduring concept of self and capable of autonomous actions.

The question of rights is quite complex on the level of definition and determining the subject of rights. When rights are interjected into the social order and made the basis of entitlements, then the picture becomes much more complex and difficult. We will encounter this difficulty in almost every topic we discuss in this introductory book.

NOTES

1. Tom L. Beauchamp and James F. Childress, *Principles of Biomedical Ethics*. New York: Oxford University Press, 1977, p. 56.

2. *Ibid.*, pp. 97ff.

3. For a thorough discussion of the principle of double effect, see the article "The Hermeneutical Function of the Principle of the Double Effect" by Peter Knauer, S.J., in *Readings in Moral Theology No. 1,* edited by Charles Curran and Richard McCormick. New York: Paulist Press, 1979.

4. Richard McCormick, S.J., *Ambiguity and Moral Choice*. Department of Theology, Marquette University, p. 93.

5. Beauchamp and Childress, *op. cit.*, pp. 135ff.

6. *Ibid.*, p. 140.

7. Beauchamp and Childress, *op. cit.*, pp. 169ff.

8. *Ibid.*, pp. 66ff.

9. James Childress, *Who Shall Decide? Paternalism in Health Care*. New York: Oxford University Press, 1982.

10. James F. Childress, *Priorities in Biomedical Ethics*. Philadelphia: The Westminster Press, 1981, p. 27.

PART ONE

ABORTION

Sissela Bok
Sidney and Daniel Callahan
Susan Nicholson
Thomas A. Shannon

1 *Ethical Problems of Abortion*

SISSELA BOK

This is a very sensitive and thorough analysis of some critical issues in the ethics of abortion. Bok presents an excellent evaluation of issues such as the relation of mother and fetus, the purposes of the attempt to distinguish human from non-human, and the reasons for protecting human life. The article concludes with an examination of the delicate problem of ethical line drawing. Bok forces the reader to become critically involved in the issues and to re-evaluate one's own position in the light of a thoughtfully developed position.

Dr. Sissela Bok, Ph.D., teaches at Brandeis University, Waltham, MA.

The recent Supreme Court decisions[1] have declared abortions to be lawful in the United States during the first trimester of pregnancy. After the first trimester, the state can restrict them by regulations protecting the pregnant woman's health; and after 'viability' the state may regulate or forbid abortions except where the medical judgment is made that an abortion is necessary to safeguard the life or the health of the pregnant woman. But it would be wrong to conclude from these decisions that no *moral* distinctions between abortions can now be made—that what is lawful is always justifiable. These decisions leave the moral issues of abortion open, and it is more important than ever to examine them.

While abortion is frequently rejected for religious reasons,[2] arguments against it are also made on other grounds. The most forceful one holds that if we grant that a fetus possesses humanity, we must accord it human rights, including the right to live. Another argument invokes the danger to *other* unborn humans, should abortion spread and perhaps even become obligatory in certain cases, and the danger to newborns, the retarded, and the senile should society begin to take the lives of those considered expendable. A third argument stresses the danger that physicians and nurses and those associated with the act of abortion might lose their traditional protective attitude toward life if they become inured to taking human lives at the request of mothers.

Among the arguments made in favor of permitting abortion, one upholds the right of the mother to determine her own fertility, and her right to the use of her own body. Another stresses, in cases of genetic defects of a severe variety, a sympathetic understanding of the suffering which might accompany living, should the fetus not be aborted. And a third reflects a number of social concerns, ranging from the problem of overpopulation *per se* to the desire to reduce unwantedness, child abuse, maternal deaths through illegal abortions, poverty and illness.

In discussing the ethical dilemmas of abortion, I shall begin with the basic conflict—that between a pregnant woman and the unborn life she harbors.

I. MOTHER AND FETUS

Up to very recently, parents had only limited access to birth prevention. Contraception was outlawed or treated with silence. Sterilization was most often unavailable and abortion was left to those desperate enough to seek criminal abortions. Women may well be forgiven now, therefore, if they mistrust the barrage of arguments concerning abortion, and may well suspect that these are rear-guard actions in an effort to tie them still longer to the bearing of unwanted children.

Some advocates for abortion hold that women should have the right to do what they want with their own bodies, and that removing the fetus is comparable to cutting one's hair or removing a disfiguring growth. This view simply ignores the fact that abortion involves more than just one life. The same criticism holds for the vaguer notions which defend abortion on the grounds that a woman should have the right to control her fate, or the right to have an abortion as she has the right to marry. But no one has the clear-cut right to control her fate where others share it, and marriage requires consent by two persons, whereas the consent of the fetus is precisely what cannot be obtained. How, then, can we weigh the rights and the interests of mother and fetus, where they conflict?

The central question is whether the life of the fetus should receive the same protection as other lives—often discussed in terms of whether killing the fetus is to be thought of as killing a human being. But before asking that question, I would like to ask whether abortion can always be thought of as *killing* in the first place. For abortion can be looked upon, also, as the withdrawal of bodily life support on the part of the mother.

A. *Cessation of Bodily Life Support*

Would anyone, before or after birth, child or adult, have the right to continue to be dependent upon the bodily processes of another against that person's will? It can happen that a person will require a sacrifice on the part of another in order not to die; does he therefore have the *right* to this sacrifice?

Judith Thomson has argued most cogently that the mother who finds herself pregnant, as a result of rape or in spite of every precaution, does not have the obligation to continue the pregnancy:

> I am arguing only that having a right to life does not guar-
> antee having either a right to be given the use of or a right
> to be allowed the continued use of another person's body—
> even if one needs it for life itself.[3]

Abortion, according to such a view, can be thought of as the cessation of continued support. It is true that the embryo cannot survive alone, and that it dies. But this is not unjust killing, any more than when Siamese twins are separated surgically and one of them dies as a result. Judith Thomson argues that at least in those cases where the mother is involuntarily pregnant, she can cease her support of the life of the fetus without infringing its right to live. Here, viability—the capability of living independently from the body of the mother—becomes important. Before that point, the unborn life will end when the mother ceases her support. No one else can take over the protection of the unborn life. After the point where viability begins, much depends on what is done by others, and on how much assistance is provided.

It may be, however, that in considering the ethical implications of the right to cease bodily support of the fetus we must distinguish between causing death indirectly through ceasing such support and actively killing the fetus outright. The techniques used in abortion differ significantly in this respect.[4] A method which prevents implantation of the fertilized egg or which brings about menstruation is much more clearly cessation of life support than one which sucks or scrapes out the embryo. Least like cessation of support is abortion by saline solution, which kills and begins to decompose the fetus, thus setting in motion its expulsion by the mother's body. This method is the one most commonly used in the second trimester of pregnancy. The alternative method possible at that time is a hysterotomy, or "small Ceasarean," where the fetus is removed intact, and where death very clearly does result from the interrution of bodily support.

If we learn how to provide life support for the fetus outside the natural mother's body, it may happen that parents who wish to adopt a baby may come into a new kind of conflict with those who wish to have an abortion. They may argue that *all* the aborting mother has a right to is to cease supporting a fetus with her own body. They may insist, if the pregnancy is already in the second trimester, that she has no right to choose a technique which also kills the baby. It would be wrong for the natural parents to insist at that point that the severance must be performed in such a way that others cannot take over the care and support for the fetus. But a conflict could arise if the mother were asked to postpone the abortion in order to improve the chances of survival and well-being of the fetus to be adopted by others.

Are there times where, quite apart from the technique used to abort, a woman has a *special* responsibility to continue bodily support of a fetus? Surely the many pregnancies which are entered upon voluntarily are of such a nature. One might even say that, if anyone ever did have special obligations to continue life support of another, it would be the woman who had *voluntarily undertaken* to become pregnant. For she has then brought about the situation where the fetus has come to require her support, and there is no one else who can take over her responsibility until after the baby is viable.

To use the analogy of a drowning person, one can think of three scenarios influencing the responsibility of a bystander to leap to the rescue. First, someone may be drowning and the bystander arrives at the scene, hesitating between rescue and permitting the person to drown. Secondly, someone may be drowning as a result of the honestly mistaken assurance by the bystander that swimming would be safe. Thirdly, the bystander may have pushed the drowning person out of a boat. In each case the duties of the bystander are different, but surely they are at their most stringent when he has intentionally caused the drowning person to find himself in the water.

These three scenarios bear some resemblance, from the point of view of the mother's responsibility to the fetus, to: first, finding out that she is pregnant against her wishes; second, mistakenly trusting that she was protected against pregnancy; and third, intentionally becoming pregnant.

Every pregnancy which has been intentionally begun creates special responsibilities for the mother.[5] But there is one situation in which these dilemmas are presented in a particularly difficult form. It is where two parents deliberately enter upon a pregnancy, only to find that the baby they are expecting has a genetic disease or has suffered from damage in fetal life, so that it will be permanently malformed or retarded. Here, the parents have consciously brought about the life which now requires support from the body of the mother. Can they now turn about and say that this particular fetus is such that they do not wish to continue their support? This is especially difficult when the fetus is already developed up to the 18th or 20th week. Can they acknowledge that they meant to begin a human life, but not *this* human life? Or, to take a more callous example, suppose, as sometimes happens, that the parents learn that the baby is of a sex they do not wish?[6]

In such cases the justification which derives from wishing to cease life support for a life which had not been intended is absent, since this life *had* been intended. At the same time, an assumption of responsibility which comes with consciously beginning a pregnancy is much weaker than the corresponding assumption between two adults, or the social assumption of responsibility for a child upon birth for reasons which will be discussed in the next section.

To sum up at this point, ceasing bodily life support *of a fetus or of anyone else* cannot be looked at as a breach of duty except where such a duty has been assumed in the first place. Such a duty is closer to existing when the pregnancy has been voluntarily begun. And it does not exist at all in cases of rape. Certain *methods* of abortion, furthermore, are more difficult to think of as cessation of support than others. Finally, pregnancy is perhaps unique in that cessation of support means death for the fetus up to a certain point of its development, so that nearness *to* this point in pregnancy argues against abortion.

I would like now to turn to the larger question of whether the life of the fetus *should* receive the same protection as other lives—whether killing the fetus, by whatever means, and for whatever reason, is to be thought of as killing a human being.

A long tradition of religious and philosophical and legal thought has attempted to answer this question by determining if there is human life before birth, and, if so, when it *becomes* human. If human life is present from conception on, according to this tradition, it must be protected as such from that moment. And if the embryo *becomes* human at some point during a pregnancy, then that is the point at which the protection should set in.

B. *Humanity*

The point in a pregnancy at which a human individual can be said to exist is differently assigned. John Noonan generalizes the predominant Catholic view as follows:

> If one steps outside the specific categories used by the theologians, the answer they gave can be analyzed as a refusal to discriminate among human beings on the basis of their varying potentialities. Once conceived, the being was recognized as a man

because he had man's potential. The criterion for humanity, thus, was simple and all-embracing: If you are conceived by human parents, you are human.[7]

Once conceived, he holds, human life has about an 80% chance to reach the moment of birth and develop further. *Conception*, therefore, represents a point of discontinuity, after which the probabilities for human development are immensely higher than for the sperm or the egg before conception.

Others have held that the moment when *implantation* occurs, 6-7 days after conception, is more significant from the point of view of humanity and individuality than conception itself. This permits them to allow the intrauterine device and the 'morning after pill' as not taking human life, merely interfering with implantation.

Another view is advanced by Jérôme Lejeune, who suggests that unity and uniqueness, "the two headings defining an individual" are not definitely established until between two and four weeks after conception.[8] Up to that time it is possible that two eggs may have collaborated to build together one embryo, known as a "chimera," whereas after that time such a combination is no longer possible. Similarly, up to that time, a fertilized egg from which twins may result may not yet have split in two.

Still another approach to the establishing of humanity is to say that *looking* human is the important factor. A photo of the first cell having divided in half clearly does not depict what most people mean when the use the expression "human being." Even the four-week-old embryo does not look human, whereas the six-week-old one is beginning to. Recent techniques of depicting the embryo and the fetus have remarkably increased our awareness of the "human-ness" at this early stage; this new *seeing* of life before birth may come to increase the psychological recoil from aborting those who already look human— thus adding a powerful psychological factor to the medical and personal factors already influencing the trend to earlier and earlier abortions.

Others reason that the time at which electrical impulses are first detectable from the brain, around the eighth week, marks the line after which human life is present. If brain activity is advocated as the criterion for human life among the dying, they argue, then why not use it also at the very beginning?[9] Such a use of the criterion for human life has been interpreted by some to indicate that abortion would not be killing before electrical impulses are detectable, only afterwards. Such an analogy would seem to possess a symmetry of sorts, but it is only superficially plausible. For the lack of brain response at the end of life has to be shown to be *irreversible* in order to support a conclusion that life is absent. The lack of response from the embryo's brain, on the other hand, is temporary and precisely not irreversible.

Another dividing line, once more having to do with our perception of the fetus, is that achieved when the mother can feel the fetus moving. *Quickening* has traditionally represented an important distinction, and in some legal traditions such as the common law, abortion has been permitted before quickening, but is a misdemeanor, "a great misprision," afterwards, rather than homicide. It is certain that the first felt movements represent an awe-inspiring change for the mother, and perhaps, in some primitive sense, a 'coming to life' of the being she carries.

Yet another distinction occurs when the fetus is considered *viable*. According to this view, once the fetus is capable of living independently of its mother, it must be regarded as a human being and protected as such. The United States Supreme Court decisions on abortion established viability as the "compelling" point for the state's "important and legitimate interest in potential life," while eschewing the question of when 'life' or 'human life' begins.[10]

A set of later distinctions cluster around the process of birth itself. This is the moment when life begins, according to some religious traditions, and the point at which 'persons' are fully recognized in the law, according to the Supreme Court.[11] The first breaths taken by newborn babies have been invested with immense symbolic meaning since the earliest gropings toward understanding what it means to be alive and human. And the rituals of acceptance of babies and children have often served to define humanity to the point where the baby could be killed if it were not named or declared acceptable by the elders of the community or by the head of the household, either at birth or in infancy. Others have mentioned as factors in our concept of humanity the ability to experience, to remember the past and envisage the future, to communicate, even to laugh at oneself.

In the positions here examined, and in the abortion debate generally, a number of concepts are at times used as if they were interchangeable. 'Humanity,' 'human life,' 'life,' are such concepts, as are 'man,' 'person,' 'human being,' or 'human individual.' In particular, those who hold that humanity begins at conception or at implantation often have the tendency to say that at that time a human being or a person or a man exists as well, whereas others find it impossible to equate them.

Each of these terms can, in addition, be used in different senses which overlap but are not interchangeable. For instance, humanity and human life, in one sense, are possessed by every cell in our bodies.

Many cells have the full genetic makeup required for asexual reproduction—so-called cloning—of a human being. Yet clearly this is not
the sense of those words intended when the protection of humanity or
of human life is advocated. Such protection would press the reverence
for life to the mad extreme of ruling out haircuts and considering
mosquito bites murder.

It may be argued, however, that for most cells which have the potential of cloning to form a human being, extraordinarily complex
measures would be required which are not as yet sufficiently perfected
beyond the animal stage. Is there, then, a difference, from the point of
view of human potential, between these cells and egg cells or sperm
cells? And is there still another difference in potential between the
egg cell before and after conception? While there is a statistical difference in the *likelihood* of their developing into a human being, it
does not seem possible to draw a clear line where humanity definitely
begins.

The different views as to when humanity begins are not dependent upon factual information. Rather, these views are representative
of different worldviews, often of a religious nature, involving deeply
held commitments with moral consequences. There is no disagreement
as to what we now know about life and its development before and
after conception; differences arise only about the names and moral
consequences we attach to the changes in this development and the
distinctions we consider important. Just as there is no point at which
Achilles can be pinpointed as catching up with the tortoise, though
everyone knows he does, so too everyone is aware of the distance
traveled, in terms of humanity, from before conception to birth,
though there is no one point at which humanity can be agreed upon as
setting in. Our efforts to pinpoint and to define reflect the urgency
with which we reach for abstract labels and absolute certainty in facts
and in nature; and the resulting confusion and puzzlement are close to
what Wittgenstein described, in *Philosophical Investigations*, as the
"bewitchment of our intelligence by means of language."

Even if some see the fertilized egg as possessing humanity and as
being "a man" in the words used by Noonan, however, it would be
quite unthinkable to act upon all the consequences of such a view. It
would be necessary to undertake a monumental struggle against all
spontaneous abortions—known as miscarriages—often of severly malformed embryos expelled by the mother's body. This struggle would
appear increasingly misguided as we learn more about how to preserve
early prenatal life. Those who could not be saved would have to be
buried in the same way as dead infants. Those who engaged in abortion would have to be prosecuted for murder. Extraordinary practical

complexities would arise with respect to the detection of early abortion, and to the question of whether the use of abortifacients in the first few days after conception should also count as murder. In view of these inconsistencies, it seems likely that this view of humanity, like so many others, has been adopted for limited purposes having to do with the prohibition of induced abortion, rather than from a real belief in the full human rights of the first few cells after conception.

II. Purposes for Seeking to Distinguish Human and Non-Human

A related reason why there are so many views and definitions of humanity is that they have been sought for such different *purposes*. I indicated already that many of the views about humanity developed in the abortion dispute seem to have been worked out for one such purpose—that of defending a preconceived position on abortion, with little concern for the other consequences flowing from that particular view. But there have been so many other efforts to define humanity and to arrive at the essence of what it means to be human—to distinguish men from angels and demons, plants and animals, witches and robots. The most powerful one has been the urge to know about the human species and to trace the biological or divine origins and the essential characteristics of mankind. It is magnificently expressed beginning with the very earliest creation myths; in fact, this consciousness of oneself and wonder at one's condition has often been thought one of the essential distinctions between men and animals.

A separate purpose, both giving strength to and flowing from these efforts to describe and to understand humanity, has been that of seeking to define what a *good* human being is—to delineate human aspirations. What ought fully human beings to be like, and how should they differ from and grow beyond their immature, less perfect, sick or criminal fellow men? Who can teach such growth—St. Francis or Nietzsche, Buddha or Erasmus? And what kind of families and societies give support and provide models for growth?

Finally, definitions of humanity have been sought in order to try to set limits to the protection of life. At what level of developing humanity can and ought lives to receive protection? And who, among those many labelled less than human at different times in history—slaves, enemies in war, women, children, the retarded—should be denied such protection?

Of these three purposes for defining 'humanity,' the first is classificatory and descriptive in the first hand (though it gives rise to normative considerations). It has roots in religious and metaphysical thought, and has branched out into biological and archeological and anthropological research. But the latter two, so often confused with the first, are primarily *normative* or prescriptive. They seek to set norms or guidelines for who is fully human, and who is at least minimally human—so human as to be entitled to the protection of life. For the sake of these normative purposes, definitions of 'humanity' established elsewhere have been sought in order to determine action—and all too often the action has been devastating for those excluded.

It is crucial to ask at this point why the descriptive and the normative definitions have been thought to coincide; why it has been taken for granted that the line between human and non-human or not-yet-human is identical with that distinguishing those who may be killed from those who are to be protected.

One or both of two fundamental assumptions are made by those who base the protection of life upon the possession of 'humanity.' The first is that all human beings are not only different from, but *superior* to all other living matter. This is the assumption which changes the definition of humanity into an evaluative one. It lies at the root of Western religious and social thought, from the Bible and the Aristotelian concept of the 'ladder of life,' all the way to Teilhard de Chardin's view of mankind as close to the intended summit and consummation of the development of living beings.

The second assumption holds that the superiority of human beings somehow justifies their using what is non-human as they see fit, dominating it, even killing it when they wish to. St. Augustine, in *The City of God*,[12] expresses both of these anthropocentric assumptions when he holds that the injunction "Thou shalt not kill" does not apply to killing animals and plants, since, having no faculty of reason,

> therefore by the altogether righteous ordinance of the Creator both their life and death are a matter subordinate to our needs.

Neither of these assumptions is self-evident. And the results of acting upon them, upon the bidding to subdue the earth, to subordinate its many forms of life to human needs, are no longer seen by all to be beneficial.[13] The very enterprise of *basing* normative conclusions on such assumptions and distinctions can no longer be taken for granted.

Despite these difficulties, many still try to employ definitions of 'humanity' to do just that. And herein lies by far the most important reason for abandoning such efforts: the monumental misuse of the concept of 'humanity' in so many practices of discrimination and atrocity throughout history. Slavery, witchhunts and wars have all been justified by their perpetrators on the grounds that they held their victims to be less than fully human. The insane and the criminal have for long periods been deprived of the most basic necessities for similar reasons, and excluded from society. A theologian, Dr. Joseph Fletcher, has even suggested recently that someone who has an I.Q. below 40 is "questionably a person" and that those below the 20-mark are not persons at all.[14] He adds that:

This has bearing, obviously, on decision making in gynecology, obstetrics, and pediatrics, as well as in general surgery and medicine.

Here a criterion for 'personhood' is taken as a guideline for action which could have sinister and far-reaching effects. Even when entered upon with the best of intentions, and in the most guarded manner, the enterprise of basing the protection of human life upon such criteria and definitions is dangerous. To question someone's humanity or personhood is a first step to mistreatment and killing.

We must abandon, therefore, this quest for a definition of humanity capable of showing us who has a right to live. To do so must not, however, mean any abandon of concern with the human condition—with the quest for knowledge about human origins and characteristics and with aspirations for human goodness. It is only the use of the concept of 'humanity' as a criterion of *exclusion* which I deplore.

In recent decades, philosophers have devoted much thought to the nature of ethical principles, to the kind of statement they make, and to their internal grammar. Much has been written about the requirement that these principles be universal—that they hold for all mankind, all moral persons, all rational beings. As a rough distinction, such a simple characterization of the *extent* to which ethical principles should hold is undoubtedly natural and relatively unproblematic. It would rule out, for example, the denial of basic rights to some persons while according them to others, whereas it would not prohibit the employment of plant fiber in clothing or lumber in furniture. But I submit that in the many borderline cases where humanity is questioned by some—the so-called 'vegetables,' the severely retarded, or the embryo—even the seemingly universal yardsticks of 'humanity' or rationality are dangerous.

But if we rule out the appeal to a standard of 'humanity' in deciding about the protection of life in such difficult cases, may we not have lost the only criterion of objective decisions? Or could there be other criteria less dangerous and vague than that connected with 'humanity'?

In order to seek such criteria, it is crucial to arrive at an understanding of the harm that comes from the taking of life. Why do we hold life to be sacred? Why does it require protection beyond that given to anything else? The question seems unnecessary at first—surely most people share what has been called "the elemental sensation of vitality and the elemental fear of its extinction," and what Hume termed "our horrors at annihilation."[15] Many think of this elemental sensation as incapable of further analysis. They view any attempt to say *why* we hold life sacred as an instrumentalist rocking of the boat which may endanger this fundamental and unquestioned respect for life. Yet I believe that such a failure to ask what the respect for life ought to protect lies at the root of the confusion about abortion and many other difficult decisions concerning life and death. I shall try, therefore, to list the most important reasons which underlie the elemental sense of the sacredness of life. Having done so, these reasons can be considered as they apply or do not apply to the embryo and the fetus.

III.   REASONS FOR PROTECTING LIFE

1. Killing is viewed as the greatest of all dangers *for the victim*.
- The knowledge that there is a threat to life causes intense anguish and apprehension.
- The actual taking of life can cause great suffering.
- The continued experience of life, once begun, is considered so valuable, so unique, so absorbing, that no one who has this experience should be unjustly deprived of it. And depriving someone of this experience means that all else of value to him will be lost.
2. Killing is brutalizing and criminalizing *for the killer*. It is a threat to others, and destructive to the person engaged therein.
3. Killing often causes *the family of the victim and others* to experience grief and loss. They may have been tied to the dead person by affection or economic dependence; they may have given of themselves in the relationship, so that its severance causes deep suffering.
4. *All of society*, as a result, has a stake in the protection of life. Permitting killing to take place sets patterns for victims, killers, and survivors, that are threatening and ultimately harmful to all.

These are neutral principles governing the protection of life. They are shared by most human beings reflecting upon the possibility of dying at the hands of others. It is clear that these principles, if applied in the absence of the confusing terminology of 'humanity,' would rule out the kinds of killing perpetrated by conquerors, witch-hunters, slave-holders, and Nazis. Their victims feared death and suffered; they grieved for their dead; and the societies permitting such killing were brutalized and degraded.

Turning now to abortions once more, how do these principles apply to the taking of the lives of embryos and fetuses?

A. *Reasons to Protect Life in the Prenatal Period*

Consider the very earliest cell formations soon after conception. Clearly, most of these *reasons* for protecting human life are absent here.

This group of cells cannot suffer in death, nor can it fear death. Its experiencing of life has not yet begun; it is not yet conscious of the loss of anything it has come to value in life and is not tied by bonds of affection to other human beings. If the abortion is desired by both parents, it will cause no grief such as that which accompanies the death of a child. Almost no human care and emotion and resources have been invested in it. Nor is a very early abortion brutalizing for the person voluntarily performing it, or a threat to other members of the human community.[16] The only factor common to these few cells and, say, a soldier killed in war or a murdered robbery victim is that of the *potential* denied, the interruption of life, the deprivation of the possibility to grow and to experience, to have the joys and sorrows of existence.

For how much should this one factor count? It should count *at least* so much as to eliminate the occasionally voiced notion that pregnancy and its interruption involve only the mother in the privacy of her reproductive life, that to have an abortion is somehow analogous with cutting one's finger nails.

At the same time, I cannot agree that it should count enough so that one can simply equate killing an embryo with murder, even apart from legal considerations or the problems of enforcement. For it *is* important that most of the reasons why we protect lives are absent here. It does matter that the group of cells cannot feel the anguish or pain connected with death, that it is not conscious of the interruption of its life, and that other humans do not mourn it or feel insecure in their own lives if it dies.

But, it could be argued, one can conceive of other deaths with those factors absent, which nevertheless would be murder. Take the killing of a hermit in his sleep, by someone who instantly commits suicide. Here there is no anxiety or fear of the killing on the part of the victim, no pain in dying, no mourning by family or friends (to whom the hermit has, in leaving them for good, already in a sense 'died'), no awareness by others that a wrong has been done; and the possible brutalization of the murderer has been made harmless to others through his suicide. Speculate further that the bodies are never found. Yet we would still call the act one of murder. The reason we would do so is inherent in the act itself, and depends on the fact that his life was taken, and that he was denied the chance to continue to experience it.

How does this privation of potential differ from abortion in the first few days of pregnancy? I find that I cannot use words like 'deprived,' 'deny,' 'take away,' and 'harm' when it comes to the group of cells, whereas I have no difficulty in using them for the hermit. Do these words require, if not a person conscious of his loss, at least someone who at a prior time has developed enough to be or have been conscious thereof? Because there is no semblance of human form, no conscious life or capability to live independently, no knowledge of death, no sense of pain, one cannot use such words meaningfully to describe early abortion.

In addition, whereas it is possible to frame a rule permitting abortion which causes no anxiety on the part of others covered by the rule —other embryos or fetuses—it is not possible to frame such a rule permitting the killing of hermits without threatening other *hermits*. All hermits would have to fear for their lives if there were a rule saying that hermits can be killed if they are alone and asleep and if the agent commits suicide.

The reasons, then, for the protection of lives are minimal in very early abortions. At the same time, some of them are clearly present with respect to *infanticide*, most important among them the brutalization of those participating in the act and the resultant danger for all who are felt to be undesirable by their families or by others. This is not to say that acts of infanticide have not taken place in our society; indeed, as late as the nineteenth century, newborns were frequently killed, either directly or by giving them into the care of institutions such as foundling hospitals, where the death rate could be as high as 90 percent in the first year of life.[17] A few primitive societies, at the edge of extinction, without other means to limit families, still practice infanticide. But I believe that the *public acceptance* of infanticide in all other societies is unthinkable, given the advent of modern methods of contraception and early abortion, and of institutions to which parents can give their children, assured of their survival and of the high likelihood that they will be adopted and cared for by a family.

B. *Dividing Lines*

If, therefore, very early abortion does not violate these principles of protection for life, but infanticide does, we are confronted with a new kind of continuum in the place of that between less human and more human: that of the growth in strength, during the prenatal period, of these principles, these reasons for protecting life. In this second continuum, it would be as difficult as in the first to draw a line based upon objective factors. Since most abortions can be performed earlier or later during pregnancy, it would be preferable to encourage early abortions rather than late ones, and to draw a line before the second half of the pregnancy, permitting later abortions only on a clear showing of need. For this purpose, the two concepts of *quickening* and *viability*—so unsatisfactory in determining when humanity begins —can provide such limits.

Before quickening, the reasons to protect life are, as has been shown, negligible, perhaps absent altogether. During this period, therefore, abortion could be permitted upon request. Alternatively, the end of the first trimester could be employed as such a limit, as is the case in a number of countries.

Between quickening and viability, when the operation is a more difficult one medically and more traumatic for parents and medical personnel, it would not seem unreasonable to hold that special reasons justifying the abortion should be required in order to counterbalance this resistance; reasons not known earlier, such as the severe malformation of the fetus. After viability, finally, all abortions save the rare ones required to save the life of the mother,[18] should be prohibited, because the reasons to *protect* life may now be thought to be partially present; even though the viable fetus cannot fear death or suffer consciously therefrom, the effects on those participating in the event, and thus on society indirectly, could be serious. This is especially so because of the need, mentioned above, for a protection against infanticide. In the unlikely event, however, that the mother should first come to wish to be separated from the fetus at such a late stage, the procedure ought to be delayed until it can be one of premature birth, not one of harming the fetus in an abortive process.

Medically, however, the definition of 'viability' is difficult. It varies from one fetus to another. At one stage in pregnancy, a certain number of babies, if born, will be viable. At a later stage, the percentage will be greater. Viability also depends greatly on the state of our knowledge concerning the support of life after birth, and on the nature of the support itself. Support can be given much earlier in a modern hospital than in a rural village, or in a clinic geared to doing abortions only. It may some day even be the case that almost any human life will be considered viable before birth, once artificial wombs are perfected.

As technological progress pushes back the time when the fetus can be helped to survive independently of the mother, a question will arise as to whether the cutoff point marked by viability ought also be pushed back. Should abortion then be prohibited much earlier than is now the case, because the medical meaning of 'viability' will have changed, or should we continue to rely on the conventional meaning of the word for the distinction between lawful and unlawful abortion?

In order to answer this question it is necessary to look once more at the reasons for which 'viability' was thought to be a good dividing-line in the first place. Is viability important because the baby can survive outside of the mother? Or because this chance of survival comes at a time in fetal development when the *reasons* to protect life have grown strong enough to prohibit abortion? At present, the two coincide, but in the future, they may come to diverge increasingly.

If the time comes when an embryo *could* be kept alive without its mother and thus be 'viable' in one sense of the word, the reasons for protecting life from the point of view of victims, agents, relatives and society would still be absent; it seems right, therefore, to tie the obligatory protection of life to the present conventional definition of 'viability' and to set a socially agreed upon time in pregnancy after which abortion should be prohibited.

To sum up, the justifications a mother has for not wishing to give birth can operate up to a certain point in pregnancy; after that point, the reasons society has for protecting life become sufficiently weighty so as to prohibit late abortions and infanticide.

IV. MORAL DISTINCTIONS

But moral distinctions ought nevertheless to be made by the mother considering an abortion even during the period when she may lawfully obtain one. In addition to those having to do with the *method* of abortion and the degree to which the pregnancy was voluntary or involuntary (as discussed previously), the *time* in pregnancy, the weightiness of the *reasons* for wanting the abortion, the desires of the *father*, and the possibility of alternatives such as adoption, must all be considered.

1. The *time* in pregnancy at which the abortion takes place is a very important factor. Very early in pregnancy, the reasons for protecting life are clearly absent. Few will have to face the questions which come with aborting a 4 or 5-month-old fetus when early abortions are generally available. But *in* such late abortions, it is especially important to consider what the reasons are for desiring the abortion.

2. Among all of the reasons why a pregnancy is unwanted, it is possible to perceive a gradation from reasons all would recognize as very compelling, such as a threat to the mother's life, to reasons most would think of as frivolous, such as a determination that only a fetus

of a desired sex should be allowed to be born. This gradation among the reasons for wishing not to have a baby will be part of any judgment concerning the *morality* of acts to prevent births. It is also possible to divide the innumerable reasons for not wanting a pregnancy into two main categories. The first one, sometimes called 'selective' unwantedness, refers to those pregnancies which are desired, often planned, by the parents, but during the course of which evidence comes to light concerning a risk, or even a certainty of abnormality in the fetus. If, for example, the mother has Rubella, or German Measles, in the first trimester, there is a probability of fetal abnormality. And it is now possible to learn, through prenatal diagnosis, whether the fetus suffers from a chromosomal abnormality, the most common of which causes mongolism, or from one of a number of genetic diseases which can cause malformation or mental retardation.[19] In all of these cases the parents, while they might ordinarily welcome a pregnancy, may come to the conclusion that they do not wish to give birth in this particular case.

But the determination of such defects through amniocentesis can only be made when the amniotic fluid is present to a sufficient degree, and the final results of the tests may not be available until the fifth month of pregnancy. Only *late* abortions are possible after amniocentesis, and this makes the decision for parents and doctors a much more difficult one.

The reasons for not wanting a malformed baby differ with the capacities of the parents and the severity of the abnormality. Some parents, and families, cope admirably and with great love with children who would prove burdensome and even destructive to other families. A severely disabled fetus, likely to suffer greatly once born and perhaps to die in childhood, could be 'unwanted' out of concern for its own welfare, as well as for the welfare of the family. A great deal depends on the help available from the community, in terms of financial assistance, special schooling, medical resources, and general support. Other factors which can be important are the pride of the family, or even parental prejudice, e.g., parents' wish for an abortion after learning that the fetus is of one sex rather than another.

Perhaps most difficult from a moral point of view are the situations where the parents know beforehand that they are carriers of genetic defects, and where they enter upon a pregnancy determined in advance to abort any fetus which is found to exhibit the defect. I say this with the greatest humility, knowing the strength of the urge to have one's own babies. But I see no difference between starting another human life with such plans, and creating 'test-tube' fetuses only to throw away those deemed undesirable. In cases such as these, other ways of bringing children into the lives of parents must be worked out. At times artificial insemination may provide an answer,[20] at other times adoption, or working with children in the many capacities where help is needed, may be preferable.

But there are many cases where these distinctions cannot be so clearly made. It may be difficult to know whether there was an intention to have a baby, or to risk becoming pregnant. It might be argued that someone who engaged in sexual activity, even using contraceptives, ought to be willing to take the responsibility for a human life which results. Whereas to abort under such circumstances, or even after a voluntarily begun pregnancy, is not murder, it ought not to be taken lightly. For the same reason, it is insensitive to omit contraceptive measures and to rely on the availability of abortion in the case of pregnancy. (Though the availability of methods making abortions possible in the very earliest days of pregnancy and the hazy line between such abortions and contraception may make such a distinction less pointed.)

Another set of criteria which will be difficult to work out when considering reasons for abortion is that which should govern abortions for the sake of the welfare of the fetus. For while almost all would agree about the extreme cases I have mentioned, there will be disagreement as to what to do in those cases where the affliction is not totally debilitating, or where there is merely a *risk* of disease, not a certainty. What if the risk is small? A recent newspaper article stated that there is one chance out of a hundred that a baby will be born retarded if the mother has had the flu in the first trimester of her pregnancy. Whether or not this particular concern turns out to be correct, it is going to be increasingly possible to specify odds of this kind, sometimes with a very low probability of danger. It has been suggested that parents will come to want to take very few chances of defects, so long as the choice is open to them of having abortions.

Even if it is possible, however, to work out criteria concerning the welfare of the baby, there are times when the cost at which this welfare is to be purchased must be weighed against the welfare of other human beings. If for example, a fetus is diagnosed as having a disease which can be controlled after birth so as not to cause suffering, but only at staggering costs to the family or the community—say of millions of dollars each day—abortion would clearly be called for in spite of the theoretical possibility of carrying the baby to term and treating it. The other possibility would be not aborting, and permitting the baby to suffer in the absence of such expensive relief, and then once more, the magnitude of the suffering might have argued in favor of abortion.

All these cases, where certain births are unwanted because of the characteristics of the fetus, differ crucially from those in the second category where no children at all are wanted at the time of the pregnancy. In this larger group are the more familiar cases where there is danger to the mother's physical health or her emotional stability, or where there is not enough food, clothing, or shelter to cope with yet another child. Here, too, are cases where there has been rape, or incest, or where a very young girl is pregnant. There are also the frequent cases where the mother feels she is beyond the age best suited for child-caring, or does not want to accept the great changes in life—the restriction, the financial pinch, and the feeling of being tied down—which often accompany the birth of a child. These changes affect mothers most powerfully in our society of nuclear families where the burdens of child-rearing often fall on them alone. In all of these cases, contraception could have avoided the pregnancy, and an early abortion is possible as a last resort. Adoption is an alternative resort which should always be considered. It must be remembered, however, that with prevailing attitudes it would be exceedingly difficult for a married woman with existing children to give a baby up for adoption.

The distinction between the two *kinds* of reasons for not wanting a pregnancy is crucial. For while the first group of conceptions—unwanted because of the characteristics of the fetus—often require abortions if births are to be prevented (and often late abortions, since prenatal diagnosis takes time and can rarely begin until the second trimester of pregnancy), the second group can usually be prevented through contraception, sterilization, abstinence, or protection of the mother from sexual assault. Abortion is necessary here only as a last resort, where other methods have failed, and an *early* abortion is possible, presenting fewer medical, ethical, and emotional problems than a later one.

3. At times, there are conflicts between mothers and fathers of the unborn. According to one study,[21] about one-half of the pregnancies unwanted by one or both parents were unwanted by *only one* parent. Very often such disagreements are settled amicably, usually in favor of having the baby. But who should make the decision when the mother wishes to have an abortion, and the father wants to restrain her?[22] In a recent Canadian case,[23] a judge prohibited an abortion desired by a mother. The father had brought suit on his own behalf and on that of the 'infant plaintiff.'

It is difficult to see how such a disagreement can be anything but disruptive for the relationship between the two parents, as well as very harmful for the child after birth. Whoever 'wins' in such a conflict will have won a Pyrrhic victory indeed.

Early in pregnancy, the mother has at her disposal methods of abortion which need not involve the father's knowledge of her condition. The same is true if he does not learn of the pregnancy as it progresses. But barring such eventualities, who would decide in the event of a conflict?

In such a conflict, while it is important to ascertain the father's views when possible, there ought not to be a *requirement* that both parents consent to an abortion, as is now often the case.[24] The mother has the burden of pregnancy, and most often of caring for the baby she bears. The decision to interrupt her pregnancy should therefore be hers. But into her decision should go the awareness of the heavy price she will have to pay in the relationship with the father, if she aborts their unborn child against his wishes. And the father's reasons for wishing to continue the pregnancy should be given due weight, so as to counterbalance in her judgment all but the most pressing reasons she has for wishing to have the abortion.

The father's wishes should be given great weight, especially if he wants not only to preserve the life of his unborn child, but also to share responsibility and care after birth. At a future time, when it may be possible to remove a fetus relatively early in pregnancy and protect it artificially until 'birth,' fathers, just as adoptive parents, ought to have the right to declare their intentions to take responsibility for the baby. Mothers at that time, while severing their connections with the fetus, should not be able to demand its death.

Furthermore, if we look back on the reasons for protecting life, one of them concerns the grief felt by family members when someone is killed. If, therefore, a father feels such grief, and if he supports his contention by promising to assume the burdens of child-rearing after birth, this ought to be an important consideration, persuasive to the mother or to her physician or to both. Our society has been moving in the direction of recognizing that men as well as women can provide care and nurturance for children. To permit a father to prevent the abortion of his child on the condition that he bring it up later would seem to be a move in the same direction. If he is unwilling to make such a commitment, however, his grief at the impending death of the fetus is less entitled to respect.

4. The alternatives to abortion differ depending upon whether birth prevention is considered before or after conception. The alternatives open before conception—abstinence, different methods of contraception, and sterilization—do not raise the particular moral problems connected with taking the life of the fetus, or of rejecting the baby after birth.

Once conception *has* occurred, the alternatives to abortion are to accept responsibility for the baby after birth, or to relinquish it to the state or to adoptive parents. It is extremely important to consider these alternatives in the case of each unwanted pregnancy, and only to have recourse to abortion after discarding them. Many pregnant women, whether they are seeking abortions or not, are ambivalent, struggling within themselves in order to reconcile the tenderness normally evoked by the thought of a baby, with fears connected with their pregnancy. The fears may have to do with the future of the baby, or with the future of the family unit into which the baby will come. Sometimes there is no such family unit, and sometimes the relationship with the baby's father is such as to threaten the future of the baby. The decisive point comes when the choice is made to prevent a pregnancy or a birth. And this choice in turn is strongly influenced by social attitudes towards means of birth prevention, and by their availability.

The fact of having children has always been considered 'natural,' and someone not wishing a child, or any children, has been expected to produce reasons in support of such an attitude. It may be that we are now coming closer to a time when choosing not to have a child will be seen to reflect, not necessarily a hostile and niggardly attitude, a 'denial of life,' but a respect for the living, and a correct estimate of what kind of life a baby can be given. In that case, reasons will come to be expected *before* giving birth to a new baby, and thoughts for the welfare of the child to be will come to be seen as an important aspect of child-bearing.

In order for such choices to be possible at all, however, *information* is necessary. All those who are physically able to become parents must have wise and full advice regarding family life, sexual life, and birth prevention. From a moral point of view, contraception is greatly preferable to abortion. The *knowledge* about contraceptive alternatives to childbirth, or to abortion, is therefore crucial to all potential parents. Withholding information in order to preserve 'innocence' among the young is a self-defeating and unjustifiable exercise of paternalistic power, contributing to the birth of unwanted children and to shattered lives.

I have argued that it may be moral to have an abortion under certain circumstances, but that the range of morally justifiable abortions is more restricted than that of those abortions declared lawful by the Supreme Court. But some argue that such views of morality and legality, if widely followed, could lead to great dangers for society.

V.   PROBLEMS OF LINE-DRAWING

A.   *Can We Allow Abortion Without Risking Infanticide?*

Foes of abortion argue that a society which permits abortion may not be able to hold the line against infanticide.[25] Once we admit *reasons* for abortions such as fetal malformation or simply not wanting another child, they say, what is to prevent people from acting upon these very same reasons after birth?[26] A baby just before birth, they argue, is identical to one just after birth. What, then, will provide the discontinuity?

I have argued, on the contrary, that another set of *reasons*—the reasons for protecting human life—gain in strength during pregnancy and are such as to prohibit abortions after a certain point and therefore also to prohibit infanticide. While it is true that no theoretical line can be drawn which distinguishes between a baby just before birth and one just after birth, there is no difficulty in distinguishing an aborted embryo from a newborn baby. A time must therefore be set in pregnancy well before birth for the cutting-off point. The discontinuity will then exist between abortion and infanticide. The argument that the reason *for* aborting may still exist at childbirth does not take into account the reasons *against* killing, and the threat which would be felt by all if infanticide as a parental option were thought to be possible.[27]

How can one *know* whether such a discontinuity can be observed in practice? The only way to know is to consider those societies which have already permitted abortion for considerable lengths of time. These countries do not in fact experience tendencies toward infanticide. The infant mortality statistics in Sweden and Denmark are extremely low, and the protection and care given to all living children, including those born with special problems, is exemplary.

Moreover, Nazi Germany, which is frequently cited as a warning of what is to come once abortion becomes lawful, had *very strict laws prohibiting abortion.* In 1943, Hitler's regime made the existing penalties for women having abortions, and those performing them, even more severe by removing the limit on imprisonment and by including the possibility of "hard labor" for "especially serious cases."[28]

The fear of slipping from abortion towards infanticide, therefore, while understandable, does not seem to be grounded in fact.

B. *Is There a Risk of Compulsory Abortion?*

A second type of line-drawing problem is the following: if a beginning is made by permitting amniocentesis and abortion in cases where the mother learns she is expecting a grossly malformed baby, might there not come to be a *requirement* for others to undergo amniocentesis, and to induce abortion if the fetus is found to be defective? And once abortion is no longer reprehensible, might a community not require abortions where expectant mothers are heavily addicted, and where it is not only likely that they will harm or neglect their children after birth, but where they are demonstrably severely harming them even before birth? Might it not be increasingly easy for parents to force their daughters to have abortions should they become pregnant while they are too young, or unmarried?[29] Or even for husbands to require abortions where they judge their wives to be unstable or perhaps ill? And finally, if abortion is permitted for indigent mothers, in part out of sympathy for mother and child, and in part out of a computation of the likely costs to the community of enforcing the births of unwanted children, might there not in the long run be a requirement for abortion where mothers on welfare are concerned, or any others who are judged unable to provide, materially or emotionally or intellectually, for the needs of their children?

One can readily concede that it is important to be vigilant against any such developments. Any inroads upon a pregnant woman's physical integrity, against her will, are very serious and we need strong protection for the control she should be able to exercise over her own body. Great risks of abuse would obviously accompany any provision for obligatory abortion. But to forbid voluntary abortion because of the danger of involuntary abortion would be like forbidding voluntary adoptions on the grounds that they might lead to involuntary adoption policies. The battle against coercion must be fought at all times, with respect to many social options, but this is no reason to prohibit the options themselves.

Conclusion

There are many reasons which may lead a mother not to wish to give birth, but to have an abortion instead. They range from the most compelling to the most trivial. In early pregnancy, society's reasons for protecting life—the suffering and harm to the victim, to the agent, to the family and friends, and to society as a whole—do not apply, either to the zygote or to the embryo. Abortion, for whatever reasons, should then be available upon request. Preventing birth before conception or just after conception, however, presents fewer ethical conflicts than later abortions.

As pregnancy progresses, the social reasons for preventing killing are more and more applicable to the fetus. At the stage where a fetus is viable—capable of independent life outside the mother's body—these reasons begin to be as substantial as at birth and thereafter. In addition, viability represents the time when cessation of bodily support by the mother need not result in fetal death; as a result a viable fetus is capable of protection by others. For these reasons, I believe that after the established time of possible viability, methods separating fetus and mother so as to kill the fetus should be prohibited. But an earlier time

—perhaps 18 rather than 24 weeks—is preferable for all but exceptional cases (such as those occurring after prenatal diagnosis of severe malformation).

Even though abortion may be *lawful* up to this time, however, it is not necessarily an act which an individual may consider right or justifiable. This discrepancy results, I believe, from the fact that the *social* reasons for protecting life may also be looked upon in each case as *individual* reasons. Society may not find that abortion harms either victim or agent, family or social practices. But the individual parent or physician may see risks to himself as a person from such acts and look at them as breaches of personal responsibility toward the unborn. They may then regard abortion as personally distasteful, even though it is lawful.

Some physicians, for example, do feel that they cannot participate in abortions without personal danger of brutalization and without sharing responsibility for killing. This may be especially true when they are called in, as in large hospitals, to perform one abortion after another without any chance to consult with the women involved and to hear their case histories. There should never be a requirement that a physician or nurse must participate in an abortion. Even if women have a right to abortion, they have not therefore the right to force others to perform such acts.

In the same way, a mother or a father may feel personal grief over the death of a fetus, and responsibility for killing it, quite apart from the legality of the act. This grief and this responsibility, which would be present as a matter of course where parents wish for the birth of their baby, may also accompany an unwanted pregnancy. The following factors should then be weighed by the mother before she can be confident that abortion is the right way out of her dilemma, and one she will not come to regret or view with guilt:

- whether or not the pregnancy was voluntarily undertaken.
- the importance and validity of the *reasons* for wanting the abortion.
- the technique to be used in the abortion; the extent to which it can be regarded as 'cessation of bodily life support,' rather than as outright killing.
- the time of pregnancy.
- whether or not the father agrees to the abortion.
- whether or not all other alternatives have been considered, such as adoption.
- her religious views.

And the father, if he weighs these factors differently, may feel the grief and responsibility differently too, and wish to take over the care of the baby after birth.

Abortion is a last resort, and must remain so. It is much more problematic than contraception, yet it is sometimes the only way out of a great dilemma. Neither individual parents nor society should look at abortion as a policy to be encouraged at the expense of contraception, sterilization, and adoption. At the same time, there are a number of circumstances in which it can justifiably be undertaken, for which public and private facilities must be provided in such a way as to make no distinction between rich and poor.

NOTES

1. Roe v. Wade, *United States Law Week 41*, 1973, pp. 4213-33. Doe v. Bolton, *Ibid.*, pp. 4233-40.

2. See *The Morality of Abortion*, ed. by John T. Noonan, Jr. (Cambridge: Harvard University Press, 1970), and G. H. Williams, "Religious Residues and Presuppositions in the American Debate on Abortion," *Theological Studies* 31 (1970), 10-75.

3. Judith Thomson, "A Defense of Abortion," *Philosophy and Public Policy* 1 (1971), 47-66.

4. See Selig Neubardt and Harold Schulman, *Techniques of Abortion* (Boston: Little, Brown and Company, 1972).

5. But lines are hard to draw here. There are many intermediate cases between the pregnancy intentionally begun and, for instance, that resulting from carelessness with contraceptives.

6. See Morton A. Stenchever, "An Abuse of Prenatal Diagnosis," *Journal of the American Medical Association* 221 (July 24, 1972), 408.

7. Noonan, *Morality of Abortion*, p. 51. For a thorough discussion of this and other views concerning the beginnings of human life, see Daniel Callahan, *Abortion: Law, Choice and Morality* (New York: Macmillan Company, 1970).

8. Jérôme Lejeune, "On the Nature of Man," (Lecture at the American Society of Human Genetics at San Francisco, October 2-4, 1969).

9. Paul Ramsey, "Feticide/Infanticide upon Request," *Religion in Life* 39 (July, 1970), 170-86. Arthur J. Dyck, "Perplexities for the Would-Be Liberal in Abortion," *Journal of Reproductive Medicine* 8 (June, 1972), 351-54.

10. Roe v. Wade, *United States Law Week 41*, pp. 4227, 4229.

11. *Ibid.*, p. 4227. For further discussion see L. Tribe, "Foreword: Toward a Model of Roles in the Due Process of Life and Law," *Harvard Law Review* 87 (1973), 1-54.

12. Augustine, *The City of God Against the Pagans*, Book I. Ch. XX (Cambridge: Harvard University Press, 1957).

13. C. D. Stone, "Should Trees Have Standing? Toward Legal Rights for Natural Objects," *Southern California Law Review* 45, 450-501, provides an interesting analysis of the extension of rights to those not previously considered persons, such as children, and a discussion of possible future extensions to natural objects.

14. Joseph Fletcher, "Indicators of Humanhood: A Tentative Profile of Man," *The Hastings Center Report* 2 (November, 1972), 1-4.

15. Edward Shils, "The Sanctity of Life," in *Life or Death: Ethics and Options*, ed. by D. H. Labby (Seattle: University of Washington Press, 1968), p. 12. David Hume, "Of the Immortality of the Soul," *Essays: Moral, Political, and Literary* (London: Longmans, Green, and Co., 1882), II, p. 405.

16. This question will be taken up in detail in Part V. It is because all of the reasons for protecting life are *present* when someone considered to be a slave is murdered that the spate of recent sensationalistic comparisons of abortion and slavery do not make sense, even though it is true that in both cases there are denials of the humanity of the victims. Once again, a confusion in the use of the word humanity' is at fault.

17. William L. Langer, "Checks on Population Growth: 1750-1850," *Scientific American* 226 (February, 1972).

18. Every effort must be made by physicians and others to construe the Supreme Court's statement "If the State is interested in protecting fetal life after viability, it may go so far as to proscribe abortion during that period except when it is necessary to preserve the life or health of the mother" to concern, in effect, only the life or threat to life of the mother. See Alan Stone, "Abortion and the Supreme Court: What Now?" *Modern Medicine*, April 30, 1973, pp. 33-37, for a discussion of this question and what it means for physicians.

19. Theodore Friedmann, "Prenatal Diagnosis of Genetic Disease," *Scientific American* 225 (November, 1971), 34-42 and A. Milunsky, *et al.*, "Prenatal Genetic Diagnosis," *New England Journal of Medicine* 283 (December 17, 1970), 1370-81; (December 24, 1970), 1441-47; (December 31, 1970), 1498-1504.

20. Especially when genetic evaluation of *donors* becomes a common practice. See Walter Wadlington, "Artificial Insemination: The Dangers of a Poorly Kept Secret," *Northwestern University Law Review* 64 [6] (1970), 777-807.

21. See Edward Pohlman, "Unwanted Conceptions: Research on Undesirable Consequences," *Eugenics Quarterly* 14 [2] (June, 1967), 144.

22. I discuss the reverse situation, where the father wishes to force the mother to have an abortion, in the next section.

23. See *New York Times*, Saturday, January 28, 1972.

24. "When abortion is recommended by a physician, the indications should be stated in the patient's records, and informed consent obtained from the patient and her husband, or herself if she is unmarried, or from her nearest relative or guardian if she is under the age of consent." From *Policy on Abortion*, issued in August, 1970 by the Executive Board of the American College of Obstetricians and Gynecologists. See Tribe, *Harvard Law Review*, 38-41.

25. See for example, Noonan, *Morality of Abortion*, p. 258.

26. Some have used the same argument for the opposite conclusion. Since, or if, we allow abortion, they say, we *should* allow infanticide under certain conditions. See Michael Tooley, "Abortion and Infanticide," *Philosophy and Public Affairs* 2 (Fall, 1972), 37-65, and John M. Freeman and Robert E. Cooke, "Is There a Right to Die— Quickly?", *Journal of Pediatrics* 80 (Spring, 1972), 940-5. Once again, such a conclusion fails to take into account the powerful social reasons against infanticide.

27. It is important to be clear here about the differences between active killing of infants and the fact that the battle for life, in those rare cases where an infant is born with a severe malformation, such as the absence of a brain, is not undertaken or not carried as far as it would otherwise be. There *are* difficult borderline cases, but nothing suggests that killing actively in early pregnancy opens the door to the active killing of infants.

28. See *Reichsgesetzblatt*, 1926, Teil I, Nr. 28, 25 May 1926, ¶ 218, and 1943, Teil I, 9 March 1943, Art. I, "Angriffe auf Ehe, Familie, und Mutterschaft."

29. See the Maryland case *in Re Smith* reported in *41 U.S. Law Week* 2202, 1972, where a 16-year-old girl was jailed at the request of a Circuit Court judge in order to undergo the abortion she refused, but which her mother insisted upon. At the last moment, a higher court freed the girl.

2 *Breaking Through the Stereotypes*

SIDNEY AND DANIEL CALLAHAN

This article reports on and summarizes a Hastings Center research project on views of abortion. The purpose of the project was to situate this debate within the discussants' more general value framework and attempt to transcend the stalemated moral and legal debate. Thus the project attempted to discover elements which united, rather than divided, areas of mutual concern, and points of contact that could lead to the building of consensus.

Sidney Callahan is Associate Professor of Psychology at Mercy College

Daniel Callahan is Director of the Hastings Center

Apart from some of the nastier reasons people impute to each other, just why is it that there are such profound differences about abortion? For at least twenty years now we have asked that question of each other, just as we have asked how our own differences and those of others might be reconciled. Ever since the topic of abortion became of interest to us, in the 1960s, we have disagreed. Well over half of our thirty years of marriage have been marked (though rarely marred) by an ongoing argument. For all of that period, one of us (Daniel) has taken a pro-choice position and the other (Sidney) a pro-life position (to use, somewhat reluctantly, the common labels).

At one time, while Daniel was writing a book on the subject, we talked about it every day for four years. Thereafter, Sidney wrote a number of articles on abortion, some of which would be xeroxed and distributed by pro-life protestors at Daniel's lectures. Whether observers made the connection between the two Callahans was not always clear, but we experienced the conflict first-hand. Over the years, every argument, every statistic, every historical example cited in the literature has been discussed between us. As Eliza Doolittle of *My Fair Lady* says about "words": "There's not a one I haven't heard."

Yet we continue to disagree. How can that be? Our desire to better

understand our own differences and those of others led us not long ago
to organize a small research project at The Hastings Center, supported
by a grant from the Ford Foundation. As a social pyschologist, Sidney
had earlier investigated the differing views and personal characteristics
people have about the making and keeping of promises. She found that
the moral stance one takes on that common moral problem reflects
deep and pervasive premises about the self and the world. In Daniel's
work on biomedical ethics, he has similarly observed that people bring
to specific moral issues their broad outlooks toward themselves and
the world; but those outlooks are often not immediately apparent on
the surface of their conventional arguments and moral stances.

Why not, we thought, look at the problem by considering the
different ways in which abortion opponents understand themselves
and the world? How do they bring that wider and deeper understanding to bear on this difficult, divisive issue? Many people, we reluctantly suspect, are not greatly interested in understanding in some sympathetic way why abortion is so divisive an issue. To recall Karl Marx's
expression, they want to change the world not understand it. In the
larger political arena, it is victory that counts. But given the depth and
apparent intractability of abortion differences, we think that in the
long run most persons in the society will have to find a way to live
with differences.

Our project, therefore, sought to see if we could provide some
better insight into how individuals weigh and order their values when
dealing with abortion. Though they came up from time to time, we did
not directly deal with the most common issues in the abortion debate—when does life begin? What should the law be? and so on—but
instead with the way in which abortion as a problem is situated within
the terrain of a person's general, more encompassing values. We hoped
that, if we could not entirely escape the common forms of sociological or psychological reductionism, we might at least bring to them
some greater complexity and penetration. We sought only understanding, not a compromise solution, a consensus position, or a political
recommendation.

A few other decisions gave the project its final shape. With the
exception of Daniel, all of the other participants would be women.
They would be equally drawn from the pro-choice and the pro-life
side. And they would focus their discussion on four broad themes:
feminism, the family, childbearing and childrearing, and the political
and cultural nature of our society. Those topics, we believe, provide for
many in our society the background framework of values that often
shape abortion attitudes.

Finally, although we wanted a group that was evenly divided on the moral and political issues, we also wanted one that could effectively talk and work together. Thus there was no pretense that the group would be representative of all the ethnic, religious, political, and cultural groups active in the abortion debate. But it was to be representative of one important, if sometimes overlooked, group—those women who, though they differ, are willing to talk with those on the other side, willing to make the effort to empathize with those who hold opposing views, and willing to see if they can find some shared ground to keep their dialogue alive. The results of our discussion were sufficient to persuade us that a more complex, nuanced, and fruitful argument is possible. That argument is more fully laid out in the book we edited as an outcome of the project *Abortion: Understanding Differences* (Plenum Press, 1984).

The general debate has seen an effort, on all sides, to make abortion fit into some overall coherent scheme of values, one that combines personal convictions and consistency with more broadly held social values. Abortion poses a supreme test in trying to achieve that coherence. It stands at the juncture of a number of value systems, all of which continually joust with each other for dominance, but none of which by itself can do full justice to all the values that, with varying degrees of insistence and historical rootedness, clamor for attention and respect. Here we will try to present a composite picture of the positions presented at our meetings. Not all of the participants may have perceived the discussion the way we did, but we think the following account would gain general support.

The values that sustain and give theoretical legitimacy to both the pro-life and pro-choice movements are commonplace and command widespread respect. Neither has invented unusual moral principles nor idiosyncratic values. Consider first the pro-life position. It is committed to respect for an individual's right to life, even if that right is uncertain or in doubt in borderline cases (or even if there is doubt about whether it is "life"); the need to protect the weak and powerless, at the least in order to preserve them from the harm that can be done by the more powerful, and at the most to provide them with an opportunity to develop their full potential; the legitimacy of writing moral convictions and principles into law, particularly when that seems necessary to protect the rights of others (as in the civil rights movement); the value, not of fatalism but of accepting accidents and mischance as a part of life, and a denial of violent solutions as a way out of such vicissitudes; an obligation on the part of the community, whether through mediating institutions or the state, to provide support for those whose troubles (for example, an unwanted pregnancy) might lead them to forced, destructive choices; and, finally, the conviction that moral values and ideals toward nascent life should be upheld even at the cost of individual difficulties and travail.

The values that were identified as integral to the pro-life position are a mixture of those ordinarily labeled "liberal" and "conservative." The pro-life movement cannot, in its essence, be reduced to a simple conservative nostalgia or backlash, however much that may characterize some of its activist leaders and many of its mainline features. In the formulations of some, it can just as well go in a recognizably liberal direction. What probably most distinguishes it in that rendering from the more garden varieties of liberalism is its willingness to live with— and accept—externally imposed tragedy as a part of life. That has not been a traditional part of secular liberalism, which has always been far more inclined toward instrumental rationality than the version that has surfaced in the pro-life movement. The liberal community itself, however, has engaged in some sharp criticism of the part of its tradition that has stressed "rationalization" (a rational socially engineered solution to personal and political problems) and "emancipation" (freedom from the restraint of society and rejection of moral traditions). Hence, not only can the pro-life movement make a strong claim to upholding many traditional liberal values, it can also (in some important formulations) lay claim to reflecting some recent developments intrinsic to liberalisms' self-definition.

The pro-choice movement can lay an equally strong claim to an important piece of the American and Western tradition. By stressing freedom of choice, it gives centrality to the sovereignty of the individual conscience, especially in cases of moral doubt. It also recognizes a closely related principle: that those who must personally bear the burden of their moral choices ought to have the right to make those choices. By its emphasis on the unique burden of women in pregnancy and childrearing it has fostered the enfranchisement of women in controlling their own destinies. In its polity, the pro-choice movement is at one with that recently emergent tradition that would free procreational choices from the control of the state and, more generally, give the benefit of uncertainty in matters of conscience to the individual rather than the government. Its recognition of the injustice inherent in the known pattern of illegal abortions—that of *de facto* discrimination in favor of the affluent and the powerful—makes an important contribution to a more just society. Through its concern for choice and control in procreation, it has focused attention on parental responsibility, helping to remove childbearing from the realm of biological chance and sexual inevitability. By sundering a once necessary relationship between sexual activity and procreation, it helps provide an adaptation to a world that no longer needs, nor can afford, unlimited childbearing.

Just as the pro-life movement can be said to have its conservative and liberal wings, the same is true of the pro-choice movement. In its libertarian formulation, it is heavily weighted toward the maximization of individual choice and the privatization of moral judgment. The basic concern is not so much with the social and economic conditions under which choices are made, or with the ethical criteria by which they ought to be made, but solely with preserving the right to make a choice. But that is not the only pro-choice formulation. In a different rendering—what might be called liberal communitarianism—the pro-choice movement recognizes that a socially forced choice in favor of abortion is not a fully free choice; that a lack of communal, economic, and social support often coerces an abortion that would not be necessary in a more just society; that private moral choices are subject to moral judgments and standards; and that what ought to be an inherently difficult tragic choice can easily be trivialized and routinized— tacitly sanctioned and advanced by a society that promotes narcissism, prefers technological fixes to structural change, and is all too happy to see abortion put to the service of reducing welfare burdens.

There are, we think, two different abortion debates now taking place, one of them tense, open and familiar, the other more relaxed, less public, and surprising in some of its features. At one level, there is a fairly primitive, monochromatic struggle that takes place between the most public and vociferous activists on both sides. Kristin Luker's research on those groups (presented in our project before its appearance in book form in *Abortion and the Politics of Motherhood*) has vividly laid out the background values and assumptions that animate their convictions. There is a pro-life movement dedicated to the preservation of the nuclear family, the centrality of childbearing in the life of women, and a religious rather than a secular view of life. As a mirror image of that movement, there is a pro-choice ideology dedicated to female emancipation from the body and a repressive nuclear family, a subordination of childbearing to other personal goals, a celebration of rational control of self in place of the acceptance of fate, and a secular rather than a religious view of life.

At that level, the debate admits of no accommodation. It is a living out, in bold relief, of the struggle between modernity and traditionalism that has been waged since at least the age of the Enlightenment. For both the pro-choice modernizers and the pro-life traditionalists, abortion serves as a perfect symbol for such pervasive issues as the roles and rights of the sexes, the family, the relationship between law and morality, the nature and malleability of social reality, and the place of reason and choice in human life. But by choosing to cast the issues in those fundamental terms, and by making abortion carry the weight of a Manichean-life struggle between the good (evil) past and the good (evil) present, each side has doomed itself to an utter inability to talk with the other side, the likelihood that neither side can wholly triumph in the future, and the disheartening prospect of never-ending, never-decided civil strife for everyone else.

For all of those reasons, it is the debate at the other level that bears attention, cultivation, and development. Our own project discussions manifested some traits significantly different from those sketched above. Four features of that discussion are worth noting.

The first, already alluded to, is that participants from each side combined both liberal and conservative, modernizing and traditional-ist, ingredients in their respective positions. Each side is uncomfortable with the more stark options and tight combinations of values pursued at the extremes of the debate. They thus felt free—and indeed, in many ways, compelled—to appropriate and adapt from both poles, to fashion a different kind of synthesis. Both, strikingly, borrow from the various civil-rights struggles of the recent past. The pro-life groups point out that a fundamental aim of the civil rights efforts was to protect and give voice to those without power—to give them an equal moral standing in the community. For them, the task is to extend to the fetus the rights won by women and racial minority groups; fetal rights are not inherently hostile to women's rights. The pro-choice groups, sensitive to the deprivations of women who are given no options in their reproductive lives, want to provide women with a choice about something central to their lives. Yet, though they may differ about the meaning of the various civil-rights struggles, those battles serve as a common reference point for both. Most critically, neither side finds the understanding and interpretation of the other outlandish or implausible.

Second, both sides tended to share a distrust of that form of libertarianism that would wholly sunder the individual from the com-munity, setting up the private self as an isolated agent bound by no moral standards other than those perceived or devised by the agent. In this, they not only share some of the conservative and neoconservative critiques of liberalism, but share as well a similar questioning that has become part of the liberal tradition itself, whether from Marxist or other sources. They are, however, hardly less distrustful of that form of traditionalism that believes the past must be preserved in all of its purity. They want to be able to use the past selectively, preserving what remains valuable, rejecting what has been either harmful or wholly overtaken by time, and in general seeing the past as a resource requiring constant adjustment and adaptation for life in the present.

Third, they are uncomfortable with the labels *pro-life* and *pro-choice*. Those terms, they are well aware, were devised for polemical and political purposes, not for carefully nuanced distinctions. *Pro-life* is misleading because it begs the question of what actually serves human life and welfare; *pro-choice* is not less misleading because it begs the question of whether freedom of choice ought to be made an ultimate moral value, regardless of the nature of the choice to be exercised. Put another way, *pro-life* begs the question of moral means. The labels are also disliked because of a suggestion that one must be wholly one or the other. But the more complex reality is that many in the pro-life group will not condemn out of hand all women who have abortions; and many in the pro-choice group are repelled by the banal moral arguments used to justify many abortions. Neither group, in short, is happy when *pro-life* or *pro-choice* seem to require a *reductio ad absurdum,* or inflexible, insensitive moral rules, to be pursued regardless of consequence.

Fourth, both sides are concerned about the conditions that lead or drive women to abortions, and about the social, economic, and cultural contexts of abortion decisions. They rejected, on the one hand, that rendering of the pro-life position that construes all choices in favor of abortion as merely personal convenience or crass expediency; and, on the other, that version of the pro-choice position that is interested only in the easy availability of abortion, regardless of cause or motivation. They are willing to pursue together an understanding of ways to limit a forced choice of abortion because of poverty or the oppression of women, or lack of social support for childbearing; and they are no less willing to pursue together those social reforms that would be more supportive of troubled pregnancies.

Why, then, sharing so much in their beliefs about how the abortion problem should be understood, and sharing some mutual criticisms of the assumptions and premises of those who fight at what we have called the first level, do they still differ? In part, they can differ because of the relative weight they give to various considerations; ever so faintly tilting one way or another can be decisive when the political and legal choices are so narrow. But in the end it came down, we think, to what is perhaps one of the most profound and subtle value differences of all. That is the matter of one's general hopes and beliefs about the world, human nature, and reality. Put simply, for many who are pro-choice, abortion is a necessary evil, one that must be tolerated and supported until such time as better sex education, more effective contraception, and a more just social order make possible fewer troubled pregnancies. And even then, there will still be some justifiable reasons for abortion; it will never disappear. For the pro-life group, it is a ban on abortion that must be the necessary evil, one that must be advanced as a long-term step in devising a social order that is more supportive of women and childbearing, more dedicated to an eradication of violence as a solution to personal or social threats.

Both sides, then, are prepared to agree that abortion is undesirable, a crude solution to problems that would better be solved by other means. The crucial difference, however, is that those on the pro-choice side believe that the world as it is must be acknowledged, and not just as it might or ought to be. Here and now, in our present social reality, there are women who need or desire abortions. Future solutions to the general problem of abortion, at some unspecified date, will do them no good. They have to live with the reality they encounter. They cannot be asked to bear personally the burden of helping to create a better future, which, even if possible, is not within their individual power to bring about. By contrast, the pro-life group believes that a better future cannot be achieved unless we begin now to live the ideals that we want to achieve, unless we are prepared to make present sacrifices toward future goals, and unless aggression toward the fetus is denied, however high the individual cost of denying it. The acceptance of reality as it is implicitly legitimates the *status quo,* undercuts efforts to bring about social change, and sanctions violence as an acceptable method of coping with problems.

Differences of that kind run deeply, pitting fundamentally discrepent attitudes and predispositions against each other. The dichotomies are expressed in our ordinary language when "idealists" are contrasted with "realists," or when the "hard-nosed" are pitted against the "starry-eyed." The liberal pro-life group, it sometimes seems, favors the equivalent of unilateral disarmament on abortion, and is willing to bear the hazards of a stance that will put many women at risk of disaster. They are willing to make a moral bet that the violence inherent in abortion will, in the long run, be repudiated. The public, they think, will eventually respond to the principled witness of those who reject it. The pro-choice group, for its part, is hesitant to indulge hopes of that kind. They are unwilling to ask women to give up a viable solution to their present problems in the name of a yet-to-be future, one that might never come.

Perhaps the most striking outcome of our project was the way it broke many stereotypes. Too often it is assumed that a commitment to feminism entails a pro-choice position; but that is only one version of feminism, not necessarily its essence. Too often it is assumed that a commitment to the family as an enduring value entails a prohibition of abortion; but that does not follow either. Too often it is assumed that a pro-choice stand entails treating children as disposable goods, of value only if wanted. But that is too often a parody of the genuine affirmation of the value of children that can be a central part of a pro-choice position. Too often it is assumed that a society which values the rights of individuals must deny the value of community and thus any social restrictions on abortion choices; but in some renderings a denial of abortion can be a way of affirming rights.

There is no suggestion here that the differences are any less sharp than ever, or to deny that even slight differences can have a significant social impact. It is only to suggest that the relationship of abortion to such deeper values as feminism, the family, childrearing, and the political culture are open to more flexible, interesting possibilities than has been apparent in much of the public debate. If our own domestic wrangles have not led to a general shift in position for either of us, it has nonetheless been valuable. Neither of us has remained unchanged by the other.

3 Abortion: On Fetal Indications

SUSAN NICHOLSON

The problem of aborting a fetus because of fetal indications presents a specific problem in morality; for in this situation the intent of the abortion is to insure the death of the fetus, which may not be part of an abortion for other reasons which could result only in the separation of the fetus from the mother. In this provocative article, Nicholson argues that fetal euthanasia can be compared to the withdrawal of support from congenitally handicapped newborns. On the basis of this analogy, Nicholson argues that it is consistent with Roman Catholic morality to approve fetal euthanasia. In addition to the development of this argument, Nicholson also provides an interesting commentary on the Roman Catholic moral tradition of the obligation to preserve life and the distinction between the use of ordinary and extraordinary means of treatment.

Susan Nicholson is a member of the Department of Philosophy at Simmons College

Preceding sections have argued that it is morally permissible for a woman to terminate bodily life-support of a fetus resulting from rape, or where continuation of support is incompatible with her own life. Abortion in such circumstances is morally justifiable even though it predictably results in the death of what has been assumed to be a human being. In such abortions, fetal death is not the course aimed at. Hence, the preceding arguments would not justify fetal killing in circumstances in which development of an artificial uterus made possible termination of bodily life-support *without* killing the fetus.

In this section we consider a justification offered for abortion which, if accepted, *would* permit fetal killing even in a technologically advanced age of artificial uteruses. I refer to what is sometimes called the "fetal indication" for abortion, namely, that the fetus is seriously malformed. A woman who seeks an abortion on fetal indications typically terminates fetal life-support because she wants the fetus dead. If an artificial uterus were available, she would not want the fetus transferred to it. For a variety of reasons she feels that it would be better not just that the bodily connection between herself and the fetus be terminated, but that the fetus *die.*

The purpose of this section is to attempt to answer with regard to abortion on fetal indications questions raised previously with regard to rape and therapeutic abortion—namely, whether or not Roman Catholic doctrine on abortion is consistent with other aspects of Catholic moral theology, and whether or not it properly commands support from secular morality.

As in preceding sections, the structure of my argument is analogical and I assume, for the sake of argument, the human status of the fetus. I argue that the Roman Catholic condemnation of abortion on fetal indications is incompatible with the principle of Roman Catholic medical ethics permitting omission or termination of extraordinary measures for prolonging life. The logical implications of this principle, while disavowed by Roman Catholic moralists, are surprisingly liberal. In fact, they are so liberal that it is quite possible that Roman Catholic moral theology here goes beyond what is generally approved in our secular society.

This last point is a speculative one. Since the principles involved in determining the morality of abortion on fetal indications are much more controversial than those relevant to therapeutic abortion and abortion of pregnancies resulting from rape, it is not possible to specify the relationship between the Roman Catholic position and secular morality with much assurance.

The technique of *amniocentesis,* developed within the last decade, has made possible identification of a fetus as malformed. Available from approximately 16 weeks of pregnancy onwards, amniocentesis consists of injecting a needle through the woman's abdomen into the amniotic sac and withdrawing some of the fluid which surrounds the fetus. This amniotic fluid contains fetal cells, and a chromosomal analysis is capable at present of detecting the presence of all the major chromosomal abnormalities and more than 60 rare biochemical diseases (Powledge, 1976:7). It is anticipated that further development of amniocentesis and other new methods for monitoring fetal development will add to this list. Amniocentesis replaces the statistical knowledge of fetal anomalies available through genetic analyses with the kind of information hitherto possible only at birth.

95. Several reasons might be given for aborting a fetus whose malformities have been detected by amniocentesis. Broadly speaking, the reasons may be social, familial, or fetal. Social reasons include a

eugenic concern for the "health" of the gene pool, as well as a concern for the social costs involved in the care, support, and education of a severely handicapped person during her/his lifetime. A familiar reason involves concern for the stresses on the particular person or persons to whom the disabled person is related. A "fetal" reason would be concern for the emotional and physical suffering which will be experienced by a person with the chronic, incurable condition detected *in utero.*

I wish to consider the strongest possible case which can be made for abortion on fetal indications. Hence I will not attempt to defend the abortion of a malformed fetus which is performed for social or familial reasons. This simplification will reduce considerably the complexity of the moral issues involved.

In particular, abortion for social or familial reasons involves whether or not an individual's presumed interest in living may justifiably be overridden in the interests of society or the family. If the fetus is aborted because it is believed that it is in an individual's *own* best interests not to live a disabled life, this issue does not arise. The question I wish to address, then, is whether or not it could ever be morally justified to abort a malformed fetus for the fetus' own sake.

96. It is evident that we are confronted here with the question of the morality of *euthanasia,* and of *fetal euthanasia* in particular. Euthanasia will be taken in this study to refer to acts or omissions which result in death, which are aimed at death, and which are motivated primarily by compassion for the person who dies.[1]

Roman Catholic doctrine unequivocally condemns fetal euthanasia. The following passage, taken from an essay on abortion by Congressman Fr. Robert F. Drinan (1973:130) is typical of Roman Catholic opinion:

> But can one logically and realistically claim that a defective nonviable fetus may be destroyed without also conceding the validity of the principle that, at least in some extreme cases, the taking of a life by society may be justified by the convenience or greater overall happiness of the society which takes the life of an innocent but unwanted and troublesome person?
>
> I submit that it is illogical and intellectually dishonest for anyone to advocate as morally permissible the destruction of a defective, nonviable fetus but to deny that this concession is not a fundamental compromise with what is surely one of the moral-legal absolutes of Anglo-American law—the principle that the life of an innocent human being may not be taken away simply because, in the judgment of society, nonlife for the particular individual would be better than life.

It is intellectually dishonest to maintain that a defective, non-viable fetus may be destroyed unless one is also prepared to admit that society has the right to decide that for certain individuals, who have contracted physical and/or mental disabilities, nonexistence is better than existence.

Drinan's remarks against fetal euthanasia are telling in that they conjure up visions of physicians who carry out social policy by administering fatal air injections over the protests of disabled persons who want to go on living. This picture is misleading, however, in several respects.

97. In the first place fetal euthanasia, as defined above, is not carried out *on behalf of* societal interests, but on behalf of the person who would otherwise live with the defects detected *in utero.* Nor is the judgment that nonlife for that person would be better than life a judgment made *by* society. Rather, the judgment is generally made by the person's parents.

98. In the second place, fetal euthanasia never brings about the fetus' death contrary to fetal wishes. Even those who believe that the fetus is a human being must acknowledge that the fetus lacks the capacity to desire life or death.

It is true that fetal euthanasia, since it occurs without the fetus' consent, is nonvoluntary euthanasia. Voluntary euthanasia is defined as euthanasia which occurs with the patient's consent; nonvoluntary euthanasia as that which occurs without the consent. However, some distinctions within this category of nonvoluntary euthanasia are called for. Nonvoluntary euthanasia consists of situations in which (1) the patient is considered competent to give consent and withholds it, wishing to live; (2) the patient is not considered competent to give consent, although capable of wanting to live or to die; (3) the patient is presently incapable of wishing either to live or to die. Within this third category we may make still another distinction. Some persons presently incapable of desiring either to live or to die have nonetheless lived long enough to enable close others to offer a judgment, based on their acquaintance with the patient's personality and values, of what the patient would want. With other presumed persons, such as fetuses, this is of course impossible.

It is important to make these distinctions because objections made to nonvoluntary euthanasia may not be applicable to all varieties of it. In particular, some objections to euthanasia which occurs *contrary* to the patient's wishes are not applicable to euthanasia which occurs *in the absence of such wishes.*

For instance, euthanasia which occurs contrary to a patient's desire to go on living involves overriding the patient's judgment of what will advance her/his own interests, or at the very least involves the greatest frustration on a person's desires imaginable. These objectionable features do not characterize fetal euthanasia. It is possible to maintain that a patient's judgment or desires concerning her/his life or death should not be overridden but that when the patient is incapable of either judgment or desire, someone else should make a judgment on the patient's behalf.[2]

99. In the third place, fetal euthanasia differs from Drinan's depiction in so far as it involves the withdrawal of life-support rather than the initiation of lethal measures. Consequently, abortion on fetal indications should be compared with other situations in which life-support is withdrawn in order to bring about the merciful death of the person receiving such support, where that person is incapable of making any judgments or having any wishes in the matter.

100. In accordance with this discussion, I suggest that fetal euthanasia may appropriately be compared to withdrawal of support from congenitally handicapped newborns. Recent medical literature contains discussions of instances in which treatment was withdrawn from infants born with severe handicaps, because it was believed to be in the infant's own best interests that it die.[3] The similarities with fetal euthanasia are obvious. Infants, like fetuses, are incapable of desires concerning the perpetuation or nonperpetuation of their lives, although if they live they may develop opinions as to what should or should not have been done on their behalf. Furthermore, in the case of both infants and fetuses, it is generally the parents in consultation with medical personnel who decide on behalf of their child that support should be withdrawn.

My strategy here is to set out the Roman Catholic doctrine on the steps which must be taken to preserve life. I shall argue that this doctrine entails the permissibility of a merciful withholding of treatment from infants born with severely deforming and incapacitating conditions, and hence that Roman Catholic moralists should, to be consistent, approve fetal euthanasia.

Roman Catholic doctrine on the measures which must be taken to preserve life is not developed with the rigor and thoroughness that mark Catholic doctrine on therapeutic abortion in particular, and the abortion doctrine in general. I was able to find only one book-length treatment of the subject which compares favorably with the treatment given abortion by Callahan (1970), Grisez (1970a), Granfield (1971), or Huser (1942).[4] However, several basic themes emerge from papal addresses to medical societies, Catholic texts in medical ethics,[5] and articles in Catholic theological journals. Where there is disagreement on significant details, this will be noted.

101. The two basic principles of the Catholic doctrine on the

prolongation of life are: (1) Persons are obliged to use *ordinary measures* to preserve their life and health. (2) Persons are not obliged to use *extraordinary measures* except where the preservation of their life or health is required to attain some greater good.

The duties of a physician and relatives of the patient are to provide all ordinary measures of sustaining life, in addition to whatever extraordinary measures are reasonably requested by the patient.[6] In the case of a young child the rule is that the parents are obligated to see to it that the child is provided with all ordinary means of preserving life. Parents may, if they wish, provide extraordinary measures for a child, but they are not obligated to do so. (See, e.g., Healy, 1956:80–90.)

These principles are affirmed by papal statement. According to Pope Pius XII (1957b:395–6):

> Natural reason and Christian morals say that man (and whoever is entrusted with the task of taking care of his fellowman) has the right and the duty in case of serious illness to take the necessary treatment for the preservation of life and health. . . .
>
> But normally one is held to use only ordinary means—according to circumstances of persons, places, times, and culture—that is to say, means that do not involve any grave burden for oneself or another. A more strict obligation would be too burdensome for most men and would render the attainment of the higher, more important good too difficult. Life, health, all temporal activities are in fact subordinated to spiritual ends. On the other hand, one is not forbidden to take more than strictly necessary steps to preserve life and health, as long as he does not fail in some more serious duty.

102. The most commonly used definitions of ordinary and extraordinary measures are those formulated by Kelly, and cited earlier in this study. According to Kelly (1951:550) ordinary means are

> all medicines, treatments, and operations, which offer a reasonable hope of benefit and which can be obtained and used without excessive expense, pain, or other inconvenience.

Extraordinary measures, on the other hand, are those

> which cannot be obtained or used without excessive expense, pain, or other inconvenience, or which, if used, would not offer a reasonable hope of benefit.

It may seem strange that a patient should be *required* to use ordinary measures of sustaining life. A patient would normally want to use such measures to prolong life, and where s/he didn't, why shouldn't it be permissible to dispense with them? It is the patient's own death, not someone else's, which would result from omitting such measures.

To answer this question we must refer to the Catholic view that human beings are not the owners but only the stewards of their bodily lives.[7] According to this view, God alone has complete dominion over a person's bodily life. As a good steward of someone else's possession, one may have to submit to the prolongation of a life one would just as soon relinquish. When the hardships involved in the treatments prolonging life become great enough, however, one is mercifully released from the duty of conserving that which belongs ultimately to God. Of course, one may be sufficiently attached to one's own bodily life to be willing to undergo great hardships to preserve it. In that event Roman Catholic doctrine permits one to do so, provided the effort does not detract from the attainment of higher values.

103. Prior to the development of anaesthetics and antibiotics, surgery was frequently very painful as well as dangerous, and classified by Catholic moralists as extraordinary. However, an operation or therapy which today is considered neither very dangerous nor very painful may be considered extraordinary relative to the physical condition of a particular patient.

Healy (1956:64–67) describes an appendectomy, for example, as ordinary if performed on an otherwise healthy patient, but extraordinary if performed on a patient suffering from cancer who has at most three months to live. Similarly, Kelly (1958:130) describes intravenous injections of glucose and digitalis as extraordinary treatment of a 90-year-old comatose and apparently terminally ill patient.

It is evident from these examples that the designation of a treatment as extraordinary involves a *weighing* of the benefits of the treatment against the hardships involved in the treatment. The minimum expense, inconvenience, and pain associated with intravenous feeding will not vary significantly from one patient to another, but the benefit in length of life made possible by intravenous feeding will vary considerably. This distinction between extraordinary and ordinary measures no doubt differs from the distinction made by non-Catholic physicians, who could be expected to describe intravenous therapy as ordinary treatment even where it was expected to prolong the life of a particular patient by only a very short time.[8]

Even where a treatment can be expected to prolong a patient's life for many years, it may be regarded as extraordinary if it deprives the patient of normal functioning. This is indicated by the remarks made by several Roman Catholic moralists concerning amputations or other mutilating surgery.

Sullivan (1949:65), for example, classifies amputation of both arms and both legs as an extraordinary measure. Another moralist, McFadden (1967:253), while acknowledging that modern medicine has greatly reduced the severe physical and psychological hardships of living with an amputated limb, allows that there might be circumstances in which amputation is not obligatory, as where other bodily afflictions make it impossible to develop a facile use of an artificial limb or continue as one's sole means of support. McFadden (1967:255) says that mutilating surgery is also extraordinary in cases where it is possible to "foresee with clarity the truly severe and permanent handicaps which will be the outcome of what might otherwise be called 'successful' surgery." Healy (1956:68–70) makes a similar point concerning a 40-year-old badly deformed and crippled married man who cannot survive unless his leg is amputated. According to Healy, this man is not obligated to undergo surgery. Moreover, because of the added hardship and sacrifice which would be required of his wife should he lose a leg, Healy says the man might rightly judge that he is obliged to forego the operation.

104. It is clear from these examples that the licitness of foregoing measures necessary for life does not apply solely to terminal patients. A patient may be dying, of course, in the sense that s/he will soon be dead unless preventive measures are taken, but not be dying in the stronger sense that s/he will soon be dead despite preventive measures. The patient in Healy's illustration is not dying in this stronger sense. Although he will indeed die unless his leg is amputated, if the amputation is performed he could live presumably another twenty to thirty years.

105. There are two additional aspects of the Roman Catholic doctrine which are important for our purposes. The first is that in application of the two basic principles cited above, Roman Catholic moralists make no moral distinction between failing to initiate extraordinary measures and terminating extraordinary measures. Nor do they distinguish between terminations of extraordinary measures accomplished by omissions, and those requiring the performance of acts. Kelly (1950; 1951; 1958), for example, does not differentiate between what is from the physician's point of view failure to perform a particular operation and discontinuation of intravenous feeding. Pope Pius XII (1957b) in the address quoted above states his approval of the discontinuation of mechanical respiration in certain situations. Shut-

ting off a respirator presumably requires an act. In terms of the typology described in Figure 1, Roman Catholic moralists thus approve letting die$_1$, letting die$_{2_a}$, and killing$_{2_b}$, provided that in each case the measures omitted or terminated are extraordinary. I will speak of the *withholding* of extraordinary measures to cover both the physician's failure to initiate treatment, and termination of treatment by either act or omission.

106. The second aspect of the doctrine which should be emphasized here is this: It is licit to withhold extraordinary measures from a patient without the patient's consent, provided the patient is unable to give consent. Comatose patients, for example, cannot consent to the withholding of treatment, but Catholic medical ethics nonetheless permits extraordinary measures to be withheld from them. The decision to withhold is to be made by a close relative of the patient's, or where no relatives are available, by the patient's physician. In the case of a very young child, the parents are to decide whether or not extraordinary measures will be withheld. Healy (1956:81) states that in making such decisions, the parents are obligated to do "whatever they prudently think the child would reasonably request if he were actually able to pass judgment on the matter."

107. To make this last point more concrete, consider the following example. Imagine you are told you have developed a disease which will soon claim your life unless you submit to a series of operations and other therapy which will remove or destroy arms, legs, and nerve tissue, leaving you with almost a normal life-expectancy but completely helpless, blind, deaf, subject to uncontrollable spasms, without control over your bodily functions and vulnerable to periods of intractable pain. You recognize that you would not be remiss in your duty to God to prolong your bodily life if you decided to forego

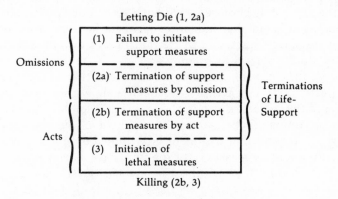

Figure 1. Killing/Letting Die Typology

such treatment, and for your own part, you would find such an existence intolerable. You therefore decide to forego treatment, even though you know that your death will be an inevitable result.

Since this is the decision you make for yourself, you may in good conscience make a similar decision on behalf of your year-old daughter when informed that she has been stricken with the same disease, and requires similar treatment to survive. You decide it is best to spare her such hardship and suffering, even though you are aware that sparing her will inevitably result in her death. You judge for her, as for yourself, that non-life is better than life accompanied by such travail.

108. Now suppose you are confronted with your newly born infant son who is *delivered* with just those same multiple deformities. Due to exposure to a certain drug during pregnancy, the infant is incurably blind and deaf, has no limbs, and will be subject throughout his life to uncontrollable spasms and periods of intractable pain. The doctor informs you that your son's life expectancy is nevertheless only slightly less than normal. Born prematurely, the infant is presently in an incubator.

You realize that you have found yourself in this situation twice before. Again you make the decision that non-life is better than life. Accordingly you request that your infant be removed from the incubator, to die.

109. Roman Catholic moralists would say that you have acted licitly in the first two instances but not in the third. How is this possible? They cannot maintain that you do not have the right to decide for your newborn that non-life is better than life, because we have seen that Catholic doctrine grants you the right to decide precisely that with regard to your year-old daughter. Nor can they object that in the present case your infant son is *killed* by the *act* of removing him from the incubator, because as we have seen, Roman Catholic doctrine makes no moral discrimination between the termination of supportive measures by act, and the termination of or failure to initiate support which occurs through omission.

What they can do, however, is point out that in the first two cases death is only a *foreseen* consequence of withholding therapy whereas in the last case death is *aimed* at. That is, in the first two cases you do *not* arrange that treatment be withheld *in order that death occur.* Rather, you request that treatment be withheld in order to avoid the use of extraordinary measures. In the third case, however, you *do* arrange that treatment be withheld *in order that death occur.* Unable to avert an intolerable existence except through death, you request that your infant be removed from the incubator *in order that he die.*

110. It is thus the *means/foresight* distinction which accounts for the moral discriminations Roman Catholic moralists would make among these three cases. In the third case, the bad effect (death), is a *means* to the good effect, whereas in the first two cases death is merely a *foreseen* consequence of dispensing with extraordinary measures of life-support.[9]

It will be recalled that the means/foresight distinction, while of no use in understanding the Roman Catholic doctrine of therapeutic abortion, is the key to many applications of the Double Effect Principle. In previous applications, the Double Effect Principle distinguished *acts* in which the bad effect is a means from *acts* in which the bad effect is merely foreseen. Here it is evident that the principle is being used to make similar distinctions among *omissions* as well.

111. It will be further recalled that except in cases of therapeutic abortion, Roman Catholic moralists regard a killing as direct if death is aimed at either as means or end, and as indirect if death is merely foreseen. Hence, except in cases of therapeutic abortion, the direct/indirect distinction is identical to what may be called the *aim/foresight* distinction. It will be observed that the means/foresight distinction is subsumed under the aim/foresight distinction.

112. It is instructive to refer to *Figure 2*. Striking a vertical line down the middle of the chart, we may distinguish acts or omissions in which death is aimed at either as means or end (left side of chart) from acts or omissions in which death is merely foreseen (right side of chart). The chart is thus divided vertically by the aim/foresight distinction, and horizontally by the killing/letting die distinction. This is done in Figure 2.

Notice that the killing/letting die distinction crosscuts the direct/indirect distinction. Acts and omissions which *aim* at death are *direct* killing and *direct* letting die, respectively. Acts and omissions which merely *foresee* death are *indirect* killing and *indirect* letting die, respectively.

Now, since euthanasia was defined in this study as acts or omissions which result in death, are aimed at death, and are motivated primarily by compassion for the person who dies, it appears on the left side of the chart. Euthanasia may involve the failure to initiate life-support (letting die$_1$), the termination of life-support by omission (letting die), or by act (killing$_{2b}$), or the initiation of lethal measures (killing$_3$). Hence it appears in all four blocks on the left side of the chart. A distinction is sometimes made between *active* or *positive* euthanasia, and *passive* or *negative* euthanasia. The distinction between active and passive euthanasia appears to parallel the distinction between killing and letting die.

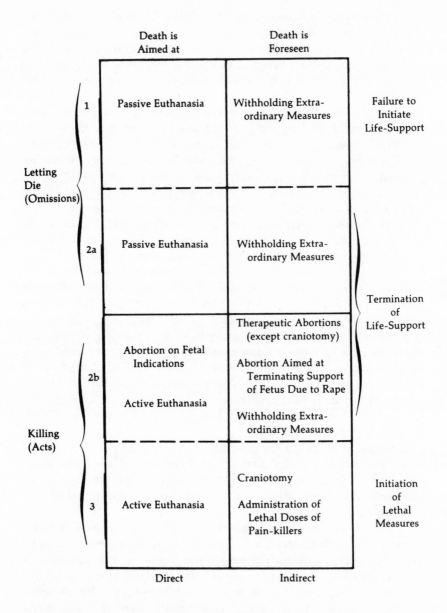

Figure 2. Typology of the Cross-Cutting of the Killing/Letting Die Distinction by the Aim/Foresight Distinction

Notice that each time euthanasia appears in Figure 2, there is a comparable type of indirect letting die or indirect killing which is approved by Catholic moral theology. This chapter presents the Catholic doctrine giving approval to the merciful withholding of extraordinary measures of prolonging life. It will be recalled that Catholic moral theology approves the compassionate initiation of increased dosages of palliatives which are predictably lethal, provided death is not aimed at but is only foreseen. This is comparable to an instance of active euthanasia such as mercifully giving a suffering patient an air injection so that s/he may die.

We may now return to the hypothetical examples of your year-old daughter to whose mutilating surgery you refuse consent, and your congenitally deformed infant son whom you order removed from the incubator. Both examples involve the merciful withholding of measures necessary for life, undertaken without the child's consent. However, the former, in which death is merely foreseen, belongs on the right side of Figure 2. The latter, in which death is a means, is a type of euthanasia, and belongs on the left side of Figure 2. It is thus by insisting on the moral relevance of the means/foresight distinction that orthodox Catholic moralists are able to approve the compassionate withholding of support measures, as well as the merciful initiation of lethal doses of palliatives, while condemning the practice of euthanasia in all its forms.[10]

Having said this, I should point out that there are traditional Catholic moralists who *do* give their approval to the withholding of extraordinary measures in order that death might occur. Sullivan is one, and Kelly, somewhat tentatively, another. Sullivan (1949:72) presents the following illustration.

A cancer patient is in extreme pain and his system has gradually established what physicians call "toleration" of any drug, so that even increased doses give only brief respites from the ever-recurring pain. The attending physician knows that the disease is incurable and that the person is slowly dying, but because of a good heart, it is possible that this agony will continue for several weeks. The physician then remembers that there is one thing he can do to end the suffering. He can cut off intravenous feeding and the patient will surely die. He does this and before the next day the patient is dead.

It is evident that in this case the physician cuts off intravenous feeding in order that the patient die. In thus approving the physician's action in this case, Sullivan clearly condones a cessation of treatment directed at ending a patient's suffering by death. Kelly (1950:219) states that on purely speculative grounds he is in agreement with Sullivan's analysis, but that on practical grounds he hesitates to recommend it lest "the abrupt ceasing to nourish a conscious patient might appear to be a sort of 'Catholic euthanasia' to many who cannot appreciate the fine distinction between omitting an ordinary means and omitting a *useless* ordinary means."

It would appear that Kelly's fears are well-founded. Sullivan has indeed approved an instance of euthanasia. The uselessness of the treatment does not alter the fact that the treatment is terminated in order that the patient die.

It is not entirely clear what Kelly has in mind when he distinguishes here between an ordinary means and a useless ordinary means.[11] Most likely he means by useless, a treatment which cannot forestall death for more than a very short period of time. In that case, "Catholic euthanasia" would be available only to those dying in the strong sense of dying discussed in section 104.

113. I submit, however, that even without Kelly's concession Roman Catholic doctrine is committed to the licitness of euthanasia, and to far more than euthanasia of the terminally ill alone. Consider again the examples of your daughter who requires mutilating surgery to live, and your congenitally deformed son in the incubator. What you want in *both* cases is to avoid subjecting your child to an existence so severely burdened that not even God requires that this bodily existence be preserved. If preserving a severely deformed bodily existence were owed to God then you could not in the first case licitly withhold mutilating treatment from your daughter while foreseeing that she would die untreated. In the second case, again your ultimate end is avoidance of a grossly disabled bodily existence. Only here it is not the therapy provided which will create such disabilities for your son. On the contrary, the disabilities are already irremediably present. Consequently, the only way to avoid such an existence is to arrange for your son's death.

Now, I do not see how the avoidance of a handicapped existence can be so desirable an end that it justifies withholding support measures with death as a foreseen result, yet fail to be a desirable enough end to justify withholding support measures in order that death occur. It would of course be immoral to use death as a means in circumstances where the end in view could be accomplished some other way. But this is not the case here. Moreover, it is similarly immoral to adopt a means in which death is a certain foreseen side-effect unless the end in view cannot be accomplished in any other way.

Note that I am not urging the general teleological principle that it is morally justifiable to adopt death as a means where doing so will increase the total good. I contend only that if two acts of omissions are similar in all relevant respects except that in one death is merely a foreseen consequence whereas in the other death is a means, then if the first is morally permissible so is the second.

It should be emphasized that this does not mean that in circumstances in which one is permitted to act or fail to act while foreseeing a person's death, one may also aim at the death of *that same person.* Consider again the parent who withholds mutilating surgery from a child while foreseeing that the child will die untreated. That this is permissible does not imply that the parent may aim at that same child's death as a means. (Similar points have been made with regard to abortion of pregnancies resulting from rape, and therapeutic abortion. A woman who aborts a fetus resulting from rape foresees but may not aim at fetal death. Should her fetus unexpectedly survive the abortion, she may not kill or let the fetus die.) It may be thought that this demonstrates the moral significance of the means/foresight distinction.

We may account for these moral judgments, however, without invoking the means/foresight distinction. The ultimate end of the parent who withholds mutilating surgery while foreseeing the child's death is avoidance of an existence intolerable to the child. The child's death is not, of course, a means to that end. Hence the parent who aims at that same child's death must have some *other* end in view. Perhaps the parent seeks the child's death in order to be rid of unwanted parental duties.

In some situations, then, the means/foresight distinction is associated with a difference which *is* morally relevant, for instance a difference in ultimate ends. This does not, of course, demonstrate that the means/foresight distinction itself possesses moral significance.

The following reflections suggest another reason why some people attribute moral significance to the means/foresight distinction. If a parent withholds mutilating treatment from a child, and the physician is mistaken in believing that the child will die untreated, then nothing is lost. The child lives, and lives without debilitating handicaps. If, on the other hand, a parent withholds treatment from a malformed child in order that the child die, and the physician is mistaken about the irremediability of the child's physical problems, then all is lost. The child could have lived without debilitating handicaps, but now is dead. Some persons may conclude that the fallibility of medical predictions provides a basis for distinguishing acts or omissions in which death is a foreseen result, from acts or omissions in which death is a means.

It would be a mistake, however, to draw this conclusion. The fallibility of medical predictions works both ways. Suppose the doctor is correct in predicting that the child will die without mutilating surgery, but wrong in estimating the severity of the disabilities which would result from the surgery. Or suppose new techniques are on the horizon for enabling persons with such disabilities to lead satisfying lives. Then if a parent withholds mutilating surgery while merely foreseeing death as a result, all is lost. The child could have lived without intolerable handicaps, and now is dead. I conclude that the fallibility of medical predictions does not provide a basis for imputing moral significance to the means/foresight distinction.

114. It is instructive at this point to consider defenses of the means/foresight distinction offered by two Roman Catholic moralists. Consider the following passage from Grisez (1970b:76).

> In this nonutilitarian moral outlook, whether or not another person's death is admitted within the scope of our intention is extremely important. A difference of intention can relate identical behavior in quite different ways to our moral attitude, and to the self being created through our moral attitude. If one intends to kill another, he accepts the identity of killer as an aspect of his moral self. If he is to be a killer through his own self-determination, he must regard himself in any situation as the lord of life and of death. The good of life must be treated as a measurable value, not as an immeasurable dignity. Others' natural attitudes toward their own lives must be regarded as an irrational fact, not as a starting point for reasonable community.

It may be argued, however, that Grisez's criticisms of direct killing are equally applicable to indirect killing.

In the first place, Grisez claims that a person who aims at death accepts the identity of killer and regards himself as the lord of life and death. Is this any less true of a doctor who deliberately administers increased dosages of a palliative to a patient while merely foreseeing the patient's death as an inevitable result? In administering dosages which s/he knows to be fatal, the physician accepts the identity of (compassionate) killer and, at least in this situation, regards her/himself as lady/lord of life.

In the second place, Grisez maintains that a person who aims at death regards life as a measurable value. But surely the permissibility of measuring life against other values is inherent in the fourth condition of the Double Effect Principle, which requires that the good intended be commensurate with the evil foreseen.

That is, the physician who administers increased dosages of a palliative while merely foreseeing that death will result has, in conformity with the Double Effect Principle, judged that the good effect of freedom from pain is commensurate with the bad effect of this particular patient's death. Similarly, a person who decides to forego extraordinary measures of life-support while foreseeing her/his own death as an inevitable result has judged that the value of avoiding burdensome life-support measures outweighs the value of continuation of her/his own life. But to weigh life and death against other values is surely to regard life as a measurable value.

Finally, it should be obvious that the attitudes of others towards their own lives may be taken into account while aiming at death, and disregarded where death is merely a foreseen result.

In a comprehensive and insightful study of the Double Effect Principle, Richard McCormick (1973) tentatively proposes the following modified understanding of the moral relevance of the means/foresight distinction. Both acts in which the bad effect is merely a foreseen consequence and acts in which the bad effect is a means may be justified by their good consequences. This is, of course, a departure from traditional Roman Catholic moral theology which forbids use of a bad means to an end, no matter how good the end. Nonetheless, McCormick does not regard the means/foresight distinction as morally superfluous. He contends that while the immediate consequences of direct and indirect killing are the same, their long-range consequences may be very different. That is, the over-all bad consequences of direct killing may be worse than those of indirect killing. Hence, the teleological assessment of the two may differ.

Why should the long-range consequences of direct killing differ from those of indirect killing? McCormick answers that the person who kills directly is more closely associated with death, more willing that death occur, than one who kills indirectly. This difference in psychological awareness of the bad effect may, in the long run, lead to significantly different consequences.

McCormick provides little elaboration or defense of his view that there is a psychological difference between aiming at death and merely foreseeing death as a result of one's actions. However, his view may derive plausibility from the following reflections.

Consider again the parent who arranges that mutilating surgery be withheld from a child while foreseeing the child's death as a result. Were the child to live without the surgery, the parent presumably would be pleased. This may be contrasted with the example of a parent who arranges that support measures be withheld from a malformed infant in order that the infant die. Were the infant to live without the support measures, the parent presumably would be displeased. Thus it may appear that the parent who merely foresees a child's death as a result of withholding support measures is less willing that death occur than the parent who, in withholding support aims at a child's death.

Observe, however, that in both instances the parent is willing that death occur *only insofar as death is associated with accomplishment of the end in view.* For a fair comparison, one must imagine the reaction of the parent of the malformed infant were s/he to learn, after support measures had been withheld, of new techniques to ameliorate the infant's disabilities. Were the infant to live without the support measures, presumably this parent too would be pleased. The point is that it would gratify both parents if the good end could be accomplished without bringing about the child's death.

115. I conclude, therefore, that if it is morally permissible for a parent to refuse mutilating surgery for a child while foreseeing that the child will die untreated, then it is morally permissible for a parent to request that a congenitally malformed infant be removed from an incubator in order that the infant die. But the case of the congenitally malformed infant was introduced as a parallel to fetal euthanasia. Hence if a parent may have a malformed infant mercifully removed from an incubator, then a woman may have a malformed fetus mercifully removed from her uterus.

It would appear, then, that the Roman Catholic doctrine of the licitness of withholding extraordinary measures of life-support entails the permissibility of fetal euthanasia. Accordingly, Roman Catholic moralists should approve of abortion on fetal indications where the abortion is performed in the best interests of the fetus. The argument I have presented here for fetal euthanasia may be summarized by a slightly altered version of the passage previously quoted from Drinan:

> It is intellectually dishonest to deny that a defective, nonviable fetus may be destroyed while admitting that parents have the right to decide that for certain very young children who have contracted physical and/or mental disabilities, nonexistence is better than existence.

It must be reiterated that since the moral principles relevant to nonvoluntary euthanasia are much more controversial than those relevant to therapeutic abortion and abortion of pregnancies due to rape, it is not claimed that the Roman Catholic doctrine is without support from a common secular morality concerning the sanctity of life. The claim made here is solely that Roman Catholic moralists cannot, in keeping with their doctrine of the prolongation of life, condemn abortion on fetal indications.

116. Two questions arise naturally from the foregoing analysis. While they cannot be dealt with here, they suggest directions for future discussion and research.

The first concerns the difference between withholding support from malformed fetuses and infants, and initiating lethal measures against them. Once it is admitted that it is permissible to withhold supportive measures from a defective fetus or infant in order that a merciful death may occur, is there any reason why lethal measures could not be initiated for the same purpose? In his study of the well-publicized Johns Hopkins case in which the parents of a Down's syndrome infant born with an intestinal blockage refused to have the blockage corrected by simple surgery, the Protestant moralist Gustafson (1973:547) raises this question.

Once a decision is made not to engage in a life-sustaining and lifesaving procedure, has not the crucial corner been turned? If that is a reasonable and moral thing to do, on what grounds would one argue that it is wrong to hasten death?

It might, in fact, be argued that it is sometimes preferable to hasten death rather than to allow death to come naturally. The Down's syndrome infant in this particular case took 15 days to die after all the supportive measures had been withdrawn. The Roman Catholic theologian Maguire (1974:11) points out that "though the death of this child *may* have been merciful, its dying was not," and suggests that this might be a case in which withholding therapy is harder to justify than initiating lethal measures.

The second question is in what circumstances can it truly be said that nonexistence is better than existence with certain disabilities? As far as I know, no longitudinal studies have been made of persons born with serious malformities. Do these people wish they had not been born? In the absence of empirical research into the conditions under which a person would prefer not to have lived, we can expect that parental perception of the manner of child it would be pleasing to rear will often fill the void. To combat this tendency, it would be necessary to establish empirically based limits on the range of malformities with reference to which a parent may choose death for a child. Until such limits have been established, a practice of infant and fetal euthanasia cannot seriously be recommended.

NOTES

1. This characterization of euthanasia is drawn from an unpublished doctoral dissertation on voluntary euthanasia by Bok (1970).

2. The same point is made by Smith (1974). A similar point is accepted, furthermore, where the use of experimental procedures is at issue. It is not considered proper to use experimental medical procedures on a competent adult without her/his consent. It is considered proper, however, for a parent to consent to the use of such procedures on a child where the parent judges this to be in the child's own best interest. See, e.g., Ramsey (1970:1–58).

3. A recent article in the *New England Journal of Medicine* describes itself as breaking a taboo of silence by disclosing that in the special care nursery of the Yale-New Haven Hospital from January 1970 to June 1972, there were 43 deaths related to decisions by physicians and parents to withhold treatment from newborns whose "prognosis for meaningful life was extremely poor or hopeless." (Duff and Campbell, 1973.) A physician responsible for an English clinic specializing in treatment of babies born with spina bifida argues that the past policy of his clinic to treat all infants is not in the interest of the patients, and urges selective treatment only. (Lorber, 1971, 1973.) For additional medical literature, consult Foltz *et al.* (1972) and Shaw (1973). For a discussion by an ethicist of the moral issues involved in the well-publicized Johns Hopkins case in which the parents of a Down's syndrome infant withheld consent to simple corrective surgery, see Gustafson (1973). Additional discussion of ethical issues occurs in Bard and Fletcher, Joseph (1968); Cooke (1972); Fletcher, John (1974); Freeman, E. (1972); Freeman, J. and Cooke (1972); Reich and Smith, H. (1973); Smith, D. (1974); and Zachery (1968).

4. This is *Death by Choice* (1974), by the theologian Daniel C. Maguire. Maguire argues for the liberalization of the orthodox Catholic doctrine. An exposition of the orthodox doctrine, presently out of print and having little depth, is given by Sullivan (1949).

5. Texts consulted were: Häring (1973); Healy (1956); Kelly (1958); Kenny (1962); Marshall (1964); McFadden (1967); and O'Donnell (1959).

6. See, e.g., Kelly (1950:216). Kelly also mentions that the physician's professional ideal may create obligations which extend beyond the duties and wishes of the patient.

7. For a good exposition of this doctrine, see Häring (1973:66–73).

8. With regard to glucose and digitalis for a 90-year-old comatose patient, Kelly (1958:130) says that moralists would generally say this was ordinary means if it were merely a matter of tiding a patient over a temporary crisis, yet "in the present case the actual benefit they confer on the patient is so slight in comparison with the continued cost and difficulty of hospitalization and care that their use should be called an *extraordinary* means of preserving life."

9. Häring (1973:146), for example, writes that he trusts the non-Catholic reader will not consider it "hairsplitting" to distinguish between cases in which the direct objective is to dispense with extraordinary measures and cases where treatment is omitted or stopped in order to allow the patient to die.

10. Kenny (1962:134), for example, claims that "the proponents of euthanasia have little, if any, conception of morality."

11. In Kelly's 1951 article, he defines ordinary means as means which, among other things, offers "a reasonable hope of benefit." Thus in this later article he appears to have incorporated the notion of usefulness into his concept of an ordinary means.

4 Abortion: A Review of Ethical Aspects of Public Policy

Thomas A. Shannon

This article presents an overview of the development of the abortion policy debate in the United States. In addition to looking at the historical and sociological dimensions of the debate, the article focuses on several aspects of the policy debate: alternatives to abortion, health care policy, religion-government relations, and pluralism.

Thomas A. Shannon is Professor of Social Ethics at Worcester Polytechnic Institute

The purpose of this paper is to review and analyze several issues related to the debate about public policy on abortion. What I hope to do in this article is review some of the ethical and political issues raised in abortion, describe some aspects of abortion policy in America, identify ethical problems raised by some of the policy questions, and then discuss some of the ethical issues involved in these policy debates. I will present some conclusions based on this material. What I hope to accomplish by this is to indicate some fundamental problems in the debate and hope that we as members of a professional society can return to our classrooms and communities and focus on some of the more substantive issues behind the debate.

I. A REVIEW OF POLICY AND INCIDENCE OF ABORTION

According to Christopher Tietze[1] as of late 1980, about 9% of the world's population lived in countries where abortion was prohibited without exception and about 19% of the world's population lived in countries where it was permitted only to save the life of a pregnant woman. Fewer than 10% live in countries where statutes authorize abortions on broader medical grounds, i.e., averting a threat to a woman's health rather than only to her life, and occasionally for eugenic or fetal indications. About 24% of the world's population were

77

able to take into account social factors such as income, housing, marital status in evaluating a woman's health. About 38% of the population live in countries which allow abortion on request without specifying a reason and this is generally limited to the first trimester of pregnancy.

These policies also have a wide range of applicability. A policy authorizing abortion to avert a threat to a pregnant woman's health could be defined narrowly or broadly. Social indications for abortion may similarly be defined. Many statutes may not be strictly enforced and, in any event, whatever statutes there are rely upon the cooperation of health care providers and delivery systems. Consequently, even though a particular country may have a liberal abortion policy which is guaranteed by statute, that does not necessarily mean that the procedure is actually available to any woman who wants an abortion.

Within the last 15 years, many countries have liberalized their abortion laws; 4 countries in Eastern Europe adopted more restrictive legislation and 3 countries liberalized their policies and then made them more restrictive.

The reasons used by proponents of less restrictive abortion legislation are summarized as follows: consideration of public health, especially the morbidity and mortality associated with illegal abortion; social justice, allowing poor women to have equal access to abortion; women's rights, including the right to control their own bodies. Only a few countries—Singapore, Indonesia, and China—have used the explicit motivation of curbing population growth in the interest of economic and social development as a reason for adopting nonrestrictive abortion policies. Ironically, many countries which permit abortions either at the request of the woman or on broadly interpreted social indications have low birth rates and some of these countries are now actively pursuing pronatalist population policies.[2]

Although highly speculative, the number of abortions internationally have been estimated at around 55,000,000 which would correspond to an abortion rate of around 70 per 1,000 women of abortion age and an abortion ratio of 300 per 1,000 known pregnancies.

The differences in abortion rates in the United States between whites and blacks are interesting. Between 1963 and 1965 among whites, the abortion rate was .19 per 1,000 and from 1966 to 1968 it was .29 per 1,000. During those same years it was .17 and .29 for blacks respectively. In 1978 the abortion rate for whites was 22.7 and 60.4 per 1,000 for blacks.[3]

II.   A Review of Policies on Abortion in the United States

In *Abortion in America* Mohr traces the history of why in 1800 there were virtually no abortion policies and in 1900 every state had an antiabortion law. While not wanting to rehearse all of the salient elements in Mohr's book, there are a few policy issues I want to emphasize.

Mohr identifies several motives why the early abortion legislation came into being. The first motive focused on preventing the mother's death through the use of an abortifacient.[4] These laws, as Mohr notes, were primarily poison control measures focusing not so much on the fetus as on the health status of the mother and the safety of the procedure that was used. These laws also had the effect of reinforcing the traditional norm of "quickening" as the dividing line between abortions which were not governed by statutes and those which were. The other two motives Mohr says contributed to the increase in abortion laws, especially coming to a climax point at the end of the nineteenth century, have to do with changes in the perception of who was receiving an abortion and who was providing them. There was a growing fear that since first generation American women were now receiving abortions at high rates, the WASP population might be outnumbered by the immigrants. This perception was related to the developing nativist movement and consequently statutes were enacted to restrict abortion, intending not the protection of the fetus, but the protection of the status and power of the established classes. Parallel to this was the growing professionalism of medicine. Physicians were interested both in developing and tightening their own standards of practice and in eliminating from medicine those described as quacks. Physicians lobbied against abortion to eliminate from the profession individuals who would not abide by its rules and as a means of controlling the standards of the members of the profession itself. The medical profession was also further able to control abortion by helping define medical conditions under which abortion might be appropriate and by providing competent individuals to perform the procedure. Thus, by the end of the nineteenth century, abortion legislation was present in all of the states and was contrary to the earlier experience of the country in which abortion was possible for those who wanted it. Again, the primary intent of this legislation was the protection of the mother and the enhancement of the social status of two different groups within society: the establishment and physicians.

Mohr also describes the pressures that led to the reevaluation of these antiabortion statutes in our own time and which in turn led to the *Roe v. Wade* decision in 1972.[5] These pressures are: 1) the fear of overpopulation; 2) a growing concern for the quality of life of the fetus as opposed to the mere preservation of life; 3) the development of the Women's Rights Movement with its emphasis on a woman's right to control her body; 4) the growing safety of abortion done under appropriate medical conditions; 5) the fact that women were getting abortions in spite of restrictive legislation. One could also add to this list the movement of several states to relax their own abortion legislation. Ultimately this led to the testing of restrictive state statutes in the Supreme Court.

What is important from this survey is that abortion legislation was developed primarily out of a variety of social issues that were not directly or quite possibly even indirectly related to concern for the fetus. The older use of the term quickening and its contemporary analogue of viability, served as a touchstone for the limits of abortion. That is, in the early nineteenth century, abortion was not considered problematic morally or medically until the point of quickening. In the view of many individuals, a similar argument is being made today from at least a medical, if not a moral point of view. And, in fact, as Mohr indicates, the *Roe* decision is based somewhat upon this older traditional view within American society: abortions before quickening or viability are not problematic. But again Mohr focuses on the social context for the development of abortion legislation and its repeal. Abortion statutes—whether pro or con—were based upon neither the sanctity of life of the fetus nor disregard of it, but rather upon other social issues and concerns.

Another important review of abortion policies comes from a recent article by Tatalovich and Daynes, entitled, "The Trauma of Abortion Politics."[6] These authors indicate three significant periods in the history of the policy debate. First, in the early 60s the basic issue was the building of a consensus toward abortion reform which focused primarily on the availability of therapeutic abortion. The authors note that the proabortion advocates shared similar assumptions, made similar arguments and held common objectives with the abortion opponents. These proponents assumed, based on the American Law Institute's recommendations, that abortion should be permitted only to a limited number of women and that it should be performed for therapeutic reasons. This position defines abortion primarily in medical terms, not moral ones. The abortion reformers were not making any radical claims. All of the abortion statutes in effect permitted therapeutic abortions when the mother's life was in danger. Some states allowed abortion when the mother's health was threatened. What the reformers were arguing for was an incremental change in the abortion laws allowing this more expanded exception. And at that point in time approximately 80% of the general population favored some abortion reform, and while this support came from both Catholics and Protestants, Catholics did not support the reform at the same level that the Protestants did.

A second critical period the authors identify is 1969 to 1970, shaped as it was by three interrelated developments. First, the proabortionists shifted towards repeal of all abortion laws (as opposed to therapeutic reform). Second, opposition to abortion began to focus on opposition to *any* change, thereby opposing not only the new movement towards total repeal of abortion laws, but even the incremental changes that were desired earlier. Third, the proponents of abortion began to shift their strategy to the use of the judiciary to achieve reform rather than expend their limited resources on attempts to change legislation state by state. This strategy culminated in *Roe*, which appeared to many to have a "winner-take-all" dimension. This court decision made it difficult for any compromise posture to be taken and helped change the nature of the debate. Interestingly, the authors point out that there were ample court precedents on either side of the issue and that the court was not inherently locked into a proabortion decision. But had the court come out the other way, there still would have been a public policy debate, with the sides reversed. A major problem is not so much the court's decision, as the perceived "winner-take-all" nature of the decision which has in effect polarized the debate.

The third issue concerns this polarization of perceptions on abortion, as well as strategies to achieve the ends of the antiabortion groups. One of the by-products of this polarization has been the legislative maneuverings of the antiabortion group. Picking up their cues for strategies for reform from the proabortion groups, the antiabortion groups have gone them one better and chose to go neither the state legislative route nor the route of the judiciary but rather are attempting to circumvent the entire judicial system by having certain kinds of legislation declared judicially off limits. The antiabortion people recognize that state by state campaigns will be costly and time consuming and they realize that a constitutional amendment may be very difficult to achieve. One effective strategy is to circumvent these processes by having congress declare certain forms of legislation off limits to judicial review. They are also attempting to devise federal legislation to restrict public monies for abortion to as few cases as possible so that those who wish abortions must pay for them themselves. Two important moves here have been: first, a statute introduced to define life as beginning at conception—thus ensuring a fetus constitutional rights, making abortion illegal, and raising constitutional problems regarding certain forms of contraception; second, the Hatch amendment, recently passed by the Senate Judiciary Subcommittee, which states that the right to an abortion is not guaranteed by the Constitution and that the states and Congress shall have power to restrict and prohibit abortions. This amendment also gives a state law precedence if it is more restrictive than federal legislation.

Thus the third major phase of the debate these authors identify consists of a conflict at a very high and intense level among groups who are violently pro or con abortion, while simultaneously denying to legislatures the ability to make compromise moves. By focusing on an either/or position, consensus is more difficult to achieve and consequently no policy is able to gain legitimacy. Our current debate is characterized by polarization and a move from a debate of the issues to personal confrontations in which parties are perceived to be liberal or conservative with respect to this particular issue.

III. OPINIONS ON ABORTION

One of the issues that is important in developing a public policy is to insure some sense of legitimacy of this policy by rooting it in the beliefs of the citizenry so that the policy at least to some degree will be acceptable and workable. I am not arguing that the morality of abortion will be settled or determined by poll taking. I do argue that we must attend to perceptions about abortion to determine if there are possible connections between the pro and con abortion groups that can effect a compromise which enables a policy to be developed.

We need to examine first what reasons for abortion people find persuasive. One important finding is that there is an average approval of 67% for six specific reasons for abortion: a woman's health is seriously endangered by the pregnancy; becoming pregnant as a result of rape; a strong chance of a serious defect in the baby; the family has a low income and cannot afford any more children; the woman is pregnant and does not want to marry the man; the women is married and does not want any more children.[7] The last three reasons are known as "soft" reasons for abortion and there is no solid social consensus on these three. The average consensus for the first three reasons, the "hard" reasons, averages about 85%, whereas it is about 50% for the soft reasons. There is clearly a strong social consensus around the broadened concept of a therapeutic abortion. There is less, but slightly increasing, support for the more social or personal reasons for wanting an abortion. It is also important to note that the average approval has changed only four percentage points since 1972. There was a jump of twenty-two points between 1965 and 1972. But there has been a remarkable stability in the approval rate since 1972.[8]

With respect to the profiles of those engaged in the debate, there are some interesting correlations. First, two relevant differences between those who are pro and con abortion are that those who are antiabortion tend to feel that obedience to authority figures is more

important and that curiosity during child development is less important than do those who are in favor of abortion. Second, a finding
which should surprise no one, the higher a person's social status, the
greater is the tendency to approve abortion. In fact one study indicated
that a formal education is the best predictor of abortion attitudes.
Third, the more one disapproves of activities such as premarital sex,
extramarital sex, and homosexuality, the less one favors abortion.
Fourth, differences between Protestants and Catholics with respect to
favoring or not favoring abortion increase in proportion to the degree
of education that the individual has had. Finally, for both Protestants
and Catholics approval of abortion decreases as religiousity indices
increase, with the notable exception of Episcopalians who are more
likely to approve of abortion the more religious they are. What is
significantly interesting and important in one study was the allegation
that the Protestant-Catholic difference accounts for only about 1% of
the variation in abortion attitudes over the years. This leads to the
interesting hypothesis that the religious differences are not the critical
differences in the abortion debate and that to cast the debate in terms
of religious preference is both mistaken and particularly counterproductive for policy debates. These studies would indicate that the
critical variables are those beyond religion and having to do with
feelings about child rearing, social practices, education, and class.[9]

A study of differences between members of the National Abortion
Rights Action League (NARAL) and the National Right to Life Com-
mitee (NRLC) showed some interesting differences with respect to
what the membership of each organization felt about abortion.[10] These
findings are of particular importance for policy making. More than
95% of NARAL members and fewer than 5% of NRLC members
approve of legal abortion when there is a strong chance of a serious
defect in the baby, when the woman is married and wants no more
children, when a woman's husband will not consent to an abortion,
when the family is too poor to afford more children, when parents will
not consent to a teenager's abortion and when an unmarried woman
wants to have an abortion. These data are not surprising, especially
insofar as they refer to the soft reasons for abortion. However, it is
interesting that 73% of NRLC members favor making abortion available to women whose life is endangered by continuation of the pregnancy. Also 15% of NRLC members approve of abortion if the pregnant woman's physical health is seriously endangered by carrying the
pregnancy to term and 7% to 8% favor legal abortion if pregnancy is
the result of rape or incest. These data indicate that members of the
NRLC do not present as monolithic and absolutistic a position on
abortion as might be assumed. While the policy that could be based on

such feelings may not be acceptable to all, nonetheless it does indicate that there are possibilities for some movement. Compromise, of course, will be called for.

Another relevant factor revealed by this survey indicates that NRLC activists are not only generally more conservative on moral issues but are also likely to describe themselves as conservatives, as Republicans, and to oppose government action to reduce income differences between rich and poor. As important as those differences are, the NRLC members are much more likely than NARAL members to give priority to their views on abortion over their views on social issues. Eighty-four percent of NRLC members as opposed to 47% of NARAL members say that abortion is so important that they would refuse to support a candidate whose position on abortion was unacceptable. This may mean that in elections or in debates of public policy, all other things being equal, there may be a strategic advantage to having a group which has the higher percentage of single issue voters on its side.

Kelley identified some general reasons why they were concerned for only one issue.[11] First, abortion stops a human life and is, therefore, a unique issue. Second, a single issue focus protects the right to life movement from being absorbed or manipulated by any political party. Third, the passage of a human life amendment to the constitution requires a political coalition of people with different ideologies and, therefore, strategically they wish to avoid being perceived as members of any other group. There seems to be a recognition that the alliance present in the prolife movement is very tenuous and that it might not be able to stand the strain of having to deal with social problems that may not be perceived as having the same importance or solution, e.g., nuclear war or social welfare programs.

It would be interesting to know how the structure and impact of the prolife movement will be affected by the interior tensions that are present, at least with respect to differences in the kinds of approvals of abortion that are tolerated by some members. The monolithic unity of the prolife movement may be a perception, not a reality. One could assume that much of the energy of the prolife movement needs to be spent in making sure that potentially disruptive issues do not enter into the dialogue and that no relationship between the ethical values surrounding the evaluation of abortion and other social issues be made, i.e., extending a prolife stance to evaluate nuclear war. One could make a reasonable case that such a position will continue to become more and more difficult as time goes on and that members of prolife groups will have to make more and more difficult choices with respect to the supporting of political candidates, especially when these candidates present viewpoints on a variety of issues that may, in fact, appeal to different populations within the prolife movement.

IV. ETHICAL DILEMMAS AND PROBLEMS IN THE PUBLIC POLICY DEBATE

In this section I will indicate some problems that are critical in the ethical dimensions of the public policy debate. These issues clearly relate to and occasionally emerge from the problems that I have already addressed. But they also go beyond these problems and form a critical context in which the issues are debated or, more realistically stated, argued.

A. *Lack of Alternatives*

There are few, if any, good alternatives to abortion. Adoption clearly is an alternative to abortion, but choosing adoption requires that the woman still carry the child to term and deal with the reality of separation from the newborn, a painful experience even if the woman is highly motivated. Even in the best of circumstances such a separation will not easily be made and when there is the suggestion of coercion or significant familial or other pressure to carry the child to term rather than abort, the separation will be much more problematic. Even for women who choose to carry a child to term in the expectation of allowing the child to be adopted, there may be lack of good or even adequate social, physical and economic support systems to make such a process easier to accomplish and to insure the health of the mother and the newborn. Thus as much as a woman may desire to have the child adopted, she may not have either the physical or social support to do so.

Also we need to keep in mind the other alternative to abortion, carrying the child to term and keeping the child. An increasing number of women, especially among the teenage population, are choosing to keep their babies. Among the issues here are the ability and appropriateness of such young mothers to care for their child, as well as problems related to adequate financial and psychological resources to provide an appropriate setting for the rearing of the child. Oftentimes teenage mothers need to interrupt their high school education. They frequently live at home with their parents. These individuals are often already on welfare or will need such assistance. In the light of economic philosophy of the Reagan administration, reliance on that particular means of provision will either be inadequate or unavailable.[12]

Thus even though many see adoption or the keeping of the child by the mother as preferable to abortion, there are many problems involved in doing this, especially in light of the unavailability of social programs to provide a context which would facilitate these kinds of decisions. Although a variety of both counseling and economic assistance programs have been made available on a private basis, these programs are simply inadequate to deal with the needs presented by those individuals who might wish to carry a child to term and then either allow the child to be adopted or keep the child.

B.   *Health Care Policies: Neutrality or Discrimination?*

The perception, if not the reality, of the discriminatory treatment of women who choose abortion[13] is another major problem. The question is: If the federal government funds both pre and post-natal services under Medicaid, should it also fund services for abortion? This position has been argued before the Supreme Court and the decision was that the government does not discriminate by refusing to provide funds for abortion under Title 19 of the Social Security Program. Such a requirement, however, means only that such funds cannot come out of the federal budget. It is possible to continue, and in fact many states have continued, to support such abortion programs out of state funds. Nonetheless Medicaid funded abortions dropped from 295,000 in FY 1977 to about 2,000 in FY 1978.

Another problem that raises the issue of discrimination is the fact that those most affected by cuts in programs will be the poor. Those individuals able to afford abortions will continue to be able to afford them, whereas individuals who either cannot afford to have an abortion or who live in states which do not provide funds for abortion may not be able to obtain them. However, one study suggested that the majority of women desiring an abortion and previously qualified for Medicaid assistance still obtained one. The fiscal, physical, and psychological costs of doing this are not known. Also, approximately one-fifth of Medicaid-eligible women were not able to receive abortions because of funding restrictions. Thus the issue is: Will a particular group in our society have to bear a disproportionate share of the burden of such funding policies? The consequence of such a policy is that the government's position is seen not as neutral but as an aggressive policy designed to decrease the number of abortions. And since it can only do that in cases where it provides the funding, of necessity such restrictions have their most significant impact on the poor and the disadvantaged.

There are several subsidiary issues in this problem, among which are determining how abortion fits into the delivery of health care services and the perception that abortion may be a cost effective method to solve many of the budgetary problems of welfare programs. It is more cost effective to provide abortions than to provide continuing welfare payments. This observation does not begin to touch or even analyze the structural arrangments of our society which insure that a certain number of individuals will always be disenfranchised both politically and economically. We also need to determine what government neutrality with respect to abortion might mean. Does this mean that the government should provide nothing in the way of funds for abortion, that the government should not interfere with anyone who wishes to obtain an abortion, or that government should help fund any health related service a person may want, including abortion?

C.   Religion-Government Relations

One of the major claims of the proabortion groups is that those involved in the antiabortion movement are trying to impose a religious solution to the problem of abortion on those who do not hold that position and that this violates their religious freedom. Daniel Callahan has made an important statement: there are religious traditions which approve abortion and, by that standard, the current policy of liberal abortion laws in this country is the imposition of a religious value on another group of people.[14] Also the claims of foul play do seem to be related only to the abortion issue. No one is arguing that the religious groups which are beginning to form coalitions and speak out on the inherent injustice of the current Reagan economic program or the immorality of our nuclear deterrence policy are violating anyone's religious liberty and that, therefore, they should not engage in these activities.

There are several important issues in this debate, however. One has to do with how religious beliefs or values are translated into language appropriate for public debate. That is, is it possible to make insights and values that come from one's religious tradition or experiences accessible to people who do not share those experiences or traditions? The problem here is twofold: being able to make oneself understandable to other individuals; and making the depth of one's convictions accessible and intelligible to individuals who do not stand within that particular tradition. Another issue has to do with ecclesiology. How is the role of a church seen with respect to the larger society? Is a church to witness its values to society or is the church to analyze and evaluate, and occasionally reject social values? If ecclesiology leads one in the first direction, then it will not be as important to devise a means of translating insights so they can be understandable in a broader arena. If one chooses the second way, it will be extremely important to develop a widely accessible language so that one can easily and helpfully engage in policy debates.

The Catholic church in particular has attempted to develop a means of speaking both within and without the church through the philosophical tradition of the natural law. While acknowledging the many theoretical and practical problems in the use of that tradition, nonetheless I think it is important to remember that it provided a means by which the church could attempt to conduct a moral and political discourse with those who did not share the same theological perspectives of the Catholic community. Using this tradition, Catholic Christians could speak to the issues of the day in a language accessible to others while maintaining insights motivated by their own faith tradition.

We must also consider the appropriateness of a particular religious group putting itself both ideologically and financially behind a particular cause. Clearly religious groups have done this in the past and will continue to do so. Important in this consideration is the history of the religion's political actions and the manner and purpose in which it is perceived to be acting now. There is a broad and generally correct perception that the abortion issue is the first time in which the Roman Catholic Church has, to so significant a degree, become involved in lobbying for a particular public policy and provided rather large sums of money to help finance different organizations.

On the other hand, there seems to be nothing inherently inappropriate about a particular religious body supporting organizations to advocate a particular point of view. Almost all religions have a social ethic by which they evaluate public policy. The labor movement, Civil Rights, the Vietnam War, and nuclear war provide examples of how various religions did this. The relevant difference in this particular debate seems to be that it is being done with respect to abortion and by the Catholic Church. Few comments are raised about groups and churches that make financial and ideological contributions to the pro-abortion half of the debate, or to other political issues. In fact, I would be willing to argue that the support of churches, both financially and ideologically, would be welcomed—if the churches supported a pro-choice stance or at least so I would infer from reading the list of sponsors of prochoice advertisements.

We need to insist upon some sense of fairness when discussing how churches take public stands on matters of significant concern either to them or to the population at large. The position of a particular church may not be a popular one, but if it is the position of that church and there are serious reasons why the church feels it should engage in fairly direct political action, then that stance of the church should at least be respected. Oftentimes the real problem is the perennial one of whose ox is being gored. For many people, I suspect, as long as a church is sympathetic to their particular position, no cause will be taken with it. But when a church says something either unpopular or problematic, then some argue that churches should not speak. Such a position is at best inconsistent and at worst requires that a church maintain an inappropriate silence on issues of moral significance and political and social consequence.

D. *The Public Debating of Abortion*

How can the abortion debate be conducted in the public arena? This question is particularly problematic when viewed from perspectives developed by MacIntyre and Hauerwas that argues that our culture has few common premises by which competing value claims can be evaluated and judged.

Alasdair MacIntyre, in his perceptive article, "How To Identify Ethical Principles,"[15] argues several theses, one of which is extremely important for the consideration of ethical issues in the public policy debate. His primary claim is that morality is at war with itself because each moral agent reaches conclusions by valid forms of inference but cannot agree about the correctness or appropriateness of the premise with which the argument begins. MacIntyre then argues that moral philosophy in general, and I would argue our culture in particular, has no procedures for weighing rival value premises.

This particular situation has two major dimensions. First, we have not inherited the social or cultural context in which we can both understand and apply a particular philosophical theory. Second, we have inherited conflicting theories of ethics or social philosophy. MacIntyre argues that the social-philosophical context out of which our country developed its political philosophy comes from Aristotle, Cicero, Locke, and Sidney. Each of these presents conflicting and even contrary claims with respect to what is good for humans and, even if one could resolve the epistemological problems, one would still have the practical problem of evaluating the various goods which they claim are in the interests of human beings and the community.

Briefly stated, MacIntyre says we have inherited two conflicting world views. First, the classical world view which asks the moral question: How might humans together realize the common good? This position assumes that community is natural and normative, there are goods that human beings can rationally identify and agree upon, and that the common pursuit of these will bring both personal and social development. The second claim focuses on the moral question: How may humans prevent each other from interfering with one another as each goes about his or her own concerns? This viewpoint assumes that the state of being autonomous is the appropriate state for human existence, that individuals may not have interests or values in common, and that liberty and the pursuit of interests will maximize individual and social goods.

Our culture and society have attempted to finesse the significant philosophical and ethical problems that come from inheriting a mixed system by developing a liberal society or a pluralistic society. This strategy attempted to take controversial issues out of the political arena and relegate them to the individual conscience. This solution has worked by and large for several generations, but primarily because there was a general acceptance of many of the norms or ideals about human behavior that came out of the classical model. That is, as long as the majority of the citizenry shared a common understanding of what was right and what was wrong and what the limits of individual behavior were, then pluralism would work. Behind pluralism stood a general understanding of the limits of behavior, even though this may not have been explicitly articulated or even socially enforced by the society.

However, we now appear to be in a situation in which people are attempting to maximize their own freedom and in which the suggestion that some values are normative appears to be restrictive, coercive, or in an extreme form, politically repressive. Individuals are pursuing their own interests limited only by noninterference with a third party or not harming an unconsenting party. Such a position generally stands behind discussions relating to issues of homosexuality, some aspects of the women's movement, the use of technologies for fetal screening, heterosexual relationships, and abortion. Consequently, we have a type of moral schizophrenia in which there is some attempt, at least culturally, to hold onto values and norms from the classical mind set, while on the other hand having our instinctual argument arise out of the more modern viewpoint which argues for the maximization of freedom. Thus, debate about the merits of a particular action or policy becomes almost impossible because of the possibly unconscious, but clearly competing, ethical premises which stand at the heart of the debate: individual autonomy vs. community standards.

Thus the political-ethical problem is how, in a culture such as ours, can we discuss substantive issues with profound social consequences? Picture our culture as a giant circuitry panel. To a certain point, the panel is capable of handling the load that is required of it. One can also assume that the panel could carry a certain amount of overload if there is a degree of creative recircuiting. The problem arises when the panel is required to carry a load greater than that for which it was designed. At that point the circuits begin to shut off and the system eventually burns out. Until a couple of generations ago, our culture was able to bear the weight of some degree of cultural diversity because the system successfully socialized the immigrants into the value system of the native population. Given the pressures engendered over the last couple of decades by the assassination of Kennedy, the Civil Rights Movement, the Vietnam War, the Feminist Movement, the Gay Rights Movement, the various urban riots precipitated both by structural racism and endemic poverty, the rise and popularity of various religious cults, and now the abortion question, perhaps the American social system is reaching the point of circuit overload. We have been successful to a certain degree in the creative recircuiting of some issues pressing upon us for many years. We can no longer avoid dealing with the assumptions and implications of these issues. But because we have no commonly accepted framework for analyzing them, we resolve the issues procedurally, using the judicial system as a means of protecting and promoting individual rights. Such a maneuver does not evaluate cases on their merits, but on procedural technicalities precisely as a way of avoiding the merits of the case. This is no longer adequate and consequently we are beginning to see the signs of a cultural backlash in which specific values, which many people may or may not agree with, are being suggested as a normative basis for socialization. We may be in danger of moving from a culture which has provided for a variability within certain limits to a culture in which all must subscribe to the same values and applications of them. The abortion debate may be the first in a series in which revised cultural values are negotiated. If that is the case, the abortion debate may be one of the most significant events of the decade.

V. Conclusions

The setting of policy on abortion will establish values, structures and behaviors. Whose values will be so enshrined, which structures will be involved and how behavior will be influenced have yet to be determined. The debate continues with different lobbies promoting their interests, no reduction in the public rancor, and little thought to how moderation or some workable compromise might be reached.

Peter Steinfels has recently made some very significant observations about how Catholics might think through a moderate abortion policy.[16] Steinfels suggests that there are two steps that should be taken, each of which involves a break with one or the other sides of the current debate. The first step argues that psychological, social, and even religious incentives that disapprove of abortion will be insufficient to restrict effectively severe attacks on the value of fetal life. This argument suggests that some legislative restrictions are necessary to protect the value of life and that some women, though Steinfels argues not all, would have to carry their pregnancies to term. Such a position will be difficult for Catholic feminists and liberals—as well as many others. This option gives a high value to fetal life and recognizes that some social supports in the form of restrictive legislation are necessary to protect that life.

The second step requires liberal Catholics to break with the prolife movement by arguing that the ethical status of the fetus is a difficult moral problem, especially in the very early stages of the development of the embryo. While one can argue that even from the earliest moments of conception the conceptus is a member of the human species and is alive, it is difficult to prove in a convincing way that at that time the developing embryo has all of the rights to the preservation and protection of life as a newborn, as a child, or as an adult. The recognition of the moral ambiguity surrounding the status of the embryo would allow room to manuever when developing a policy on abortion. But it would require a significant degree of ethical compromise for some, perhaps many, members of different churches.

What is important about Steinfels' argument is not whether or not his reading of policy on abortion is correct, but the fact that he has thought through the significant compromises that will need to be made in order to establish some kind of policy that has a viable chance. One condition of viability for a particular policy is that two specific populations, pregnant women and fetuses, will have to suffer as a consequence. Members of different groups will experience moral compromise, but clearly not as much as pregnant women and fetuses. Compromise is seldom easy, and it will be far less easy when one recognizes that a policy may require that some women carry an unwanted pregnancy to term and that some fetuses will be aborted.

In addition to compromise, it is important for the churches to recognize that in many ways the tone and style of the abortion debate is being set by extremes on both ends of the spectrum. Data about perceptions on abortion in both the National Right to Life Committee and the National Abortion Rights Action League suggest there is some room for compromise with respect to public policy. Compromise suggests, of course, that neither of these two groups gets its way. Yet we must remember that even within the NRLC there are members who will allow abortion under some circumstances and in NARAL there are individuals who do not think that all reasons for abortion are morally significant. We need to disregard the rhetoric of the groups and their claims to purity of doctrine, but attend to the real beliefs of individuals in these organizations and in churches. As long as policy is defined by either extreme or some other single interest group, no progress can be made because such policies will be so extreme that a viable coalition based on actual beliefs and practice cannot support it, nor can legislation be developed that recognizes both diversity of opinion and broad areas of consensus.

In addition to compromise and a policy based on the realistic beliefs of the population, whether political or religious, it is important for the society to begin providing structures which make it possible for individuals to act on their belief in the value of life and fetal life in particular. Such structures would require a high degree of fairness and coherence among many policies and would in effect suggest that funding be provided for both abortions and pre and postnatal care. Minimal fairness requires that provision be made for people to act out their particular choices. This position is grounded in the libertarian part of our heritage. There is a genuine problem here and a real danger for some other values may be neglected. For example, abortion is more cost effective than the provision of social services. However, I argue that it is reprehensible to use abortion as a solution to social problems related to the health care of pregnant women, the ability of families to provide adequate food, shelter and education for their children, as well as a minimal quality of life standard. Yet I need to remember that however optimally our social structures may be arranged, there always will be, I think, the need for abortion. My own hope is that a moderately restrictive policy on abortion, together with the availability of contraceptives and reasonable social policies to support women and couples who wish to have children, might permit a genuine moral debate over abortion.

Public policy on abortion must be seen as: a part of a larger policy concerning the status of individual choice within a pluralistic community; a respect for differing and often contradictory value systems professed by members of the large society, both as private individuals and as members of various voluntary associations including the churches; a recognition that there is a large enough middle ground between the extremes upon which to make a reasonable appeal for a moderate policy on abortion; a respect for fetal life which also recognizes the moral problems in establishing an inviolable right to life for the fetus; and finally, a respect for the different positions of the churches, but with the recognition that their public policy recommendations be tested against their beliefs and actions.

There can be a responsible public policy debate on abortion, but only if we are willing to bear the burden of compromise and the responsibility of realizing wherever a line is drawn, that line will entail hardship. We as a community must be willing to provide as best we can for those individuals who must bear the burden of a particular public policy.[17]

NOTES

1. Christopher Tietze, *Induced Abortion: A World Review, 1981.* N.Y.: The Population Council. P. I.

2. *Ibid.,* p. 5.

3. *Ibid.,* pp. 34–35.

4. James C. Mohr, *Abortion in America.* N.Y.: Oxford University Press, 1978. pp. 20–45.

5. *Ibid,.* pp. 250–255.

6. Raymond Tatalovich and Byron W. Daynes. "The Trauma of Abortion Politics." *Commonweal* 107 (20 Nov. 1981), pp. 644–49.

7. Donald Granberg and Beth Wellman Granberg. "Abortion Attitudes, 1965–80: Trends and Determinants." *Family Planning Perspectives.* 12 (Sept./Oct., 1980), pp. 251–52.

8. *Ibid.,* p. 252.

9. *Ibid.,* pp. 253–58.

10. Donald Granberg, "The Abortion Activists." *Family Planning Perspectives.* 13 (July/August, 1981) pp. 157–63.

11. James Kelly, "Beyond The Stereotypes." *Commonweal* 107 (20 Nov. 81), pp. 654–59.

12. Perihan A. Rosenthal, "Adolescence and Pregnancy," Department of Psychiatry, University of Massachusetts Medical Center. Unpublished manuscript. Richard P. Perkins and others, "Intensive Care in Adolescent Pregnancy." *Obstetrics and Gynecology* 52 (August, 1978), pp. 179–88.

13. The perception certainly approaches reality when one hears Senator Hyde, who sponsored legislation to restrict abortions paid for by Medicaid to those which threatened the life of the woman, say: "I certainly would like to prevent, if I could legally, anybody having an abortion, a rich woman, a middle-class woman or a poor woman. Unfortunately, the only vehicle available is the HEW Medicaid bill. A life is a life." *The Congressional Record* 17 June, 1977. p. H 6083. Quoted from Family Planning Perspectives 12 (May/June, 1980) p. 121.

14. Daniel Callahan, "Abortion: Some Ethical Issues." In *Bioethics,* Ed. T. A. Shannon. N.Y.: Paulist Press. 1981 (Revised Edition). P. 16.

15. Alasdair MacIntyre. "How to Identify Ethical Principles." *The Belmont Report,* Appendix, Volume I. DHEW Publication No. (OS) 78-0013. 10-1-41.

16. Peter Steinfels, "The Search for an Alternative." *Commonweal* 107 (20 Nov., 1981) pp. 660–64.

17. Parts of this article were originally published as "Abortion: A Review of Ethical Aspects of Public Policy" in *Abortion and the Status of the Fetus.* Edited by W. B. Bondeson, H. T. Engelhardt, J., S. F. Spicker, and D. Winship. Boston: D. Reidel Publishing Co., 1982.

Abortion/Further Reading

Bracken, Michael B., et al. "Abortion, Adoption, or Motherhood; An Empirical Study of Decision Making During Pregnancy." *American Journal of Obstetrics and Gynecology* 130 (February 1, 1978), 251–62.

Cohen, Marshall, et al., eds. *The Rights and Wrongs of Abortion.* Princeton: Princeton University Press, 1974.

Humber, James M. "Abortion, Fetal Research, and the Law." *Social Theory and Practice* 4 (Spring 1977), 127–47.

Legalized Abortion and the Public Health. Report of a study by a committee of the Institute of Medicine. Washington, D.C.; National Academy of Sciences, May 1975.

Lee, Luke T., and Paxman, John M. "Pregnancy and Abortion in Adolescence: A Comparative Legal Survey and Proposals for Reform." *Columbia Human Rights Law Review* 6 (Fall–Winter 1974–75) 307–55.

Manier, Edward; Liu, William; and Soloman, David. *Abortion: New Directions for Policy Studies.* Notre Dame: University of Notre Dame Press, 1977.

Mohr, James C. *Abortion in America: The Origins and Evolution of National Policy.* New York: Oxford University Press, 1978.

Potts, Malcolm; Diggory, Peter; and Peel, John. *Abortion.* Cambridge: Cambridge University Press, 1977.

Tribe, Laurence H. "Toward a Model of Roles in the Due Process of Life and Law." *Harvard Law Review* 87 (November 1973), 1–53.

Warren, Mary Anne. "Do Potential People Have Moral Rights?" *Canadian Journal of Philosophy* 7 (June 1977), 275–89.

PART TWO

SEVERELY HANDICAPPED CHILDREN

John Fletcher
James F. Gustafson
Raymond S. Duff
Dept. of Health and Human Services

5 *Abortion, Euthanasia, and Care of Defective Newborns*

John Fletcher, Ph.D.

Although short, Fletcher's article presents a summary statement of basic ethical issues involved in the question of selective euthanasia of the newly born infant. The core problem is will a willingness to accept arguments for genetically indicated abortion tend to influence our treatment of defective neonates. The point is an important one, and Fletcher develops his view through an evaluation of an approving view, a disapproving view, and his own middle position. The article is particularly good in indicating the social context and potential ethical implications of such decisions which present an alternative to a strict right-to-life argument.

Rev. John Fletcher is the Director of Interfaith Metropolitan Theological Education, Inc. in Washington, D.C.

The medical literature has increasingly dealt with the utility and versatility of prenatal diagnosis for the detection of a variety of inborn errors of metabolism,[1-6] chromosomal abnormalities and variants[7-12] and polygenic conditions (e.g., spina bifida anencephaly).[13-14] Most of these diagnostic procedures entail amniocentesis, but some, such as the recent maternal serum test for indexes of neural-tube abnormalities,[15,16] require confirmation by invasive technics only if the test is positive. In every instance, the information obtained about the fetus affords the parents and attending physician data that they may use to decide whether or not to abort the fetus.

Although the proper use of these diagnostic findings in deciding on elective abortion is controversial,[17,18] my purpose here is to consider a different issue: does the ethical reasoning that is applied to prenatal management bear any relation to decision-making about survival after the birth of the infant? The ethical problem facing the medical profession is simply this: how should physicians and parents now understand their obligation to care for the newborn defective infant in the light of arguments for genetically indicated abortion after amniocentesis? To be consistent, a person might ask whether the arguments that support abortion after prenatal diagnosis of genetic disease also support euthanasia of the same infants who slip through that screen and are born. The debate in ethics is at present polarized between a disapproving view, which tends to equate genetically indicated abortion with infanticide,[19-21] and an approving view, which tends toward equating the morality of abortion and selective euthanasia of the defective newborn.[22,23]

A third position, for which I argue, accentuates parental freedom to participate in life-and-death decisions independently in both the prenatal and postnatal situations, accepts abortion of a seriously defective fetus, but disapproves euthanasia of defective newborns.

Paul Ramsey, an exponent of the first view,[20] rejects arguments for abortion that are based upon a positive prenatal diagnosis of a severe fetal disease and the socioeconomic harm that will be done to the family, because he holds that the same arguments might be used under similar circumstances to justify "infanticide." Infanticide is his term for deliberately bringing about the death of a newborn defective infant. His position is built upon the presupposition that there are no clear-cut moral differences between abortion and infanticide in the same disease. In this perspective, abortion for Lesch-Nyhan syndrome, Tay-Sachs disease, or other lethal diseases would be invalid since these justifications could be used for killing the same infant born without benefit of prenatal diagnosis.

In an earlier essay, Ramsey explained that his method of testing right and wrong action in such cases was fashioned upon the ethical measure of "universalizability." This test asks, "what would be the case if everyone in a morally relevant, like situation did as I am doing" (whether there is any tendency for them to do so or not)?[24] Ramsey is primarily interested in using this method for ethical appraisal of genetically indicated abortions. He is not saying that we will necessarily begin to commit infanticide because we do abortions to prevent genetic disorders. He is saying that if we would not do the infanticides, we should not be doing the abortions. In short, there are means that are in themselves wrong regardless of the good ends that may be desired through them.

Joseph Fletcher's arguments, leading the other side of the debate, not only support abortion after prenatal diagnosis, but also advocate setting aside traditional restraints against euthanasia for defective infants. In an article on ethics and euthanasia,[25] Fletcher reasons that a decision to abort a defective fetus, which is "subhuman life," is logically of the same order as a decision to end a "subhuman life in extremis" in old age. Discussing euthanasia, he abhors moral distinctions between acts of commission and omission ("allowing to die"), whether concerned with the newborn or the terminally ill older person. His thought clearly relates the ethical arguments for genetically indicated abortion to justifications for euthanasia of newborn defective infants:

> If we are morally obliged to put an end to a pregnancy when an amniocentesis reveals a terribly defective fetus, we are equally obliged to put an end to a patient's hopeless misery when a brain scan reveals that a patient with cancer has advanced brain metastases.
>
> Furthermore . . . it is morally evasive and disingenuous to suppose that we can condemn or disapprove positive acts of care and compassion but in spite of that approve negative strategies to achieve exactly the same purpose. This contradiction has equal force whether the euthanasia comes at the fetal point on life's spectrum or at some terminal point post-natally.[25]

The bearing of Fletcher's thought on the problem here, in contrast to Ramsey's, is that if we would do abortions based on prenatal diagnosis, we should be active in ending the suffering of infants born with the same condition. To do less — to allow a newborn with severe disease to die by withholding support — is in this view hypocritical, since we would be active in ending the same life in utero.

He comes to his conclusions in ethics through the reasoning of consequentialism, for which "only the end (a proportionate good) makes sense of what we do (the means)."[22] He does not mean that any end justifies any means, and he so states earlier in the passage just quoted. When a fetus or newborn is seriously incapacitated, however, the human harm prevented and suffering relieved by abortion and euthanasia justifies these actions.

In spite of the polar difference between the two positions, the positions exhibit an interesting similarity. Each is based in part on the assumption that the prenatal and postnatal situations are so similar that ethical behavior in the former determines ethical guidance in the latter. Each ethicist, in his own terms, sees the fetus on the same level of value and dignity as he sees the newborn infant. Ramsey is unequivocal about the status of a fetus as a fellow human being whose irreducible dignity derives from God.[19,24] Fletcher's reflections on "indicators of humanhood" lead him to delay conferral of human status upon the fetus or the infant until qualitative and quantitative measures can be made.[26] In the former view, humanhood is a free gift of God; in the latter view, humanhood is a human choice. In both views, moral guidance is given to be consistent in actions before and after birth.

My task is to show that there are morally relevant differences between abortion and euthanasia, even when one considers them for the same depth of impairment. The task is complex because an understanding of human development and growth as a process militates against lifting up one sequence of development too far out of relation with another. The defective newborn infant is the same being, but at a different stage of development, as a fetal candidate for prenatal diagnosis. Yet the post-natal situation in which parents and physicians face life-and-death decisions for extremely ill infants has features of a kind different from decision making about abortion.

What are the differences? One is that the separate physical existence of the infant, apart from the mother, confronts parents, physicians and legal institutions with independent moral claims for care and support. A newborn infant is clearly a patient. The movement of the fetus prepares the parents emotionally for the acceptance of the infant as a separate individual, but before extra-uterine viability the well-being of the fetus should not be considered independently from the mother's condition. H. T. Englehardt has argued persuasively on the difference between a fetus and an infant, noting that "as soon as the fetus actualizes its potential viability, it can play a full social role and can be understood as a person."[27] A moderate ethical stance will avoid the one extreme of regarding every fetus as already a human being with rights and the other extreme of withholding human status until quality-of-life standards have been passed. The former extreme provides no rational grounds for the legitimate interests of parents, family and society to be expressed and guided in abortion decisions. The latter provides no rational ground for the interest of the newborn infant to be expressed in medical decision making. The decision of the United States Supreme Court on abortion responds to the moral imperative that new human life requires a social protection wider than prenatal and medical care, but it observes that before viability, claims for protection cannot be made compellingly without violating the privacy of the mother.[28] In law, the source of the difference between a wider parental freedom before fetal viability and a larger social responsibility after viability lies in the growing moral claims that the new human life makes upon society.

The second major difference is the fact that after birth the disease in the infant is more available to physicians for palliation or perhaps even cure. Confrontation with disease in an independently existing life requires physicians to respond within their obligations to heal and to relieve suffering. The most noteworthy disease at present that can be successfully treated in utero is erythroblastosis fetalis (Rh disease). The moral claim to relieve suffering in a diseased fetus may be more answerable in the future when genetic therapies are possible. For the present, however, the real situation for parents and physicians is that they must wait until birth to respond to the specificity of a disease with decisions to treat or not to treat.[29]

Thirdly, parental acceptance of the infant as a real person is much more developed at birth than in the earlier stages of pregnancy. The medical literature amply describes pregnancy as a crisis bringing about in the parents, especially in the mother, a series of behavioral changes that prepare them for caring for the infant.[30-33] We should expect loyalty to the developing life to grow, change, and moderate the ambivalence about the fetus usually present in the parents. An example of the depth of parental loyalty can be seen when parents of a defective newborn "mourn" the loss of the expected healthy child and reconsider acceptance of the child with a defect.[34] Since acceptance of the new life undergoes a development of its own, it should be readily apparent that increasing parental loyalty to the infant constitutes a major difference when one compares abortion of a fetus to euthanasia of an infant.

The effect of these three differences is to establish the newborn infant, even with a serious defect, as a fellow human being who deserves protection on both a legal and an ethical basis, and thus each of the differences contributes to an argument against euthanasia.

Two additional reasons round out the case for opposition to euthanasia. The first is the potential brutalization of those who participate in it. This point has been persuasively made by Bok in a discussion of infanticide,[35] and it is the source of Lorber's rejection of euthanasia as "an extremely dangerous weapon in the hands of unscrupulous individuals."[36] The second reason is the destructive social consequences of changing the ethical ambience of the birth of infants from one of thorough caring for life to one in which the public accepted a policy of euthanasia and supported its legalization. I see no way of making this social change that would not undermine the optimal moral condition for the beginning of life: the experience of trust. Erikson described the "basic trust" required between mother and infant necessary for the first task of forming healthy personality.[37] His thesis was that the task of mothering is strengthened, among other things, by a world view based on confidence that life is good, even though death and tragedy are part of life.

A society that supports acceptance of defective newborns, where reasonably possible, does more to nurture patterns of acceptance in parents and thus reinforces the child's basic trust in the world's trustworthiness.

A brief comment here is appropriate regarding the fact that physicians, parents, and ethicists are confronted with real cases of terribly damaged newborns for whom death is the desirable outcome when therapy either is not available or will only prolong the ordeal without definite ground for hope.[38] In such cases, if we would reject euthanasia because of a negative ethical assessment of the action and its consequences, what should be done? Allowing the infant to die by withholding support while relieving pain is a decision, in my view, that can be ethically justified for reasons of mercy to the infant and relief of meaningless suffering of the parents and medical team. If death is understood as a good outcome in such cases, however difficult the emotional acceptance of the infant's death, parents and physicians do not "do harm" to the infant by the decision, assuming that every reasonable therapeutic step has been taken or evaluated negatively. The crucial difference between euthanasia and allowing to die is that the self-restraint imposed by the latter choice is more consistent with ethical and legal norms that physicians and parents do no harm to the infant.

I have argued here that a decision for abortion after prenatal diagnosis does not necessarily commit parents to one course of action in the care of an infant born with the same degree of illness. The structure of my argument is based upon three differences between the fetus and the infant that are sufficiently grounded in human experience to be verified by observation. A defective newborn is a separate individual, whose disease is available for treatment, and whose parents are prepared by the process of a typical pregnancy to accept the infant. When these human experiences interact with the beliefs and values of the religious and humanistic communities that provide our culture with visions of the ultimately desirable, this interaction produces strong ethical and theologic backing for caring for the infant. If we choose to be shaped by Judeo-Christian visions of the "createdness" of life within which every creature bears the image of God, we ought to care for the defective newborn as if our relation with the Creator depended on the outcome. If we choose to be shaped by visions of the inherent dignity of each member of the human family, no matter what his or her predicament, we ought to care for this defenseless person as if the basis of our own dignity depended on the outcome. We are in a very hazardous situation ethically if we allow abortion for medical reasons in utero and then attempt to usher new life into a thoroughly caring context at birth, unless we are fully responsive to the imperatives to treat disease in the newborn when it appears.

REFERENCES

1. Milunsky A, Littlefield JW, Kanfer JN, et al: Prenatal genetic diagnosis, N Engl J Med 283:1370-1381, 1441-1447, 1498-1504, 1970

2. Gerbie AB, Nadler HL, Gerbie MV: Amniocentesis in genetic counseling: safety and reliability in early pregnancy. Am J Obstet Gynecol 109:765-770, 1971

3. Epstein CJ, Scheider EL, Conte FA, et al: Prenatal detection of genetic disorders. Am J Hum Genet 24:214-226, 1972

4. Valenti C: Antenatal detection of hemoglobinopathies: a preliminary report. Am J Obstet Gynecol 115:851-853, 1973

5. Antenatal Diagnosis. Edited by A Dorfman. Chicago, University of Chicago Press, 1972

6. Antenatal Diagnosis of Genetic Disease. Edited by AEH Emery. Edinburgh, Churchill Livingstone, 1973

7. Stelle MW, Breg WR Jr: Chromosome analysis of human amniotic-fluid cells. Lancet 1:383-385, 1966

8. Jacobson CB, Barter RH: Intrauterine diagnosis and management of genetic defects. Am J Obstet Gynecol 99:796-807, 1967

9. Nadler HL: Antenatal detection of hereditary disorders. Pediatrics 42:912-918, 1968

10. Nadler HL, Gerbie A: Present status of amniocentesis in intrauterine diagnosis of genetic defects. Obstet Cynecol 38:789-799, 1971

11. Milunsky A, Atkins L, Littlefield JW: Polyploidy in prenatal genetic diagnosis. J Pediatr 79:303-305, 1971

12. Idem: Amniocentesis for prenatal genetic studies. Obstet Gynecol 40:104-108, 1972

13. Emery AEH, Eccleston D, Scrimgeour JB, et al: Amniotic fluid composition in malformations of the central nervous system. J Obstet Gynaecol Brit Commonw 79:154-158, 1972

14. Allan LD, Ferguson-Smith MA, Donald I, et al: Amniotic-fluid alphafetoprotein in the antenatal diagnosis of spina bifida. Lancet 2:522-525, 1973

15. Brock DJH, Bolton AE, Monaghan JM: Prenatal diagnosis of anencephaly through maternal serum-alphafetoprotein measurement. Lancet 2:923-924, 1973

16. Brock DJH, Bolton AE, Scrimgeour JB: Prenatal diagnosis of spina bifida and anencephaly through maternal plasma alpha-fetoprotein measurement. Lancet 1:767-769, 1974

17. Gustafson JM: Genetic counseling and the uses of genetic knowledge—an ethical overview, Ethical Issues in Human Genetics. Edited by B Hilton, D Callahan, et al. New York, Plenum Press, 1973, pp 101-112

18. Ramsey P: Screening: an ethicist's view, Ethical Issues in Human Genetics. Edited by B Hilton, D Callahan, et al. New York, Plenum Press, 1973, pp 147-161

19. *Idem:* Feticide/Infanticide upon request. Religion in Life 39:170-186, 1970

20. *Idem:* Abortion. Thomist 37:174-226, 1973

21. Dyck AJ: Perplexities for the would-be liberal in abortion. J Reprod Med 8:351-354, 1972

22. Fletcher J: The Ethics of Genetic Control. Garden City, New York, Doubleday, 1974, pp 121-123, 152-154, 185-187

23. Tooley M: Abortion and infanticide. Phil Pub Affairs 2:37-65, 1972

24. Ramsey P: Reference points in deciding about abortion, The Morality of Abortion. Edited by JT Noonan Jr. Cambridge, Harvard University Press, 1970, pp 60-100

25. Fletcher J: Ethics and euthanasia. Am J Nursing 73:670-675, 1973

26. Fletcher J: Indicators of humanhood: a tentative profile of man. Hastings Center Rep 2(5):1-4, 1972

27. Englehardt HT Jr: Viability, abortion, and the difference between a fetus and an infant. Am J Obstet Gynecol 116:429-434, 1973

28. Roe vs Wade: 410 US 113 (1973)

29. Duff RS, Campbell AGM: Moral and ethical dilemmas in the special-care nursery. N Engl J Med 289:890-894, 1973

30. Kennell JH, Klaus MH: Care of the mother of the high-risk infant. Clin Obstet Gynecol 14:926-954, 1971

31. Bibring GL: Some considerations of the psychological processes in pregnancy. Psychoanal Study Child 14:113-121, 1959

32. Caplan G: Emotional Implication of Pregnancy and Influences on Family Relationships in the Healthy Child. Cambridge, Harvard University Press, 1960

33. Nadelson C: "Normal" and "special" aspects of pregnancy. Obstet Gynecol 41:611-620, 1973

34. Solnit AJ, Stark MH: Mourning and the birth of a defective child. Psychoanal Study Child 16:523-537, 1961

35. Bok S: Ethical problems of abortion. Hastings Center Studies 2:33-52, 1974

36. Lorber J: Selective treatment of myelomeningocele: to treat or not to treat? Pediatrics 53:307-308, 1974

37. Erikson E: The healthy personality. Psychol Issues 1:56-65, 1959

38. McCormick RA: To save or let die: the dilemma of modern medicine. JAMA 229:172-176, 1974

6 *Mongolism, Parental Desires, and the Right To Life*

JAMES M. GUSTAFSON

This article is a reflection on the well-publicized Johns Hopkins case of a mentally retarded infant with duodenal atresia who was allowed to die because of a parent's decision not to keep the child. Gustafson presents an analysis of the parents' decision and an ethical evaluation of the elements in this decision. Attention is also paid to some of the legal issues involved. In the last half of the article, Gustafson develops two points: whether what one ought to do is determined by what one desires and whether a mentally retarded child has a right to life. Included in this is an ethical evaluation of suffering which adds a new dimension to the general debate.

Dr. James M. Gustafson, Ph.D., is University Professor of Theological Ethics at the University of Chicago

The Problem

THE FAMILY SETTING

Mother, 34 years old, hospital nurse.
Father, 35 years old, lawyer.
Two normal children in the family.

In late fall of 1963, Mr. and Mrs. ——— gave birth to a premature baby boy. Soon after birth, the child was diagnosed as a "mongoloid" (Down's syndrome) with the added complication of an intestinal blockage (duodenal atresia). The latter could be corrected with an operation of quite nominal

107

risk. Without the operation, the child could not be fed and would die.

At the time of birth Mrs. ――― overheard the doctor express his belief that the child was a mongol. She immediately indicated she did not want the child. The next day, in consultation with a physician, she maintained this position, refusing to give permission for the corrective operation on the intestinal block. Her husband supported her in this position, saying that his wife knew more about these things (i.e., mongoloid children) than he. The reason the mother gave for her position—"It would be unfair to the other children of the household to raise them with a mongoloid."

The physician explained to the parents that the degree of mental retardation cannot be predicted at birth—running from very low mentality to borderline subnormal. As he said: "Mongolism, it should be stressed, is one of the milder forms of mental retardation. That is, mongols' IQs are generally in the 50-80 range, and sometimes a little higher. That is, they're almost always trainable. They can hold simple jobs. And they're famous for being happy children. They're perennially happy and usually a great joy." Without other complications, they can anticipate a long life.

Given the parents' decision, the hospital staff did not seek a court order to override the decision (see "Legal Setting" below). The child was put in a side room and, over an 11-day period, allowed to starve to death.

Following this episode, the parents undertook genetic counseling (chromosome studies) with regard to future possible pregnancies.

The Legal Setting

Since the possibility of a court order reversing the parents' decision naturally arose, the physician's opinion in this matter—and his decision not to seek such an order—is central. As he said: "In the situation in which the child has a known, serious mental abnormality, and would be a burden both to the parents financially and emotionally and perhaps to society, I think it's unlikely that the court would sustain an order to operate on the child against the parents' wishes." He went on to say: "I think one of the great difficulties, and I hope [this] will be part of the discussion relative to this child, is what happens in a family where a court order is used as the means of correcting a congenital abnormality. Does that child ever really become an accepted member of the family? And what are all of the feelings, particularly guilt and coercion feelings that the parents must have following that type of extraordinary force that's brought to bear upon them for making them accept a child that they did not wish to have?"

Both doctors and nursing staff were firmly convinced that it was "clearly illegal" to hasten the child's death by the use of medication.

One of the doctors raised the further issue of consent, saying: "Who has the right to decide for a child anyway? . . . The whole way we handle life and death is the reflection of the long-standing belief in this country that children don't have any rights, that they're not citizens, that their parents can decide to kill them or to let them live, as they choose."

The Hospital Setting

When posed the question of whether the case would have been taken to court had the child had a normal IQ, with the parents refusing permission for the intestinal operation, the near unanimous opinion of the doctors: "Yes, we would have tried to override their decision." Asked why, the doctors replied: "When a retarded child presents us with the same problem, a different value system comes in; and not only does the staff acquiesce in the parent's decision to let the child die, but it's probable that the courts would also. That is, there is a different standard. . . . There is this tendency to value life on the basis of intelligence. . . . [It's] a part of the American ethic."

The treatment of the child during the period of its dying was also interesting. One doctor commented on "putting the child in a side room." When asked about medication to hasten the death, he replied: "No one would ever do that. No one would ever think about it, because they feel uncomfortable about it. . . . A lot of the way we handle these things has to do with our own anxieties about death and our own desires to be separated from the decisions that we're making."

The nursing staff who had to tend to the child showed some resentment at this. One nurse said she had great difficulty just in entering the room and watching the child degenerate—she could "hardly bear to touch him." Another nurse, however, said: "I didn't mind coming to work. Because like I would rock him. And I think that kind of helped me some—to be able to sit there and hold him. And he was just a tiny little thing. He was really a very small baby. And he was cute. He had a cute little face to him, and it was easy to love him, you know?" And when the baby died, how did she feel?—"I was glad that it was over. It was an end for him."

The Resolution

This complex of human experiences and decisions evokes profound human sensibilities and serious intellectual examination. One sees in and beyond it dimensions that could be explored by practitioners of various academic disciplines. Many of the standard questions about the ethics of medical care are pertinent, as are questions that have been long discussed by philosophers and theologians. One would have to write a full-length book to plow up, cultivate, and bring to fruition the implications of this experience.

I am convinced that, when we respond to a moral dilemma, the way in which we formulate the dilemma, the picture we draw of its salient features, is largely determinative of the choices we have. If the war in Vietnam is pictured as a struggle between the totalitarian forces of evil seeking to suppress all human values on the one side, and the forces of righteousness on the other, we have one sort of problem with limited choice. If, however, it is viewed as a struggle of oppressed people to throw off the shackles of colonialism and imperialism, we have another sort of problem. If it is pictured as more complex, the range of choices is wider, and the factors to be considered are more numerous. If the population problem is depicted as a race against imminent self-destruction of the human race, an ethics of survival seems to be legitimate and to deserve priority. If, however, the population problem is depicted more complexly, other values also determine policy, and our range of choices is broader.

One of the points under discussion in this medical case is how we should view it. What elements are in the accounts that the participants give to it? What elements were left out? What "values" did they seem to consider, and which did they seem to ignore? Perhaps if one made a different montage of the raw experience, one would have different choices and outcomes.

Whose picture is correct? It would not be difficult for one moral philosopher or theologian to present arguments that might undercut, if not demolish, the defenses made by the participants. Another moralist might make a strong defense of the decisions by assigning different degrees of importance to certain aspects of the case. The first might focus on the violation of individual rights, in this case the rights of the infant. The other might claim that the way of least possible suffering for the fewest persons over the longest range of time was the commendable outcome of the account as we have it. Both would be accounts drawn by external observers, not by active, participating agents. There is a tradition that says that ethical reflection by an ideal external observer can bring morally right answers. I have an observer's perspective, though not that of an "ideal observer." But I believe that it is both charitable and intellectually important to try to view the events as the major participants viewed them. The events remain closer to the confusions of the raw experience that way; the passions, feelings, and emotions have some echo of vitality remaining. The parents were not without feeling, the nurses not without anguish. The experiences could become a case in which x represents the rights of the infant to life, y represents the consequences of continued life as a mongoloid person, and z represents the consequences of his continued life for the family and the state. But such abstraction has a way of oversimplifying experience. One would "weigh" x against y and z. I cannot reproduce the drama even of the materials I have read, the interviews with doctors and nurses, and certainly even those are several long steps from the thoughts and feelings of the parents and the staff at that time. I shall, however, attempt to state the salient features of the dilemma for its participants; features that are each value laden and in part determinative of their decisions. In the process of doing that for the participants, I will indicate what reasons might justify their decisions. Following that I will draw a different picture of the experience, highlighting different values and principles, and show how this would lead to a different decision. Finally, I shall give the reasons why I, an observer, believe they, the participants, did the wrong thing. Their responsible and involved participation, one must remember, is very different from my detached reflection on documents and interviews almost a decade later.

The Mother's Decision

Our information about the mother's decision is secondhand. We cannot be certain that we have an accurate account of her reasons for not authorizing the surgery that could have saved the mongoloid infant's life. It is not my role to speculate whether her given reasons are her "real motives"; that would involve an assessment of her "unconscious." When she heard the child was probably a mongol, she "expressed some negative feeling" about it, and "did not want a retarded child." Because she was a nurse she understood what mongolism indicated. One reason beyond her feelings and wants is given: to raise a mongoloid child in the family would not be "fair" to the other children. That her decision was anguished we know from several sources.

For ethical reflection, three terms I have quoted are important: "negative feeling," "wants" or "desires," and "fair." We need to inquire about the status of each as a justification for her decision.

What moral weight can a negative feeling bear? On two quite different grounds, weight could be given to her feelings in an effort to sympathetically understand her decision. First, at the point of making a decision, there is always an element of the rightness or wrongness of the choice that defies full rational justification. When we see injustice being done, we have strong negative feelings; we do not need a sophisticated moral argument to tell us that the act is unjust. We "feel" that it is wrong. It might be said that the mother's "negative feeling" was evoked by an intuition that it would be wrong to save the infant's life, and that feeling is a reliable guide to conduct.

Second, her negative response to the diagnosis of mongolism suggests that she would not be capable of giving the child the affection and the care that it would require. The logic involved is an extrapolation from that moment to potential consequences for her continued relationship to the child in the future. The argument is familiar; it is common in the literature that supports abortion on request—"no unwanted child ought to be born." Why? Because unwanted children suffer from hostility and lack of affection from their mothers, and this is bad for them.

The second term is "wants" or "desires." The negative feelings are assumed to be an indication of her desires. We might infer that at some point she said, "I do not want a retarded child." The status of "wanting" is different, we might note, if it expresses a wish before the child is born, or if it expresses a desire that leads to the death of the infant after it is born. No normal pregnant woman would wish a retarded child. In this drama, however, it translates into: "I would rather not have the infant kept alive." Or, "I will not accept parental responsibilities for a retarded child." What is the status of a desire or a want as an ethical justification for an action? To discuss that fully would lead to an account of a vast literature. The crucial issue in this case is whether the existence of the infant lays a moral claim that supersedes the mother's desires.

If a solicitor of funds for the relief of refugees in Bengal requested a donation from her and she responded, "I do not want to give money for that cause," some persons would think her to be morally insensitive, but none could argue that the refugees in Bengal had a moral claim on her money which she was obligated to acknowledge. The existence of the infant lays a weightier claim on her than does a request for a donation. We would not say that the child's right to surgery, and thus to life, is wholly relative to, and therefore exclusively dependent upon, the mother's desires or wants.

Another illustration is closer to her situation than the request for a donation. A man asks a woman to marry him. Because she is asked, she is under no obligation to answer affirmatively. He might press claims upon her—they have expressed love for each other; or they have dated for a long time; he has developed his affection for her on the assumption that her responsiveness would lead to marriage. But none of these claims would be sufficient to overrule her desire not to marry him. Why? Two sorts of reasons might be given. One would refer to potential consequences: a marriage in which one partner does not desire the relationship leads to anxiety and suffering. To avoid needless suffering is obviously desirable. So in this case, it might be said that the mother's desire is to avoid needless suffering and anxiety: the undesirable consequences can be avoided by permitting the child to die.

The second sort of reason why a woman has no obligation to marry her suitor refers to her rights as an individual. A request for marriage does not constitute a moral obligation, since there is no prima facie claim by the suitor. The woman has a right to say no. Indeed, if the suitor sought to coerce her into marriage, everyone would assert that she has a right to refuse him. In our case, however, there are some differences. The infant is incapable of expressing a request or demand. Also, the relationship is different: the suitor is not dependent upon his girl friend in the same way that the infant is dependent upon his mother. Dependence functions in two different senses; the necessary conditions for the birth of the child were his conception and *in utero* nourishment—thus, in a sense the parents "caused" the child to come into being. And, apart from instituting adoption procedures, the parents are the only ones who can provide the necessary conditions for sustaining the child's life. The infant is dependent on them in the sense that he must rely upon their performance of certain acts in order to continue to exist. The ethical question to the mother is, Does the infant's physical life lay an unconditioned moral claim on the mother? She answered, implicitly, in the negative.

What backing might the negative answer be given? The most persuasive justification would come from an argument that there are no unconditioned moral claims upon one when those presumed claims go against one's desires and wants. The claims of another are relative to my desires, my wants. Neither the solicitor for Bengal relief nor the suitor has an unconditioned claim to make; in both cases a desire is sufficient grounds for denying such a claim. In our case, it would have to be argued that the two senses of dependence that the infant has on the mother are not sufficient conditions for a claim on her that would morally require the needed surgery. Since there are no unconditioned claims, and since the conditions in this drama are not sufficient to warrant a claim, the mother is justified in denying permission for the surgery.

We note here that in our culture there are two trends in the development of morality that run counter to each other: one is the trend that desires of the ego are the grounds for moral and legal claims. If a mother does not desire the fetus in her uterus, she has a right to an abortion. The other increasingly limits individual desires and wants. An employer might want to hire only white persons of German ancestry, but he has no right to do so.

The word "fair" appeals to quite different warrants. It would not be "fair" to the other children in the family to raise a mongoloid with them. In moral philosophy, fairness is either the same as justice or closely akin to it. Two traditional definitions of justice might show

how fairness could be used in this case. One is "to each his due." The other children would not get what is due them because of the inordinate requirements of time, energy, and financial resources that would be required if the mongoloid child lived. Or, if they received what was due to them, there would not be sufficient time, energy, and other resources to attend to the particular needs of the mongoloid; his condition would require more than is due him. The other traditional definition is "equals shall be treated equally." In principle, all children in the family belong to a class of equals and should be treated equally. Whether the mongoloid belongs to that class of equals is in doubt. If he does, to treat him equally with the others would be unfair to him because of his particular needs. To treat him unequally would be unfair to the others.

Perhaps "fairness" did not imply "justice." Perhaps the mother was thinking about such consequences for the other children as the extra demands that would be made upon their patience, the time they would have to give the care of the child, the emotional problems they might have in coping with a retarded sibling, and the sense of shame they might have. These consequences also could be deemed to be unjust from her point of view. Since they had no accountability for the existence of the mongoloid, it was not fair to them that extra burdens be placed upon them.

To ask what was due the mongoloid infant raises harder issues. For the mother, he was not due surgical procedure that would sustain his life. He was "unequal" to her normal children, but the fact of his inequality does not necessarily imply that he has no right to live. This leads to a matter at the root of the mother's response which has to be dealt with separately.

She (and as we shall see, the doctors also) assumed that a factual distinction (between normal and mongoloid) makes the moral difference. Factual distinctions do make moral differences. A farmer who has no qualms about killing a runt pig would have moral scruples about killing a deformed infant. If the child had not been mongoloid and had an intestinal blockage, there would have been no question about permitting surgery to be done. The value of the infant is judged to be relative to a quality of its life that is predictable on the basis of the factual evidences of mongolism. Value is relative to quality: that is the justification. Given the absence of a certain quality, the value is not sufficient to maintain life; given absence of a quality, there is no right to physical life. (Questions about terminating life among very sick adults are parallel to this instance.)

What are the qualities, or what is *the* quality that is deficient in this infant? It is not the capacity for happiness, an end that Aristotle and others thought to be sufficient in itself. The mother and the doctors knew that mongoloids can be happy. It is not the capacity for pleasure, the end that the hedonistic utilitarians thought all men seek, for mongoloids can find pleasure in life. The clue is given when a physician says that the absence of the capacity for normal intelligence was crucial. He suggested that we live in a society in which intelligence is highly valued. Perhaps it is valued as a quality in itself, or as an end in itself by some, but probably there is a further point, namely that intelligence is necessary for productive contribution to one's own well-being and to the well-being of others. Not only will a mongoloid make a minimal contribution to his own well-being and to that of others, but also others must contribute excessively to his care. The right of an infant, the value of his life, is relative to his intelligence; that is the most crucial factor in enabling or limiting his contribution to his own welfare and that of others. One has to defend such a point in terms of the sorts of contributions that would be praiseworthy and the sorts of costs that would be detrimental. The contribution of a sense of satisfaction to those who might enjoy caring for the mongoloid would not be sufficient. Indeed, a full defense would require a quantification of qualities, all based on predictions at the point of birth, that would count both for and against the child's life in a cost-benefit analysis.

The judgment that value is relative to qualities is not implausible. In our society we have traditionally valued the achiever more than the nonachievers. Some hospitals have sought to judge the qualities of the contributions of patients to society in determining who has access to scarce medical resources. A mongoloid is not valued as highly as a fine musician, an effective politician, a successful businessman, a civil rights leader whose actions have brought greater justice to the society, or a physician. To be sure, in other societies and at other times other qualities have been valued, but we judge by the qualities valued in our society and our time. Persons are rewarded according to their contributions to society. A defense of the mother's decision would have to be made on these grounds, with one further crucial step. That is, when the one necessary condition for productivity is deficient (with a high degree of certitude) at birth, there is no moral obligation to maintain that life. That the same reasoning would have been sufficient to justify overtly taking the infant's life seems not to have been the case. But that point emerges later in our discussion.

The reliance upon feelings, desires, fairness, and judgments of qualities of life makes sense to American middle-class white families, and anguished decisions can very well be settled in these terms. The choice made by the mother was not that of an unfeeling problem-solving machine, nor that of a rationalistic philosopher operating from these assumptions. It was a painful, conscientious decision, made apparently on these bases. On can ask, of course, whether her physicians should not have suggested other ways of perceiving and drawing the contours of the circumstances, other values and ends that she might consider. But that points to a subsequent topic.

The Father's Decision

The decision of the father is only a footnote to that of the mother. He consented to the choice of not operating on the infant, though he did seek precise information about mongolism and its consequences for the child. He was "willing to go along with the mother's wishes," he "understood her feelings, agreed with them," and was not in a position to make "the same intelligent decision that his wife was making."

Again we see that scientific evidence based on professional knowledge is determinative of a moral decision. The physician was forthright in indicating what the consequences would be of the course of action they were taking. The consequences of raising a mongoloid child were presumably judged to be more problematic than the death of the child.

The Decision of the Physicians

A number of points of reference in the contributions of the physicians to the case study enable us to formulate a constellation of values that determined their actions. After I have depicted that constellation, I shall analyze some of the points of reference to see how they can be defended.

The constellation can be stated summarily. The physicians felt no moral or legal obligation to save the life of a mongoloid infant by an ordinary surgical procedure when the parents did not desire that it should live. Thus, the infant was left to die. What would have been a serious but routine procedure was omitted in this instance on two conditions, both of which were judged to be necessary, but neither of which was sufficient in itself: the mongolism and the parents' desires. If the parents had desired the mongoloid infant to be saved, the surgery would have been done. If the infant had not been mongoloid and the parents had refused permission for surgery to remove a bowel obstruction, the physicians would at least have argued against them and probably taken legal measures to override them. Thus, the value-laden points of reference appear to be the desires of the parents, the mongolism of the infant, the law, and choices about ordinary and extraordinary medical procedures.

One of the two most crucial points was the obligation the physicians felt to acquiesce to the desires of the parents. The choice of the parents not to operate was made on what the physicians judged to be adequate information: it was an act of informed consent on the part of the parents. There is no evidence that the physicians raised questions of a moral sort with the parents that they subsequently raised among themselves. For example, one physician later commented on the absence of rights for children in our society and in our legal system and on the role that the value of intelligence seems to have in judging worthiness of persons. These were matters, however, that the physicians did not feel obligated to raise with the distressed parents. The physicians acted on the principle that they are only to do procedures that the patient (or crucially in this case, the parents of the patient) wanted. There was no overriding right to life on the part of a mongoloid infant that led them to argue against the parents' desires or to seek a court order requiring the surgical procedure. They recognized the moral autonomy of the parents, and thus did not interfere; they accepted as a functioning principle that the parents have the right to decide whether an infant shall live.

Elaboration of the significance of parental autonomy is necessary in order to see the grounds on which it can be defended. First, the physicians apparently recognized that the conscientious parents were the moral supreme court. There are grounds for affirming the recognition of the moral autonomy of the principal persons in complex decisions. In this case, the principals were the parents: the infant did not have the capacities to express any desires or preferences he might have. The physicians said, implicitly, that the medical profession does not have a right to impose certain of its traditional values on persons if these are not conscientiously held by those persons.

There are similarities, but also differences, between this instance and that of a terminal patient. If the terminally ill patient expresses a desire not to have his life prolonged, physicians recognize his autonomy over his own body and thus feel under no obligation to sustain his life. Our case, however, would be more similar to one in which the terminally ill patient's family decided that no further procedures ought to be used to sustain life. No doubt there are many cases in which the patient is unable to express a preference due to his physical conditions, and in the light of persuasive medical and familial reasons the physician agrees not to sustain life. A difference between our case and that, however, has to be noted in order to isolate what seems to be the crucial point. In the case of the mongoloid infant, a decision is made at the beginning of his life and not at the end; the effect is to cut off a life which, given proper care, could be sustained for many years, rather than not sustaining a life which has no such prospects.

Several defenses might be made of their recognition of the parents' presumed rights in this case. The first is that parents have authority over their children until they reach an age of discretion, and in some respects until they reach legal maturity. Children do not have recognized rights over against parents in many respects. The crucial difference here, of course, is the claimed parental right in this case to determine that an infant shall not live. What grounds might there be for this? Those who claim the moral right to an abortion are claiming the right to determine whether a child shall live, and this claim is widely recognized both morally and legally. In this case we have an extension of that right to the point of birth. If there are sufficient grounds to indicate that the newborn child is significantly abnormal, the parents have the same right as they have when a severe genetic abnormality is detected prenatally on the basis of amniocentesis. Indeed, the physicians could argue that if a mother has a right to an abortion, she also has a right to determine whether a newborn infant shall continue to live. One is simply extending the time span and the circumstances under which this autonomy is recognized.

A second sort of defense might be made: that of the limits of professional competence and authority. The physicians could argue that in moral matters they have neither competence nor authority. Perhaps they would wish to distinguish between competence and authority. They have a competence to make a moral decision on the basis of their own moral and other values, but they have no authority to impose this upon their patients. Morals, they might argue, are subjective matters, and if anyone has competence in that area, it is philosophers, clergymen, and others who teach what is right and wrong. If the parents had no internalized values that militated against their decision, it is not in the province of the physicians to tell them what they ought to do. Indeed, in a morally pluralistic society, no one group or person has a right to impose his views on another. In this stronger argument for moral autonomy no physician would have any authority to impose his own moral values on any patient. A social role differentiation is noted: the medical profession has authority only in medical matters—not in moral matters. Indeed, they have an obligation to indicate what the medical alternatives are in order to have a decision made by informed consent, but insofar as moral values or principles are involved in decisions, these are not within their professional sphere.

An outsider might ask what is meant by authority. He might suggest that surely it is not the responsibility (or at least not his primary responsibility) or the role of the physician to make moral decisions, and certainly not to enforce his decisions on others. Would he be violating his role if he did something less determinative than that, namely, in his counseling indicate to them what some of the moral considerations might be in choosing between medical alternatives? In our case the answer seems to be yes. If the principals desire moral counseling, they have the freedom to seek it from whomsoever they will. In his professional role he acknowledges that the recognition of the moral autonomy of the principals also assumes their moral self-sufficiency, that is, their capacities to make sound moral decisions without interference on his part, or the part of any other persons except insofar as the principals themselves seek such counsel. Indeed, in this case a good deal is made of the knowledgeability of the mother particularly, and this assumes that she is morally, as well as medically, knowledgeable. Or, if she is not, it is still not the physician's business to be her moral counselor.

The physicians also assumed in this case that the moral autonomy of the parents took precedence over the positive law. At least they felt no obligation to take recourse to the courts to save the life of this infant. On that issue we will reflect more when we discuss the legal point of reference.

Another sort of defense might be made. In the order of society, decisions should be left to the most intimate and smallest social unit involved. That is the right of such a unit, since the interposition of outside authority would be an infringement of its freedom. Also, since the family has to live with the consequences of the decision, it is the right of the parents to determine which potential consequences they find most desirable. The state, or the medical profession, has no right to interfere with the freedom of choice of the family. Again, in a formal way, the argument is familiar; the state has no right to interfere with the determination of what a woman wishes to do with her body, and thus antiabortion laws are infringements of her freedom. The determination of whether an infant shall be kept alive is simply an extension of the sphere of autonomy properly belonging to the smallest social unit involved.

In all the arguments for moral autonomy, the medical fact that the infant is alive and can be kept alive does not make a crucial difference. The defense of the decision would have to be made in this way: if one grants moral autonomy to mothers to determine whether they will bring a fetus to birth, it is logical to assume that one will grant the same autonomy after birth, at least in instances where the infant is abnormal.

We have noted in our constellation of factors that the desire of the parents was a necessary but not a sufficient condition for the decisions of the physicians. If the infant had not been mongoloid, the physicians would not have so readily acquiesced to the parents' desires. Thus, we need to turn to the second necessary condition.

The second crucial point is that the infant was a mongoloid. The physicians would not have acceded to the parents' request as readily if the child had been normal; the parents would have authorized the surgical procedure if the child had been normal. Not every sort of abnormality would have led to the same decision on the part of the physicians. Their appeal was to the consequences of the abnormality of mongolism: the child would be a burden financially and emotionally to the parents. Since every child, regardless of his capacities for intelligent action, is a financial burden, and at least at times an emotional burden, it is clear that the physicians believed that the quantity or degree of burden in this case would exceed any benefits that might be forthcoming if the child were permitted to live. One can infer that a principle was operative, namely, that mongoloid infants have no inherent right to life; their right to life is conditional upon the willingness of their parents to accept them and care for them.

Previously we developed some of the reasons why a mongoloid infant was judged undesirable. Some of the same appeals to consequences entered into the decisions of the physicians. If we are to seek to develop reasons why the decisions might be judged to be morally correct, we must examine another point, namely, the operating definition of "abnormal" or "defective." There was no dissent to the medical judgment that the infant was mongoloid, though precise judgments about the seriousness of the child's defect were not possible at birth.

Our intention is to find as precisely as possible what principles or values might be invoked to claim that the "defectiveness" was sufficient to warrant not sustaining the life of this infant. As a procedure, we will begin with the most general appeals that might have been made to defend the physician's decision in this case. The most general principle would be that any infant who has any empirically verifiable degree of defect at birth has no right to life. No one would apply such a principle. Less general would be that all infants who are carriers of a genetic defect that would have potentially bad consequences for future generations have no right to life. A hemophiliac carrier would be a case in point. This principle would not be applicable, even if it were invoked with approval, in this case.

Are the physicians prepared to claim that all genetically "abnormal" infants have no claim to life? I find no evidence that they would. Are they prepared to say that where the genetic abnormality affects the capacity for "happiness" the infant has no right to live?

Such an appeal was not made in this case. It appears that "normal" in this case has reference to a capacity for a certain degree of intelligence.

A presumably detectable physical norm now functions as a norm in a moral sense, or as an ideal. The ideal cannot be specified in precise terms, but there is a vague judgment about the outer limits beyond which an infant is judged to be excessively far from the norm or ideal to deserve sustenance. Again, we come to the crucial role of an obvious sign of the lack of capacity for intelligence of a certain measurable sort in judging a defect to be intolerable. A further justification of this is made by an appeal to accepted social values, at least among middle- and upper-class persons in our society. Our society values intelligence; that value becomes the ideal norm from which abnormality or deficiencies are measured. Since the infant is judged not to be able to develop into an intelligent human being (and do all that "normal" intelligence enables a human being to do), his life is of insufficient value to override the desires of the parents not to have a retarded child.

Without specification of the limits to the sorts of cases to which it could be applied, the physicians would probably not wish to defend the notion that the values of a society determine the right to life. To do so would require that there be clear knowledge of who is valued in our society (we also value aggressive people, loving people, physically strong people, etc.), and in turn a procedure by which capacities for such qualities could be determined in infancy so that precise judgments could be made about what lives should be sustained. Some members of our society do not value black people; blackness would obviously be an insufficient basis for letting an infant die. Thus, in defense of their decision the physicians would have to appeal to "values generally held in our society." This creates a different problem of quantification: what percentage of dissent would count to deny a "general" holding of a value? They would also have to designate the limits to changes in socially held values beyond which they would not consent. If the parents belonged to a subculture that valued blue eyes more than it valued intelligence, and if they expressed a desire not to have a child because it had hazel eyes, the problem of the intestinal blockage would not have been a sufficient condition to refrain from the surgical procedure.

In sum, the ideal norm of the human that makes a difference in judging whether an infant has the right to life in this case is "the capacity for normal intelligence." For the good of the infant, for the sake of avoiding difficulties for the parents, and for the good of society, a significant deviation from normal intelligence, coupled with the appropriate parental desire, is sufficient to permit the infant to die.

A third point of reference was the law. The civil law and the courts figure in the decisions at two points. First, the physicians felt no obligation to seek a court order to save the life of the infant if the parents did not want it. Several possible inferences might be drawn from this. First, one can infer that the infant had no legal right to life; his legal right is conditional upon parental desires. Second, as indicated in the interviews, the physicians believed that the court would not insist upon the surgical procedure to save the infant since it was a mongoloid. Parental desires would override legal rights in such a case. And third (an explicit statement by the physician), if the infant's life had been saved as the result of a court order, there were doubts that it would have been "accepted" by the parents. Here is an implicit appeal to potential consequences: it is not beneficial for a child to be raised by parents who do not "accept" him. The assumption is that they could not change their attitudes.

If the infant had a legal right to life, this case presents an interesting instance of conscientious objection to law. The conscientious objector to military service claims that the power of the state to raise armies for the defense of what it judges to be the national interest is one that he conscientiously refrains from sharing. The common good, or the national interest, is not jeopardized by the granting of a special status to the objector because there are enough persons who do not object to man the military services. In this case, however, the function of the law is to protect the rights of individuals to life, and the physician-objector is claiming that he is under no obligation to seek the support of the legal system to sustain life even when he knows that it could be sustained. The evidence he has in hand (the parental desire and the diagnosis of mongolism) presumably provides sufficient moral grounds for his not complying with the law. From the standpoint of ethics, an appeal could be made to conscientious objection. If, however, the appropriate law does not qualify its claims in such a way as to (a) permit its nonapplicability in this case or (b) provide for exemption on grounds of conscientious objection, the objector is presumably willing to accept the consequences for his conscientious decision. This would be morally appropriate. The physician believed that the court would not insist on saving the infant's life, and thus he foresaw no great jeopardy to himself in following conscience rather than the law.

The second point at which the law figures is in the determination of how the infant should die. The decision not to induce death was made in part in the face of the illegality of overt euthanasia (in part, only, since also the hospital staff would "feel uncomfortable" about hastening the death). Once the end or purpose of action (or inaction) was judged to be morally justified, and judged likely to be free from legal censure, the physicians still felt obliged to achieve that purpose within means that would not be subject to legal sanctions. One can only speculate whether the physicians believed that a court that would not order an infant's life to be saved would in turn censure them for overtly taking the life, or whether the uncomfortable feelings of the hospital staff were more crucial in their decision. Their course of decisions could be interpreted as at one point not involving obligation to take recourse to the courts and at the other scrupulously obeying the law. It should be noted, however, that there is consistency of action on their part; in neither instance did they intervene in what was the "natural" course of developments. The moral justification to fail to intervene in the second moment had to be different from that in the first. In the first it provides the reasons for not saving a life; in the second, for not taking a life. This leads to the last aspect of the decisions of the physicians that I noted, namely, that choices were made between ordinary and extraordinary means of action.

There is no evidence in the interviews that the language of ordinary and extraordinary means of action was part of the vocabulary of the medical staff. It is, however, an honored and useful distinction in Catholic moral theology as it applies to medical care. The principle is that a physician is under no obligation to use extraordinary means to sustain life. The difficulty in the application of the principle is the choice of what falls under ordinary and what under extraordinary means. Under one set of circumstances a procedure may be judged ordinary, and under another extraordinary. The surgery required to remove the bowel obstruction in the infant was on the whole an ordinary procedure; there were no experimental aspects to it, and there were no unusual risks to the infant's life in having it done. If the infant had had no other genetic defects, there would have been no question about using it. The physicians could make a case that when the other defect was mongolism, the procedure would be an extraordinary one. The context of the judgment about ordinary and extraordinary was a wider one than the degree of risk to the life of the patient from surgery. It included his other defect, the desires of the family, the potential costs to family and society, etc. No moralists, to my knowledge, would hold them culpable if the infant were so deformed that he would be labeled (nontechnically) a monstrosity. To heroically maintain the life of a monstrosity as long as one could would be most extraordinary. Thus, we return to whether the fact of mongolism and its consequences is a sufficient justification to judge the livesaving procedure to be extraordinary in this instance. The physicians would argue that it is.

The infant was left to die with a minimum of care. No extraordinary means were used to maintain its life once the decision not to operate had been made. Was it extraordinary not to use even ordinary procedures to maintain the life of the infant once the decision not to operate had been made? The judgment clearly was in the negative. To do so would be to prolong a life that would not be saved in any case. At that point the infant was in a class of terminal patients, and the same justifications used for not prolonging the life of a terminal patient would apply here. Patients have a right to die, and physicians are under no moral obligation to sustain their lives when it is clear that they will not live for long. The crucial difference between a terminal cancer patient and this infant is that in the situation of the former, all procedures which might prolong life for a goodly length of time are likely to have been exhausted. In the case of the infant, the logic of obligations to terminal patients takes its course as a result of a decision not to act at all.

To induce death by some overt action is an extraordinary procedure. To justify overt action would require a justification of euthanasia. This case would be a good one from which to explore euthanasia from a moral point of view. Once a decision is made not to engage in a life-sustaining and lifesaving procedure, has not the crucial corner been turned? If that is a reasonable and moral thing to do, on what grounds would one argue that it is wrong to hasten death? Most obviously it is still illegal to do it, and next most obviously people have sensitive feelings about taking life. Further, it goes against the grain of the fundamental vocation of the medical profession to maintain life. But, of course, the decision not to operate also goes against that grain. If the first decision was justifiable, why was it not justifiable to hasten the death of the infant? We can only assume at this point traditional arguments against euthanasia would have been made.

The Decisions of the Nurses

The nurses, as the interviews indicated, are most important for their expressions of feelings, moral sensibilities, and frustrations. They demonstrate the importance of deeply held moral convictions and of profound compassion in determining human responses to ambiguous circumstances. If they had not known that the infant could have survived, the depth of their frustrations and feelings would have not been so great. Feelings they would have had, but they would have been compassion for an infant bound to die. The actual range of decision for them was clearly circumscribed by the role definitions in the medical professions; it was their duty to carry out the orders of the physicians. Even if they conscientiously believed that the orders they were executing were immoral, they could not radically reverse the course of events; they could not perform the required surgery. It was their lot to be the immediate participants in a sad event but to be powerless to alter its course.

It would be instructive to explore the reasons why the nurses felt frustrated, were deeply affected by their duties in this case. Moral convictions have their impact upon the feelings of persons as well as upon their rational decisions. A profound sense of vocation to relieve suffering and to preserve life no doubt lies behind their responses, as does a conviction about the sanctity of human life. For our purposes, however, we shall leave them with the observation that they are the instruments of the orders of the physicians. They have no right of conscientious objection, at least not in this set of circumstances.

Before turning to another evaluative description of the case, it is important to reiterate what was said in the beginning. The decisions by the principals were conscientious ones. The parents anguished. The physicians were informed by a sense of compassion in their consent to the parents' wishes; they did not wish to be party to potential suffering that was avoidable. Indeed, in the way in which they formulated the dilemma, they did what was reasonable to do. They chose the way of least possible suffering to the fewest persons over a long range of time, with one exception, namely, not taking the infant's life. By describing the dilemma from a somewhat different set of values, or giving different weight to different factors, another course of action would have been reasonable and justified. The issue, it seems to me, is at the level of what is to be valued more highly, for one's very understanding of the problems he must solve are deeply affected by what one values most.

The Dilemma from a Different Moral Point of View

Wallace Stevens wrote in poetic form a subtle account of "Thirteen Ways of Looking at a Blackbird." Perhaps there are 13 ways of looking at this medical case. I shall attempt to look at it from only one more way. By describing the dilemma from a perspective that gives a different weight to some of the considerations that we have already exposed, one has a different picture, and different conclusions are called for. The moral integrity of any of the original participants is not challenged, not because of a radical relativism that says they have their points of view and I have mine, but out of respect for their conscientiousness. For several reasons, however, more consideration ought to have been given to two points. A difference in evaluative judgments would have made a difference of life or death for the infant, depending upon: (1) whether what one ought to do is determined by what one desires to do and (2) whether a mongoloid infant has a claim to life.

To restate the dilemma once again: If the parents had "desired" the mongoloid infant, the surgeons would have performed the operation that would have saved its life. If the infant had had a bowel obstruction that could be taken care of by an ordinary medical procedure, but had not been a mongoloid, the physicians would probably have insisted that the operation be performed.

Thus, one can recast the moral dilemma by giving a different weight to two things: the desires of the parents and the value or rights of a mongoloid infant. If the parents and the physicians believed strongly that there are things one ought to do even when one has no immediate positive feelings about doing them, no immediate strong desire to do them, the picture would have been different. If the parents and physicians believed that mongoloid children have intrinsic value, or have a right to life, or if they believed that mongolism is not sufficiently deviant from what is normatively human to merit death, the picture would have been different.

Thus, we can redraw the picture. To be sure, the parents are ambiguous about their feelings for a mongoloid infant, since it is normal to desire a normal infant rather than an abnormal infant. But (to avoid a discussion of abortion at this point) once an infant is born its independent existence provides independent value in itself, and those who brought it into being and those professionally responsible for its care have an obligation to sustain its life regardless of their negative or ambiguous feelings toward it. This probably would have been acknowledged by all concerned if the infant had not been mongoloid. For example, if the pregnancy had been accidental, and in this sense the child was not desired, and the infant had been normal, no one would have denied its right to exist once it was born, though some would while still *in utero*, and thus would have sought an abortion. If the mother refused to accept accountability for the infant, alternative means of caring for it would have been explored.

To be sure, a mongoloid infant is genetically defective, and raising and caring for it put burdens on the parents, the family, and the state beyond the burdens required to raise a normal infant. But a mongoloid infant is human, and thus has the intrinsic value of humanity and the rights of a human being. Further, given proper care, it can reach a point of significant fulfillment of its limited potentialities; it is capable of loving and responding to love; it is capable of realizing happiness; it can be trained to accept responsibility for itself within its capacities. Thus, the physicians and parents have an obligation to use all ordinary means to preserve its life. Indeed, the humanity of mentally defective children is recognized in our society by the fact that we do not permit their extermination and do have policies which provide, all too inadequately, for their care and nurture.

If our case had been interpreted in the light of moral beliefs that inform the previous two paragraphs, the only reasonable conclusion would be that the surgery ought to have been done.

The grounds for assigning the weights I have to these crucial points can be examined. First, with reference simply to common experience, we all have obligations to others that are not contingent upon our immediate desires. When the registrar of my university indicates that senior grades have to be in by May 21, I have an obligation to read the exams, term papers, and senior essays in time to report the grades, regardless of my negative feelings toward those tasks or my preference to be doing something else. I have an obligation to my students, and to the university through its registrar, which I accepted when I assumed the social role of an instructor. The students have a claim on me; they have a right to expect me to fulfill my obligations to them and to the university. I might be excused from the obligation if I suddenly become too ill to fulfill it; my incapacity to fulfill it would be a temporarily excusing condition. But negative feelings toward that job, or toward any students, or a preference for writing a paper of my own at that time, would not constitute excusing conditions. I must consider, in determining what I do, the relationships that I have with others and the claims they have on me by virtue of those relationships.

In contrast to this case, it might be said that I have a contractual obligation to the university into which I freely entered. The situation of the parents is not the same. They have no legal contractual relationship with the infant, and thus their desires are not bound by obligations. Closer to their circumstances, then, might be other family relationships. I would argue that the fact that we brought our children into being lays a moral obligation on my wife and me to sustain and care for them to the best of our ability. They did not choose to be; and their very being is dependent, both causally and in other ways, upon us. In the relationship of dependence, there is a claim of them over against us. To be sure, it is a claim that also has its rewards and that we desire to fulfill within a relationship of love. But until they have reached an age when they can accept full accountability (or fuller accountability) for themselves, they have claims upon us by virtue of our being their parents, even when meeting those claims is to us financially costly, emotionally distressing, and in other ways not immediately desirable. Their claims are independent of our desires to fulfill them. Particular claims they might make can justifiably be turned down, and others can be negotiated, but the claim against us for their physical sustenance constitutes a moral obligation that we have to meet. That obligation is not conditioned by their IQ scores, whether they have cleft palates or perfectly formed faces, whether they are obedient or irritatingly independent, whether they are irritatingly obedient and passive or laudably self-determining. It is not conditioned by any predictions that might be made about whether they will become the persons we might desire that they become. The infant in our case has the same sort of claim, and thus the parents have a moral obligation to use all ordinary means to save its life.

An objection might be made. Many of my fellow Christians would say that the obligation of the parents was to do that which is loving toward the infant. Not keeping the child alive was the loving thing to do with reference both to its interests and to the interests of the other members of the family. To respond to the objection, one needs first to establish the spongy character of the words "love" or "loving." They can absorb almost anything. Next one asks whether the loving character of an act is determined by feelings or by motives, or whether it is also judged by what is done. It is clear that I would argue for the latter. Indeed, the minimal conditions of a loving relationship include respect for the other, and certainly for the other's presumption of a right to live. I would, however, primarily make the case that the relationship of dependence grounds the claim, whether or not one feels loving toward the other.

The dependence relationship holds for the physicians as well as the parents in this case. The child's life depended utterly upon the capacity of the physicians to sustain it. The fact that an infant cannot articulate his claim is irrelevant. Physicians will struggle to save the life of a person who has attempted to commit suicide even when the patient might be in such a drugged condition that he cannot express his desire—a desire expressed already in his effort to take his life and overridden by the physician's action to save it. The claim of human life for preservation, even when such a person indicates a will not to live, presents a moral obligation to those who have the capacity to save it.

A different line of argument might be taken. If the decisions made were as reliant upon the desires of the parents as they appear to be, which is to say, if desire had a crucial role, what about the desire of the infant? The infant could not give informed consent to the nonintervention. One can hypothesize that every infant desires to live, and that even a defective child is likely to desire life rather than death when it reaches an age at which its desires can be articulated. Even if the right to live is contingent upon a desire, we can infer that the infant's desire would be for life. As a human being, he would have that desire, and thus it would constitute a claim on those on whom he is dependent to fulfill it.

I have tried to make a persuasive case to indicate why the claim of the infant constitutes a moral obligation on the parents and the physicians to keep the child alive. The intrinsic value or rights of a human being are not qualified by any given person's intelligence or capacities for productivity, potential consequences of the sort that burden others. Rather, they are constituted by the very existence of the human being as one who is related to others and dependent upon others for his existence. The presumption is always in favor of sustaining life through ordinary means; the desires of persons that run counter to that presumption are not sufficient conditions for abrogating that right.

The power to determine whether the infant shall live or die is in the hands of others. Does the existence of such power carry with it the moral right to such determination? Long history of moral experience indicates not only that arguments have consistently been made against the judgment that the capacity to do something constitutes a right to do it, or put in more familiar terms, that might makes right. It also indicates that in historical situations where persons have claimed the right to determine who shall live because they have the power to do so, the consequences have hardly been beneficial to mankind. This, one acknowledges, is a "wedge" argument or a "camel's nose under the tent" argument. As such, its limits are clear. Given a culture in which humane values are regnant, it is not likely that the establishment of a principle that some persons under some circumstances claim the right to determine whether others shall live will be transformed into the principle that the right of a person to live is dependent upon his having the qualities approved by those who have the capacity to sustain or take his life. Yet while recognizing the sociological and historical limitations that exist in a humane society, one still must recognize the significance of a precedent. To cite an absurd example, what would happen if we lived in a society in which the existence of hazel eyes was considered a genetic defect by parents and physicians? The absurdity lies in the fact that no intelligent person would consider hazel eyes a genetic defect; the boundaries around the word defect are drawn by evidences better than eye color. But the precedent in principle remains; when one has established that the capacity to determine who shall live carries with it the right to determine who shall live, the line of discussion has shifted from a sharp presumption (of the right of all humans to live) to the softer, spongier determination of the qualities whose value will be determinative.

Often we cannot avoid using qualities and potential consequences in the determination of what might be justifiable exceptions to the presumption of the right to life on the part of any infant—indeed, any

person. No moralist would insist that the physicians have an obligation to sustain the life of matter born from human parents that is
judged to be a "monstrosity." Such divergence from the "normal"
qualities presents no problem, and potential consequences for its continued existence surely enter into the decision. The physicians in our
case believed that in the absence of a desire for the child on the part of
the parents, mongolism was sufficiently removed from an ideal norm
of the human that the infant had no overriding claim on them. We are
in a sponge. Why would I draw the line on a different side of mongolism than the physicians did? While reasons can be given, one must
recognize that there are intuitive elements, grounded in beliefs and
profound feelings, that enter into particular judgments of this sort. I
am not prepared to say that my respect for human life is "deeper,"
"profounder," or "stronger" than theirs. I am prepared to say that the
way in which, and the reasons why, I respect life orient my judgment
toward the other side of mongolism than theirs did.

First, the value that intelligence was given in this instance appears to me to be simplistic. Not all intelligent persons are socially
commendable (choosing socially held values as the point of reference
because one of the physicians did). Also, many persons of limited intelligence do things that are socially commendable, if only minimally
providing the occasion for the expression of profound human affection and sympathy. There are many things we value about human
life; that the assumption that one of them is the *sine qua non*, the necessary and sufficient condition for a life to be valued at all, over-
simplifies human experience. If there is a *sine qua non*, it is physical
life itself, for apart from it, all potentiality of providing benefits for
oneself or for others is impossible. There are occasions on which other
things are judged to be more valuable than physical life itself; we
probably all would admire the person whose life is martyred for the
sake of saving others. But the qualities or capacities we value exist in
bundles, and not each as overriding in itself. The capacity for self-determination is valued, and on certain occasions we judge that it is
worth dying, or taking life, for the sake of removing repressive limits
imposed upon persons in that respect. But many free, self-determining
persons are not very happy; indeed, often their anxiety increases with
the enlargement of the range of things they must and can determine
for themselves. Would we value a person exclusively because he is
happy? Probably not, partly because his happiness has at least a
mildly contagious effect on some other persons, and thus we value
him because he makes others happy as well. To make one quality we
value (short of physical life itself, and here there are exceptions) determinative over all other qualities is to impoverish the richness and vari-

ety of human life. When we must use the sponge of qualities to determine exceptions to the presumption of the right to physical life, we need to face their variety, their complexity, the abrasiveness of one against the other, in the determination of action. In this case the potentialities of a mongoloid for satisfaction in life, for fulfilling his limited capacities, for happiness, for providing the occasions of meaningful (sometimes distressing and sometimes joyful) experience for others are sufficient so that no exception to the right to life should be made. Put differently, the anguish, suffering, embarrassment, expenses of family and state (I support the need for revision of social policy and practice) are not sufficiently negative to warrant that a mongoloid's life not be sustained by ordinary procedures.

Second, and harder to make persuasive, is that my view of human existence leads to a different assessment of the significance of suffering than appears to be operative in this case. The best argument to be made in support of the course of decisions as they occurred is that in the judgment of the principals involved, they were able to avoid more suffering and other costs for more people over a longer range of time than could have been avoided if the infant's life had been saved. To suggest a different evaluation of suffering is not to suggest that suffering is an unmitigated good, or that the acceptance of suffering when it could be avoided is a strategy that ought to be adopted for the good life, individually and collectively. Surely it is prudent and morally justifiable to avoid suffering if possible under most normal circumstances of life. But two questions will help to designate where a difference of opinion between myself and the principals in our drama can be located. One is, At what cost to others is it justifiable to avoid suffering for ourselves? On the basis of my previous exposition, I would argue that in this instance the avoidance of potential suffering at the cost of that life was not warranted. The moral claims of others upon me often involve emotional and financial stress, but that stress is not sufficient to warrant my ignoring the claims. The moral and legal claim of the government to the right to raise armies in defense of the national interest involves inconvenience, suffering, and even death for many; yet the fact that meeting that claim will cause an individual suffering is not sufficient ground to give conscientious objection. Indeed, we normally honor those who assume suffering for the sake of benefits to others.

The second question is, Does the suffering in prospect appear to be bearable for those who have to suffer? We recognize that the term "bearable" is a slippery slope and that fixing an answer to this question involves judgments that are always hypothetical. If, however, each person has a moral right to avoid all bearable inconvenience or suffering that appears to run counter to his immediate or long-range self-interest, there are many things necessary for the good of other individuals and for the common good that would not get done. In our case, there appear to be no evidences that the parents with assistance from other institutions would necessarily find the raising of a mongoloid child to bring suffering that they could not tolerate. Perhaps there is justifying evidence to which I do not have access, such as the possibility that the mother would be subject to severe mental illness if she had to take care of the child. But from the information I received, no convincing case could be made that the demands of raising the child would present intolerable and unbearable suffering to the family. That it would create greater anguish, greater inconvenience, and greater demands than raising a normal child would is clear. But that meeting these demands would cause greater suffering to this family than it does to thousands of others who raise mongoloid children seems not to be the case.

Finally, my view, grounded ultimately in religious convictions as well as moral beliefs, is that to be human is to have a vocation, a calling, and the calling of each of us is "to be for others" at least as much as "to be for ourselves." The weight that one places on "being for others" makes a difference in one's fundamental orientation toward all of his relationships, particularly when they conflict with his immediate self-interest. In the Torah we have that great commandment, rendered in the New English Bible as "you shall love your neighbour as a man like yourself" (Lev. 19:18). It is reiterated in the records we have of the words of Jesus, "Love your neighbor as yourself" (Matt. 22:39, and several other places). Saint Paul makes the point even stronger at one point: "Each of you must regard, not his own interests, but the other man's" (1 Cor. 10:24, NEB). And finally, the minimalist saying accredited both to Rabbi Hillel and to Jesus in different forms, "Do unto others as you would have others do unto you."

The point of the biblical citations is not to take recourse to dogmatic religious authority, as if these sayings come unmediated from the ultimate power and orderer of life. The point is to indicate a central thrust in Judaism and Christianity which has nourished and sustained a fundamental moral outlook, namely, that we are "to be for others" at least as much as we are "to be for ourselves." The fact that this outlook has not been adhered to consistently by those who professed it does not count against it. It remains a vocation, a calling, a moral ideal, if not a moral obligation. The statement of such an outlook does not resolve all the particular problems of medical histories such as this one, but it shapes a bias, gives a weight, toward the well-being of the other against inconvenience or cost to oneself. In this case, I believe that all the rational inferences to be drawn from it, and all the emotive power that this calling evokes, lead to the conclusion that the ordinary surgical procedure should have been done, and the mongoloid infant's life saved.

7 Guidelines for Deciding Care of Critically Ill or Dying Patients

RAYMOND S. DUFF, M.D.

This article proposes a critical examination of medical technology in light of the author's perception of its being intrusive, occasionally cruel, sometimes of little value, and expensive. The author proposes guidelines for the evaluation of technology in the light of patient and family values and their autonomy as well as those of physicians, nurses and social workers.

Raymond S. Duff, M.D. is in the Department of Pediatrics at Yale University School of Medicine

The guidelines for deciding care of critically ill or dying patients presented in this article were offered in response to a request for an editorial on the article by Frader published in this issue of *Pediatrics.*[1] Some comments about Dr. Frader's report and about the origin of the guidelines will be given first.

The difficulties in providing intensive care as described by Frader come as no surprise to those familiar with trends in the development of modern medicine. The problem can be stated as follows. Technology increasingly "reigns"[2] while discourse about disease and about patient, family, and staff experiences and values is restrained.[3] These conditions result from the public's and the profession's feelings that professionally designated, aggressive intervention to defeat disease and death is far superior to patient and family accommodations to disease and ultimately acceptance of defeat. Preston[4] refers to these respective approaches as "aspirational" and "humble" heroisms and argues that in modern medicine a "balanced" heroism involving both is essential to ensure that patients receive the technical and personal care they need (the ends of medicine) as determined by careful deliberation of both lay and professional values. But, maintaining this balance may bring

135

little reward to health professionals even though the potential for reward is very great.[5] Available rewards may be consumed in support of technology, and technologists may inappropriately win over those with a "general" interest in patient care, an observation made by Henderson more than 40 years ago.[6] A further complication is that the demands of any science may conflict with particular human needs, and scientists tend to ignore such conflicts.[7] Finally, some patients, families, or health professionals faced with the ambiguities and uncertainties of crisis may be unwilling or unable to participate in determining or providing well-appointed care. Instead, they may demand cure and relief from technology even though in particular situations the chance of achieving benefit may be low or nil and the risk of harm may be great.

These problems, present throughout medicine, are especially evident in intensive care units. Here, according to Frader, systematic, disciplined, dispassionate professionalism characterizes discussions of technical aspects of care. No doubt, children benefit from this aspirational heroism and some important educational experiences are ensured. However, when patient- or family-centered issues of a personal, ethical, or legal nature are involved, escapism and clumsiness are common. This is observed most often when choices are difficult, the prognosis is poor, or the patient is dying or dead. Then, because humble heroism is left out, personal aspects of child and family care may be neglected, technical care may be misdirected, and staff members may be tense or confused; in addition, education is both incomplete and flawed. From his interpretation of the Quinlan tragedy, the Saikewicz case, and other "public and legal battles," Frader is pessimistic about restructuring decision-making to remedy these difficulties.

Questions regarding the intensive care issues that Frader studied were raised more than two years ago in our own department. As a result of this and as a result of concerns about the Quinlan decision, Dr. Howard Pearson (Chairman, Department of Pediatrics) requested that a position paper and guidelines concerning the care of critically ill or dying patients be drawn up by a committee "not stacked against any philosophy." In accordance with this, persons who served on the committee were selected to represent several disciplines and many persuasions. Beginning in the fall of 1976, the entire committee or subcommittees met on numerous occasions before writing its final report dated April 30, 1977. In a memorandum of the transmittal, the chairman wrote:

Although we acknowledge substantial and uncomfortable disagreement among us, we feel little inclination to seek more harmony because there is risk of tyranny in that, as there is in anarchy. . . .[8] Throughout this effort I have tried to guide our deliberations and to forge our report so as to favor no particular philosophy found in our committee or in the literature. However, there is a bias. In its emphasis on patient and family autonomy, the report is more Jeffersonian or Populist than Hamiltonian or aristocratic. In view of the probable implications of this bias for serving and guiding the public and for creating a noble profession, the committee, I believe, has no regret and offers no apology.

The thinking behind that remark, developed in part elsewhere,[9] is something like the following. Since service for patients and families evaluated largely on their own terms is the primary aim of medicine, modified egalitarianism, which recognizes the importance of the views, contributions, and adaptations of patients and families rather than professional elitism, should be the foundation of our ethics. This approach, given recent philosophical support by Ladd,[10] emphasizes an opinion of man stated by Rousseau: "Cast your eyes over all the nations of the world, run through the histories of all people, among so many inhuman and strange cults, among that prodigious diversity of manners and characters, you will find everywhere the same principles of morality, everywhere the same notions of good and evil. . . . Tell me if there is some land on earth where it is a crime to keep faith, to be merciful, beneficient, generous; where the man of honor is despised and the perfidious man honored. . . . We can be men without being scholars; freed from the necessity of consuming our lives in the study of ethics, we have at less effort a more sure guide in this immense labyrinth of human opinions. [We have in conscience a] sure guide of an ignorant and limited being, but intelligent, infallible judge of good and evil making man like God." In the guidelines which follow, some degree of professional paternalism[11] or ethical elitism balancing the extreme egalitariansim of Rousseau just stated is recognized. This is necessary to prevent decision-making based on ignorance or folly.

Ethical elitism, often signalled in medicine by the comment, "Doctor, you know best," as a primary guide for decision making fosters dependency. It may erode patient and family feelings of control and make them helpless, truly a disservice.[12] It may be associated with patient noncompliance, a common problem,[13] which may frustrate the finest efforts of professionals. It may impoverish. It cannot be consistently caring since caring always requires consideration of the values and contributions of those cared for.[14] Ethical elitism may often violate such dictates as *primum non nocere* (first, do no harm) or *guerir quelquefois, soulager souvent, consoler toujours* (to cure sometimes, to relieve often, to comfort always).

In practical terms, regardless of the eventual results for patients (healthy, handicapped, or dead), the best services for patients and the best education for patients, families, and staff in any situation require concerted efforts, which for the ICU can be described briefly as follows. ICUs must have medical, nursing, and other talents to diagnose and treat diseases and injuries. Since such services must be adapted to meet present and anticipated particular human needs of child and family, one by one, knowledge of each child and family is as essential as that about disease and its treatment. To prevent unnecessary physiologic, personal, and social malfunction, to cope with weaknesses, and to build on strengths, the care of patients and the support and guidance of parents and siblings require orchestrated decisions and actions based on knowledge of diseases and persons; and both kinds of knowledge are essential from the moment care begins.[15]

Physicians, nurses, and social workers probably are best prepared to assume primary leadership in disease management, child care, and coping with the more complex human aspects of illness, respectively; and of course there is frequent overlapping of these roles. Accordingly, these professionals must work together as allies with children and families in a collegial atmosphere of respectful, supportive interdependence. Most rounds in the ICU and many teaching sessions about patient management should include disciplined discourse on pertinent child, parent, sibling, and staff feelings and adaptations. It is essential that children and/or families be participants in many of these dialogues so that staff may learn directly from them as well as each other both specific and general approaches to recovery, living with handicap, or grief.

In order to ensure that decisions are based on thorough deliberation of complete information, the medical leadership proposed in the guidelines below must be accompanied by equally strong leadership from nurses and social workers. From the development of these disciplines in the 20th century, such leadership is increasingly evident. Not only for patients and families but for health professions as well, the time has come for full acceptance and enhancement of this leadership. If this is done and if staff grow in their respective roles, our limited experience indicates that most of the ethical and legal issues and the problems of human relationships described by Frader and others[16] will be resolved.

The guidelines given below have been presented, discussed and used in selected situations in the Pediatric Department at Yale. In addition, they have been discussed in numerous forums in New Haven and elsewhere. In general, comments from physicians, nurses, social workers, chaplains, administrators, lawyers, philosophers, psychologists, theologians, and many laymen have been favorable. Most agreed that the approach to patient care was in harmony with the finest traditions of caring for people. Emphasis on individual and family responsibilities and interests probably would maximize chances for adaptation and growth of all individuals including health professionals. Most of all, since the social bonds (sometimes described as sacred) between persons would be used and strengthened, in general, life could be more abundant.

The guidelines are presented in two parts: "Preamble" and "Specifics." The remainder of this article is the work of the Committee.

PREAMBLE

The results of using medical technology to treat or control diseases in situations of poor prognosis for life or quality of life may be marginal at best and sometimes harmful. Costs in money, and suffering and inconvenience of patients and families are usually greatest when expected results are least. To decide each person's care in these situations, patients (when able), families, and physicians (theoretically in that order of importance) have a long tradition of trying to do what seems prudent. Their choices are known to vary widely and occasionally may include an early death if this is considered the least tragic outcome. Herein is the basis of much controversy commonly noted in debates over proxy consent, quality of life, legal problems, moral persuasions, medical ideologies, and related issues. At times, attention has focused more on the resulting turmoil than on sick persons, families, and their respective interests. This committee was created because of recognition that these problems account for deterioration of care of some patients who, though few in number at any given time, need protection.

This committee, like others which have considered the question of guidelines for patient care, finds the issues are delicate, ponderous, and vastly complex with respect to disease, personal and family considerations, the interests of health professionals, and the concerns of society. We are convinced that consensus regarding specific guidelines in deciding care is impossible. Moreover, it is undesirable because variations in decisions for care are essential: the moral choices of individual persons and their families must be honored in order to avoid tyranny. Nevertheless, specifying the persons who should decide care and the general procedures they should follow is necessary in order to exercise ordinary virtues of compassion, prudence, and occasionally heroism when these are most needed in tragic situations. The goal of medicine is not always to extend or to preserve biologic life. Respect of persons, families, and the values they hold may dictate another choice. Both the public and health professionals should understand this fact of modern medicine so that the patients, families, and health professionals may be protected against the scenes of caring becoming even more an arena of conflicting ideologies.

Determining care in tragic situations is not new. In earlier times it was decided in the privacy of homes where there was little chance for public observation. Now, advanced technology poses more choices and more dilemmas; and since most care requires a large team of professionals working in a semipublic place, the age of presumed innocence is passed.

Each hospitalized patient of any age has by custom *one* physician who is responsible for his care and is accountable to him, his family, the hospital, and the law. This physician, often called the *physician of record* or the *responsible physician,* has responsibility for coordinating the efforts of all persons concerned with the care of his or her patient. Such persons include the patient (when able to participate in decisions on care) and the family. Also, consulting physicians, nurses, house staff, social workers, and appropriate others may be included as occasion requires. When involved with care, each of these persons must have access to the responsible physician to clarify confusion or resolve differences. It is essential that the physician of record inform children, as appropriate (see below), and families, always, about the child's problems, the proposed care including its probable risks and benefits, and divisions of opinion regarding care. This procedure works more or less well in situations where controversy and urgency for decisions and action are minimal. However, this procedure breaks down often when it is most needed, as in intensive care situations and when the patient has a poor prognosis or is dying.

There are two common causes of breakdown, both involving medical leadership. The first is that the physician of record is not identifiable. For example, a pediatrician may have admitted a child who soon is cared for by another physician or physicians whose skills are necessary. Such physicians may be general surgeons, neurosurgeons, urologists, orthopedists, plastic surgeons, hematologists, neurologists, neonatologists, or others. The second cause of breakdown is failure of the physician of record to perform as he should. At times he may be unavailable, or his task may be extremely difficult as in situations where many persons of varied opinions are caring for the patient; then, he may have too little control. Conversely, he may exercise excessive control by presuming that his central role in developing decisions requires that he primarily decides on care. The physician of record and others may fail to decide on important issues of care or may make choices inconsistent with each other. Moreover, discussion of care to ensure informed consent and selection of care in keeping with patient and family preferences may be abridged or omitted. In such situations, house staff and nurses usually are left at the child's side to do the best they can without the guidance of deliberated choices that could have been made. They and the children and families in their care are then deeply troubled because of their intimate associations with the ironies of care.

Two special problems in the care of children concern what information is to be given to them and the degree to which they may decide their own treatment. Although infants and very young children cannot directly help in determining their own care, those who make these decisions should always take into account the child's signals of pleasure and distress. At all ages, children should have their questions answered in ways most helpful to them. If there is disagreement on this point, parents should decide. However, by age 16, children have the legal right to know. Regarding treatment, at the age of 7 years, it is conceivable, although unlikely, that a child's thoughts and wishes might be decisive. After the age of 11 years, it becomes increasingly likely that a child's thoughts and wishes can be decisive, provided the child is in a reasonable state of competence. Children over the age of 14 ordinarily are capable of making their own decisions about treatment, including the decision to live or die. However, the legal responsibility for deciding care resides with the parents until the adolescent is 18 years of age.

Another issue repeatedly raised in our deliberations concerns "allowing" or "helping" people to die. We recognize that many people are allowed to die. Presumably, most health professionals support this course. A problem arises if we behave so as to help people to die when that seems most sensible. Some persons are content with present homicide laws which hold that active killing regardless of motive is murder or manslaughter. They fear that permitting death by choice in the medical context may be abused possibly even to the extent noted in Nazi Germany. Others view this opinion as simplistic and oppressive They point out that death elected by an individual and his family and physician is vastly different from death decided by and for the state. In addition, given the circumstances of technologic control over living and dying, the distinction between "active" and "passive" killing is increasingly blurred. Holding to this distinction leads to the creation of fictions that hide the real issues. Most of all, since those who decide care have the fear that criminal charges may be brought against them even if they discuss the real issues, caring for the sick or dying may generally be compromised. According to this second view, neither coercive living nor coercive dying has any place in a free society; and one can be as oppressive as the other. The committee, like society at large, is divided philosophically (as expected) on this issue, and there is no hope for agreement among us. Numerous writings could be cited to support different positions.[17] However, because of the law, the specific guidelines given below are not to be construed as recommending or condoning "active" euthanasia. Some coercive living under oppressive conditions must be endured unless individuals prompted by compassion and conscience engage in risky acts of disobedience.

There was sharp debate as to whether economic costs and suffering and inconvenience of families, in addition to that of patients, should be recognized as appropriate influences upon decisions for care. We acknowledge that these factors commonly influence choices for care. In the nature of things, this is inevitable and is consistent with the notion of patient and family autonomy. Yet, sometimes this autonomy must be limited since poor decisions may arise from misguided altruism or unchecked selfishness. In particular, we caution that great care be given to defining "hopelessness" biologically. Also, treatment should be assessed by its probable consequences (valuable, useless, or harmful), not by economic costs. Such issues should be deliberated primarily in the dialogue of the patient, the family, and the responsible physician.

After lengthy discussion of these problems, the committee proposed procedural guidelines. We believe these are needed now. They or modifications of them will be needed even more as medical technology advances. In view of the ever increasing control that health professionals have over life and dying, presuming innocence in these matters or neglecting them is naive, dangerous, and unreasonable. It is assumed that generally the guidelines will place patient and family interests first and institutionalized interests second. However, there are risks that this may not be the case. For example, with conflicts between patient interests and teaching and research as they are, the responsible physician (a pivotal person in the whole scheme of care) may experience conflict of interest. Agony is always possible; it may be severe in some situations. Hence, the physician of record may benefit by sharing his trials with others, especially those who from maturity or experience have faced similar issues. However, despite agony aggravated by uncertainty, he must bear responsibility for his patients and do his best. As noted by LaBarre,[18] this is a "a loyalty that is [his] burden, his glory, and his cross."

SPECIFICS

1. When a child is admitted to Yale-New Haven Hospital, the resident in pediatrics will ensure that a notation is made in the child's record designating the name of the responsible physician for that child during the period of hospitalization. If the family does not already know the responsible physician, they should be given the name of that physician and at the earliest practical time he should communicate with the family.

2. The responsible physician may be a pediatrician in private practice, a pediatric specialist such as a hematologist, neonatologist, etc., a pediatric attending physician on a given patient care division, or a member of another clinical service such as surgery, neurosurgery, plastic surgery, orthopedics, urology, etc. It will usually be evident who the responsible physician is. In case of doubt, the pediatric resident will consult with the physicians directly involved. If this attempt to designate the responsible physician fails, he willl ask the Chief of Pediatrics to resolve the question. If the Chief of Pediatrics is unable to resolve the question, he will consult with the relevant chiefs of the other services involved and if necessary with the chief of the medical staff. The family and, when appropriate, the child will have input into the choice of the responsible physician. (Hereafter, when describing the child's role in deciding care, we mean the child when appropriate in terms stated in the preamble.) They may request that a change be made following established procedures. Such requests should be considered promptly and usually will be honored. If a change in responsible physician is found desirable or necessary after admission of a child, such change shall be made only after discussion and agreement among the two physicians and the child and the family. This change will be entered clearly in the record. When a child's management and care requires the skills of one or more specialists especially in intensive care units where swift action and coordination of multiple hospital services are essential, the physician of record may be full-time in the medical center and assigned as attending in the intensive care unit or appropriate other full-time or community physician. This choice should be worked out by the referring physician or family pediatrician, the attending physician in the intensive care unit, and the child and family. Whatever choice is made, the physician of record must ensure that decisions for care reflect child and family values and that supports of child and family as well as technical care are excellent. Superior competence in providing both technical and supportive care may rarely be found in one physician. Family pediatricians may possess superior knowledge and skills in some aspects of

care, and full-time physicians may have unique skills in others. They need each other. Children and families need both, usually with equal urgency. Administrative arrangements should reflect these realities.

3. The child's own feelings, thoughts, values, and wishes as well as those of the parents must be considered at all times and at all ages (See Preamble).

4. The duties of the responsible physician include exercise of his or her judgment in evaluating the patient's problems and in exchanging information about the child's condition regularly with the child and family and with those appropriately involved in the care of the child. But the responsible physician's role is more than one of leadership or director. He must function most often as a team member with the child, family, house officers, nurses, and social workers. These other persons often possess knowledge and skills essential for deciding care as well as for providing it in hospital or later. They must be free to decide some questions regarding care and to communicate with others on the team. If the child and family cannot be team members (as will sometimes be the case), the responsible physician often must rely heavily on the house officer, nurse, and social worker. This may be true especially in some critical situations when value conflicts or disagreements about care may arise among the child, family, and health professionals (responsible physician, family pediatrician, referring physician, consulting physicians, nurses, social workers, chaplains, and possibly others). In such case, the responsible physician with the team and appropriate consultants will attempt to define issues, outline options, and decide care. Generally, the choices should be made in accordance with the values of the child, his family, the physician of record, and others on the team in that order of importance. Usually this team will assess the child's problem and prognosis and develop major recommendations for a course of action before communicating with the child and family. Then, a full review of the situation will be carried out by the physician of record with the child and family before actually taking a course of action. Of course, the acuteness of some problems may mandate immediate action (to protect the child) before these deliberations can occur. If so, these deliberations should take place as soon as possible and should include review of the reasons for taking prompt action and the results of doing so.

5. In the event of major disagreements among senior physicians or other senior persons especially nurses and social workers involved in the care, the responsible physician must present the conflicting recommendations to the child and family who may then help to resolve the conflict. The responsible physician, child, or family may request fur-

ther consultations from physicians, nurses, social workers, clergymen, or other persons.

6. If questions of care still are not resolved, a conference of the contending parties, at times including the child and family, shall be convened by the Chief of the Pediatric Service or his delegate at the request of the chief resident or the responsible physician. Such a conference serves to share information and opinions. The power to decide rests as before: first with the child and family and second with the responsible physician.

7. If the child or parents disagree with the proposed course of action, their decision must be reviewed in light of: the diagnosis; the expected outcome with and without treatment, including the quality of life for the child and family; the degree of certainty of outcome; the risks of psychological burdens; and the probability of benefits from treatment. Of course, parents may seek legal counsel and court assistance at any time to resolve conflicts with medical authorities. Medical authorities through the hospital may do likewise especially if the parents or child insist on a choice viewed as detrimental to the child. The decision for the best interest of the child may then be made by whomever the court designates.

8. Some health professionals, because of their interpretation of professional norms or prognostic indicators or because of their own values or conscience, may object to a choice that the child, family, and physician of record prefer. Such dissenting persons can and should make their views known to the physician of record. This physician in turn will discuss the issues with objecting persons and appropriate others before deciding whether to discuss them with the child and family. The guiding principle here is primarily loyalty to the child and family in light of their values and realities. Paternalistic acts of whatever benevolent intent must not be imposed unless there is convincing reason to believe the preferred choice is inferior and an alternate one is superior. No other course will enhance or even permit respect of persons we try to help in tragedies. If the physician of record objects to a child and family choice that is supported by another physician or physicians, he must make his views known to the child and family. He or those dissenting others just mentioned may be replaced without prejudice.

9. House staff, nurses, and, often, social workers are usually close to patients. They give much direct care and provide essential support to patients and families. They are better able to provide optimal care for critically ill patients and their families when they understand specifically the plans for care and generally the motives and values of

the responsible physician, child, and family. To facilitate this, the responsible physician should classify his critically ill or dying patients or those with a very poor prognosis in one of the following categories. He should record this and supporting and dissenting opinions in the medical record. As changes in patients' conditions take place, regular reassessment of persons in all groups is required in order to ensure that classification is appropriate. Patients in any class may be reclassified into any other. Classes are:

Class A: Maximal Therapeutic Effort without Reservation. In general, patients in this group are likely to benefit enough from aggressive treatment that those deciding care believe the impositions associated with care are justified.

Class B: Selective Limitation of Therapeutic Measures. Those deciding care believe that patients in this group will not benefit over-all from applying maximal therapeutic efforts. The responsible physician must clearly state the reasons for initiating any major new procedure so that all care givers despite some inevitable disagreement may be united and supportive in their interactions with these patients and their families. Patients in this group along with their families should be made comfortable and not abused by inappropriate resuscitative measures.

Class C: Discontinuance of Life-Sustaining Therapy. Most of these patients are dying and usually can be made comfortable. In keeping with the highest principles of caring for persons in ways that they and their families desire, the child, family, responsible physician, and others will work out patient by patient how they will proceed. Recognizing this terminal phase of life, their primary aim is to ease dying as conscience, prudence, and kindness dictate.

The Committee on Guidelines consisted of 12 physicians: R. Duff (Chairman), I. Gross, J. Leventhal, R. J. Levine, M. Lewis, L. Margolis, G. Seashore, B. Shaywitz, C. Stashwick, R. Touloukian, M. Wessel, and one who chose not to be named; four nurses: K. Fallon, P. Johnson, R. O'Grady, and B. Smith; three social workers: R. Breslin, C. Cooper, and J. London; Chaplain D. Duncombe; Attorney A. Holder; and an administrator (*ex officio*).

ACKNOWLEDGMENT

The author wishes to thank members of the committee and numerous others who have commented on this manuscript.

REFERENCES

1. Frader JE: Difficulties in providing intensive care. *Pediatrics* 64:10, 1979

2. Reiser SJ: *Medicine and the Reign of Technology.* London, Cambridge University Press, 1978

3. Foucault M: *The Birth of the Clinic,* New York, Vintage Books, 1975

4. Preston R: *Human Ambiguity and Nursing,* PhD dissertation. Yale University, New Haven, 1977

5. Fox T: Purposes of medicine. *Lancet* 2:801, 1965

6. Henderson LJ: The practice of medicine as applied sociology. *Trans Assoc Am Physicians* 51:8, 1936

7. Holton G: Scientific optimism and societal concerns. *Hastings Cent Rep* 5:39, 1975

8. Sisk JP: The tyranny of harmony. *The American Scholar* 46:193, 1977

9. Duff R: On deciding the use of the family commons, in Bergsma D, Pulver AE (eds): *Developmental Disabilities: Psychologic and Social Implications.* New York, Alan R Liss, 1976, pp 73–84

10. Ladd J: Egalitarianism and elitism in ethics, *L'Égalité* 5:297, 1977

11. Gert B, Culver CM: Paternalistic behavior. *Philosophy and Public Affairs* 6:45, 1976

12. Seligman MEP: *Helplessness: On Depression, Development, and Death.* San Francisco, WH Freeman and Co, 1975

13. Davis MS: Physiologic, psychological and demographic factors in patient compliance with doctor's orders. *Med Care* 6:115, 1968

14. Mayeroff M: *On Caring.* New York, Harper and Row, 1971

15. Breslin R: Family crisis care. *Clin Perinatol* 3:447, 1976

16. Howard J, Davis F, Pope C, et al: Humanizing health care: The implications of technology, centralization, and self-care. *Med Care* 15 (suppl):11, 1977

17. Gorovitz S: Dealing with dying, in Bayles MD, High DM (eds): *Medical Treatment of the Dying: Moral Issues.* Cambridge, Schenkman Publishing Co, 1978, pp 29–45

18. LaBarre W: *The Human Animal.* Chicago, University of Chicago Press, 1954, p 221

8 Child Abuse and Neglect Prevention and Treatment

DEPARTMENT OF HEALTH AND HUMAN SERVICES

These Federal Regulations set forth the standard for treatment of infants with birth defects. The Regulations represent the culmination of several years of debate in the Agency, following the well publicized Infant Doe cases in which newborns were refused treatment or in which less invasive treatments were chosen. The purpose of the Regulations is to prevent child neglect or abuse through a denial of medical treatment. The Regulations were rejected by the Supreme Court.

SUBPART A—GENERAL PROVISIONS

SUBPART B—GRANTS TO STATES

SUBPART C—DISCRETIONARY GRANTS AND CONTRACTS

APPENDIX—INTERPRETATIVE GUIDELINES REGARDING 45 CFR 1340.15—SERVICES AND TREATMENT FOR DISABLED INFANTS.

2. The authority citation for Part 1340 is revised to read as follows:

Authority: Child Abuse Prevention and Treatment Act. Pub. L. 93–247, 88 Stat. 4; Pub. L. 95–266, 92 Stat. 205, Sections 609–610; Pub. L. 97–35, 95 Stat. 488; Pub. L. 98-457, 98 Stat. 1749 (42 U.S.C. 5101 et seq. and 42 U.S.C. 5101 note).

3. The introductory text of § 1340.14. Eligibility requirements is revised to read as follows:

§ 1340.14   ELIGIBILITY REQUIREMENTS.

In order for a State to qualify for an award under this subpart, the State must meet the requirements of § 1340.15 and satisfy each of the following requirements:

4. A new § 1340.15 is added to Subpart B—Grants to States, to read as follows:

§ 1340.15   SERVICES AND TREATMENT FOR DISABLED INFANTS.

(a) *Purpose.* The regulations in this section implement certain provisions of the Child Abuse Amendments of 1984, including section 4(b)(2)(K) of the Child Abuse Prevention and Treatment Act governing the protection and care of disabled infants with the life-threatening conditions.

(b) *Definitions:* (1) The term "medical neglect" means the failure to provide adequate medical care in the context of the definitions of "child abuse and neglect" in section 3 of the Act and § 1340.2(d) of this part. The term "medical neglect" includes, but is not limited to, the withholding of medically indicated treatment from a disabled infant with a life-threatening condition.

(2) The term "withholding of medically indicated treatment" means the failure to respond to the infant's life-threatening conditions by providing treatment (including appropriate nutrition, hydration,

and medication) which, in the treating physician's (or physicians') reasonable medical judgment, will be most likely to be effective in ameliorating or correcting all such conditions, except that the term does not include the failure to provide treatment (other than appropriate nutrition, hydration, or medication) to an infant when, in the treating physician's (or physicians') reasonable medical judgment any of the following circumstances apply:

(i) The infant is chronically and irreversibly comatose:

(ii) The provision of such treatment would merely prolong dying, not be effective in ameliorating or correcting all of the infant's life-threatening conditions, or otherwise be futile in terms of the survival of the infant; or

(iii) The provision of such treatment would be virtually futile in terms of the survival of the infant and the treatment itself under such circumstances would be inhumane.

(3) Following are definitions of terms used in paragraph (b)(2) of this section:

(i) The term "infant" means an infant less than one year of age. The reference to less than one year of age shall not be construed to imply that treatment should be changed or discontinued when an infant reaches one year of age, or to affect or limit any existing protections available under State laws regarding medical neglect of children over one year of age. In addition to their applicability to infants less than one year of age, the standards set forth in paragraph (b)(2) of this section should be consulted thoroughly in the evaluation of any issue of medical neglect involving an infant older than one year of age who has been continuously hospitalized since birth, who was born extremely prematurely, or who has a long-term disability.

(ii) The term "reasonable medical judgment" means a medical judgment that would be made by a reasonably prudent physician, knowledgeable about the case and the treatment possibilities with respect to the medical conditions involved.

(c) *Eligibility Requirements.* (1) In addition to the other eligibility requirements set forth in this Part, to qualify for a grant under this section, a State must have programs, procedures, or both, in place within the State's child protective service system for the purpose of responding to the reporting of medical neglect, including instances of withholding of medically indicated treatment from disabled infants with life-threatening conditions.

(2) These programs and/or procedures must provide for:

(i) Coordination and consultation with individuals designated by and within appropriate health care facilities;

(ii) Prompt notification by individuals designated by and within appropriate health care facilities of cases of suspected medical neglect (including instances of the withholding of medically indicated treatment from disabled infants with life-threatening conditions); and

(iii) The authority, under State law, for the State child protective service system to pursue any legal remedies, including the authority to initiate legal proceedings in a court of competent jurisdiction, as may be necessary to prevent the withholding of medically indicated treatment from disabled infants with life-threatening conditions.

(3) The programs and/or procedures must specify that the child protective services system will promptly contact each health care facility to obtain the name, title, and telephone number of the individual(s) designated by such facility for the purpose of the coordination, consultation, and notification activities identified in paragraph (c)(2) of this section, and will at least annually recontact each health care facility to obtain any changes in the designations.

(4) These programs and/or procedures must be in writing and must conform with the requirements of section 4(b)(2) of the Act and § 1340.14 of this part.

In connection with the requirement of conformity with the requirements of section 4(b)(2) of the Act and § 1340.14 of this part, the programs and/or procedures must specify the procedures the child protective services system will follow to obtain, in a manner consistent with State law:

(i) Access to medical records and/or other pertinent information when such access is necessary to assure an appropriate investigation of a report of medical neglect (including instances of withholding of medically indicated treatment from disabled infants with life threatening conditions); and

(ii) A court order for an independent medical examination of the infant, or otherwise effect such an examination in accordance with processes established under State law, when necessary to assure an appropriate resolution of a report of medical neglect (including instances of withholding of medically indicated treatment from disabled infants with life threatening conditions).

(5) The eligibility requirements contained in this section shall be effective October 9, 1985.

(d) *Documenting eligibility*. (1) In addition to the information and documentation required by and pursuant to § 1340.12(b) and (c), each State must submit with its application for a grant sufficient information and documentation to permit the Commissioner to find that the State is in compliance with the eligibility requirements set forth in paragraph (c) of this section.

(2) This information and documentation shall include:

(i) A copy of the written programs and/or procedures established by, and followed within, the State for the purpose of responding to the reporting of medical neglect, including instances of withholding of medically indicated treatment from disabled infants with life-threatening conditions:

(ii) Documentation that the State has authority, under State law, for the State child protective service system to pursue any legal remedies, including the authority to initiate legal proceedings in a court of competent jurisdiction, as may be necessary to prevent the withholding of medically indicated treatment from disabled infants with life-threatening conditions. This documentation shall consist of:

(A) A copy of the applicable provisions of State statute(s); or

(B) A copy of the applicable provisions of State rules or regulations, along with a copy of the State statutory provisions that provide the authority for such rules or regulations; or

(C) A copy of an official, numbered opinion of the Attorney General of the State that so provides, along with a copy of the applicable provisions of the State statute that provides a basis for the opinion, and a certification that the official opinion has been distributed to interested parties within the State, at least including all hospitals; and

(iii) Such other information and documentation as the Commissioner may require.

(e) *Regulatory construction.* (1) No provision of this section or part shall be construed to affect any right, protection, procedures, or requirement under 45 CFR Part 84, Nondiscrimination on the Basis of Handicap in Programs and Activities Receiving or Benefitting from Federal Financial Assistance.

(2) No provision of this section or part may be so construed as to authorize the Secretary or any other governmental entity to establish standards prescribing specific medical treatments for specific conditions, except to the extent that such standards are authorized by other laws or regulations.

5. 45 CFR Part 1340 is further amended by adding at the end thereof the following Appendix:

APPENDIX TO PART 1340

Interpretative Guidelines Regarding 45 CFR 1340.15—Services and Treatment for Disabled Infants

This appendix sets forth the Department's interpretative guidelines regarding several terms that appear in the definition of the term "withholding of medically indicated treatment" in section 3(3) of the Child Abuse Prevention and Treatment Act, as amended by section 121(3) of the Child Abuse Amendments of 1984. This statutory definition is repeated in § 1340.15(b)(2) of the final rule.

The Department's proposed rule to Implement those provisions of the Child Abuse Amendments of 1984 relating to services and treatment for disabled infants included a number of proposed clarifying definitions of several terms used in the statutory definition. The preamble to the proposed rule explained these proposed clarifying definitions, and in some cases used examples of specific diagnoses to elaborate on meaning.

During the comment period on the proposed rule, many commenters urged deletion of these clarifying definitions and avoidance of examples of specific diagnoses. Many commenters also objected to the specific wording of some of the proposed clarifying definitions, particularly in connection with the proposed use of the word "imminent" to describe the proximity in time at which death is anticipated regardless of treatment in relation to circumstances under which treatment (other than appropriate nutrition, hydration and medication) need not be provided. A letter from the six principal sponsors of the "compromise amendment" which became the pertinent provisions of the Child Abuse Amendments of 1984 urged deletion of "imminent" and careful consideration of the other concerns expressed.

After consideration of these recommendations, the Department decided not to adopt these several proposed clarifying definitions as part of the final rule. It was also decided that effective implementation of the program established by the Child Abuse Amendments would be advanced by the Department stating its interpretations of several key terms in the statutory definition. This is the purpose of this appendix.

The interpretative guidelines that follow have carefully considered comments submitted during the comment period on the proposed rule. These guidelines are set forth and explained without the use of specific diagnostic examples to elaborate on meaning.

Finally, by way of introduction, the Department does not seek to establish these interpretative guidelines as binding rules of law, nor to prejudge the exercise of reasonable medical judgment in responding to specific circumstances, Rather, this guidance is intended to assist in interpreting the statutory definiton so that it may be rationally and thoughtfully applied in specific contexts in a manner fully consistent with the legislative intent.

1. *In general; the statutory definition of "withholding of medically indicated treatment."*

Section 1340.15(b)(2) of the final rule defines the term "withholding of medically indicated treatment" with a definition identical to that which appears in section 3(3) of the Act (as amended by section 121(3) of the Child Abuse Amendments of 1984).

This definition has several main features. First, it establishes the basic principle that all disabled infants with life-threatening conditions must be given medically indicated treatment, defined in terms of action to respond to the infant's life-threatening conditions by providing treatment (including appropriate nutrition, hydration or medication) which, in the treating physician's (or physicians') reasonable medical judgment, will be most likely to be effective in ameliorating or correcting all such conditions.

Second, the statutory definition spells out three circumstances under which treatment is not considered "medically indicated." These are when, in the treating physician's (or physicians') reasonable medical judgment:
—The infant is chronically and irreversibly comatose:
—The provision of such treatment would merely prolong dying, not be effective in ameliorating or correcting all of the infant's life-threatening conditions, or otherwise be futile in terms of survival of the infant; or
—The provision of such treatment would be virtually futile in terms of survival of the infant and the treatment itself under such circumstances would be inhumane.

The third key feature of the statutory definition is that even when one of these three circumstances is present, and thus the failure to provide treatment is not a "withholding of medically indicated treatment," the infant must nonetheless be provided with appropriate nutrition, hydration, and medication.

Fourth, the definition's focus on the potential effectiveness of treatment in ameliorating or correcting life-threatening conditions makes clear that it does not sanction decisions based on subjective opinions about the future "quality of life" of a retarded or disabled person.

The fifth main feature of the statutory definition is that its operation turns substantially on the "reasonable medical judgment" of the treating physician or physicians. The term "reasonable medical judgment" is defined in § 1340.15(b)(3)(ii) of the final rule, as it was in the Conference Committee Report on the Act, as a medical judgment that would be made by a reasonably prudent physician, knowledgeable about the case and the treatment possibilities with respect to the medical conditions involved.

The Department's interpretations of key terms in the statutory definition are fully consistent with these basic principles reflected in the definition. The discussion that follows is organized under headings that generally correspond to the proposed clarifying definitions that appeared in the proposed rule but were not adopted in the final rule. The discussion also attempts to analyze and respond to significant comments received by the Department.

2. *The term "life-threatening condition"*.

Clause (b)(3)(ii) of the proposed rule proposed a definition of the term "life-threatening condition." This term is used in the statutory definition in the following context:

[T]he term "withholding of medically indicated treatment" means the failure to respond to the infant's *life-threatening conditions* by providing treatment (including appropriate nutrition, hydration, and medication) which, in the treating physician's or physicians' reasonable medical judgment, will be most likely to be effective in ameliorating or correcting all such conditions [, except that * * * [Emphasis supplied].

It appears to the Department that the applicability of the statutory definition might be uncertain to some people in cases where a condition may not, strictly speaking, by itself be life-threatening, but where the condition significantly increases the risk of the onset of complications that may threaten the life of the infant. If medically indicated treatment is available for such a condition, the failure to provide it may result in the onset of complications that, by the time the condition becomes life-threatening in the strictest sense, will eliminate or reduce the potential effectiveness of any treatment. Such a result cannot, in the Department's view, be squared with the Congressional intent.

Thus, the Department interprets the term "life-threatening condition" to include a condition that, in the treating physician's or physicians' reasonable medical judgment, significantly increases the risk of the onset of complications that may threaten the life of the infant.

In response to comments that the proposed rule's definition was potentially overinclusive by covering any condition that one could argue "may " become life-threatening, the Department notes that the statutory standard of "the treating physician's or physicians' reasonable medical judgment" is incorporated in the Department's interpretation, and is fully applicable.

Other commenters suggested that this interpretation would bring under the scope of the definition many irreversible conditions for which no corrective treatment is available. This is certainly not the intent. The Department's interpretation implies nothing about whether, or what, treatment should be provided. It simply makes clear that the criteria set forth in the statutory definition for evaluating whether, or what, treatment should be provided are applicable. That is just the start, not the end, of the analysis. The analysis then takes fully into account the reasonable medical judgment regarding potential effectiveness of possible treatments, and the like.

Other comments were that it is unnecessary to state any interpretation because reasonable medical judgment commonly deems the conditions described as life-threatening and responds accordingly. HHS agrees that this is common practice followed under reasonable medical judgment, just as all the standards incorporated in the statutory definition reflect common practice followed under reasonable medical judgment. For the reasons stated above, however, the Department believes it is useful to say so in these interpretative guidelines.

   3. *The term "treatment" in the context of adequate evaluation.*

Clause (B)(3)(ii) of the proposed rule proposed a definition of the term "treatment." Two separate concepts were dealt with in clause (A) and (B), respectively, of the proposed rule. Both of these clauses were designed to ensure that the Congressional intent regarding the issues to be considered under the analysis set forth in the statutory definition is fully effectuated. Like the guidance regarding "life-threatening condition," discussed above, the Department's interpretations go to the applicability of the statutory analysis, not its result.

The Department believes that Congress intended that the standard of following reasonable medical judgment regarding the potential effectiveness of possible courses of action should apply to issues regarding adequate medical evaluation, just as it does to issues regarding adequate medical intervention. This is apparent Congressional intent because Congress adopted, in the Conference Report's definition of "reasonable medical judgment," the standard of adequate knowledge about the case and the treatment possibilities with respect to the medical condition involved.

Having adequate knowledge about the case and the treatment possibilities involved is, in effect, step one of the process, because that is the basis on which "reasonable medical judgment" will operate to make recommendations regarding medical intervention. Thus, part of the process to determine what treatment, if any, "will be most likely to be effective in ameliorating or correcting" all life-threatening conditions is for the treating physician or physicians to make sure they have adequate information about the condition and adequate knowledge about treatment possibilities with respect to the condition involved. The standard for determining the adequacy of the information and knowledge is the same as the basic standard of the statutory definition: reasonable medical judgment. A reasonably prudent physician faced with a particular condition about which he or she needs additional information and knowledge of treatment possibilities would take steps to gain more information and knowledge by, quite simply, seeking further evaluation by, or consultation with, a physician or physicians whose expertise is appropriate to the condition(s) involved or further evaluation at a facility with specialized capabilities regarding the condition(s) involved.

Thus, the Department interprets the term "treatment" to include (but not be limited to) any further evaluation by, or consultation with, a physician or physicians whose expertise is appropriate to the condition(s) involved or further evaluation at a facility with specialized capabilities regarding the condition(s) involved that, in the treating physician's or physicians' reasonable medical judgment, is needed to assure that decisions regarding medical intervention are based on adequate knowledge about the case and the treatment possibilities with respect to the medical conditions involved.

This reflects the Department's interpretation that failure to respond to an infant's life-threatening conditions by obtaining any further evaluations or consultations that, in the treating physician's reasonable medical judgment, are necessary to assure that decisions regarding medical intervention are based on adequate knowledge about the case and the treatment possibilities involved constitutes a "withholding of medically indicated treatment." Thus, if parents refuse to consent to such a recommendation that is based on the treating physician's reasonable medical judgment that, for example, further evaluation by a specialist is necessary to permit reasonable medical judgments to be made regarding medical intervention, this would be a matter for appropriate action by the child protective services system.

In response to comments regarding the related provision in the proposed rule, this interpretative guideline makes quite clear that this interpretation does not deviate from the basic principle of reliance on reasonable medical judgment to determine the extent of the evaluations necessary in the particular case. Commenters expressed concerns that the provision in the proposed rule would intimidate physicians to seek transfer of seriously ill infants to tertiary level facilities much more often than necessary, potentially resulting in diversion of the limited capacities of these facilities away from those with real needs for the specialized care, unecessary separation of infants from their parents when equally beneficial treatment could have been provided at the community or regional hospital, inappropriate deferral of therapy while time-consuming arrangements can be affected, and other counterproductive ramifications. The Department intended no intimidation, prescription or similar influence on reasonable medical judgment, but rather, intended only to affirm that it is the Department's interpretation that the reasonable medical judgment standard applies to issues of medical evaluation, as well as issues of medical intervention.

4. *The term "treatment" in the context of multiple treatments.*

Clause (b)(3)(iii)(B) of the proposed rule was designed to clarify that, in evaluating the potential effectiveness of a particular medical treatment or surgical procedure that can only be reasonably evaluated in the context of a complete potential treatment plan, the "treatment" to be evaluated under the standards of the statutory definition includes the multiple medical treatments and/or surgical procedures over a period of time that are designed to ameliorate or correct a life-threatening condition or conditions. Some commenters stated that it could be construed to require the carrying out of a long process of medical treatments or surgical procedures regardless of the lack of success of those done first. No such meaning is intended.

The intent is simply to characterize that which must be evaluated under the standards of the statutory definition, not to imply anything about the results of the evaluation. If parents refuse consent for a particular medical treatment or surgical procedure that by itself may not correct or ameliorate all life-threatening conditions, but is recommended as part of a total plan that involves multiple medical treatments and/or surgical procedures over a period of time that, in the treating physician's reasonable medical judgment, will be most likely to be effective in ameliorating or correcting all such conditions, that would be a matter for appropriate action by the child protective services system.

On the other hand, if, in the treating physician's reasonable medical judgment, the total plan will, for example, be virtually futile and inhumane, within the meaning of the statutory term, then there is no "withholding of medically indicated treatment." Similarly, if a treatment plan is commenced on the basis of a reasonable medical judgment that there is a good chance that it will be effective, but due to a lack of success, unfavorable complications, or other factors, it becomes the treating physician's reasonable medical judgment that further treatment in accord with the prospective treatment plan, or alternative treatment, would be futile, then the failure to provide that treatment would not constitute a "withholding of medically indicated treatment." This analysis does not divert from the reasonable medical judgment standard of the statutory definition; it simply makes clear the Department's interpretation that the failure to evaluate the potential effectiveness of a treatment plan as a whole would be inconsistent with the legislative intent.

Thus, the Department interprets the term "treatment" to include (but not be limited to) multiple medical treatments and/or surgical procedures over a period of time that are designed to ameliorate or correct a life-threatening condition or conditions.

5. *The term "merely prolong dying."*

Clause (b)(3)(v) of the proposed rule proposed a definition of the term "merely prolong dying," which appears in the statutory definition. The proposed rule's provision stated that this term "refers to situations where death is imminent and treatment will do no more than postpone the act of dying."

Many commenters argued that the incorporation of the word "imminent," and its connotation of immediacy, appeared to deviate from the Congressional intent, as developed in the course of the lengthy legislative negotiations, that reasonable medical judgments can and do result in nontreatment decisions regarding some conditions for which treatment will do no more than temporarily postpone a death that will occur in the near future, but not necessarily within days. The six principal sponsors of the compromise amendment also strongly urged deletion of the word "imminent."

The Department's use of the term "imminent" in the proposed rule was not intended to convey a meaning not fully consonant with the statute. Rather, the Department intended that the word "imminent" would be applied in the context of the condition involved, and in such a context, it would not be understood to specify a particular number of days. As noted in the preamble to the proposed rule, this clarification was proposed to make clear that the "merely prolong dying" clause of the statutory definition would not be applicable to situations where treatment will not totally correct a medical condition but will give a patient many years of life. The Department continues to hold to this view.

To eliminate the type of misunderstanding evidenced in the comments, and to assure consistency with the statutory definition, the word "imminent" is not being adopted for purposes of these interpretative guidelines.

The Department interprets the term "merely prolong dying" as referring to situations where the prognosis is for death and, in the treating physician's (or physicians') reasonable medical judgment, further or alternative treatment would not alter the prognosis in an extension of time that would not render the treatment futile.

Thus, the Department continues to interpret Congressional intent as not permitting the "merely prolong dying" provision to apply where many years of life will result from the provision of treatment, or where the prognosis is not for death in the near future, but rather the more distant future. The Department also wants to make clear it does not intend the connotations many commenters associated with the word "imminent." In addition, contrary to the impression some commenters appeared to have regarding the proposed rule, the Department's interpretation is that reasonable medical judgments will be formed on the basis of knowledge about the condition(s) involved, the degree of inevitability of death, the probable effect of any potential treatments, the projected time period within which death will probably occur, and other pertinent factors.

6. *The term "not be effective in ameliorating or correcting all of the infant's life threatening conditions" in the context of a future life-threatening condition.*

Clause (b)(3)(vi) of the proposed rule proposed a definition of the term "not be effective in ameliorating or correcting all the infant's life-threatening conditions" used in the statutory definition of "withholding of medically indicated treatment."

The basic point made by the use of this term in the statutory definition was explained in the Conference Committee Report:

Under the definition, if a disabled infant suffers from more than one life-threatening condition and, in the treating physician's or physicians' reasonable medical judgment, there is no effective treatment for one of those conditions, then the infant is not covered by the terms of the amendment (except with respect to appropriate nutrition, hydration, and medication) concerning the withholding of medically indicated treatment. H. Conf. Rep. No. 1038, 98th Cong., 2d Sess. 41 (1980).

This clause of the proposed rule dealt with the application of this concept in two contexts: first, when the nontreatable condition will not become life-threatening in the near future, and second, when humaneness makes palliative treatment medically indicated.

With respect to the context of a future life-threatening condition, it is the Department's interpretation that the term "not be effective in ameliorating or correcting all of the infant's life-threatening conditions" does not permit the withholding of treatment on the grounds that one or more of the infant's life-threatening conditions, although not life-threatening in the near future, will become life-threatening in the more distant future.

This clarification can be restated in the terms of the Conference Committee Report excerpt, quoted just above, with the italicized words indicating the clarification, as follows: Under the definition, if a disabled infant suffers from more than one life-threatening condition, and in the treating physician's or physicians' reasonable medical judgment, there is no effective treatment for one of these conditions *that threatens the life of the infant in the near future,* then the infant is not covered by the terms of the amendment (except with respect to appropriate nutrition, hydration, and medication) concerning the withholding of medically indicated treatment; *but if the nontreatable condition will not become life-threatening until the more distant future, the infant is covered by the terms of the amendment.*

Thus, this interpretative guideline is simply a corollary to the Department's interpretation of "merely prolong dying," stated above, and is based on the same understanding of Congressional intent, indicated above, that if a condition will not become life-threatening until the more distant future, it should not be the basis for withholding treatment.

Also for the same reasons explained above, the word "imminent" that appeared in the proposed definition is not adopted for purposes of this interpretative guideline. The Department makes no effort to draw an exact line to separate "near future" from "more distant future." As noted above in connection with the term "merely prolong dying," the statutory definition provides that it is for reasonable medical judgment, applied to the specific condition and circumstances involved, to determine whether the prognosis of death, because of its nearness in time, is such that treatment would not be medically indicated.

7. *The term "not be effective in ameliorating or correcting all life-threatening conditions" in the context of palliative treatment.*

Clause (b)(3)(iv)(B) of the proposed rule proposed to define the term "not be effective in ameliorating or correcting all life-threatening conditions" in the context where the issue is not life-saving treatment, but rather palliative treatment to make a condition more tolerable. An example of this situation is where an infant has more than one life-threatening condition, at least one of which is not treatable and will cause death in the near future. Palliative treatment is available, however, that will, in the treating physician's reasonable medical judgment, relieve severe pain associated with one of the conditions. If it is the treating physician's reasonable medical judgment that this palliative treatment will ameliorate the infant's *overall* condition, taking all individual conditions into account, even though it would not ameliorate or correct *each* conditon, then this palliative treatment is medically indicated. Simply put, in the context of ameliorative treatment that will make a condition more tolerable, the term "not be effective in ameliorating or correcting *all* life-threatening conditions" should not be construed as meaning *each and every* conditon, but rather as referring to the infant's *overall* condition.

HHS believes Congress did not intend to exclude humane treatment of this kind from the scope of "medically indicated treatment." The Conference Committee Report specifically recognized that "it is appropriate for a physician, in the exercise of reasonable medical judgment, to consider that factor (humaneness) in selecting among effective treatments," H. Conf. Rep. No. 1038, 98th Cong., 2d Sess. 41 (1984). In addition, the articulation in the statutory definition of circumstances in which treatment need not be provided specifically states that "appropriate nutrition, hydration, and medication" must nonetheless be provided. The inclusion in this proviso of medication, one [but not the only] potential palliative treatment to relieve severe pain, corroborates the Department's interpretation that such palliative treatment that will ameliorate the infant's overall condition, and that in the exercise of reasonable medical judgment is humane and medically indicated, was not intended by Congress to be outside the scope of the statutory definition.

Thus, it is the Department's interpretation that the term "not be effective in ameliorating or correcting all of the infant's life-threatening conditions" does not permit the withholding of ameliorative treatment that, in the treating physician's or physicians' reasonable medical judgment, will make a condition more tolerable, such as providing palliative treatment to relieve severe pain, even if the overall prognosis, taking all conditions into account, is that the infant will not survive.

A number of commenters expressed concerns about some of the examples contained in the preamble of the proposed rule that discussed the proposed definition relating to this point, and stated that, depending on medical complications, exact prognosis, relationships to other conditions, and other factors, the treatment suggested in the examples might not necessarily be the treatment that reasonable medical judgment would decide would be most likely to be effective. In response to these comments, specific diagnostic examples have not been included in this discussion, and this interpretative guideline makes clear that the "reasonable medical judgment" standard applies on this point as well.

Other commenters argued that an interpretative guideline on this point is unnecessary because reasonable medical judgment would commonly provide ameliorative or palliative treatment in the circumstances described. The Department agrees that such treatment is common in the exercise of reasonable medical judgment, but believes it useful, for the reasons stated, to provide this interpretative guidance.

8. *The term "virtually futile."*

Clause (b)(3)(vii) of the proposed rule proposed a definition of the term "virtually futile" contained in the statutory definition. The context of this term in the statutory definition is:

[T]he term "withholding of medically indicated treatement" * * * does not include the failure to provide treatment (other than appropriate nutrition, hydration, or medication) to an infant when, in the

treating physician's or physicians' reasonable medical judgment, * * *
the provision of such treatment would be *virtually futile* in terms of
the survival of the infant and the treatment itself under such circumstances would be inhumane. Section 3(3)(C) of the Act [emphasis
supplied].

The Department interprets the term "virtually futile" to mean that
the treatment is highly unlikely to prevent death in the near future.

This interpretation is similar to those offered in connection with
"merely prolong dying" and "not be effective in ameliorating or correcting all life-threatening condtions" in the context of a future life-
threatening condition, with the addition of a characterization of likelihood that corresponds to the statutory word "virtually." For the
reasons explained in the discussion of "merely prolong dying," the
word "imminent" that was used in the proposed rule has not been
adopted for purposes of this interpretative guideline.

Some commenters expressed concern regarding the words "highly
unlikely," on the grounds that such certitude is often medically impossible. Other commenters urged that a distinction should be made
between generally utilized treatments and experimental treatments.
The Department does not believe any special clarifications are needed
to respond to these comments. The basic standard of reasonable medical judgment applies to the term "virtually futile." The Department's
interpretation does not suggest an impossible or unrealistic standard of
certitude for any medical judgment. Rather, the standard adopted in
the law is that there be a "reasonable medical judgment." Similarly,
reasonable medical judgment is the standard for evaluating potential
treatment possibilities on the basis of the actual circumstances of the
case. HHS does not believe it would be helpful to try to establish
distinctions based on characterizations of the degree of general usage,
extent of validated efficacy data, or other similar factors. The factors
considered in the exercise of reasonable medical judgment, including
any factors relating to human subjects experimentation standards, are
not disturbed.

9. *The term "the treatment itself under such circumstances would be
inhumane."*

Clause (b)(3)(viii) of the proposed rule proposed a definition of
the term "the treatment itself under such circumstances would be
inhumane," that appears in the statutory definition. The context of
this term in the statutory definition is that it is not a "withholding of
medically indicated treatment" to withhold treatment (other than appropriate nutrition, hydration, or medication) when, in the treating
physician's reasonable medical judgment, "the provision of such treatment would be virtually futile in terms of the survival of the infant

and the treatment itself under such circumstances would be inhumane." § 3(3)(C) of the Act.

The Department interprets the term "the treatment itself under such circumstances would be inhumane" to mean the treatment itself involves significant medical contraindications and/or significant pain and suffering for the infant that clearly outweigh the very slight potential benefit of the treatment for an infant highly unlikely to survive. (The Department further notes that the use of the term "inhumane" in this context is not intended to suggest that consideration of the humaneness of a particular treatment is not legitimate in any other context; rather, it is recognized that it is appropriate for a physician, in the exercise of reasonable medical judgment, to consider that factor in selecting among effective treatments.)

Other clauses of the statutory definition focus on the expected *result* of the possible treatment. This provision of the statutory definition adds a consideration relating to the *process* of possible treatment. It recognizes that in the exercise of reasonable medical judgment, there are situations where, although there is some slight chance that the treatment will be beneficial to the patient (the potential treatment is considered *virtually* futile, rather than futile), the potential benefit is so outweighed by negative factors relating to the process of the treatment itself that, under the circumstances, it would be inhumane to subject the patient to the treatment.

The Department's interpretation is designed to suggest the factors that should be taken into account in this difficult balance. A number of commenters argued that the interpretation should permit, as part of the evaluation of whether treatment would be inhumane, consideration of the infant's future "quality of life."

The Department strongly believes such an interpretation would be inconsistent with the statute. The statute specifies that the provision applies only where the treatment would be "virtually futile in the terms of the survival of the infant," and the "treatment *itself* under such circumstances would be inhumane." [Emphasis supplied.] The balance is clearly to be between the very slight chance that treatment will allow the infant to survive and the negative factors relating to the process of the treatment. These are the circumstances under which reasonable medical judgment could decide that the treatment itself would be inhumane.

Some commenters expressed concern about the use of terms such as "clearly outweigh" in the description of this balance on the grounds that such precision is impractical. Other commenters argued that this interpretation could be construed to mandate useless and painful treatment. The Department believes there is no basis for these worries because "reasonable medical judgment" is the governing standard. The interpretative guideline suggests nothing other than application of this standard. What the guideline does is set forth the Department's interpretation that the statute directs the reasonable medical judgment to considerations relating to the slight chance of survival and the negative factors regarding the process of treatment and to the balance between them that would support a conclusion that the treatment itself would be inhumane.

Other commenters suggested adoption of a statement contained in the Conference Committee Report that makes clear that the use of the term "inhumane" in the statute was not intended to suggest that consideration of the humaneness of a particular treatment is not legitimate in any other context. The Department has adopted this statement as part of its interpretative guideline.

10. *Other terms.*

Some comments suggested that the Department clarify other terms used in the statutory definition of "withholding of medically-indicated treatment," such as the term "appropriate nutrition, hydration or medication" in the context of treatment that may not be withheld, notwithstanding the existence of one of the circumstances under which the failure to provide treatment is not a "withholding of medically indicated treatment." Some commenters stated, for example, that very potent pharmacologic agents, like other methods of medical intervention, can produce results accurately described as accomplishing no more than to merely prolong dying, or be futile in terms of the survival of the infant, or the like, and that, therefore, the Department should clarify that the proviso regarding "approporiate nutrition, hydration or medication" should not be construed entirely independently of the circumstances under which other treatment need not be provided.

The Department has not adopted an interpretative guideline on this point because it appears none is necessary. As noted above in the discussion of palliative treatment, the Department recognizes that there is no absolutely clear line between medication and treatment other than medication that would justify excluding the latter from the scope of palliative treatment that reasonable medical judgment would find medically indicated, notwithstanding a very poor prognosis.

Similarly, the Department recognizes that in some circumstances, certain pharmacologic agents, not medically indicated for palliative purposes, might, in the exercise of reasonable medical judgment, also not be indicated for the purpose of correcting or ameliorating any particular condition because they will, for example, merely prolong dying. However, the Department believes the word "appropriate" in this proviso of the statutory definition is adequate to permit the exercise of reasonable medical judgment in the scenario referred to by these commenters.

At the same time, it should be clearly recognized that the statute is completely unequivocal in requiring that all infants receive "appropriate nutrition, hydration, and medication," regardless of their condition or prognosis.

Dated: March 29, 1985.

Dorcas R. Hardy,
Assistant Secretary for Human Development Services.
Approved: April 5, 1985.

Margaret M. Heckler,
Secretary.

Severely Handicapped Children Further Reading

Duff, Raymond S. "On Deciding the Care of Severely Handicapped or Dying Persons: With Particular Reference to Infants." *Pediatrics* 57 (April 1976) 487–92.

Frankel, Lawrence S.; Damme, Catherine J.; and Van Eys, Jan. "Childhood Cancer and the Jehovah's Witness Fate." *Pediatrics* 60 (December 6, 1977), 916–.

Garland, Michael J. "Care of the Newborn: The Decision Not to Treat." *Perinatology/Neonatology* 1 (September–October 1977), 14ff.

Heymann, Philip B., and Holz, Sarah. "The Severely Defective Newborn: The Dilemma and the Decision Process." *Public Policy* 23 (Fall 1975), 381–418.

Jonsen, A. R., and Garland, Michael, eds. *Ethics of Newborn Intensive Care.* San Francisco and Berkeley: University of California School of Medicine and Institute of Governmental Studies, 1976.

Robertson, John A. "Involuntary Euthanasia of Defective Newborns: A Legal Analysis." *Stanford Law Review* 27 (January 1975), 213–67.

Shaw, Anthony; Randolf, Judson G.; and Manard, Barbara. "Ethical Issues in Pediatric Surgery: A Nationwide Survey of Pediatricians and Pediatric Surgeons." *Pediatrics* 60 (October 1977, 588–99).

Swinyard, Chester A., ed. *Decision Making and the Defective Newborn.* Springfield, Illinois.: Charles C. Thomas, publisher, 1977.

Veatch, Robert M. "The Technical Criteria Fallacy," *Hastings Center Report* 7 (August 1977), 15–16.

Weber, Leonard J. *Who Shall Live? The Dilemma of Severely Handicapped Children and Its Meaning for Other Moral Questions.* New York: Paulist Press 1976.

PART THREE

DEATH AND DYING

Frank J. Veith
Hans Jonas
William J. Curran
Gilbert Meilaender
Thomas A. Shannon
Steven Neu
Carl M. Kjellstrand

9 *Brain Death*

Frank J. Veith and others

Many debates on brain death have occurred over the past decade. Some debates were brought about by the fact of the use of medical technology which would allow circulation and respiration to be artificially maintained even though the person's brain is destroyed; other debates have focused around the utility of a brain death definition so that organs could be harvested for transplantation more readily; also a revised definition of brain death would ease many of the dilemmas associated with turning off life support systems. This article summarizes information on clinical and laboratory criteria for brain death; argues that the concept of brain death is in accord with philosophy and three major western religions; shows the need for legislation that would allow the use of brain death as a criterion of death; and reviews the present status of judicial and statutory law relating to the determination of death. The authors provide a variety of perspectives which help us come to terms with many of the critical issues in accepting or rejecting the use of a particular definition of brain death as a useful criterion for determining death.

Frank J. Veith, M.D., is with the Department of Surgery Montefiore Hospital, New York

Brain Death is a term commonly used to describe a condition in which the brain is completely destroyed and in which cessation of function of all other organs is imminent and inevitable. The concept of brain death is important to consider, since advances in medical technology have resulted in the artificial prolongation of the overall process of dying. In the past, cessation of heartbeat and spontaneous respiration always produced prompt death of the brain, and, similarly, destruction of the brain resulted in prompt cessation of respiration and circulation. In this context, it was reasonable that absence of pulse and respiration became the traditional criteria for pronouncement of death. Recently, however, technological advances have made it possible to sustain brain function in the absence of spontaneous respiratory and cardiac function, so that the death of a person can no longer be equated with the loss of these latter two natural vital functions. Furthermore, it is now possible that a person's brain may be completely destroyed even though his circulation and respiration are being artificially maintained by mechanical devices.

I. A Status Report of Medical and Ethical Considerations

A number of authors have argued persuasively that a person whose brain is totally destroyed is in fact dead,[1-4] and this premise has gained considerable acceptance throughout the world from the public and from professionals in various relevant fields. Accordingly, the pronouncement of death on the basis of irreversible cessation of all brain function has become common. Nevertheless, this use of the concept of brain death has caused considerable controversy among physicians, lawyers, legislators, philosophers, and theologians. This controversy is founded partly on the failure of some to accept the concept that death may be pronounced on brain-related criteria,[5] and partly on the contention that statutory recognition of such pronouncements is neither necessary nor desirable.[6,7] Groups subscribing to either one or both of these positions actively oppose passage of statutory definitions of death and render enactment of such legislation difficult in the 32 states presently without such laws.

The purposes of this communication are to contribute to a resolution of the controversy and thereby to facilitate passage of statutes recognizing brain death by accomplishing several objectives. First, it will summarize information that establishes the ability to determine the state of complete destruction of the brain with certainty on the basis of available clinical and laboratory criteria. Second, it will demonstrate that total destruction of the brain constitutes a determinant of death that is not in conflict with sound secular philosophic considerations, Orthodox Judaic law, traditional Catholic ethics, or the mainstream of Protestant theology. Third, it will document the need for legislative recognition that death may be pronounced on the basis of complete and irreversible destruction of the brain. And fourth, it will review the present status of judicial and statutory law relating to the determination of death in the United States (in a later issue).

Validity of Criteria for Determining Complete Destruction of the Brain

Any ethical or legal considerations concerning pronouncements of death on a neurologic basis must be founded on the certainty that a person who meets the clinical and laboratory criteria has had actual complete destruction of the brain. In 1968, guidelines were formulated by an Ad Hoc Committee of the Harvard Medical School to permit the determination of irreversible coma.[8] These Harvard criteria require that neurologic examinations disclose unreceptivity, unresponsiveness, absence of spontaneous movements and breathing, absent reflexes, fixed dilated pupils, and persistence of all these findings over a 24-hour period in the absence of intoxicants or hypothermia. A persistently isoelectric EEG over the same period is also required to confirm the clinical examination. Since 1968, the validity of these widely used criteria has been established in several ways.

These validations include the substantial morphologic evidence that, when the criteria have been fulfilled, there is widespread destruction of the brain. Richardson has found that the brains of 128 patients meeting the Harvard criteria showed extensive destructive changes (oral communication, March 1976).[9] In a larger series of autopsy studies, however, the exact nature and distribution of these fatal morphologic lesions in the brain were also shown to be dependent on the etiology and on the interval between fulfillment of the Harvard criteria and pathologic examination.[10] The latter observation is consistent with the well-known finding in other organs that time must often elapse before morphologic evidence of cellular destruction can be detected.

In addition, patients who fulfill the Harvard criteria have been shown by isotopic techniques to have no significant intracranial blood flow,[11] and absent intracranial blood flow over a 10- to 15-minute interval is uniformly associated with subsequent necrosis and liquefaction of the brain.[12] The latter finding is based on autopsy studies from several Scandinavian hospitals of more than 120 patients who had nonvisualization of intracranial arteries after cerebral angiography with contrast injections repeated over a 10- to 15-minute interval. In related studies from several centers, clinical and EEG evidence of complete brain destruction was almost always associated with angiographic evidence of cessation of intracranial blood flow.[13-16]

Another validation of the Harvard criteria derives from cooperative studies of the value of EEG and neurologic examination in the determination of complete brain destruction.[17,18] In these studies, members of the American Electroencephalographic Society and of EEG societies in Europe were questioned. Of the 2,642 cases under study, there was no instance of recovery in a patient who fulfilled the Harvard criteria. Furthermore, since 1970, there have been no adequately documented examples in which the Harvard criteria could be considered invalid.[19] Moreover, many authorities presently consider these criteria too strict in at least two regards.[19-24] First, it has been shown that spinal reflexes including withdrawal movements may persist after complete destruction of the brain. Second, it is believed that certain determination that the brain is totally destroyed can be made even when the period of clinical and EEG evidence of absent brain function is reduced to less than 24 hours. The latter is consistent with the opinion that methods for measuring intracranial blood flow will allow a sure determination of complete brain destruction to be made with periods of observation less than the 24 hours proposed in the original Harvard criteria.[11-16,22] In this regard, it should be noted that the immature brain is more resistant to all forms of insult. Therefore, altered, less restrictive criteria for determining total brain destruction in patients under 14 years of age may differ from those in adults.

Further support for the use of less restrictive criteria is provided by the recently completed Collaborative Study on Cerebral Survival, which was based on an analysis of 503 unresponsive apneic patients. From this experience it was concluded that, if all appropriate diagnostic and therapeutic procedures had been performed to exclude reversible conditions, brain destruction was always present if certain criteria were observed for at least 30 minutes six hours or more after the cerebral insult had occurred. The specified criteria were unresponsivity, apnea, dilated pupils and absent cephalic reflexes, electrocerebral (EEG) silence, and confirmation of absent cerebral blood flow by angiography, isotopic bolus techniques, or echo encephalography.[23,25,26] The confirmatory test for absent cerebral blood flow was not deemed necessary in cases where the obvious etiologic factor was known to be a nontreatable condition, such as massive brain trauma.

Although some groups have indicated that EEG is not required to determine that brain death has occurred,[21,27] and although many neurologists and neurosurgeons would agree that brain death can safely be pronounced in the absence of electrocerebral silence in the occasional patient, the recommendation that EEG criteria be met before brain death is pronounced is probably best for general usage.[22-25,28] This recommendation appears advisable at present in light of a report that a patient who ultimately recovered had met the clinical criteria of brain death but never had electrocerebral silence,[28] and in view of the current trend toward increasingly frequent medical malpractice suits.

A final validation of the criteria for measuring total destruction of the brain has been an attempt on our part to explore purported anecdotal exceptions. In every instance where recovery of brain function was claimed, the criteria had not been fulfilled. Thus, the validity of the criteria must be considered to have been established with as much certainty as is possible in biology or medicine.

Philosophical and Religious Acceptability

It is one thing to know that we now possess the technical capacity to determine accurately that a human brain has been completely and irreversibly destroyed. It is quite another matter to make the social policy judgment that it is acceptable to use complete and irreversible destruction of the human brain as a basis for treating the person as a whole as if he or she were dead. We are convinced that society now has sufficient philosophical certainty, based on the main stands of secular philosophical thought and the major Western religious traditions, to use destruction of the brain as an indicator that the person has died.

It has been suggested that *one* reason for changing society's concept of death to one oriented to brain function is that it would provide desperately needed organs for transplantation and other useful medical purposes. However, the fact that someone would be useful to others if pronounced dead should not alone be a sufficient reason for considering that person dead and cannot be the sole basis for changing to the use of brain-oriented criteria. Rather, there must be sound reasons independent of that if society is going to alter its definition of death.

The principal reason for deciding that a person is dead should be based on a fundamental understanding of the nature of man. Our present conceptualization of man almost reflexly draws a distinction between a person whose organs are under nervous system influence and the remnant of a person or his corpse in which residual and nonhomeostatic functions may or may not have completely ceased. Without a brain, the body becomes the convenient medium in which the energy-requiring states of organs run down and the organs decay. These residual activities do not confer an iota of humanity or personality. Thus, in the circumstance of brain death, neither a human being nor a person any longer exists.

Although all members of society will not be able to agree precisely on an acceptable formulation of man's nature, fortunately all that is necessary to establish a public policy is agreement on some widely acceptable, general statements about the nature of man. Almost all segments of society will agree that some capacity to think, to perceive, to respond, and to regulate and integrate bodily functions is essential to human nature. Thus, if none of these brain functions are present and will ever return, it is no longer appropriate to consider a person as a whole as being alive.

If there were no offense, no moral or social costs in treating dead persons as if they were alive, then the safer course would be to continue to do so. Quite clearly, however, this is not the case. In addition to reflecting an inadequate understanding of the nature of man, it is an affront to the individual person or that person's memory to treat a human being who has irreversibly lost all brain function as if he were alive. It confuses the person with his corpse and is morally wrong.

Furthermore, maintenance of a dead person on life support systems for no reason is an irresponsible squandering of our economic and social resources. Such a practice places an unnecessary financial burden on society and an additional emotional burden on the person's family and is thereby also morally wrong. Thus, even without consideration of the use of the body or its organs for transplantation or other altruistic purposes, there are sound moral and social reasons for treating a body that has lost significant thinking, perceiving, responding, regulating, and integrating capacities as dead. Of course, it is a waste of human resources and a further wrong to continue treating a corpse as if it were alive when such treatment may deprive other living persons of needed organs. Thus, from a moral and ethical perspective, persons who have lost all brain function and who are certainly dead should be treated accordingly. Before adopting this conclusion as a public policy, however, it is important to examine how such a position accords with the major religious traditions of our society.

The Orthodox Jewish response to the premise that death may be pronounced on brain-related criteria is, like much of the moral conscience of Western civilization, based on biblical and talmudic ethical imperatives. According to these, it is axiomatic that human life is of infinite worth. A corollary of this is that a fleeting moment of life is of inestimable worth because a piece of infinity is also infinite. The taking or shortening of a human life is, therefore, ethically wrong, and premature termination of life or euthanasia is no less murder for the good intentions that were the motivation for the immoral act.

The indices of life are many. Which of them can be viewed, in ethical or religious terms, as the definition or sine qua non of the living state rather than a mere confirmation that the patient is still living? It is first important to point out that absent heartbeat or pulse was *not* considered a significant factor in ascertaining death in any early religious sources.[30] Furthermore, the scientific fact that cellular death does not occur at the same time as the death of the human being is well recognized in the earliest biblical sources. The twitching of a lizard's amputated tail or the death throes of a decapitated man were never considered residual life but simple manifestations of cellular life that continued after death of the entire organism had occurred.[31] In the situation of decapitation, death can be defined or determined by the decapitated state itself as recognized in the Talmud and the Code of Laws.[31-33] Complete destruction of the brain, which includes loss of all integrative, regulatory, and other functions of the brain, can be considered physiological decapitation and thus a determinant per se of death of the person.

Loss of the ability to breathe spontaneously is a crucial criterion for determining whether complete destruction of the brain has occurred. Earliest biblical sources recognized the ability to breathe independently as a prime index of life.[30,34] The biblical verse in Genesis records: "And the Lord had fashioned man of dust of the earth and instilled in his nostrils the breath of life and man became a living creature."[34] Spontaneous respiration is thus an indicator of the living state. However, it cannot be considered its definition, since a respirator patient whose sole defect is paralysis of the motor neurons to the muscles of respiration due to neurologic disease is surely fully alive despite his inability to breathe spontaneously. Therefore, to define death in biblical terms, loss of respiration must be combined with other more obvious evidence of the nonliving state. Such evidence would be provided by the clinical and laboratory criteria that allow a physician to determine that complete and irreversible destruction of the brain or physiological decapitation has occurred.

The higher integrative functions of the brain are carried out by portions of the brain other than the brainstem. Irreversible loss of these functions, signifying destruction of corresponding parts of the brain, does not alone constitute a determinant of death in biblical terms. Coincident loss of vegetative functions, represented by loss of spontaneous respiration and indicating destruction of the brainstem, is also a requisite. Thus, destruction of the entire brain or brain death, and only that, is consonant with biblical pronouncements on what constitutes an acceptable definition of death, i.e. a patient who has all the appearances of lifelessness and who is no longer breathing spontaneously. Patients with irreversible total destruction of the brain fulfill this definition even if heart action and circulation are artificially maintained. This definition is also fulfilled in patients who die with or from irreversible cessation of heart action, because this results in a failure to perfuse the brain, which produces total brain destruction. Thus, cessation of heart action is a cause of death rather than a component of its definition. In the light of these considerations, the Harvard criteria or other neurologic criteria for determining death can be viewed as the scientific expression of those observations that, until recently, were the actual way a patient was known to be dead.

The tumult that has greeted the suggestion that brain death be given legal recognition is partly the reaction of an uninformed public who envisions the possibility that a man who can move, feel, and think or can possibly recover these functions could be declared dead.

The realization that brain death is only professional jargon to describe a patient who exhibits a permanent loss of signs of life, such as spontaneous movement and responsivity, and has permanently lost the ability to breathe spontaneously would facilitate society's acceptance of the concept of brain death and would help to gain public support for legislation recognizing that death may be pronounced on the basis of total and irreversible destruction of the brain.

Since the distinction between cellular and organismal death is valid, once death of the person has occurred and can be determined, there is no biblical obligation to maintain treatment or artificial support of the corpse. Thus, according to M. Feinstein, there is no religious imperative to continue to use a respirator to inflate and deflate the lungs and thus maintain the cellular viability of other organs in an otherwise dead patient (written communication, May 5, 1976).

This Orthodox Jewish position is not alone among major Western religious traditions in supporting a concept of death based on irreversible loss of brain function. In the Roman Catholic Church, there is no definitive, authoritative pronouncement, but Catholic theologians interested in moral questions associated with the definition of death issue have generally accepted a concept of death based on brain function. The traditional Roman Catholic understanding of the moment of real death has been based on the time of departure of the soul from the body. Since this separation is not an observable phenomenon, it must be related to physically measurable signs defining apparent death. Because the only certain signs have been the appearance of rigor mortis and the beginning of bodily decomposition, it has been recognized that real death may not coincide with apparent death. Use of such signs as cessation of heartbeat and breathing places the moment of apparent death in greater proximity to the time of true theological death. For practical reasons, theologians have accepted these signs of apparent death as reasonably accurate indicators of irreversible cessation of all vital bodily functions adequate for allowing such processes as embalming and autopsy. When artificial life support systems are used to maintain heart and lung function and when the brain is irreversibly destroyed, there is also no reasonable hope of restoring vital bodily functions to a person. Accordingly, "it would seem that death is more certain under these conditions than it was at the [time of] cessation of spontaneous heart and lung function. If theologians were willing to accept the latter as signs of apparent death, they should be more willing to accept the irreversible cessation of brain function."[35]

A similar position has been reached by the Catholic theologian, Rev. Bernard Haring,[3] who after analysis of the theological arguments concludes, "I feel that the arguments for the equation of the total death of the person with brain death are fully valid." In the same vein, the prominent author on Roman Catholic interpretations of medical ethics, Charles J. McFadden, argues that "once the fact of brain death has been established, *the person is dead*, even though heart beat and respiration are continued by mechanical means."[36] These statements are consistent with the discourse of Pope Pius XII who, in discussing patients who are terminally unconscious, said

> one can refer to the usual concept of separation . . . of the soul from the body; but on the practical level, one needs to be mindful of the connotation of the terms "body" and "separation". . . . As to the pronouncement of death in certain particular cases, the answer cannot be inferred from religious and moral principles, and consequently, it is an aspect lying outside the competence of the Church.[37]

We understand the papal point to be that determination of the criteria for deciding the moment of death requires technical measures that can only be established by those with the appropriate medical expertise.

Among Protestant theologians, there are no consistent positions on questions of medical ethics including the definition of death. However, leading spokesmen of widely diverging traditions accept brain-related criteria for pronouncing death.[2,38-43] The body is an essential element of the person according to Christian theology; but, as many of these authors emphasize, mere cellular and organ system activity alone is not sufficient to treat a human body as if it were alive. Even more conservative thinkers such as Paul Ramsey accept the use of brain-oriented criteria for pronouncement of death. He recognizes proposals for updating the definition of death as, in reality,

> proposals for updating our procedures for determining that death has occurred, for rebutting the belief that machines or treatments are the patient, for withdrawing the notion that artificially sustained signs of life are in themselves signs of life, for telling when we should stop ventilating and circulating the blood of an unburied corpse because there are no longer any vital functions really alive or recoverable in the patient.[2]

Thus, the complete and permanent absence of any brain-related vital bodily function is recognized as death by Jewish, Roman Catholic, and Protestant scholars even if they may disagree among themselves on the precise theoretical foundations of this judgment.

II. A Status Report of Legal Considerations

Part I of this article established the scientific validity of current clinical and laboratory criteria for determining complete destruction of the brain or brain death. It also showed that total destruction of the brain constitutes a determinant of death, which is in accord with secular philosophy and the three major Western religions. In part II, legal issues that arise from use of brain-related criteria to pronounce death are considered.

Need For Statutory Recognition of Brain Death

The fact that physicians can recognize total and irreversible destruction of the brain on the basis of clinical and laboratory criteria is accepted and commonly utilized in many areas of the world. The need to make such pronouncements is based primarily on the requirement of society to respond appropriately to two recent advances in medical technology. The first is the hardware that can artificially maintain lung and heart action in the absence of spontaneous respiration and circulation. Although these devices may be lifesaving in many situations, their use in maintaining respiration and circulation in a human body that is dead by virtue of total destruction of the brain serves no useful purpose. In such instances it is reasonable to terminate these artificial support systems.

The second advance that requires pronouncement of death on brain-related criteria is cadaver organ transplantation. Most suitable donor organs come from patients who die from injury or disease of the brain. Only in such patients may the donor's circulation be artificially maintained after death so that needed organs can be removed with minimal ischemic damage. Since destruction of the brain is the cause of the donor's death, there is no reason not to remove these organs before cessation of the donor's artificially maintained circulation. This requires recognition that destruction of the brain is the basis for death of the donor and pronouncement of death on brain-related criteria.

Since the responsibility for pronouncing death resides with physicians, it has been suggested that no statute giving legal recognition to any particular criterion for determining death is necessary or desirable.[1] However, there is a potential dilemma in the absence of legal recognition of the medically accepted practice of pronouncing death on neurologic criteria. Physicians who pronounce death on this basis may be disputed in a judicial proceeding with the contention that death occurs only when spontaneous respiration and heartbeat cease. This contention could be based on the common law definition of death (to follow, under "Legal Status of Brain Death")[2] which is generally held applicable to jurisdictions without specific statutes. Without statutory or case law recognition of the use of brain-related criteria for pronouncing death, it is possible that a valid medical declaration of death could be considered illegal and lead to difficulty in the prosecution of a murderer or criminal or civil liability on the part of a physician or hospital. These possibilities have made many neurologists and neurosurgeons reluctant to pronounce death on brain-related criteria and have given rise to judicial actions in several locales. These cases have been a major factor leading to the passage, in many states, of statutes recognizing the use of brain-oriented criteria for pronouncing death.

Case law recognition of the legal validity of pronouncing death on brain-related criteria, although helpful, is an inadequate solution to the dilemma that arises from the potential discrepancy between medically accepted practice and legally accepted practice for two important reasons. First, case law is fluid and subject to appeal and change by subsequent judicial action. Second, court decisions to recognize the use of brain-related criteria for pronouncing death may relate to certain special circumstances, such as transplant organ donation. A statute giving general recognition to this concept for all purposes would avoid future inconsistencies under the law and would prevent repeated anguish-producing court cases. Such a law would allow a physician to terminate artificial respiratory support for a patient who is clearly dead by accepted and validated criteria. It would obviate the possibility that the physician, other health professionals, next of kin, guardians, and institutions might be held criminally or civilly liable for actions consistent with standards of current medical practice.

In addition, even if physicians agree that brain-related criteria should be used in death pronouncements, it is still an open question what the rest of society would choose to have as its public policy. Public policy can only be determined by some public act such as legislation. Thus, a statutory definition of death would serve as a vehicle to translate a generally accepted medical standard into a form that is accepted by most if not all members of society. As such, it will help to minimize some of the burdens placed on the family and physicians of the dead person by facilitating honest relationships and communication between them in many ways.

Until such public policy recognition by legislation has occurred, the family confronted with the loss of a loved one who is dead by virtue of brain-related criteria is forced to deal with the confusing and misleading assumption, supported by an out-of-date common law, that, while the heart beats, there is life and hope of recovery. Of all the reasons for establishing a statutory definition of death, the simplest and the most important is that it will help the family of the dead patient to appreciate the reality of his death, and to reassure them that the medical determination of death is valid. Such a law will also facilitate relief of the family from financial and emotional pressures and will enable them to confront death with more dignity and understanding.

In a similar way, the physician's onerous task of conveying to the family in such a situation that their loved one is in fact dead would be aided and supported by the passage of an up-to-date statutory definition of death. This would reflect a public policy that recognizes that when the brain is dead, the person as a whole is dead and there is neither life nor hope despite the mechanically supported respiration and heartbeat. The presence of such a statute will remove from the physician the fear of unjust litigation and thereby allow him to practice medicine in a manner consistent with present scientific knowledge and standards. It will allow him to do this openly after honest discussion with the patient's family, and it will permit him to cooperate in efforts to procure cadaver organs in optimal condition for transplantation into other patients.

A further advantage of having a statutory definition of death is that it would help to guarantee that the highest standards of medical science would be used to make this determination. The recent New Jersey Supreme Court decision[3] in the Karen Quinlan case underscores the need to assure the public that pronouncements of death will be based on standardized and thoroughly validated indices. Even though Ms. Quinlan did not fulfill the criteria of brain death, the court held that her parent acting as guardian might authorize cessation of life-sustaining treatment if a physician and a hospital "ethics committee" agreed there was no reasonable possibility of recovery to a cognitive, sapient state. Although this decision and the resulting discontinuation of respiratory support did not alter Ms. Quinlan's course because she was able to breathe spontaneously, there has been substantial confusion between the issues in this case and the debate about the definition of death. Such misunderstandings could result in less than optimal nonstandardized determinations of death. These would be prevented by the existence of a statute that mandates use of the best standards of current medical practice to pronounce death.

A statutory definition of death would also have other advantages from a legal point of view. It would provide a clear and precise definition within which legal rights and relationships after death could be determined. It would facilitate the prosecution of murderers and permit the organs of murder victims to be used as transplants without jeopardizing conviction of the murderer. Such a statute would provide for consistency under the law in various jurisdictions, and it would avoid reliance on jury systems to make medical and legal decisions that might be inconsistent with present scientific knowledge.

Many physicians have suggested that the specific criteria for pronouncing brain death should not be placed in a statutory form. This is a reasonable position, since there is always the possibility that the criteria might change. This would mean that the law would have to be changed prior to utilizing any new and improved criteria. This is obviously a good reason not to legislate *specific* neurologic criteria for pronouncing death. However, it is an inadequate reason for opposing a law that, while leaving the specific criteria flexible, recognizes that death may be pronounced when irreversible cessation of brain function occurs.

Legal Status of Brain Death

Until recently, the traditional legal definition of death has been consistent with the prevailing medical concept that death is determined by cessation of the vital functions of respiration and heartbeat. This is reflected in the common law definition of death as stated in *Black's Law Dictionary*[2]: "The cessation of life; the ceasing to exist; defined by physicians as a total stoppage of the circulation of the blood, and a cessation of the animal and vital functions consequent thereon, such as respiration, pulsation, etc." With the exception of several notable recent decisions, traditional case law has similarly concentrated on the cardiovascular and respiratory functions as prime determinants of the occurrence of death.

In *Smith vs Smith*,[4] the Supreme Court of Arkansas, in a case that turned on the issue of simultaneous death, adopted *Black's* definition of death verbatim. The court took judicial notice of the fact that "one breathing, though unconscious, is not dead." Similarly, in *Thomas vs Anderson*,[5] a California District Court of Appeals also cited *Black's* definition and stated that ". . . death occurs precisely when life ceases and does not occur until the heart stops beating and respiration ends. Death is not a continuous event and is an event that takes place at a precise time." Other jurisdictions have also relied on this definition.[6,7] In addition, other cases have upheld the premise that death has not occurred until cessation of heartbeat and respiration even in circumstances where the courts have noted complete destruction of the brain.[8-10]

In all the cases cited, the determination of death was dealt with as a question of fact for a jury to decide in connection with the demise of individuals for the purposes of construing and applying "simultaneous death" clauses in testimentary documents. The factual question of the time of death in these cases was judged on the basis of circumstantial evidence relating to the cessation of heartbeat and respiration. This evidence was provided by the testimony of lay persons rather than physicians. These cases, which constitute the leading precedents in this area, predated the landmark report of the Ad Hoc Committee of the Harvard Medical School to Examine the Definition of Brain Death,[11] which is now generally regarded as the first widely recognized index that current medical concepts about the definition of death were changing.

Emerging Case Law

In contrast with these traditional opinions, several recent cases have considered the issue of death in the light of expert testimony by physicians about the irreversible cessation of brain function and have often incorporated such testimony in jury charges. These cases give explicit or implicit legal recognition to a pronouncement of death based on a determination of irreversible cessation of brain function in accordance with the customary standards of medical practice. These legal actions were relevant because the medical determination of the timing and occurrence of death in these cases were based on brain-related criteria, and legal application of traditional criteria of death would have been inappropriate. Thus, judicial action fortunately kept the law apace of scientific developments.

The first such judicial action occurred in the Oregon case, *State vs Brown*,[12] in which the defendant had been convicted on a charge of second-degree murder. On appeal, he contended that the victim's death was caused by termination of life-support systems rather than by the cranial gunshot wound that he had inflicted. The court held that the defendant's contention was without merit on the basis of expert medical testimony that the gunshot wound with resultant brain damage was the cause of death.

One year later, the impact of current medical thinking on case law was clearly evident in a Virginia case, *Tucker vs Lower*.[13] In a wrongful death action, it was alleged that an individual was not dead at the time when his heart and kidneys were removed for purposes of transplantation. The court rejected a motion for a summary judgment in favor of the defendants on the grounds that the Court was bound by the common law definition of death until it was changed by the state legislature. However, after considerable debate, the court instructed the jury that it might properly consider, as a substitute for the traditional criteria for determining the time of death, "the time of complete and irreversible loss of all function of the brain; and, whether or not the aforesaid functions [respiration and circulation] were spontaneous or were being maintained artificially or mechanically." The jury then decided that the transplant surgeons were not guilty of causing a wrongful death. Whether or not this decision was based on the jury's acceptance of the brain death concept is not known. However, this case has been widely publicized as supporting the use of brain-related criteria for pronouncing death. Furthermore, in commenting on this case, one legal scholar points out that "the jury instructions represent an admission by the courts that the old legal definition of death needs modification in the light of advances in medical science. The new definition—'brain death'—which is gaining recognition, reflects the consensus of informed medical opinion."[14]

Similarly, in a widely publicized California case, *People vs Lyons,*[15] a victim had suffered a gunshot wound of the head and had been declared neurologically dead before a transplant team headed by Norman Shumway, MD, had removed his heart. The defendant pleaded not guilty to a charge of murder, contending that the death of the victim had been caused by the removal of his heart rather than by the gunshot wound inflicted by the defendant. On the basis of expert testimony, the jury was instructed as a matter of law that "the victim was legally dead before removal of the organs from his body." The court thereby removed from the jury its traditional task of having to determine the exact time of death. The brain death standard was explicitly accepted.

However, a contrasting ruling was made in the initial phase of another California criminal prosecution, emphasizing the inconsistency that can occur with case law. In this case the defendant, who had been driving on the wrong side of a freeway while intoxicated, had caused an accident that severely injured a 13-year-old girl. She was pronounced dead on brain-related criteria, and her heart was used as a transplant. On the basis of these facts, a municipal court judge at a preliminary hearing did not hold the defendant to answer to a manslaughter charge, apparently determining that the pronouncement of death on neurologic criteria and the subsequent removal of the heart created substantial doubt as to the proximate cause of death. The Court concluded that "the evidence is not certain as to the cause of death of Colenda Ward, certain enough to charge this defendant with manslaughter."[16] On a subsequent appeal by the district attorney, the Superior Court authorized the filing of a manslaughter charge and made reference to "unimpeached medical testimony," which conclusively established "that the [victim's] heart could not beat nor could she breathe without artificial support."[16] The defendant was convicted of both manslaughter and felony drunk driving but received a sentence of less than five months. In commenting on this result, the deputy district attorney observed, "I cannot escape the firm belief that the uncertain state of the case and statutory law on the subject of brain death was a substantial factor in the imposition of such a light sentence" (written communication from Steven T. Tucker, deputy district attorney, Sonoma County, Calif., May 19, 1977).

A rather novel approach to the legal question of when does death occur was taken in 1975 in New York,[17] where a court was requested to set forth, in an action for declaratory judgment, a legal definition of the terms "death" and "time of death" as used in the New York State Anatomical Gifts Act. The court was asked to include in such definition not only the common law criteria of cardiac and respiratory failure, but also the concept of "brain death." Following extensive uncontroverted testimony concerning brain death criteria, the court held that "death" as used in the Anatomical Gifts Act "implies a definition consistent with the generally accepted medical practice of doctors primarily concerned with effectuating the purposes of this statute." Having confined its decision legally recognizing brain-related criteria for pronouncing death to the Anatomical Gifts Act, the court concluded by urging the state legislature "to take affirmative action to provide a Statewide remedy for this problem."

These cases have been helpful in resolving particular controversies. However, they have probably had a greater impact by serving as a vehicle for increasing public awareness of the need for a statutory definition of death. In all but one instance in which litigation has arisen, legislation that recognizes the validity of brain death as a legally accepted standard for determining death has been enacted shortly thereafter. The single exception is New York where proposals are currently pending before the state legislature.

Legislation

At the present time, 18 states have enacted a statutory definition of death: Kansas, Maryland, Virginia, New Mexico, Alaska, California, Georgia, Michigan, Oregon, Illinois, Oklahoma, West Virginia, Tennessee, Louisiana, Iowa, Idaho, Montana, and North Carolina.[18,19] All 18 statutes recognize that death may be pronounced on the basis of irreversible cessation of brain function, and none describes in detail the specific criteria for determining brain death. However, the laws vary in certain major and minor ways. In general, they conform to one of three major types or patterns.

The first of these includes laws providing alternative definitions of death. Typical of this pattern is the first statute enacted in 1970 by Kansas:

A person will be considered medically and legally dead if, in the opinion of a physician, based on ordinary standards of medical practice, there is the absence of spontaneous respiratory and cardiac function and, because of the disease or condition which caused, directly or indirectly, these functions to cease, or because of the passage of time since these functions ceased, attempts at resuscitation are considered hopeless; and, in this event, death will have occurred at the time these functions ceased; or

A person will be considered medically and legally dead if, in the opinion of a physician, based on ordinary standards of medical practice, there is the absence of spontaneous brain function; and if based on ordinary standards of medical practice, during reasonable attempts to either maintain or restore spontaneous circulatory or respiratory function in the absence of aforesaid brain function, it appears that further attempts at resuscitation or supportive maintenance will not succeed, death will have occurred at the time when these conditions first coincide. Death is to be pronounced before artificial means of supporting respiratory and circulatory function are terminated and before any vital organ is removed for purposes of transplantation.

These alternative definitions of death are to be utilized for all purposes in this state, including the trials of civil and criminal cases, any laws to the contrary notwithstanding.

An identical statute was enacted by Maryland in 1972. In 1973, Virginia passed a similar law that differed only in that death on brain-related criteria can only be declared by two physicians, one of whom is a specialist in neurology, neurosurgery, or electroencephalography. The Virginia law also mandates that absence of spontaneous respiratory functions accompanies "absence of spontaneous brain functions." The New Mexico statute, passed in 1973, and the Alaska statute, passed in 1974, are similar to the Kansas law. The Oregon statute, enacted in 1975, is the simplest and clearest of the alternative definition type of law: "When a physician licensed to practice medicine acts to determine that a person is dead, he may make sure a determination if irreversible cessation of spontaneous respiration and circulatory function or irreversible cessation of spontaneous brain function exists."

All six of these alternative definition of death statutes suffer the disadvantage of providing two different definitions of death. The choice of which to use in a specific instance is left to the physician. The major flaw with this type of legislation is that it appears to be based on the misconception that there are two separate types of death. This is particularly unfortunate because it seems to relate to the need to establish a special definition of death for organ transplant donors. These laws could lend support to the fear that a prospective transplant organ donor would be considered dead at an earlier point in the dying process than an identical patient who was not a potential donor.

In addition, such laws suffer the legal disadvantage of possibly permitting a physician, either inadvertently or intentionally, to influence the outcome of a will. If, for example, a husband and wife are fatally injured in the same accident, survivorship and consequent inheritance may be determined by the physician's choice of which of the alternative criteria to use in the pronouncements of death.

The second major type of law was suggested by Capron and Kass to remedy this defect and to provide one definition of death that recognizes that death is a single phenomenon that can be determined by brain related criteria only in situations where artificial support of respiratory and circulatory functions is being maintained[20]:

> A person will be considered dead if in the announced opinion of a physician, based on ordinary standards of medical practice, he has experienced an irreversible cessation of spontaneous respiratory and circulatory functions. In the event that artificial means of support preclude a determination that these functions have ceased, a person will be considered dead if in the announced opinion of a physician based on ordinary practice, he has experienced an irreversible cessation of spontaneous brain functions. Death will have occurred at the time when the relevant functions ceased.

This model statute takes cognizance of the fact that the medical standards for pronouncing death may vary with circumstances. However, unlike the previous laws, it does not leave as an arbitrary decision for the physician the choice of which standard to apply, but defines under what circumstances the new or secondary brain-related criteria may be used. This bill avoids establishing a separate kind of death, brain death, and as pointed out by Capron and Kass provides "two standards gauged by different functions for measuring different manifestations of the same phenomenon. If cardiac and pulmonary functions have ceased, brain functions cannot continue; if there is no brain activity and respiration has to be maintained artificially, the same state [i.e. death] exists."[20] The Capron-Kass Bill, which clearly appears to be satisfactory if not ideal, was adopted by Michigan and West Virginia in 1975 and Louisiana in 1976. The latter law specifies that when organs are to be used as a transplant, an additional physician unassociated with the transplant team must also pronounce death. Iowa in 1976 and Montana in 1977 enacted laws based on the

Capron-Kass model with the additional requirement that brain death pronouncements must be made by two physicians.

The third major type of law follows the suggestion of the American Bar Association, which recognized the need for a standardized statutory definition of death that minimized the risk of confusion from misunderstandings of semantics, medical technology, and legal sophistication and that took into account recent developments in transplantation, supportive therapy, and resuscitation. The suggested law was developed by the Law and Medicine Committee of the American Bar Association in 1974 and approved by the House of Delegates of that organization in 1975:[21] "For all legal purposes, a human body with irreversible cessation of total brain function, according to usual and customary standards of medical practice, shall be considered dead." This Committee states[21] that the advantages of its simple, direct definition are that it (1) permits judicial determination of the ultimate fact of death, (2) permits medical determination of the evidentiary fact of death, (3) avoids religious determination of any facts, (4) avoids prescribing the medical criteria, (5) enhances changing medical criteria, (6) enhances local medical practice tests, (7) covers the three known tests (brain, beat, and breath deaths), (8) covers death as a process (medical preference), (9) covers death as a point in time (legal preference), (10) avoids passive euthanasia, (11) avoids active euthanasia, (12) covers current American and European medical practices, (13) covers both civil law and criminal law, (14) covers current American judicial decisions, and (15) avoids nonphysical sciences.

Some have objected that this simple model statute fails to recognize the still common practice of pronouncing death on the basis of cessation of heartbeat and respiration. However, in practice, death is only pronounced when the functions of circulation and respiration have ceased long enough to cause destruction of the brain and produce other signs of lifelessness. In these instances, cessation of circulation and respiration represents the specific criteria by which irreversible cessation of brain function or death is determined. Thus, this model statute recognizes traditional as well as brain-related criteria for determining death. It is, therefore, also satisfactory and has formed the basis for the California statute enacted in 1974, the Georgia statute enacted in 1975, and the Idaho statute passed in 1977. All three laws require that deaths pronounced on brain-related criteria be confirmed by a second physician. The Illinois statute, enacted in 1975, also resembles the American Bar Association's suggestion in its simplicity. It does not require concurrence of a second physician, although it has the flaw of restricting the use of brain-related criteria to instances involving the Uniform Anatomical Gift Act. It, therefore, has the disadvantage of implicitly establishing alternative types of death with special definition to be used for transplant organ donors. The Oklahoma law, enacted in 1975, also seems to be based on the American Bar Association model but is rendered confusing by the addition of a number of qualifying clauses and phrases mandating that it must also appear "that further attempts at resuscitation and supportive maintenance will not succeed." The Tennessee statute, enacted in 1976, avoids these flaws and complexities and follows exactly the recommendation of the American Bar Association.

Many factors underlie the variability between the statutes enacted in the different states and account for the difficulty in reaching agreement on what constitutes the wording of a single ideal statutory definition of death. Prominent among these factors is the present climate of public mistrust of the medical profession. This has prompted legislators to enact more complicated laws in an attempt to protect patients from erroneous or premature declarations of death.

Hopefully the present article, by summarizing the overwhelming evidence supporting the validity of brain death, will help to allay these concerns and facilitate drafting of simple, effective statutes defining death. Furthermore, by showing that pronouncements of death on brain-related criteria are in accord with secular philosophy and principles of the three major Western religions, it is hoped that the present article will help overcome opposition to legislation from those who previously failed to accept the brain death concept. And lastly, by documenting the compelling reasons to have a statutory definition of death, the present article will hopefully help to influence the American Medical Association and others, who have felt that legislation defining death is unnecessary, to adopt a supportive position, as several of the state medical societies have already done. Such support would greatly facilitate passage of appropriate statutes in the 32 states presently without them. This, in turn, would make the law in regard to brain death consistent with current medical practice throughout the entire United States.[22]

NOTES

Part I

    1. High D: Death: Its conceptual elusiveness. *Soundings* 55:438–458, 1972.

    2. Ramsey P: *The Patient as Person: Explorations in Medical Ethics.* New Haven, Conn, Yale University Press, 1970, pp. 101–112.

3. Haring B: *Medical Ethics.* Notre Dame, Ind, Fides Publishers Inc, 1973.

4. Geelhoed GW: Life and death: Who decides? *The Pharos,* January 1977, pp 7–12.

5. Jonas H: Against the stream: Comments on the definition and redefinition of death, in Jonas H (ed): *Philosophical Essays: From Ancient Creed to Technological Man.* Englewood Cliffs, NJ, Prentice Hall, 1974, pp 132–140.

6. Definition of death. *JAMA* 227:728, 1974.

7. Tobin CJ: Statement in behalf of the New York State Catholic Conference delivered at the public hearing related to death legislation held by the New York State Assembly Subcommittee on Health Care, Albany, New York, Nov 30, 1976. *Origins* 6:413–415, 1976.

8. A definition of irreversible coma, Report of the Ad Hoc Committee of the Harvard Medical School to Examine the Definition of Brain Death. *JAMA* 205:337–340, 1968.

9. Refinements in criteria for the determination of death: An appraisal, report by the Task Force on Death and Dying of the Institute of Society, Ethics and the Life Sciences. *JAMA* 221:48–53, 1972.

10. Walker AE, Diamond EL, Moseley J: The neuropathological findings in irreversible coma: A critique of the "respirator brain." *J Neuropathol Exp Neurol* 34:295–323, 1975.

11. Korein J, Braunstein P, Kricheff I, et al: Radioisotopic bolus technique as a test to detect circulatory deficit associated with cerebral death: 142 studies on 80 patients demonstrating the bedside use of an innocuous IV procedure as an adjunct in the diagnosis of cerebral death. *Circulation* 51:924–939, 1975.

12. Crafoord C: Cerebral death and the transplantation era. *Dis Chest* 55:141–145, 1969.

13. Heiskanen O: Cerebral circulatory arrest caused by acute increase of intracranial pressure: A clinical and roentgenological study of 25 cases. *Acta Neurol Scand* 40(suppl 7):1–57, 1964.

14. Bergquist E, Bergstrom K: Angiography in cerebral death. *Acta Radiol (Diagn)* 12:283–288, 1972.

15. Lofstedt S, von Reis G: Diminution or obstruction of blood flow in the internal carotid artery. *Opuscula Med* 4:345–360, 1959.

16. Greitz T, Gordon E, Kolmodin G, et al: Aortocranial and carotid angiography in determination of brain death. *Neuroradiology* 5:13–19, 1973.

17. Silverman D, Saunders MG, Schwab RS, et al: Cerebral death and the electroencephalogram, Report of the Ad Hoc Committee of the American Electroencephalographic Society on EEG Criteria for Determination of Cerebral Death. *JAMA* 209:1505–1510, 1969.

18. Silverman D, Masland RL, Saunders MG, et al: Irreversible coma associated with electrocerebral silence. *Neurology* 20:525–533, 1970.

19. Masland RL: When is a person dead? *Resident Staff Physician,* April 5, 1975, pp 49–52.

20. Korein J, Maccario M: On the diagnosis of cerebral death: A prospective study on 55 patients to define irreversible coma. *Clin Electroencephalogr* 2:178–199, 1971.

21. DeMere M, Alexander T, Auerbach A, et al: *Report on Definition of Death, From Law and Medicine Committee*. Chicago, American Bar Association, Feb 25, 1975.

22. This study was supported in part by US Public Health Service grants HL 16476 and HL 17417 and the Manning Foundation.

23. Walker AE: Cerebral death, in Tower DB (ed): *The Nervous System: The Clinical Neurosciences*. New York, Raven Press, 1975, vol 2, pp 75–87.

24. Ueki K, Takeuchi K, Katsurada K: Clinical study of brain death, presentation 286. Read before the Fifth International Congress of Neurologic Surgery, Tokyo, Oct 7–13, 1973.

25. Walker AE: The neurosurgeon's responsibility for organ procurement. *J Neurosurg* 44:1–2, 1976.

26. An appraisal of the criteria of cerebral death: A summary statement, A collaborative study. *JAMA* 237:982–986, 1977.

27. Diagnosis of brain death: Summary of Conference of Royal Colleges and Faculties of the United Kingdom. *Lancet* 2:1069–1970, 1976.

28. Molinari GF: Death: The definition: III. Criteria for death. *Encyclopedia of Bioethics*, to be published.

29. Bolton CF, Brown JD, Cholod E, et al: EEG and "brain life." *Lancet* 1:535, 1976.

30. Bab Talmud Tractate Yoma 85A.

31. Bab Talmud Tractate Chullin 21A and Mishnah Oholoth 1:6.

32. Maimonides: Tumath Meth 1:15.

33. Code of Laws: Who is considered as dead although yet living? Yoreh Deah:370:1.

34. Genesis 2:7.

35. Connery JR: Comment on the proposed act to amend the public health law of the State of New York in relation to the determination of the occurrence of death. Read before the New York State Legislature, 1975–1976 session, March 25, 1975.

36. McFadden CJ: *The Dignity of Life: Moral Values in a Changing Society*. Huntington, Ind, Our Sunday Visitor Inc, 1976, p 202.

37. Pius XII, Acta Apostolicae Sedia 45, November 1957, pp 1027–1033.

38. Nelson J: *Human Medicine: Ethical Perspective on New Medical Issues*. Minneapolis, Augsburg, 1973, pp 125–130.

39. Fletcher J: Our shameful waste of human tissue: An ethical problem for the living and the dead, in Cutler DR (ed): *Updating Life and Death: Essays in Ethics and Medicine*. Boston, Beacon Press, 1969, pp 1–30.

40. Fletcher J: New definitions of death. *Prism* 2:13ff, January 1974.

41. Vaux K: *Biomedical Ethics.* New York, Harper & Row, 1974, pp 102–110.

42. Smith H: *Ethics and the New Medicine.* Nashville, Tenn, Abingdon, 1970.

Part II

1. Definition of death. *JAMA* 227:728, 1974.

2. *Black's Law Dictionary,* ed 4. St Paul, West Publishing Co, 1968, p 488.

3. *In the matter of Karen Quinlan,* 355 A 2d 647, 1976.

4. *Smith vs Smith,* 229 Ark 579, 317 SW 2d 275, 1958.

5. *Thomas vs Anderson,* 211 P 2d 478, 1950.

6. *United Trust Co vs Pyke,* 427 P 2d 67, 1967.

7. *Schmidt vs Pierce,* 344 SW 2d 120, 1961.

8. *Vaegemast vs Hess,* 280 NW 641, 1938.

9. *Gray vs Sawyer,* 247 SW 2d 496, 1952.

10. *In Re Estate of Schmidt,* 67 Cal Reptr 847, 1968.

11. A definition of irreversible coma, Report of the Ad Hoc Committee of the Harvard Medical School to Examine the Definition of Brain Death. *JAMA* 205:337–340, 1968.

12. *State vs Brown,* 8 Oreg App 72, 1971.

13. *Tucker vs Lower,* No. 2381, Richmond Va. L & Eq Ct, May 23, 1972.

14. Kennedy I: The legal definition of death. *Medico-Legal Journal* 14:36–41, 1973.

15. *People vs Lyons,* 15 Crm L Rprt 2240, Cal Super Ct 1974.

16. *People vs Flores,* Cal Super Ct County, 7246-C, 1974, pp 1–2.

17. *New York City Health & Hosp Corp vs Sulsona,* 81 Misc 2d 1002, 1975.

18. State Laws: *Kan Stat Ann* § 77–202, Supp 1974; *Md Code Ann* § 32–364.3:1, Cum Suppl 1975; *New Mex State Ann* § 1–2–2.2, Supp 1973; *Alaska Stat* § 9.65.120, Supp 1974; *Va Code Ann* § 32–364.3:1, Supp 1975; *Cal Health and Safety Code Ann* § 7180–81, West Supp 1975; *Ill Ann Stat* Ch 3, § 552, Smith-Hurd Supp 1975; *Ga Code Ann* § 88–1715.1, 1975; *Mich Stat* PA 158, Laws 1975; *Ore Rev Stat* Ch 565, § 1, Laws 1975; Ch 91, Laws 1975, amending *Okla Stat Ann* tit 63, § 1–301 (g), 1971; *W Va Code Ann* § 16–19–1, Supp 1975; *Tenn Stat,* HB No. 1919 Ch 780, Laws 1976; *La Acts 1976,* No. 233, § 1; *Laws of 66th Iowa General Assembly,* Ch 1245, (1976 Senate File 85); Mont HB No. 371, Ch 228, Laws 1977; *1977 Idaho Session Laws,* No. 1197, Ch 30; *N Carol Laws 1977,* Ch 815, § 90–322.

19. Stuart FP: Progress in legal definition of brain death and consent to remove cadaver organs. *Surgery* 81:68–73, 1977.

20. Capron AM, Kass LR: A statutory definition of the standards for determining human death: An appraisal and a proposal. *U Penn L Rev* 121:87–118, 1972.

21. DeMere M, Alexander T, Auerbach A, et al: *Report on Definition of Death, From Law and Medicine Committee. Chicago, American Bar Association,* Feb 25, 1975.

22. This study was supported in part by US Public Health Service grants HL 16476 and HL 17417 and the Manning Foundation.

10 *The Right To Die*

HANS JONAS, PH.D

The introduction of technology into medicine has provided it with the ability to prolong the lives of individuals. Nonetheless, that ability has raised several problems that Jonas grapples with in this essay: suicide; aiding in suicide; the troublesome distinction between killing and letting die; and the right to die. Recognizing the legal rule that individuals have a right to refuse treatment, Jonas presses on to the more difficult moral dimensions of the problem and discusses issues of responsibility to one's family and society, problems surrounding a duty to force treatment on others, and the recognition of how to deal with people's autonomy in terms of informing them properly about their condition. Jonas pursues these issues by evaluating two different cases: a conscious, suffering patient who has terminal cancer, and an unconscious comatose patient. After drawing his conclusions on these cases, Jonas then concludes by evaluating the task of medicine in the light of these particular problems

Hans Jonas, Ph.D., is a member of the Graduate Faculty of The New School of Social Research

In spite of the almost commonplace ring which the title of this article has acquired in the course of recent public debate, one's first reaction should still be wonder. What an odd combination of words! How strange that we should nowadays speak of a right to *die*, when throughout the ages all talk about rights has been predicated on the most fundamental of all rights—the right to *live*. Indeed, every other right ever argued, claimed, granted, or denied can be viewed as an extension of this primary right, since every particular right concerns the exercise of some faculty of life, the access to some necessity of life, the satisfaction of some aspiration of life.

Life itself exists not by right but by natural fiat: my being alive as a sheer fact whose sole natural endorsement is its innate powers to preserve itself. But among men the fact, once there, needs the sanction of a right, because to live means to make demands on the environment and is thus conditional on being accommodated by that environment. Insofar as the environment is human, and the accommodation it accords has a voluntary element in it, such inclusive accommodation underlying all communal life amounts to an implicit granting by the many of the individual's *right* to live and his granting the same to all others. Every further right, equal or not, in natural or positive law, derives from this cardinal one and from the mutual recognition of it by its claimants. Justly, therefore, is "life" named first among the inalienable rights in the Declaration of Independence. And surely, mankind has had an arduous task, and still has, with discovering, defining, debating, obtaining, and protecting the various rights that enlarge upon the right to live.

How exceedingly odd then that we should lately find ourselves engrossed in the question of a right to die! All the more odd, since rights are espoused to secure a blessing, and death is counted as a curse or at best something to which one must be resigned. And most odd when we reflect that with death we are not making a demand on the world, where a question of right might arise, but on the contrary are quitting every possible demand. So how can the very idea of "right" here apply?

But what if my dying or not dying were to some extent in the area of choice—mine or others'? And what if not only a right but also a duty for me to live could be construed? And for others, that is, "society," not only a duty toward my right to live, but also a right to hold me to my duty to live, that is, to prevent me from dying sooner than I must, even if I so will? What, in short, if the whole syndrome of dying becomes amenable to control, and mine is arguably not the sole voice to be heard in exercising that control? Then a "right to die" does become an issue. It has in fact always been a moral and religious issue in the matter of suicide, where the element of choice is most clearly present; and there, it is also a legal issue in many systems of law that mandate or authorize various forms of intervention in this most private of all acts, some even going so far as to make suicide a crime. However, the present concern with a right to die is not about suicide, the deed of an active subject, but about a moribund patient's being passively subjected to the death-delaying ministrations of modern medicine. And although some aspects of the ethics of suicide do intrude into this question too, the presence of a fatal malady as the chief agency of death enables us to distinguish submitting to death from killing oneself, and also permitting to die from causing death.

The novel problem is this: medical technology, even when it cannot cure or relieve or purchase a further, if short-term, lease on a worthwhile life, can still put off the terminal event of death beyond the point where the patient himself may value the life thus prolonged, or even is still capable of any valuing at all. This often marks a therapeutic stage where the line between life and death wholly coincides with that between continuance and discontinuance of the treatment—in other words, where the treatment does nothing but keep the organism going, without in any sense being ameliorative, let alone curative. This case of the hopelessly suffering or comatose patient is only the extreme in a spectrum of medical knowledge which, allied to the institutional power of the hospital and backed by the law, creates situations in which it becomes a question whether the rights of the (typically powerless and somehow captive) patient are observed or violated; and among them would be a right to die. In addition, when treatment becomes identical with keeping alive, there arises for physician and hospital the spectre of killing by discontinuing treatment, for the patient the spectre of suicide with demanding it, for others that of complicity in one or the other with mercifully facilitating or not resisting it. This aspect of the matter, which alloys its purely ethical resolution with legal constraints and fears, I will discuss later. As to the rights of the patient, a novel "right to die" does seem to have emerged with these developments; and because of the novel, merely sustaining types of treatment, this right is clearly subsumed under the general right to accept or reject treatment. Let us first discuss this wider and little contested right, which always, if in a less direct manner, also includes death as a possible and perhaps certain outcome of its choices. In this, as in our whole discourse, we shall have to distinguish between legal and moral rights (and likewise duties).

The Right to Refuse Treatment

Now legally, in a free society, there is no question that everyone (except minors and incompetents) is entirely free to seek or not to seek medical advice or treatment for any illness, and equally free to withdraw from a treatment at any time other than in the midst of a critical phase.[1] The only exception is illness that poses a danger to others, as do contagious diseases and certain mental disorders: there, treatment and confinement and also preventive measures like inoculation can be made mandatory. Otherwise, without such direct implication of the public interest, my sickness or health is my wholly private affair, and I freely contract for a physician's services. This, I believe, is the *legal* position here and generally in nontotalitarian societies.

Morally, the matter is more complex. I may have responsibilities for others whose well-being depends on mine, for example, as provider for a family, mother of small children, crucial performer of a public task, which put moral restraints on my freedom to decide against treatment for myself. They are essentially the same as those that ethically restrict my right to suicide even when the religious strictures no longer count for me. With some kinds of treatment, such as the dialysis machine for kidney failure, rejection in effect amounts to suicide. Yet there is a significant difference from doing violence to oneself: others, including public powers, in fact any bystander, have the right (even considered a duty) to thwart an *active* suicide attempt by timely intervention, not excluding force. This, admittedly, is interference with a subject's most private freedom, but only a momentary one and in the longer perspective an act in behalf of that very freedom. For it will merely restore the status quo of a free agent with the opportunity for second thoughts, in which he can revise what may have been the decision of a moment's despair—or can persist in it. Persistence will in the end succeed anyhow. The time-bound intervention treats the time-bound act like an accident, from which to be saved, even against himself, and can be presumed as the victim's own more enduring, if temporarily eclipsed, wish (sometimes betrayed by the very fact of imperfect secrecy that made the intervention possible). The saved one has the power to prove the presumption wrong. I am not discussing the ethics of suicide itself, only the rights (or duties) of others to interfere with it, and there, what counts in the present discourse is just this: that counterviolence at the moment of suicidal violence will not force the subject to go on living but will merely reopen the issue.

Clearly, it is a different matter to force the hopelessly sick and suffering to keep submitting to a sustaining treatment that buys him a life he deems not worth living. Nobody has a right, let alone a duty, to do this in a protracted denial of self-determination. Temporizing restraint is required to shield the irrevocable from rashness. But beyond such brief external delay, only the inward pull of responsibilities—"I must spare myself for them"—may restrain the subject, through his own will, from doing what all by himself he would choose to do.[2] But the same kind of consideration, let us remember, can also lead to the opposite conclusion: "The treatment is financially ruinous for my family, and for their sake I quit." If a duty—albeit a nonenforceable duty—to live on for others against one's wish is asserted, then at least a right to die for them must also be conceded. But not a duty! The two opposite pulls of responsibility are not of equal moral weight, as is evident when we ask what those with a claim on a person, the objects of his responsibility, can decently plead with him for: surely only his staying alive, never his agreeing to die. Death must be the most uninfluenced of all choices; life may have its advocates, even from self-interest, certainly from love. Yet even life's case must not be pressed too hard in any such pleading. Especially love should acknowledge, against the clamor of self-interest, that no duty-to-live, though it may *overcome* in me the *desire* to die, can really nullify my right to choose death in the circumstances here assumed. Whatever the claims of the world, that right is (outside religion) morally and legally as inalienable as the right to life, although the exercise of either right may by choice—but only by free choice—be subject to other concerns. The matching of the two in a pair means that either right sees to it that the other cannot be turned into an unconditional duty: neither to live nor to die.[3]

Does public law have a place in all this? Yes, in two supportive respects: first, as part of its function to protect the right to life, it must also sanction the right to medical treatment by ensuring equal access to it; and second, given the scarcity of medical resources, it must establish equitable standards of priority for that access. This latter function of public control, as is well known from the dialysis example, can amount to decisions on who is to live and who is to die, and among the priorities governing that agonizing decision can be an individual's responsibilities for dependents, which may give him, other things being equal, an edge of eligibility over the lone individual. Thus the same thing we have found to militate from within against a person's wish or right to refuse treatment, that is, the dependence of others on him, appears now from without as an increased title to that treatment—at the cost of a third party's right to live. But what public authority can give, it can also later take away under the same principle of equity, in favor of a better claim. We shall return to this contingency as an indirect legal resort in aid of the right to die.

The dialysis example is an extreme one. Usually, the right to decline treatment or ignore doctor's orders does not involve the right to die, unless in a most abstract and indirect way, but rather the right to take risks, to gamble a bit with one's health, to trust nature and distrust medical art, to be fatalistic, or simply to come to terms with a disability, even with a shorter life expectancy, in exchange for freedom from a restrictive regimen; or just the right not to be bothered. The dialysis example was chosen because, there, continuous treatment is tantamount to keeping alive, its interruption spelling certain death, and thus opting against it is not "taking a chance" but indeed a straightforward and directly effective decision for death. It is still not quite the type of case where the "right to die" poses itself as the wor-

risome issue it has lately become. For here the patient is usually un-
impaired in his mental powers to decide for himself, and also
physically a free agent who can take himself off the machine, and nobody can force him back. Thus his right to die does not draw in the
cooperation of others and can be exercised all by himself. The same is
true for many other life-sustaining therapies, like insulin use for diabetics. In such cases, the power both to make the decision and to implement it oneself is present, and the right to die is not seriously
contested nor effectively hindered from outside, whatever its inward
ethics may be. The "worrisome" cases are those of the more or less
captive, such as the hospitalized patient with terminal illness, whose
helplessness necessarily casts others in the role of accessories to realizing his option for death, even to the point of substituting for him in
making the choice.

I shall discuss two examples: the *conscious*, suffering patient with a
disease like terminal cancer; and the irrecoverably *unconscious*, comatose patient. The latter example has been capturing the headlines
lately because of the legal drama involved, but the former is more relevant intrinsically, more common, and also more problem-ridden.

THE CONSCIOUS TERMINALLY ILL PATIENT

Consider the following scenario. The doctor says, perhaps after a
first or second operation, "We must operate again." The patient says,
"No." The doctor says, "Then you will surely die." The patient says,
"So be it." Since surgery requires the patient's consent, this would
seem to close the matter and raise neither ethical nor legal problems.
However, the reality is not quite that simple. In the first place, the
patient's refusal must be based on the same enabling condition as his
consent: it must be "informed" to be valid. In fact, a person's consent
is informed only if he also knows of the adverse prospects on which a
"no" might be based. Thus the right to die (if considered to be exercised by its competent subject himself, not by a proxy in his behalf) is
inseparable from a right to truth and is in effect voided by deception.
But such deception is almost part of medical practice, and not only for
humane but often also for outright therapeutical reasons.

Imagine the following enlargement of the above dialogue, after
the doctor has announced the necessity for another operation. Patient: "What, if successful, will it give me? How long a survival and
what sort of survival? As a chronic patient or with a return to normal
life? In pain or free from it? How long to the next onset with a repetition of the present emergency?" (Remember, we speak of an incurable, intrinsically "terminal" condition.) All these questions, to be
sure, are about reasonable *chances* according to available medical
knowledge—no more, but also no less.

Obviously the patient is entitled to an honest answer. But no less obviously, the doctor is in a quandary when honesty means cruelty. Does the patient really want the unmitigated truth? Can he face it? What will it do to his state of mind in the precious remainder of his doomed life, whether he decides for or against the temporary reprieve? And more vexing still: may the dire truth of my estimate not be self-fulfilling in that it saps the spiritual resources, the famous "will to live," with which the patient might succor my ministration, his "giving up" actually worsening the prognosis? Hope after all is a force by itself, and to stress it more than the opposite is a means not only of persuading to the therapy but also of strengthening its chances. In short, might truth not be actually injurious to the patient and deception not be beneficial in *some* sense, subjective and objective? Thus we find ourselves, in meditating on the right to die, confronted with the much older and familiar question: should the doctor tell? That question indeed arises prior to our imagined situation. Should the doctor have told the patient in the first place that his condition, short of a medical miracle, is incurable? Even "terminal" in the sense that it admits only of brief delay?

Pat answers to these questions would betray insensitivity to their complexity. For myself, I venture this statement of principle: ultimately, the patient's autonomy should be honored, that is, not be prevented by deception from making its best-informed supreme choice—unless he *wants* to be deceived. To find *this* out is part of the true physician's competence, not learned in medical school. He has to size up the person—no mean feat of intuition. Satisfied that the patient really wants the truth—his mere saying so is not proof enough—the physician is morally and contractually bound to give it to him.[4] Comforting deception, if noticeably desired, is fair; so is encouraging deception of direct therapeutical import, which anyway presupposes a situation not calling yet for the supreme choice. Otherwise, and especially if there *is* a choice to be made, the mature subject's right to full disclosure, earnestly claimed and convincingly apparent as his will, ought to have its way *in extremis,* overruling mercy and whatever custodial authority a doctor may have on behalf of the patient's presumed good.

This right to disclosure, by the way, extends beyond the needs of informed decision to a state of affairs where no decision is to be made. What is then involved is not the "right to die," an issue in the practical domain, but the contemplative right to one's death, an issue in the domain not of doing but of being. This needs some explaining. Even in the absence of therapeutical options, and thus with no "right to die" at stake, the terminal patient's right to truth is a right by itself, a sacred right for its own sake, besides its practical bearing on a person's extra-medical arrangements in response to such a truth. Taking a cue from the last sacrament of the Catholic Church, the physician should be ready to honor the essential meaning of death to finite life (against the modern debasing of it to an unmentionable misadventure) and not deny a fellow-mortal his prerogative to come to terms with its drawing near—to his very own terms of appropriation, be they submission, reconciliation, or protest, but anyway in the dignity of knowledge. Unlike the priest who acts *in loco Dei,* the physician in his purely secular role cannot thrust the knowledge on him, but must heed the patient's secret choice as he divines it. Mercy can allow the indignity of ignorance but must not inflict it. In other words, besides the "right to die," there is also the right to "own" one's death in conscious anticipation—really the seal on the right to life as one's own, which must include the right to one's own death. That right is truly inalienable, although human weakness more often than not will prefer to forego it—which again is a right to be respected and nursed along by compassionate deceit. But compassion must not become arrogance. Lying to the stricken in disregard of his credibly evinced will is cheating him of the transcendent possibility of his selfhood to be face to face with his mortality when it is about to meet him. My premise here is that mortality is an integral trait of and not a fortuitous insult to life.

But back to the right to die. Assuming then that the patient has been told and has decided against therapeutical protraction of his moribund state and in favor of letting matters take their course: in enabling him to make the decision and in abiding by it, his right to die has been respected. But then a new problem arises. The option against protracting was, among other things, an option against suffering, and thus it includes the wish to be spared suffering, either by hastening the end or by minimizing pain during the remaining span, the latter in effect sometimes amounting to the former by the heavy dosage of drugs it requires. Heeding such wishes appears to be part of what has already been granted the patient with the "right to die" as such, when his decision was first allowed. Mercy in addition joins with these wishes in proportion as the suffering is acute. But their fulfillment involves the cooperation of others, perhaps even their sole agency, and here the institutionalization of dying by hospital confinement, added to the helplessness of the patient's condition, creates problems of the gravest sort. Usually, discharge into home care is impracticable, and we need not discuss what might or might not be done in the intimate privacy of compassionate love—even this is not free of serious constraints. But the hospital, at any rate, puts the patient squarely in the public domain and under its norms and controls.

Now, as to outright hastening death by a lethal drug, the doctor cannot fairly be asked to make any of his ministrations with this *purpose,* nor the hospital staff to connive by looking the other way if someone else provides the patient the means. The law forbids it, but more so (the law being changeable) it is prohibited by the innermost meaning of the medical vocation, which should never cast the physician in the role of a dispenser of death, even at the subject's request. "Euthanasia" at the doctor's hand is arguable only in the case of a lingering, residual life with the patient's personhood already extinguished. If we rule out euthanasia at the doctor's hand, so as to preserve the integrity of his calling even at the expense of the patient's right to die, then we must add that putting the means in the patient's hands falls little short of administering them. If nothing else, it would be contrary to the premise of the physician's privileged access to such means—a privilege jeopardized by the best-meant abuse.

But there is a difference between "killing" and "permitting to die," and again between permitting to die and aiding suicide. In the case of the suffering *conscious* patient we are speaking of, permitting ought to be freed from the fears of legal or professional reproof if it consists in acceding to his steadfast request (not the request of a despairing moment) to take him off the respirator that keeps him alive with no prospect of recovery or significant improvement. Formally, the right is his, and his alone, by his status of contractual principal in a service relationship, and the jurisdictional problem arises only from the quasi-surrender of rights to institutional trusteeship implicit in hospitalization. Such surrender in matters of medical routine remains conditional on the subject's continuing primary intent and does not extend to his right of revising that intent and making another ultimate choice. As to the *morality* of complying with it by discontinuing the life-support, that is, desisting from its further use, only sophistry can in this case equate desisting with doing, thus permitting to die with killing. And after all, a patient's helplessness that puts him at the mercy of the doctor's compliance should not make his right inferior to that of the mobile patient who simply can get up and leave without hindrance. The captive patient must not be penalized by disenfranchisement for his physical impotence. If he says "enough," he should be obeyed; and social obstructions to that should be removed.[5]

But passing from desisting to doing, what can be said about administering painkillers, which is a positive act on the doctor's part? Here, the oath "not to harm" can come into conflict with the duty to relieve, when harmful doses become necessary to cope with the torture of intractable constant pain. Which duty should prevail? My intuitive answer is: in a terminal condition, the clamor for relief overrules the ban on harming and even on shortening life, and it ought to be heeded if the patient has been told the price of relief. To hasten death in this manner, as a byproduct of the quite different purpose of making the remainder of a doomed life tolerable, is morally right and should be held unimpeachable by law and professional ethics alike, even though it adds another lethal component to the given lethal condition. The latitude, thus carefully circumscribed, does not open the door to mercy killing, and it seems to me that it requires no euthanasia legislation, only a judicial refinement of the malpractice concept that removes such requested terminal alleviation from its scope. Morally and conceptually, there is no confounding this consensual trade-off between tolerableness and length of an expiring stage with "killing." (For nonterminal cases, the issue is debatable, and much depends on the kind of survival at stake.)

The Patient in Irreversible Coma

Finally, consider the patient in irreversible coma, the case of a lingering, artificially sustained residue of life, where not even an imaginary "free agent" is left whose presumed own will a deputy might carry out. Failing such a virtual agent and putative chooser in his own cause, a *right* to die is, strictly speaking, not involved, since this of all rights must be something that its owner could possibly claim, if not by himself exercise. One could not properly tell whose right is upheld or violated with any decision—that of the former person or that of the present, impersonal remainder. (As only a person can be a subject of rights, it would have to be the former person, whose "posthumous" rights, as it were, could indeed be invoked.) What is in question is rather the right or duty of others to perpetuate the given state, and alternately their right or duty to terminate it by withdrawing its artificial support. Reason, sanity, and humanity, it is safe to assert, overwhelmingly favor the second alternative: let the poor shadow of what once was a person die, as the body is ready to do, and end the degradation of its forced lingering. Yet powerful obstacles stand in the way of this counsel. There is the human reluctance to kill, as the letting die can here be construed, since it involves my ceasing to prevent it. There is the conception of the doctor's duty to be on the side of life under all circumstances. And there is the law, which forbids causing death intentionally and makes culpable even the causing it by neglect or omission. Though none of this touches properly on a right to die, and all of it at best tenuously on a right to live—there being no subject even implicitly claiming the one or the other and being hurt by its denial—yet the case of the comatose has in public argument become entangled with the right to die, and one hears this right invoked in support of one course of action, allowing to die. For this reason, I include the issue here.

There are two ways of getting out of the ethical-legal impasse I have described. One is redefining "death" so that a comatose condition of a certain kind constitutes death—the so-called "brain death" definition, which takes the whole matter (death being already an accomplished fact) out of the realm of decision and makes it a mere matter of ascertaining whether the criteria of the definition are fulfilled. If they are, withdrawal of support would appear to be not just permissible, but a matter of course and even mandatory, as it would be indefensible to waste precious medical resources on a corpse. Or would it? Might not the withdrawal, that is, making the corpse even more of a corpse, cause a waste in another direction? Is not the deceased, if residually kept functioning, a precious medical resource himself? In that case, pronouncing dead and continuing the life support would not seem contradictory; they rather would be parts of one syndrome with concerns besides the patient's. I have described in my essay "Against the Stream" (in *Philosophical Essays,* 1974) my grave misgivings about this kind of a resolution to the problem—removing it by way of a definition that is tailored to the particular situation and its practical quandary, tainted with the suspicion of expediency, and giving rise to apprehensions about the extraneous uses to which it lends itself, for example, to secure the most perfect material for organ transplants. Some of those misgivings have meanwhile come true; and the definition itself has suffered a serious setback as to its helpfulness in meeting the challenge of irreversible coma. For in the Quinlan case, where spontaneous respiration unexpectedly set in after forced respiration was discontinued by permission of the court, the girl was *not* dead by the criteria of the Harvard definition (which, incidentally, was not invoked by the court), yet still in a coma, and the question of further artificial life support (e.g., forced intravenous feeding) was posed again in all its original force. The shift from the moral to the technical ground diminishes our capacity to meet the question.

But there is another way of getting out of the impasse than by definitional semantics about life and death, namely, by squarely facing the issue of the *rightness* of continuing, solely by our artifice, what may perhaps, for all we know, still be called "life," but is only that kind of life, and this totally by grace of our artifice. Here I agree with the papal ruling that "when deep unconsciousness is judged to be permanent, extraordinary means to maintain life are not obligatory. They can be terminated and the patient allowed to die." I go a step further and say: they *ought* to be terminated because the patient *ought* to be allowed to die; stoppage of the sustaining treatment should be mandatory, not just permitted. For something like a "right to die" can, after all, be construed on behalf and in defense of the past dignity of the person that the patient once was, and the memory of which is tainted by the degradation of such a "survival." That memorial, "posthumous" right (extralegal as it is) places a duty on us, the guardians of its integrity by virtue of our mastery over it and thereby the executors of its claim. And if this is too "metaphysical" to convince our pragmatic conscience as to where our duty lies, then a down-to-earth principle of social justice, extraneous to the patient, but more likely to persuade the legislator, can come to the aid of this internal reason for mandating the termination: fair allocation of scarce medical resources (excluding the patient himself from such a classification!).

I have referred before to the life-and-death decisions necessitated by this circumstance, which is most likely to occur with respect to that elaborate apparatus whose life-preserving application must be continual. My former consideration was with the initial *admission* to such facilities when demand for them exceeds supply (the dialysis example). For the sombre choices that have to be made, priorities must be set by criteria as "just" as we can make them. The rough-and-ready battlefield "triage" system that the French adopted in the mass slaughter of World War I was the first instance of such a rule of selection. Under noncatastrophic conditions, the grading of more or less "deserving" cases becomes a complex and controversial matter, which in view of the many imponderables must often, at the upper end of the selection, be resolved arbitrarily. But although it must remain moot which is the "most" deserving case in a spectrum, at its simplifying lower end it is not moot which is the *least* deserving: the one that can least *profit* from the extraordinary treatment in short supply. This granted, the question remains whether such a selectivity extends past admission into the further course of things and can later apply to the patient's *retention* in the treatment, when a "better" candidate comes along. In general, I would deny this and recognize here a preemptive right of prior occupancy. Once underway, it would be an unconscionable cruelty to revoke the life support (still desired by the patient) for whatever extraneous interests: as with an individual once born, the place once allotted to the patient is simply not up for bidding anymore. But the irreversibly comatose is beyond the reach of cruelty as he is beyond the enjoyment of benefit, and "his" profit from the treatment is literally nil, if "his" refers to a subject capable of reaping the profit. In this unique borderline case, therefore, the criterion of "least profit" can indeed apply and ethically rule for discontinuing what has been begun, so as not to withhold from others a life-preservation from which they can profit. To me, as I have made clear, this consideration is secondary to the *internal* merits of the case which I consider sufficient and mandatory ground for termination—indeed *the* genuine ground. But as this internal aspect is, notoriously, not above controversy, distributive social justice—a more pragmatic and hence more securely entrenched principle—may be invoked to the same effect. For me to do so is what Plato called "second sailing" *(deuteros plous):* the next best way.

The Task of Medicine

Not to end with this particular subject, let me recall that my topic is "the right to die," to which the case of the comatose is marginal at best. Not only is it too rare, too extreme, and too sharply edged to serve as a representative paradigm, it is (as noted before) not properly a "rights" issue at all, with which, however, it is conflated in the public imagination. The real locus of that right to agonize about is the much more common and treacherous shadow land of the conscious terminal sufferer. It is he, not the body already lost to all conscious life, whose plight poses the ethically troubling problems. What the two have nonetheless in common is this: that beyond the compass of "rights," they pose the question as to the ultimate *task* of medical art. They force us to ask: is merely keeping a naturally doomed body this side of expiring among the genuine goals or duties of the physician? As to actual goals served by the art we must note that, at one end of the spectrum, the once severe definition of medicine's goals has become much loosened and now includes services (mostly surgical) that are not "medically indicated" at all: contraception, abortion and sterilization on nonmedical grounds, sex change, not to speak of cosmetic surgery for vanity or occupational advantage. Here, "service to life" has been extended beyond the ancient tasks of healing and alleviating to performing functions of a general "body technician" for diverse ends of social or personal choice.

But at the upper end of the spectrum, where our "right to die" issue is located, the august and ancient commitments still determine the doctor's task. It is therefore important to define the underlying "commitment to life" itself and thereby the lengths to which medical art must or must not go in honoring this commitment. Now we have already laid it down as a rule that even a transcendent duty to live on the patient's side does not justify a coercion to life on the doctor's side. But at present, the doctor himself is forced into such a coercion, partly by the ethics of the profession, partly by existing law or judicial usage. Through the institutionalization of sickness and especially of dying, once the doctor has plugged the patient into the machine at the hospital, he too is plugged in. It is notoriously easier to get a court ruling for imposing treatment (children of Jehovah's Witnesses) than one for breaking off treatment (Quinlan). To defend the right to die, therefore, the real vocation of medicine must be reaffirmed, so as to free both patient and physician from their present bondage. The novel condition of the patient's impotence coupled with the power of life-prolonging technologies prompts such a reaffirmation. I suggest that the trust of medicine is the wholeness of life. Its commitment is to keep the flame of life burning, not its embers glimmering. Least of all is it the infliction of suffering and indignity. How to translate such a statement of principle into legally viable policy is another matter, and however well it is done, we cannot hope it will eliminate twilight zones with anxious choices. But with the principle as such affirmed, there is hope that the doctor can become again a humane servant instead of the tyrannical and himself tyrannized master of the patient.

It is thus ultimately the concept of *life,* not the concept of death, which rules the question of the "right to die." We have come back to the beginning, where we found the right to life standing as the basis of all rights. Fully understood, it also includes the right to death.

NOTES

1. A "critical phase" would be that between two linked operations or during post-operative care, or similar situations where only the complete therapeutical sequence is medically sane. It must then be considered contracted for as an indivisible whole. Physician and hospital would not have performed the first steps without the patient's commitment to the remainder.

2. If a believer, he might even "all by himself" reject the choice as falling within the sin of suicide. I would deny that it does (surrender to the sentence already pronounced is no more suicide than the prisoners on death-row ceasing to seek further reprieve), but we are here considering only the secular ethics of these questions, without preempting their possible theological aspects.

3. Secular and religious ethics here agree. No religion, however strongly it condemns suicide as sin because it holds life to be a duty toward God, makes thereby the preservation of one's own life an unconditional duty—which would indeed lead to horrendous moral consequences.

4. Dr. Eric Cassell gave me this point as being his own policy, with his conviction from experience that the requisite discernment of will is possible.

5. The present state of the law seems to be that such an "enough" by the patient, given his competence, can indeed not be denied but would also, given present "malpractice" policy, force the doctor to resign from the case. As this would deprive the patient of further medical and hospital care (which he still needs for dying tolerably), the threat effectively blocks the option.

11 Defining Appropriate Medical Care: Providing Nutrients and Hydration for the Dying

WILLIAM J. CURRAN

This essay summarizes and reviews a New Jersey Supreme Court decision which determined that criteria for the removal of a feeding tube should be viewed similarly to those for other medical treatments provided to the elderly in nursing homes. The Court established three standards to use in determining whether incompetent, terminal patients need be fed as well as utilizing an ombudsman program to investigate the physical and mental abuse of elderly in nursing homes. By permitting the removal of such feeding tubes, the Court has made a substantive contribution to this new debate.

William J. Curran is Frances Glessner Lee Professor of Legal Medicine at the Harvard Medical School and School of Public Health

The New Jersey Supreme Court first attained national prominence in medicolegal issues of obligations to critically ill patients in the Karen Ann Quinlan case. The high court in New Jersey issued an eminently sensible opinion in that case, allowing the patient's guardian, her father, to use his discretion in removal of life support from his daughter, who was then irreversibly comatose.[1] The court directed that in future cases, the attending physician and the family be advised in such matters by a hospital-based ethics or prognosis committee, which could avoid a case-by-case judicial review. It was expected that the patient would die soon after removal of the respirator, but she did not. Although the hospital physicians, still opposed to the court's decision that she be allowed to die, removed the respirator, Ms. Quinlan remained alive for nine years in a New Jersey nursing home.

The same high court has rendered a new decision in an even more troubling area: the obligation to provide nutrition and water to elderly patients in nursing homes who are greatly impaired and dying. The difficulties in these cases are manifold. The patients have often lost all control of bodily functions, cannot communicate, are experiencing varying degrees of pain and discomfort, and must be fed intravenously or by a nasogastric tube in order to survive in an extremely feeble condition. The patients are maintained by nursing staff and are rarely seen by physicians except in the event of radical changes in their condition. When, if ever, are the staff and the supervising physician justified in withdrawing (or withholding) nutrition and hydration, allowing the patient to die quietly rather than linger on in such a condition?

There has been a concern that the failure to provide food and water is, in some deeply symbolic way, different from the cessation of medical treatment, whether described as "ordinary" or "extraordinary." Food and water seem to be a key part of the care given in medical and nursing services. In the latest version of the federal government's efforts to prevent "child abuse" in the case of severely impaired infants (the Baby Doe law and regulations), the law does not allow removal of nutritional and hydration care under any circumstances.[2,3]

In a case named *In the Matter of Claire Conroy*,[4] the New Jersey court has determined that removal of the nasogastric tube should be viewed in the same way as other medical and nursing treatment provided to elderly patients in nursing homes. Removal of the tube was found to be legally proper under detailed judicial guidelines. A comprehensive review of the decision is not possible in this limited space, but the highlights can be outlined.

The patient was an 85-year-old woman with irreversible physical and mental impairments, including arteriosclerotic heart disease, hypertension, and diabetes. She could not speak or move on her own and responded only by moaning or smiling in response to certain stimuli. She was essentially unaware of her surroundings. She had no control of her excretory functions and required nasogastric feeding. She was not brain-dead or in a coma. Her guardian since 1979 had been a nephew who visited her each week. She had no other living relatives. The nephew had earlier opposed any efforts to end life support, and he had nothing to gain financially by her death. He petitioned the court to allow removal of the nasogastric tube. The physician in charge opposed removal, since he considered it "unacceptable medical practice."

During the litigation, the patient died with the nasogastric tube in place.

The trial court ruled in favor of the petitioner, but an intermediate appellate court reversed that ruling. The Supreme Court, although the patient had died, retained jurisdiction in order to make its own decision. The case by this time had received considerable publicity. In the appeal to the high court, national attention was enhanced through amicus curiae briefs filed by several groups, including the New Jersey Hospital Association, a group of former members and professional staff of the President's Commission for the Study of Ethical Problems in Medicine and Biomedical and Behavioral Research, the National Citizen's Coalition for Nursing Home Reform, Concern for the Dying, and the New Jersey Concerned Taxpayers.

In their latest ruling, the New Jersey Court established three separate tests or standards under which patients like Ms. Conroy (those in nursing homes who are suffering from "serious and permanent mental and physical impairment," will "probably die within approximately one year" even with treatment, are incompetent to make decisions about life support, and are unlikely ever to regain competence) need not be given nasogastric feeding and other forms of life support.

The first test was described as a "subjective standard" under which the wish of the patient not to receive further treatment or feeding would be followed. The evidence of this refusal could be found, said the court, in specific communications, such as a "living will" stating the person's wish not to be treated or sustained under certain circumstances; in an "oral directive" to a family member, friend, or health-care provider; or in a durable power of attorney or appointment of a proxy or representative to make such decisions on the person's behalf.

The second and third tests would be used if it was not clear that the patient had expressed a specific desire not to be treated or fed under the circumstances. These tests would apply the *parens patriae* power of the state to act in the best interests of an incompetent person. The second test was described as a "limited objective standard" to be applied if there was only "some trustworthy evidence" that the patient would have refused treatment and feeding. This evidence could include casual comments to family and friends, the life style of the person, attitudes and actions of independence, and the person's concern for dignity and the ability to sustain his or her own capacity. According to the majority opinion, however, the patient would have to be suffering from unavoidable pain, thus making continued life too heavy a burden to bear.

In the absence of any reliable evidence of the patient's wishes, the court indicated that a third test could be applied, a "pure objective standard" under which feeding and life-support systems could be removed. In such a situation, a stricter standard of the patient's unbearable life would need to be indicated. The net burdens of continued life should "clearly and markedly" outweigh any benefits. This would be the case if the patient met all the conditions stated above and suffered from recurring, unavoidable pain that was so severe that administering life-sustaining treatment or feeding would be "inhumane." The court expressly denied authority under this third test to remove life support from any patient on a "quality of life" basis other than extreme pain or on the ground that the patient's "value to society" was negligible.

One might have expected that the high court would end its opinion at this point, except to indicate that guardians could exercise these new standards under the guidance of ethics or prognosis committees set up in New Jersey hospitals and in some nursing homes as well, under the *Quinlan* decision and a procedure formulated by the New Jersey attorney general's office.[5,6] In a move that came as a surprise to most observers of the decision in the lower courts, the Supreme Court took no notice at all of the ethics–prognosis committee approach so strongly supported in the *Quinlan* opinion. Instead, the majority of the court recognized another administrative system, set up in New Jersey in recent years, as seemingly more acceptable for nursing home oversight. This is the state ombudsman program established to investigate physical and mental abuse of patients in nursing homes. The court determined that this program should be called on to examine all indentified cases in nursing homes in which life support, including feeding and hydration, would be withheld or withdrawn under any of the three tests described above and in which the request to investigate was instituted by a guardian, family, friends, or the attending physician or nursing home. (An independent person could also make a complaint to the ombudsman concerning a case in which these guidelines were not followed and abuse of the patient was suspected.)

The ombudsman would be required to conduct an immediate review of the matter and report within 24 hours to the commissioner of human services and other appropriate authorities. The ombudsman would seek appointment of two physicians not associated with the facility to examine the patient and provide an opinion on his or her condition and prognosis. In order to authorize that life support, feeding, and hydration be whithheld or withdrawn, the ombudsman would have to agree that the applicable standard was met and obtain the concurrence of the two examining physicians, the attending doctor, the guardian, if any, and the patient's family or next of kin. It was pointed out in a footnote that in the *Quinlan* case the court had allowed the guardian to replace a reluctant or unwilling attending physician with another physician of his choice who was willing to support the guardian's wishes to remove life support. If all these steps were taken and recorded, the authorization of the ombudsman would, in the absence of bad faith, immunize all participants from civil and criminal liability for actions taken.

The importance of this decision in the growing court literature on medical obligation to the dying cannot be overstated. It is the most far-reaching of the judicial opinions in laying down general guidelines for the care of patients in nursing homes. The court's position in allowing removal of nutrition and hydration as well as other forms of life support is without precedent in the American courts. Equally impressive is the willingness of the court to articulate three separate legal standards that can support and justify such removal. Other courts have tended to rely only on the first type of standard, the subjective test, or "substituted judgment," in which a guardian may act only when there is clear evidence of a previously indicated desire on the part of the patient that life support be removed or treatment withheld, under the circumstances prevailing at the time. There has been less support recently for a "best interests" test, no matter how expressed, despite a long history of use of the *parens patriae* doctrine in English and American common law. The *Conroy* case reinforces the legitimacy of this traditional doctrine and supports the actions of guardians who, in good faith and without a conflict of interest, determine that the patient's best interests will not be served by prolonging a painful, hopeless existence.

The *Conroy* opinion is thoughtful and well constructed, not only in the breadth and clarity of its guidelines but in the accomplishment of the court in bringing six of seven judges to full concurrence in the opinion. Only one justice dissented in part. This justice would, in fact, have gone further than the majority by allowing removal or withholding of life support, including nutrition and hydration, on the basis of a "best interests" determination, without the stricter qualifications in regard to pain and suffering. The result, therefore, is a strong position and a firm consensus of the court on the basic philosophy to allow termination of life support in stated circumstances.

The wisdom of the *Conroy* decision in actual operation, however, has yet to be measured. The involvement of a state ombudsman may prove to be a useful and welcome alternative to the continuous involvement of courts and may be more suited to the environment of nursing homes than the ethics–prognosis committees in hospitals. On the other hand, the legislature, in its parsimony, may never provide adequate funds to allow the program to operate effectively. Even if the ombudsman program is broadly successful, New Jersey will have two different systems functioning to deal with similar clinical situations in nursing homes and hospitals, since the *Conroy* guidelines are specifically applicable only to nursing homes. Legislative action to clarify problems of interpretation across the systems is advisable; otherwise, further high-level judicial involvement, no matter how much the New Jersey Supreme Court would like to avoid it, seems inevitable.

REFERENCES

1. In re Karen Ann Quinlan, 70 N.J. 10 (1976).

2. Child Abuse Amendments Act of 1984, Public Law 98–457.

3. Proposed Rule and Interim Guidelines, 45 CFR Part 1340. December 10, 1985.

4. In the matter of Claire Conroy, 98 N.J. 321 (1985).

5. New Jersey Guidelines for Health Care Facilities to Implement Procedures Concerning the Care of Comatose Non-Cognitive Patients. January 27, 1977.

6. McIntyre RL, Buchalter DN. Institutional committees: the New Jersey experience. In: Cranford RE, Doudera AE, eds. Institutional ethics committees and health care decision making. Ann Arbor, Mich: Health Administration Press, 1984:106–17.

12 On Removing Food and Water: Against the Stream

GILBERT MEILAENDER

This article argues against withholding or withdrawing food or water from dying, incompetent patients. The author considers whether or not providing food should be considered medical treatment, whether or not withholding food is analogous to withholding a useless treatment, and whether or not such feeding constitutes a burden for the patient. Essentially, for Meilaender, withholding food is too close an aiming at death to be morally justified.

Gilbert Meilaender is Professor of Religion at Oberlin College

As infants we were given food and drink when we were too helpless to nourish ourselves. And for many of us a day will come before we die when we are once again too helpless to feed ourselves. If there is any way in which the living can stand by those who are not yet dead, it would seem to be through the continued provision of food and drink even when the struggle against disease has been lost. To continue to nourish the life of one who has been defeated in that battle is the last evidence we can offer that we are more than frontrunners, that we are willing to love to the very point of death.

Today this intuitive reaction is being challenged. The President's Commission for the Study of Ethical Problems in Medicine and Biomedical and Behavioral Research has suggested that for patients with permanent loss of consciousness artificial feeding interventions need not be continued.[1] A group of physicians writing in the *New England Journal of Medicine* has counseled doctors that for irreversibly ill patients whose condition warrants nothing more aggressive than general nursing care, "naturally or artificially administered hydration and nutrition may be given or withheld, depending on the patient's comfort."[2]

Court decisions in cases like those of Claire Conroy in New Jersey or Clarence Herbert in California or Mary Hier in Massachusetts are contradictory,[3] but a consensus is gradually building toward the day when what we have already done in the case of some nondying infants with birth defects who were "allowed to die" by not being fed will become standard "treatment" for all patients who are permanently unconscious or suffering from severe and irreversible dementia. Those who defend this view stand ready with ethical arguments that nutrition and hydration are not "in the best interests" of such patients, but Daniel Callahan may have isolated the energizing force that is driving this consensus: "A denial of nutrition," he says, "may in the long run become the only effective way to make certain that a large number of biologically tenacious patients actually die."[4]

To the degree that this is true, however, the policy toward which we are moving is not merely one of "allowing to die": it is one of aiming to kill. *If* we are in fact heading in this direction, we should turn back before this policy corrupts our intellect and emotions and our capacity for moral reasoning. That stance I take to be a given, for which I shall not attempt to argue. Here I will consider only whether removal of artificial nutrition and hydration really does amount to no more than "allowing to die."

WHY FEEDING IS NOT MEDICAL CARE

The argument for ceasing to feed seems strongest in cases of people suffering from a "persistent vegetative state," those (like Karen Quinlan) who have suffered an irreversible loss of consciousness. Sidney Wanzer and his physician colleagues suggest that in such circumstances "it is morally justifiable to withhold antibiotics and artificial nutrition and hydration, as well as other forms of life-sustaining treatment allowing the patient to die." The President's Commission advises: "Since permanently unconscious patients will never be aware of nutrition, the only benefit to the patient of providing such increasingly burdensome interventions is sustaining the body to allow for a remote possibility of recovery. The sensitivities of the family and of care giving professionals ought to determine whether such interventions are made." Joanne Lynn, a physician at George Washington University, and James Childress, a professor of religious studies at the University of Virginia, believe that "in these cases, it is very difficult to discern how any medical intervention can benefit or harm the patient."[5] But we need to ask whether the physicians are right to suggest that they seek only to allow the patient to die; whether the President's

Commission has used language carefully enough in saying that nutrition and hydration of such persons is merely sustaining a *body;* whether Lynn and Childress may too readily have assumed that providing food and drink is *medical* treatment.

Should the provision of food and drink be regarded as *medical* care? It seems, rather, to be the sort of care that all human beings owe each other. All living beings need food and water in order to live, but such nourishment does not itself heal or cure disease. When we stop feeding the permanently unconscious patient, we are not withdrawing from the battle against any illness or disease; we are withholding the nourishment that sustains all life.

The President's Commission does suggest that certain kinds of care remain mandatory for the permanently unconscious patient: "The awkward posture and lack of motion of unconscious patients often lead to pressure sores, and skin lesions are a major complication. Treatment and prevention of these problems is standard nursing care and should be provided." Yet it is hard to see why such services (turning the person regularly, giving alcohol rubs, and the like) are standard nursing care when feeding is not. Moreover, if feeding cannot benefit these patients, it is far from clear how they could experience bed sores as harm.

If this is true, we may have good reason to question whether the withdrawal of nutrition and hydration in such cases is properly characterized as stopping medical treatment in order to allow a patient to die. There are circumstances in which a plausible and helpful distinction can be made between killing and allowing to die, between an aim and a foreseen but unintended consequence. And sometimes it may make excellent moral sense to hold that we should cease to provide a now useless treatment, foreseeing but not intending that death will result. Such reasoning is also useful in the ethics of warfare, but there its use must be strictly controlled lest we simply unleash the bombs while "directing our intention" to a military target that could be attacked with far less firepower. Careful use of language is also necessary lest we talk about unconscious patients in ways that obscure our true aim.

Challenging those who have argued that it is no longer possible to distinguish between combatants and noncombatants in war, Michael Walzer has pointed out that "the relevant distinction is not between those who work for the war effort and those who do not, but between those who make what soldiers need to fight and those who make what they need to live, like the rest of us."[6]

Hence, farmers are not legitimate targets in war simply because they grow the food that soldiers need to live (and then to fight). The soldiers would need the food to live, even if there were no war. Thus, as Paul Ramsey has observed, though an army may march upon its belly, bellies are not the target. It is an abuse of double-effect reasoning to justify cutting off the food supply of a nation as a way of stopping its soldiers. We could not properly say that we were aiming at the soldiers while merely foreseeing the deaths of the civilian population.

Nor can we, when withdrawing food from the permanently unconscious person, properly claim that our intention is to cease useless treatment for a dying patient. These patients are not dying, and we cease no treatment aimed at disease; rather, we withdraw the nourishment that sustains all human beings whether healthy or ill, and we do so when the only result of our action can be death. At what, other than that death, could we be aiming?

One might argue that the same could be said of turning off a respirator, but the situations are somewhat different. Remove a person from a respirator and he may die—but then, he may also surprise us and continue to breathe spontaneously. We test to see if the patient can breathe. If he does, it is not our task—unless we are aiming at his death—now to smother him (or to stop feeding him). But deprive a person of food and water and she will die as surely as if we had administered a lethal drug, and it is hard to claim that we did not aim at her death.

I am unable—and this is a lack of insight, not of space—to say more about the analogy between eating and breathing. Clearly, air is as essential to life as food. We might wonder, therefore, whether provision of air is not also more than medical treatment. What justification could there be, then, for turning off a respirator? If the person's death, due to the progress of a disease, is irreversibly and imminently at hand, then continued assistance with respiration may now be useless. But if the person is not going to die from any disease but, instead, simply needs assistance with breathing because of some injury, it is less clear to me why such assistance should not be given. More than this I am unable to say. I repeat, however, that to remove a respirator is not necessarily to aim at death; one will not go on to kill the patient who manages to breathe spontaneously. But it is difficult for me to construe removal of nutrition for permanently unconscious patients in any other way. Perhaps we only wish them dead or think they would be better off dead. There are circumstances in which such a thought is understandable. But it would still be wrong to enact that wish by aiming at their death.

Separating Personhood and Body

Suppose that we accept the view that provision of food and water is properly termed medical treatment. Is there good reason to withhold this treatment from permanently unconscious patients? A treatment refusal needs to be justified either on the ground that the treatment is (or has now become) useless, or that the treatment (though perhaps still useful) is excessively burdensome for the patient. Still taking as our focus the permanently unconscious patient, we can consider, first, whether feeding is useless. There could be occasions on which artificial feeding would be futile. Lynn and Childress offer instances of patients who simply cannot be fed effectively, but they are not cases of permanently unconscious patients.

Yet for many people the uselessness of feeding the permanently unconscious seems self-evident. Why? Probably because they suppose that the nourishment we provide is, in the words of the President's Commission, doing no more than "sustaining the body." But we should pause before separating personhood and body so decisively. When considering other topics (care of the environment, for example) we are eager to criticize a dualism that divorces human reason and consciousness from the larger world of nature. Why not here? We can know people—of all ranges of cognitive capacity—only as they are embodied; there is no other "person" for whom we might care. Such care is not useless if it "only" preserves bodily life but does not restore cognitive capacities. Even if it is less than we wish could be accomplished, it remains care for the embodied person.

Some will object to characterizing as persons those who lack the capacity or, even, the potential for self-awareness, for envisioning a future for themselves, for relating to other selves. I am not fully persuaded that speaking of "persons" in such contexts is mistaken, but the point can be made without using that language. Human nature has a capacity to know, to be self-aware, and to relate to others. We can share in that human nature even though we may not yet or no longer exercise all the functions of which it is capable. We share in it simply by virtue of being born into the human species. We could describe as persons all individuals sharing our common nature, all members of the species. Or we could ascribe personhood only to those human beings presently capable of exercising the characteristic human functions.

I think it better—primarily because it is far less dualistic—to understand personhood as an endowment that comes with our nature, even if at some stages of life we are unable to exercise characteristic human capacities. But the point can be made, if anyone wishes, by talking of embodied human beings rather than embodied persons. To be a human being one need not presently be exercising or be capable of exercising the functions characteristic of consciousness. Those are capacities of human nature; they are not functions that all human beings exercise. It is human beings, not just persons in that more restricted sense, whose death should not be our aim. And if this view is characterized as an objectionable "speciesism," I can only reply that at least it is not one more way by which the strong and gifted in our world rid themselves of the weak, and it does not fall prey to that abstraction by which we reify consciousness and separate it from the body.

The permanently unconscious are not dying subjects who should simply be allowed to die. But they will, of course die if we aim at their death by ceasing to feed them. If we are not going to feed them because that would be nothing more than sustaining a body, why not bury them at once? No one, I think, recommends that. But if, then, they are still living beings who ought not be buried, the nourishment that all human beings need to live ought not be denied them. When we permit ourselves to think that care is useless if it preserves the life of the embodied human being without restoring cognitive capacity, we fall victim to the old delusion that we have failed if we cannot *cure* and that there is, then, little point to continued *care*. David Smith, a professor of religious studies at the University of Indiana, has suggested that I might be mistaken in describing the comatose person as a "nondying" patient. At least in some cases, he believes lapsing into permanent coma might be a sign that a person is trying to die. Thus, though a comatose state would not itself be sufficient reason to characterize someone as dying, it might be one of several conditions whiffl, taken together, would be sufficient. This is a reasonable suggestion, and it might enable us to distinguish different sorts of comatose patients—the dying, for whom feeding might be useless; the nondying, for whom it would not. Even then, however, I would still be troubled by the worry I raised earlier: whether food and drink are really medical treatment that should be withdrawn when it becomes useless.

Even when care is not useless it may be so burdensome that it should be dispensed with. When that is the case, we can honestly say—and it makes good moral sense to say—that our aim is to relieve the person of a burden, with the foreseen but unintended effect of a hastened death. We should note, however, that this line of argument *cannot* be applied to the cases of the permanently unconscious. Other patients—those, for example, with fairly severe dementia—may be made afraid and uncomfortable by artificial nutrition and hydration. But this can hardly be true of the permanently unconscious. It seems unlikely that they experience the care involved in feeding them as burdensome.

Even for severely demented patients who retain some consciousness, we should be certain that we are considering the burden of the treatment, not the burden of continued existence itself. In the case of Claire Conroy, for example, the trial judge suggested that her life (not simply the intervention needed to feed her) had become "impossibly and permanently burdensome." That is a judgment, I think, that no one should make for another; indeed, it is hard to know exactly how one would do so. Besides, it seems evident that if the burden involved is her continued life, the point of ceasing to feed is that we aim at relieving her of that burden—that is, we aim to kill.

Having said that, I am quite ready to grant that the burden of the feeding itself may sometimes be so excessive that it is not warranted. Lynn and Childress offer examples, some of which seem persuasive. If, however, we want to assess the burden of the treatment, we should certainly not dispense with nutrition and hydration until a reasonable trial period has demonstrated that the person truly finds such care excessively burdensome.

In short, if we focus our attention on irreversibly ill adults for whom general nursing care but no more seems appropriate, we can say the following: *First,* when the person is permanently unconscious, the care involved in feeding can hardly be experienced as burdensome. Neither can such care be described as useless, since it preserves the life of the embodied human being (who is not a dying patient). *Second,* when the person is conscious but severely and irreversibly demented, the care involved in feeding, though not useless, *may* be so burdensome that it should cease. This requires demonstration during a trial period, however, and the judgment is quite different from concluding that the person's life has become too burdensome to preserve. *Third,* for both sorts of patients the care involved in feeding is not, in any strict sense, medical treatment, even if provided in a hospital. It gives what all need to live; it is treatment of no particular disease; and its cessation means certain death, a death at which we can only be said to aim, whatever our motive.

That we should continue to feed the permanently unconscious still seems obvious to some people, even as it was to Karen Quinlan's father at the time he sought removal of her respirator. It has not always seemed so to me, but it does now. For the permanently unconscious person, feeding is neither useless nor excessively burdensome. It is ordinary human care and is not given as treatment for any life-threatening disease. Since this is true, a decision not to offer such care can enact only one intention: to take the life of the unconscious person.

I have offered no arguments here to prove that such a life-taking intention and aim would be morally wrong, though I believe it is and that to embrace such an aim would be corrupting. If we can face the fact that withdrawing the nourishment of such persons is, indeed, aiming to kill. I am hopeful (though not altogether confident) that the more fundamental principle will not need to be argued. Let us hope that this is the case, since that more basic principle is not one that can be argued *to;* rather, all useful moral argument must proceed *from* the conviction that it is wrong to aim to kill the innocent.

REFERENCES

1. The President's Commission for the Study of Ethical Problems in Medicine and Biomedical and Behavioral Research, *Deciding to Forego Life-Sustaining Treatment* (Washington, DC: Government Printing Office, 1982), p. 190.

2. Sidney H. Wanzer, M.D., et al., "The Physician's Responsibility Toward Hopelessly Ill Patients," *New England Journal of Medicine,* 310 (April 12, 1984) 958.

3. See a discussion of the first two cases in Bonnie Steinbock, "The Removal of Mr. Herbert's Feeding Tube," *Hastings Center Report,* 13 (October 1983) 13-16; also see George J. Annas, "The Case of Mary Hier: When Substituted Judgment Becomes Sleight of Hand," *Hastings Center Report* 14 (August 1984), 23-25.

4. Daniel Callahan, "On Feeding the Dying," *Hastings Center Report,* 13 (October 1983) 22.

5. Joanne Lynn and James Childress, "Must Patients Always Be Given Food and Water?" *Hastings Center Report,* 13 (October 1983) 18.

6. Michael Walzer, *Just and Unjust Wars* (New York: Basic Books, Inc., 1977), p. 146.

13 Keeping Dead Mothers Alive During Pregnancy: Ethical Issues

THOMAS A. SHANNON

This article argues that mothers who are brain dead should not necessarily be kept alive until the fetus is viable. Several issues are examined in developing this argument: the implications for the definition of death, the cost of maintaining the life support system, respect for the cadaver, the status of the fetus, implications on the social status of women, the rights of the father, and the consent of the mother, and the issue of extra-ordinary care. While few such cases have been reported, the problem raised is critical and provides an opportunity to discuss several important ethical questions.

Thomas A. Shannon is Professor of Social Ethics in the Department of Humanities at Worcester Polytechnic Institute

Since 1982, there have been three cases reported in which pregnant women declared brain dead have been maintained on life support systems until the fetus could be safely delivered. In one case the fetus was maintained this way for sixty-four days. [A,E] Such a possibility arises because the maintenance of physiological functions through advanced life support systems is not incompatible with the criterion of brain death.

In this article I wish to raise and evaluate several ethical problems associated with this phenomenon. Although the cases are few, the problems these cases present overlap with some of the most difficult ones in health care ethics: abortion, resource allocation, defining death, and the withdrawal of life support systems.

I. General Issues

For several decades there has been a debate about the validity of brain criteria for determining whether or not an individual is dead. The 1981 Presidential Commission recommended the acceptance of the death of the entire brain, including the brain stem, as an appropriate criterion for death. [D] Additionally, definitions of death incorporating this criterion are in effect in at least thirty states which have either statutory or case law recognizing such a definition. Thus there is broad consensus regarding the use of this criterion.

Several issues surround the use of the criterion of brain death. The first is perceptual in that the person declared dead is typically on a life support system and one sees the person breathing and knows that the heart is still beating. Thus, although the person has been declared dead, he or she may not be perceived to be dead. Our perceptions do not cohere with our definitions.

Second, cadavers are frequently kept on life support systems to preserve organs that will be donated. Typically cadavers are maintained for several days while the tissue typing and recipient search is conducted. Here is a practice which recognizes that a person is dead but maintains the life support system to preserve organs for transplantation. This practice is reminiscent of a proposal made eleven years ago by Willard Gaylin, the President of the Hastings Center. Gaylin considered maintaining cadavers, now called neomorts, for various purposes: research, professional training, or as an organ bank. [B] Holding a cadaver on a life support system until the fetus is viable is perhaps only an extension of current practice in organ donation.

Third, these practices raise the question of respect for the cadaver. Once this body was an individual's self-presentation to the world or the person's incarnation within the world. The cadaver still bears a relation to that presence. The objectification, and perhaps commodification, of the cadaver engendered by these practices call us to a reevaluation of how we respect the cadaver. In speaking of organ transplantation, William May observed the following:

> The detached organ or member becomes, in a sense, a fit object for ridicule. It has lost its raison d'être and therefore its centeredness. It has become an eccentricity, an embarrassment, an obscenity. It seems to have committed the indecency of refusing to vanish along with the self, while simultaneously failing effectively to remind us of what has vanished. The severance of death has been crazily compounded by a different order of severance that leaves the community charged with picking up leftovers rather than laying to rest remains. [C]

Later in the same article, May makes this observation:

The development of a system of routine salvaging of organs would tend to fix on the hospital a second association with death—as devourer. In the course of life a breakdown in health is often accompanied by a sense that one has been exhausted and burned out by a world that has consumed all one's resources. The hospital traditionally offered a respite from a devouring world and the possibility of restoration. The healing mission of the hospital is obscured, however, if the hospital itself becomes the arch-symbol of the world that devours. Categorical salvaging of organs suggests that eventually and ultimately the process of consumption that dominates the outer world must now be consummated in the hospital. One's very vitals must be inventoried, extracted and distributed by the state on behalf of the social order. What is left over is an utterly unusable husk.

While the procedure of routine salvaging may, in the short run, furnish more organs for transplants, in the long run its systemic effect on the institutions of medical care would seem to be depressing and corrosive of that trust upon which the arts of healing depend. [C]

While these observations refer primarily to a proposal to harvest organs routinely, nonetheless they offer some interesting insight into the case of a brain dead pregnant woman maintained on a life support system. For example, does this practice constitute a reduction of an individual to a specific biological function? May's argument is quite relevant here. Instead of a detached organ's being the source of embarrassment, the entire body is. Although the person is dead, the body has a new status, albeit a confusing one: an incubator. The community may be uncertain of how to react to that status. Even though one could argue that saving fetal life is an important social value, one also has to recognize that such maintenance is a further extension of the objectification of the person into medical practice.

Fourth is a consideration of the allocation of scarce resources. Assumedly such a brain dead pregnant woman could be preserved only in an intensive or acute care unit. Careful monitoring of the cadaver is required to make sure that the appropriate physiological conditions are maintained so the fetus obtains appropriate amounts of oxygen and nourishment. These procedures are expensive, require a substantive use of hospital resources, and come at a time of increasing social demands to control health costs.

Who, then, will bear the cost? Should third party payers maintain cadavers on life support systems? No benefit is being derived by the cadaver. Can one justify third party payments to maintain a fetus in a cadaver? This raises the question of what benefits ought to be provided for a fetus in a particularly sharp way.

There are, then, four general problems that surround the discussion of a pregnant brain dead woman: the meaning of our perceptions of brain death; the practice of maintaining cadavers on life support systems; the objectification of the body and the reduction of an individual to particular biological functions; the allocation of resources. These issues set a context in which other concerns can be examined.

II. The Woman

Clearly, the females of all species are the ones who bear the offspring. Many cultures see this as the primary function of the female and the basis of her status within society. On the other hand, many argue that reducing a woman to this biological function is degrading. Such biological reductionism makes the woman and her social status depend on only one element and contributes to her objectification and a devaluing of her person.

The maintenance of a female cadaver to salvage the fetus can contribute to such a reduction of the woman to her reproductive function. Such a practice is an important symbolic statement about women and their role within society. One can also imagine this practice's being extended so that maintained cadavers could be the incubator for a non-coitally conceived child, thus eliminating the need for artificial uteruses or surrogate mothers. Such potential applications should make us pause considerably before continuing such applications.

A second question is under what conditions a woman would be required to undergo heroic measures to support the life of her fetus. This is, of course, complicated by the fact that here the woman is dead and one is asking what kinds of measures can be enforced on a cadaver.

Generally speaking, most ethical commentators argue that no one is required to undergo heroic measures to support one's own life, let alone the life of another.[1] There are four reasons for this. First, extraordinary measures are recognized as transcending any moral duty we have to preserve our own life. Second, a mother is morally permitted to have surgery or take medications that, while benefiting her, may directly or indirectly compromise the life of the fetus. Third, the common duty of beneficence has limits, some of which may be derived from harm to third parties, i.e., economic harm to an extant family or causing a living person to be deprived of a life support system. Fourth, this practice implements the technological imperative: "We can do it;

therefore, we ought to do it." While this capacity provides us with options otherwise unattainable, nonetheless one must still evaluate morally the consequences of such a capacity.

III. THE FETUS

The status of pre-viable fetal life with respect to its preservation in a maintained cadaver must also be taken into account. At issue is the justification or establishment of the rights of a pre-viable fetus.

Legally, the fetus has no rights until viability. Thus the only legal basis for such maintainance would be viability.

Morally, the status of the fetus is under sharp debate. Some argue that the fetus is a human person from the moment of conception and is entitled to any and all rights that other human persons have. Within this context, one would make a strong argument that the cadaver's bodily functions be maintained so that the fetus can continue to enjoy its right to life. Others would argue that because the fetus has attained a certain genetic and developmental level, it is entitled to some rights, though not all that an adult human person would have. Still others would argue that because the fetus is in a process of development its moral status is unclear or, in some cases, absent.

Medical developments further complicate the moral analysis. Because of advances in both gene therapy and intra-uterine surgery, the fetus is becoming a patient. Also, the growing practices of in vitro fertilization and embryo transfer suggest that the embryo has value, at least as a desired future person.

If the fetus is a patient, does it have rights and on what basis? Do all beings who are patients have rights because of that classification? Does a fetus have rights because it is desired? Or does the fetus have rights because it is a person who also happens to be a patient? Thus the accessibility of the fetus—whether through the externalization of conception or accessibility through surgery—and its potential new status as patient further complicate our moral evaluation of fetal rights.

Finally, we can consider the post-natal situation of the fetus. First, the unusual circumstances of such a process of gestation may constitute a family secret that could be disruptive in the rearing of the child. Second, if others learn of this experience, the child could be stigmatized and suffer psychological harm. Third, because of the unusual circumstances surrounding the period of gestation, there may be media attention which could be exploited and again the child could suffer as a result of this.

These final concerns are speculative and need closer scrutiny. Perhaps our experience with "test tube babies" may provide guidance for considering these issues.

IV. THE FATHER

Fathers have typically been perceived in a variety of ways ranging from the traditional stereotype of the absentee parent to that of a totally involved, nurturing, primary care giver. If one turns to the legal literature on abortion, one discovers quickly that the father has no veto rights over an abortion during the first trimester and probably also none during the second as well. One can argue, therefore, that the father has no say whatsoever unless the fetus is viable. On the other hand, one could argue that since the pregnancy has been allowed to continue, the father has a very strong interest in the fetus and would be the one to exercise proxy consent on its behalf.

One can also argue that the next of kin typically makes decisions with respect to the disposition of the cadaver or its parts and, by analogy, the husband would be the one to decide about the continuation or withdrawal of a life support system to maintain the fetus' life. If, however, the father is not also a husband, he does not qualify technically as the next of kin and, therefore, his status as a decision-maker for the disposition of the cadaver—and fetus—is unclear.

In any event, the father may have a strong ethical interest in the survival of the fetus. How that interest may be protected is unclear given the legal situation and the uncertain status of the fetus. Having rejected the image of the child as property of the parents, society has not as yet articulated or accepted another model that can clarify the father's moral interest in a pre-viable fetus.

V. SPECIFIC ETHICAL ISSUES

Up to this point I have focused on general problems. I now turn to specific ethical issues that argue against the maintenance of a pregnant cadaver.

This first issue is the already mentioned technological imperative: if we can do something, we should do it. When this imperative is uncritically followed, we do things simply because we have a technical capacity to do so. We avoid considering whether what we are doing is appropriate or not. We act simply because we can. The justification is capacity, not moral obligation. We maintain the cadaver because we can—thus avoiding any ethical discussion of whether or not we ought to do this.

A second issue, related to the technological imperative, is the inappropriate use of technology. Life support systems and intensive care units have a clear clinical purpose of aiding patients with massive trauma or who are recovering from major surgery.

Is the maintenance of a cadaver on a life support system an inappropriate use of a technology designated to be a temporary support system? I argue that it is because no benefit can be gained by the cadaver, the breathing is being supported for no purpose with respect to the cadaver, and we are being guided by the technological imperative.

A third issue centers on the use of brain criteria for declaration of death. The use of the absence of brain activity as a criterion for death is clearly gaining acceptance in our country. Maintaining a cadaver declared dead by virtue of such criteria will undermine this definition, for we will have criteria that are not universally applicable. Using this criterion to declare someone dead but then ignoring the consequences of this declaration will only undercut the appropriateness of this definition.[F]

Fourth, in the general tradition of medical ethics, there has been a strong common acceptance of the principle that no one is ever required to use extraordinary means to preserve one's own life or the life of another. The basis of this judgment is that no one is bound to be heroic and that the virtue of beneficence has a limit when an individual is put at a disproportionate amount of risk.

Maintaining a cadaver with life support systems for several months is, I argue, a clear case of extraordinary means because no benefit is derived by the cadaver and because of the cost. With respect to beneficence, one might argue that since the individual in question is a cadaver, she is not being placed at risk. However, the risks of the potential maltreatment of the cadaver, the social symbolism of the image of the woman as only or primarily an incubator, and the impact on the definition of brain death are sufficient to reject supporting a cadaver on a life support system.

Two other critical issues remain to be discussed. First, did the mother consent to this procedure? If the mother had the opportunity to discuss the situation with her spouse or the father and the medical team and she consented to being so maintained after death, then I would argue that this situation is sufficiently analogous to organ donation to permit her being maintained. The consent of the mother is critical because it is her body that will be maintained. Her consent to the procedure thus substantially qualifies many of the problems I have raised.

Second, how close to viability is the fetus? Even if the mother had not consented but the fetus is very close to viability, then I argue that viability should be the relevant issue for deciding what to do. First, if the fetus is almost viable, we are not talking about a protracted period of maintaining a cadaver. Second, large sums of money will not be expended. This is an important consideration because we do not know the source of payment. Third, it is unlikely that someone else might need the life support system during the short period the cadaver is being maintained.

Obviously the phrase "very close to viability" is vague. In fetal development, one or two weeks can make a huge difference with respect to viability. If the fetus is close to that situation, preserving the life support system so the fetus can be born is supportable. But once one moves beyond a week or two, I find it difficult to continue the support system for all the reasons developed above.

VI. CONCLUSIONS

In this article I have raised several problems surrounding the maintainence of a cadaver on a life support system to allow a fetus to come to term. In this conclusion I will highlight the issues I find most critical for making a decision in this most critical situation.

First, we need to take into account the status of the fetus. Minimally, the fetus is a living, developing member of the human species. Legally, until viability, the fetus cannot make any binding claims, especially that of maintaining someone on a life support system. Morally speaking, even adult human beings cannot make that claim on their behalf. Thus, even if one argues that the fetus is entitled to all human rights, the fetus' moral status could not require maintaining the cadaver on the life support system so it could attain viability. And if the fetus' moral standing is not equal to other persons', the argument for maintaining the cadaver as an incubator is all the more difficult.

Second, maintaining a cadaver on a life support system for a prolonged period of time will give rise to confusion about the status and value of brain criteria as an appropriate definition of death. Generally speaking once a person is dead, there is no obligation to maintain the cadaver. The obligations we have to the cadaver are based on respect for the person who was present through the now dead body. Such maintenance of this cadaver on a life support system is a form of disrespect and a mutilation of that body.

Finally such maintenance of a cadaver which is carrying a fetus contributes to the reduction of women to their reproductive role. This uncritically puts women at the disposal of the technological imperative and allows technology to be used on them in an inappropriate way. Although women are in a unique position because of their role in reproduction, nonetheless to reduce women to the role of reproduction denies their own unique personhood and makes their rights and value as persons, as well as the respect owed their cadavers, subservient to values that may be alien to them and may poorly serve the role of women in society.

Two factors may challenge this argument against such maintenance of a cadaver: the prior consent of the mother and/or closeness to viability. But absent these two factors, I argue that there is no moral obligation to maintain a pregnant cadaver on a life support system so that the fetus can survive.[2]

NOTES

1. A striking exception to this tradition can be found in the recently released "Guidelines for Legislation on Life Sustaining Treatment." (10 November 1984) The Committee for Pro-Life Activities of the National Conference of Catholic Bishops suggests that proposed legislation relating to the withdrawal of life support systems "provide that life sustaining treatment should not be withdrawn or withheld from a pregnant woman if continued treatment may benefit her unborn child." (Origins 14 (24 January 1985): 528.

This recommendation certainly departs from the tradition of the optional use of extraordinary treatment in the Roman Catholic tradition. It also does not fit easily with the accepted tradition of allowing a woman to obtain an indirect abortion in the case of uterine cancer or ectopic pregnancy. For if a woman can obtain an indirect abortion in these cases to benefit her, surely treatment could be withdrawn from her when it provides no benefit to her. Finally, as phrased, the recommendation assumes that the life support system is a treatment. Assumedly the reason why it is proposed to have it withdrawn is precisely that it is not a treatment in that it is only prolonging the dying process.

2. I wish to thank the members of the Writing Seminar at the Psychiatry Department at the University of Massachusetts and Roger Gottlieb, my colleague in the Humanities Department at WPI, for the assistance they provided me in writing this paper.

REFERENCES

A. "Baby Is Born to Brain Dead Woman." *The Evening Gazette* (Worcester, MA) 31 March 1983, p. 6.

B. Willard Gaylin, M.D., "Harvesting the Dead." *Harper's Magazine,* September 1974.

C. William May, "Attitudes Toward the Newly Dead." The Hastings Center *Studies* Vol. 1 (1973) 3ff.

D. President's Commission for the Study of Ethical Problems in Medicine and Biomedical and Behavioral Research. *Defining Death.* U.S. Government Printing Office, Washington, D.C.

E. Mark Siegler, M.D., and Daniel Wikler, Ph.D., "Brain Death and Live Birth." *Journal* of the American Medical Association 248 (3 Sept. 1982) 1101-02.

F. Robert Veatch, Ph.D., "Maternal Brain Death: An Ethicist's Thoughts." *Journal* of the American Medical Association 248 (3 Sept. 1982) 1102-03.

14 Stopping Long-Term Dialysis: An Empirical Study of Withdrawal of Life-Supporting Treatment

STEVEN NEU
CARL M. KJELLSTRAND

Discussions about discontinuing treatment frequently end in generalities or in statements reflecting one's own biases. This study examines the practice of discontinuing treatment in a dialysis center. In the center studied, discontinuance of dialysis accounted for 22% of all deaths. The authors conclude that withdrawal of treatment is a common mode of death among the old and those with complicating degenerative diseases. As such, the authors provide a helpful empirical basis on which to develop further examination of the issues involved.

Steven Neu and Carl M. Kjellstrand are physicians in the Regional Kidney Disease Program in the Department of Medicine in Hennepin County Medical Center in Minneapolis.

Abstract: Dialysis was discontinued in 155 (9 percent) of 1766 patients being treated for end-stage renal disease, accounting for 22 percent of all deaths. Treatment was withdrawn more frequently in older than in younger nondiabetic patients, and more often in young diabetic patients than in young nondiabetic patients. Withdrawal was twice as common in nondiabetic patients with other degenerative disorders (P < 0.005); in patients receiving intermittent peritoneal dialysis (P < 0.025); and in patients living in nursing homes (P < 0.025). Half the patients were competent when the decision to withdraw was made, and 39 percent of this group had no new preceding medical complications. Among incompetent patients,

the physician initiated the decision for withdrawal in 73 percent, and the patient's family in 27 percent; all patients had recent medical complications. In the early 1970s the physician initiated the decision in 66 percent of all patients; in the early 1980s this figure had decreased to 30 percent (P < 0.0005).

We conclude that stopping treatment is a common mode of death in patients receiving long-term dialysis, particularly in those who are old and those who have complicating degenerative diseases. Because of the increasing age of patients on dialysis, withdrawal of treatment will probably become more common in the future. (N Engl J Med 1986; 314:14-20.)

Withholding or withdrawing life-supporting treatment is one of the most important ethical issues for medicine in the late 20th century. At least six physicians have been accused of murder for withdrawing or withholding such treatment.[1-5]

Decisions involving the withholding or withdrawing of life-sustaining treatment are common, both as a result of the rapid advances in medical technology and the increasing age of patients. It has been estimated that at least 6 percent of decisions made on a medical ward involve considerations of this kind.[6] Many articles of a normative or anecdotal character have been written about this subject. It is a difficult subject to analyze empirically because a death due to termination of treatment is usually recorded under the disease being treated, rather than withdrawal of treatment.[7]

Treatment with long-term renal dialysis offers unique opportunities for the empirical analysis of this problem: dialysis is regular and ongoing; death is a clear and inevitable consequence when dialysis is stopped; the treatment is an example of medical high technology; and the patient population mirrors that encounterd at any hospital.[8,9]

In this report we analyze the practice of discontinuing dialysis before biologic death among patients on long-term dialysis.

METHODS

The Regional Kidney Disease Center, with its hub at Hennepin County Medical Center, is the largest center for long-term dialysis in Minnesota. Established in 1966, it serves most of the area of Minnesota, North Dakota, and South Dakota through a system of satellite dialysis units. Its organization has been described previously.[10]

When a patient is admitted with chronic end-stage renal failure, he or she is seen by a team of physicians, nurses, social workers, and financial counselors. All options for treatment, including avoiding dialysis, are explained and explored. After the first outpatient dialysis, the patient is regarded as a long-term patient. Fewer than 0.5 percent of patients evaluated for dialysis are excluded, and fewer than 1 percent die before their first outpatient treatment.

Approximately 15 percent of the patients receive dialysis at home. Before 1981, such treatment consisted almost exclusively of hemodialysis, but later hemodialysis was increasingly replaced by continuous ambulatory peritoneal dialysis. In the vast rural area served, 20 percent of patients are treated at satellite facilities. Since 1982, intermittent peritoneal dialysis has virtually been replaced by continuous dialysis. Each patient accepted for long-term dialysis is assigned a staff physician and a nurse practitioner, who usually remain with the patient throughout the treatment period.

Study Population

Our study began with 1766 patients who entered the dialysis program between its initiation—January 1, 1966—and July 1, 1983. Observation was ended on July 1, 1984; all patients were observed for a minimum of one year or until their death. We obtained the names of patients who died but who had lived for more than three days after their last dialysis (i.e., the maximum time between two dialyses; dialysis was performed two or three times per week) and in whom the cause of death was recorded as uremia, failure to thrive, dementia, or central nervous system problems. Of 704 patients dying, 280 (39.8 percent) fell into this category. We read all charts, and in approximately 20 percent of the cases we reviewed the charts with the attending physicians or nurse practitioners. In 106 patients it was clear that a lethal somatic complication either caused death or contraindicated further dialysis. Examples of such complications were brain death, rapidly progressive brain damage with herniation, myocardial infarction or infection and resistant hypotension, or intractable arrhythmia. The exact cause of death could not be determined in 19 patients. Data on the remaining 155 patients form the basis of this study. Technically, these patients had been able to undergo dialysis, but they had died because dialysis was stopped before a biologic cause of death supervened.

We attempted to determine the mental competence of these 155 patients by reading the usually long notes in the charts regarding the decision to stop dialysis. In 66 cases it was clear that the patients were competent, since they had participated in extensive discussions and understood that death was the consequence of cessation of dialysis. In 66 other cases it was equally clear that the patients were incompetent: 23 were comatose, 37 had advanced arteriosclerotic or dialysis dementia (diagnosis established by electroencephalogram, brain scan, neurologic consultation, and repeated clinical examinations), and 6 had severe memory or intellectual deficits that were secondary to strokes. The competence of 23 patients could not be established.

Statistical Analysis

Statistical analysis was performed with the chi-square test. Any difference for which the probability value was below 5 percent was accepted as statistically significant. When specific study periods were analyzed, all patients entering a period—including both those who had been placed on dialysis before the period but survived into it, and those who were placed on dialysis during the period—were regarded as patients at risk for discontinuation of dialysis. Thus, percentages of patients discontinuing dialysis during specific study periods were slightly lower than percentages for the whole study periods.

Results

Study Population

Of 1766 patients (915 male and 851 female) accepted for long-term hemodialysis, 704 (39.9 percent) died. Of these, 155 (8.8 percent of all patients, and 22 percent of all patients who died) died because dialysis was stopped (76 men vs. 79 women, P not significant). Two hundred of the 453 patients with diabetes died, 45 of them (9.9 percent of all diabetic patients and 22.5 percent of all diabetics who died) because of treatment withdrawal. Among the 1313 patients with other diagnoses, 110 died (8.4 percent of all nondiabetic patients and 21.8 percent of all nondiabetic patients who died) because dialysis was stopped (P not significant for all comparisons of diabetic patients with other patients).

Changes with Time, Age, and Diagnosis

Two risk factors—the presence of diabetes and increasing age — are analyzed in Table 1 over three periods. Dialysis was discontinued in 7 of 444 (1.6 percent) of the young patients (< 46 years old) without diabetes, and in 87 of 519 (16.8 percent) of the nondiabetic patients over 60 years of age (P < 0. 0005). A similar trend occurred among the diabetic patients, but this difference did not reach statistical significance. In all age groups except the oldest, the practice of stopping dialysis was three to five times more common among patients with diabetes (P < 0.001). When the two risk factors of age and diabetes were controlled, there was no evidence that dialysis was stopped more often in the 1980s than in the early 1970s.

Table 1. Discontinuation of Dialysis among Diabetic and Nondiabetic Patients, According to Age Group and Study Period.*

	1970–1975	1976–1979	1980–1983	Total†
	patients discontinuing dialysis/patients on dialysis (percent)			
Diabetics				
< 46 yr	4/50 (8.0)	6/73 (8.2)	2/99 (2.0)	12/160 (7.5)
46–60 yr	4/29 (13.8)	4/40 (10.0)	8/96 (8.3)	16/136 (11.8)
> 60 yr	3/11 (27.3)	2/41 (4.9)	12/111 (10.8)	17/141 (12.1)
	11/90 (12.2)	12/154 (7.8)	22/306 (7.2)	45/437 (10.3)
Nondiabetics				
< 46 yr	2/176 (1.1)	2/179 (1.1)	3/190 (1.6)	7/444 (1.6)
46–60 yr	4/164 (2.4)	10/165 (6.1)	2/163 (1.2)	16/366 (4.4)
> 60 yr	12/139 (8.6)	28/243 (11.5)	47/318 (14.8)	87/519 (16.8)
	18/479 (3.8)	40/587 (6.8)	52/671 (7.7)	110/1329 (8.3)
Total	*29/569 (5.1)*	*52/741 (7.0)*	*74/977 (7.6)*	*155/1766 (8.8)*

*The number of patients discontinuing dialysis did not differ significantly between the diabetic group and the nondiabetic group. Within the diabetic group the number stopping dialysis in any age group did not differ significantly from the number in any other age group; within the nondiabetic group the number stopping dialysis did differ significantly among the age groups ($P < 0.0005$). Comparison of the age groups within the diabetic group with those within the nondiabetic group revealed the following P values: patients less than 46 years old, $P < 0.001$; patients 46 to 60 years, $P < 0.001$; patients over 60 years, P not significant.

†Totals for "patients on dialysis" are not sums of values for the study periods; for explanation, see Statistical Analysis under Methods.

Decision Makers

Notes describing the competence of patients and the decision-making process were present in 132 charts. Half the patients were competent, and half were not. Of the 66 competent patients, 58 made the decision on their own. In two other cases families appeared to bring up the subject of discontinuation of dialysis first, as did the physicians in six cases, but of course the patients acquiesced in all instances. There was no apparent somatic complication that triggered the decision in 26 (39.4 percent) of the competent patients, but new medical complications preceded the decision on withdrawal in all the incompetent patients. The physicians first brought up the subject of discontinuation to the families of 47 (73.4 percent) of the 64 incompetent patients for

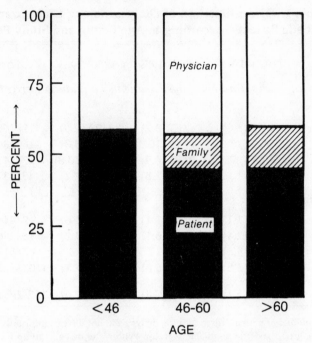

Figure 1. Distribution of Decision Makers Initiating Discontinuation of Dialysis, According to Patient Age Group.

In all age groups, physicians made initial contact in 40 percent of cases. In the two older age groups, families increasingly made the first contact in 10 to 15 percent of cases. Initial decision making by patients in the two older groups was not significantly less than in the younger group.

whom definite information regarding decision making was available. The families of 17 patients (26.6 percent) took the initiative. It was unclear who initiated the discussion concerning two patients.

Figure 1 shows the percentages of decision makers in relation to the age of the patients. Irrespective of patient age, physicians tended to take the initiative approximately 40 percent of the time. However, among patients who were middle-aged (46 to 60) or older, the families assumed this role 10 to 15 percent of the time (P not significant for the change in the number of patients making decisions).

Patients and families increasingly assumed the role of decision makers since 1970. In the early 1970s physicians initiated the decision to stop treatment in 66 percent of cases, but by the early 1980s this figure had decreased to approximately 30 percent (P < 0.005) (Fig. 2).

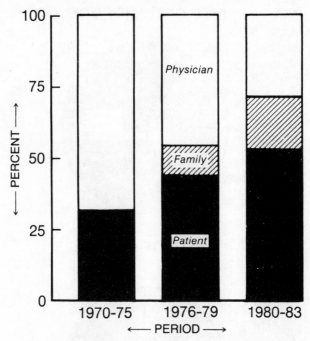

Figure 2. Distribution of Decision Makers Initiating Discontinuation of Dialysis, According to Study Period.

In the early 1970s physicians initiated discontinuation in 66 percent of cases. In the early 1980s families and patients initiated
discontinuation in 70 percent of cases; decision making by physicians had declined significantly (P<0.005).

Site of Residence and Death

The site of residence could be ascertained for 98 of the 155
patients (Fig. 3). The percentage for nursing-home residence among
patients in whom dialysis was terminated (19 percent) was higher than
among all patients over 70 years old (7 percent) (P < 0.025).[8]

The site of death could be determined for 145 patients. Most died
in hospitals (Fig. 3).

Type and Duration of Dialysis and Time to Death

The mode of dialysis could be determined for 148 of the 155
patients, who were compared with all 1064 patients started on dialysis
between 1978 and 1983. When dialysis was stopped, 108 (73 percent)
were on in-center hemodialysis, 17 (11.5 percent) were on home hemodialysis, and 3 (2 percent) were on ambulatory peritoneal dialysis (P

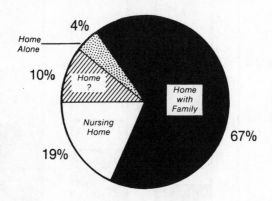

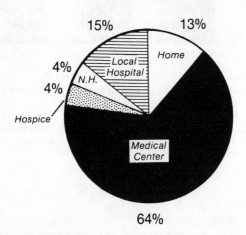

Figure 3. Site of Residence and Site of Death at Time of Discontinuation of Dialysis.

Eighty-one percent of the patients lived at home, and 19 percent at a nursing home (N.H.). Two thirds of the patients lived with a family member. Four fifths of the patients died in a hospital, and only 13 percent at home. Four percent of the patients entered hospices.

not significant for all comparisons with all other patients). Twenty (13.5 percent) of the 148 were on intermittent peritoneal dialysis, as opposed to 81 of 1064 (7.6 percent) on dialysis from 1978 to 1983 (P < 0.025). There was no difference in mode of dialysis between patients with diabetes and those with other diagnoses.

The decision to discontinue dialysis was made after a mean treatment period of 30 months (range, 1 to 134). Only 10 percent of the patients discontinued dialysis after three years, but four patients, including one with diabetes, had been on dialysis for over nine years when they made the decision to discontinue treatment.

Patients survived a mean of 8.1 days (SD, 5.3; range, 1 to 29) after dialysis was stopped.

Complications Present at Initiation of Dialysis

Table 2 lists the recorded medical complications of patients at initiation of dialysis. Dementia was not recorded, but even if it had been, there might have been difficulty in initially distinguishing between permanent organic brain disease and the symptoms of untreated uremia. Only 4 (8.9 percent) of 45 diabetic patients, and 19 (17.3 percent) of 110 nondiabetic patients were free of recorded complications before dialysis was begun (P not significant). Thirty-five percent of the diabetic patients had three or more complications, as compared with 18 percent of the nondiabetic patients (P < 0.05). However, no complications were significantly more frequent among the diabetics whose treatment was stopped than among those whose treatment was

Table 2. Medical Complications Present at Initiation of Dialysis in Diabetics and Nondiabetics.

COMPLICATION	DIABETES		OTHER CAUSES OF RENAL FAILURE	
	DIALYSIS STOPPED (N = 45)	DIALYSIS CONTINUED (N = 408)	DIALYSIS STOPPED (N = 110)	DIALYSIS CONTINUED (N = 1203)
	no. of patients (percent)		*no. of patients (percent)*	
Artherosclerotic heart disease	19 (42)	120 (29)	42 (38)	223 (19)*
Cerebrovascular accident	5 (11)	28 (7)	9 (8)	60 (5)
Hypertensive cardiac hypertrophy	10 (22)	55 (13)	13 (12)	107 (9)
Peripheral vascular disease	7 (16)	89 (22)	22 (20)	98 (8)*
Cancer	3 (7)	32 (8)	22 (20)	113 (9)*
Chronic pulmonary disease	3 (7)	43 (11)	22 (20)	124 (10)*
Uncontrolled high blood pressure	22 (49)	158 (39)	28 (25)	440 (37)
Peptic ulcer	5 (11)	52 (13)	14 (13)	152 (13)
Cirrhosis	1 (2)	5 (1)	0 (0)	9 (1)

*Significantly different from the number of patients in whom dialysis was stopped (P < 0.005, chi-square test).

continued. Among the patients with other causes of renal failure, arteriosclerotic heart disease, peripheral vascular disease, cancer, and chronic pulmonary disease were significantly more common in those in whom treatment was withdrawn than in those in whom it was continued. Blindness was present in 14 (31.1 percent) of the 45 diabetic patients in whom dialysis was stopped and in 99 (24.3 percent) of the 408 other diabetic patients (P not significant).

Complications Emerging during Dialysis

Brain disease was the most common complication leading to withdrawal of dialysis. Forty-four (28.3 percent) of the 155 patients had dementia, and 19 (12.3 percent) had a cerebrovascular accident (Table 3). Catastrophic acute illness, occurring in 22 (14.2 percent) of the 155 patients, was the next most common emerging complication. In 26 (16.8 percent) of the patients we could find no complication that accounted for the patients' decision to discontinue dialysis.

Except for records of amputations and blindness in diabetic pa-

Table 3. Most Important Emerging Complications at Time of Death in Patients Whose Dialysis Treatment Was Stopped.*

COMPLICATION	DIABETES (N = 45)	OTHER CAUSES OF RENAL FAILURE (N = 110)
	no. of patients (percent)	
Dementia	11 (24)	33 (30)
Cerebrovascular accident	7 (16)	12 (11)
Catastrophic acute illness	7 (16)	15 (14)
Fractures, pain	1 (2)	10 (9)
Weakness, depression	7 (16)	8 (7)
Cancer	2 (4)	5 (5)
Liver failure	—	4 (4)
Peripheral vascular disease (amputations)	1 (2)	3 (3)
Failure of transplant	2 (4)	1 (1)
No complication	7 (16)	19 (17)
	45 (100)	110 (100)

*The number of patients with diabetes who belong to any category under "Complication" was not significantly different from the number with other causes of renal failure.

tients, information about emerging complications was not available for all patients who continued dialysis. Amputations were performed in 1 (2.2 percent) of the 45 diabetic patients in whom dialysis was stopped, and in 20 (4.9 percent) of the 408 diabetic patients who continued treatment (P not significant). Blindness occurred in 5 (16.1 percent) of the 31 patients with sight at the start of dialysis who discontinued treatment. Among the diabetic patients who continued to receive dialysis, blindness occurred in 21 (6.8 percent) of 309 (P not significant) (Whitley K: personal communication).

Discontinuing Treatment for Other Reasons

In only one case did discontinuation of treatment lead to court action. A 63-year-old woman treated by intermittent peritoneal dialysis became increasingly confused and vigorously resisted treatment. Three years after dialysis was begun, the decision to discontinue dialysis was made by the physician and the patient's husband. The husband died of a myocardial infarction six months later. Three years later, the patient's children brought a charge of wrongful death against the attending physician. A jury found the physician innocent.

Even though a bioethics committee was established at Hennepin County Medical Center as early as 1972, it has never reviewed any case involving discontinuation of dialysis.

Three of the patients discontinued their dialysis by committing suicide: a 36-year-old woman previously treated for depression, after 27 months of dialysis; a 58-year-old man, after 18 months of home dialysis; and a 56-year-old blind man with diabetes, after 3 months of dialysis.

DISCUSSION

Our study shows that stopping long-term dialysis is not uncommon. It occurred in 1 of every 11 patients, and in 1 of every 6 over the age of 60. Twenty-two percent of all deaths among dialysis patients were due to stopping treatment. Our experience is not unique. A similar study in Canada found an almost identical incidence.[11] Of 80 deaths among patients on long-term dialysis in that study, 22 (28 percent) occurred because dialysis was stopped. In one third of these deaths the patient made the decision, and in two thirds the impetus came from either the dialysis staff or patients' families. One patient committed suicide.

Large registries show lower figures. Thus, of 114 patients who died during dialysis in Minnesota in 1981, only 7 (6 percent) were registered as having withdrawn—a figure only one fourth of our percentage.

However, the causes of 56 percent of the deaths were classified as miscellaneous or unknown and included such diagnoses as uremia.[12] The European Dialysis and Transplant Association reported that in 1979, 2.3 percent of all deaths were due to stopping dialysis, 0.8 percent were due to suicide, and 10.4 percent were due to undetermined or unknown causes.[13] The Canadian registry for 1983 recorded a much higher incidence[14]: 9.3 percent of the deaths were due to "social cause" (i.e., resulting from withdrawal [Posen G: personal communication]), and 27.4 percent were due to miscellaneous or unknown causes. Since the Minnesota register includes our patients and the Canadian register includes hospitals in Toronto, we believe that discontinuation of the dialysis is under-reported as a cause of death. Plough and Salem[7] have shown that causes of deaths perceived as reflecting badly on the dialysis team are regularly reported under a heading acceptable to the team. Thus, these authors found that only 1 of 22 deaths caused by stopping dialysis, suicide, dialysis-related accidents, or dietary indiscretion was correctly classified; the other 21 were reported as cardiac deaths.

We found age and diabetes to be the most important risk factors for discontinuation. Among diabetic patients, no other complications present at initiation of dialysis seem to be important. On the contrary, among nondiabetic patients, diseases of degeneration such as heart and vascular disease, chronic lung disease, and cancer were significantly more common in those who ultimately died because dialysis was stopped. The practice of stopping dialysis has increased over time but correlates with an increase in the proportion of older and diabetic patients receiving dialysis.

In general, the patients in our study fell into three groups: half were incompetent because of dementia, strokes, or coma and could therefore not comprehend the benefits of dialysis treatment, but those who were conscious experienced and suffered from uncomfortable side effects. The decision to discontinue treatment was made by their families and physicians. The competent patients fell into the other two groups: those who had no medical complication that seemed to trigger the decision to discontinue dialysis, and those who made the decision when a complication occurred.

It is difficult to evaluate the role of these complications, because they are common in all dialysis patients. When we had firm data for comparison, as for amputation and blindness in diabetic patients, we could find no difference between the occurrence of these complications in patients in whom dialysis was stopped and in those who remained on dialysis. In 39 percent of the competent patients who chose to discontinue dialysis, and in the three patients who committed suicide, there were no obvious new medical complications before withdrawal. The incidence of suicide in our study is similar to that in the European Dialysis and Transplant Registry[13] and is 15 times higher than that reported for the population in general.[15] The patients choosing discontinuation made deliberate decisions, having spent almost three years on dialysis before treatment was stopped.

Loneliness does not seem to be an important factor in making the decision to stop dialysis. Only 4 percent of the patients lived alone. Most lived at home with spouses, children, or parents. When the decision to stop was made, almost 80 percent of the patients were already in or were then admitted to an acute care hospital, where they died. Only 4 percent entered a hospice, and only 13 percent died at home. These figures correspond to the figures for the sites of death of cancer patients.[16]

There was an obvious decline over time in the percentage of physicians initiating the decision to stop dialysis. One contributing factor may be the increasing awareness of patients' and families' rights, as in such cases as that of Karen Ann Quinlan. Another may be a lessening of paternalistic attitudes of physicians toward patients.

Whether one is allowed to stop life-supporting treatment or not has always been and remains a matter of intense debate. We believe that most would agree that the competent patient has the right to reject such treatment.[17] Most major religions agree that if a treatment is burdensome, a patient may withdraw from it. Such withdrawal is not suicide, and the physician is blameless.[18-21] Recently, however, that right has been violated, and patients have needed to take court action to discontinue treatment with respirators or dialysis.[17,22,23]

On the other hand, there is profound disagreement about discontinuation of treatment in the incompetent patient. Although most religions[18-21] and some courts, as in the Quinlan case,[24] have accepted substituted judgment and stated that families and physicians should make these decisions, this is by no means universally accepted. In the cases of Fox,[25] Saikewicz,[24] and Spring,[26] the courts demanded that the decision be made by a court. The trial judge in the Fox case even argued that life-supporting treatment should never be withdrawn from an incompetent patient. He said that such decisions, however well intended, are "ritualistic exercises, necessarily doomed to failure."[25] Physicians also hold different opinions on this issue.[27] Some argue that these decisions are not made in the patients' interest but because physicians, families, and staff become tired, demoralized, and discouraged about taking care of demented, old, or senile patients. It is pointed out that suffering can always be eradicated by the heavy use of analgesics or sedatives.[28] Other physicians believe that there is too much meaningless life support and that the best decision in many instances is to do nothing.[28-30] Some physicians, such as Stenn, who suffered from a painful peritoneal sarcoma and experienced much discomfort from the analgesics and sedatives used, have even argued for active euthanasia.[31]

Our study cannot answer these questions; it is only an empirical observation of what has been done. We believe that it reflects norms currently followed by physicians and families.[6,7,11,13,14,32]

The chart notes describing how people dealt with the problems of terminating treatment clearly showed the agony and difficulty for everyone involved. This is as it should be. If such decisions are ever made quickly or easily, patients and society should indeed worry over what goes on inside hospitals.

Some may wish to use the observations presented here as arguments for severe restrictions on the number of elderly patients and patients with diabetes who are selected for long-term dialysis. We distance ourselves from such arguments. Because there are no reliable markers foretelling the success or failure of dialysis[8,9] in old or diabetic patients, we advocate a liberal policy for the selection of such patients. But patients, physicians, and families should also be willing to consider discontinuing treatment when its main effects are only discomfort and pain. However, such a decision is obviously to be regarded as a deeply regrettable step, taken only as a last resort, at the request of the competent patient or, if the patient is incompetent, at the family's behest. Paradoxically, the trend in the United States is to do just the opposite. Prospective payment, by rewarding nontreatment, will certainly decrease the willingness of both physicians and hospitals to start potentially expensive long-term treatment. At the same time involvement in any legal decision to *discontinue* treatment, as exemplified by the Baby Doe case, will make this decision, too, even more difficult. If these trends continue, they will force patients and their families to fight both for access to, and relief from, the medical system.

We are indebted to the attending physicians, nurse practitioners, fellows, nurses, and residents of the Regional Kidney Disease Program and the Hennepin County Medical Center who have grappled with these difficult questions over the years; to Dr. Fred Shapiro and Ms. Nancy Buckney, who classified and kept track of the patients; to Dr. Roberta Simmons, Dr. Richard Simmons, and Professor John Dolan, who gave invaluable help to our analysis; and to Ms. Angela Henriksen, who gave fine editorial assistance.

REFERENCES

1. Maguire DC. Death, legal and illegal. In: Fulton R, Markusen E, Owen G, Scheiber JL, eds. Death and dying: challenge and change. Reading, Mass.: Addison-Wesley, 1978:313-5.

2. Kirunadomen i sin helhet. Lakartidningen 1965; 62:500-4.

3. Culliton BJ. The Haemmerli affair: is passive euthanasia murder? Science 1975; 190:1271-5.

4. Brahams D. Acquittal of paediatrician charged after death of infant with Down syndrome. Lancet 1981; 2:1101-2.

5. Lo B. The death of Clarence Herbert: withdrawing care is not murder. Ann Intern Med 1984; 101:248-51.

6. Lo B, Schroeder SA. Frequency of ethical dilemmas in a medical inpatient service. Arch Intern Med 1981; 141:1062-4.

7. Plough AL, Salem S. Social and contextual factors in the analysis of mortality in end-stage renal disease patients: implications for health policy. Am J Public Health 1982; 72:1293-5.

8. Westlie L, Umen A, Nestrud S, Kjellstrand CM. Mortality, morbidity, and life satisfaction in the very old dialysis patient. Trans Am Soc Artif Intern Organs 1984; 30:21-30.

9. Shapiro FL, Umen A. Risk factors in hemodialysis patient survival. ASAIO J 1983; 6:176-84.

10. Shapiro F, McLaughlin D. Planning, developing, and operating a regional dialysis program. In: Drukker W, Parsons FM, Maher JC, eds. Replacement of renal function by dialysis. The Hague: Martinus Nijhoff, 1978:405-17.

11. Rodin GM, Chmara J, Ennis J, Fenton S, Locking H, Steinhouse K. Stopping life-sustaining medical treatment: psychiatric considerations in the termination of renal dialysis. Can J Psychiatry 1981; 26:540-4.

12. Carlson D, Duncan DA, Naessens JM, Johnson WJ. Hospitalization in dialysis patients. Mayo Clin Proc 1984; 59:769-75.

13. Brynger H, Brunner FP, Chantler C, et al. Combined report on regular dialysis and transplantation in Europe, X, 1979. Proc Eur Dial Transplant Assoc 1980; 17:2-86.

14. Schriel J, Silins J, Hauser J, Posen GA, Coll EA. Canadian renal failure register: 1983 report. Ottawa, Ont.: Kidney Foundation of Canada, 1984:56.

15. Stengel E. Suicide and attempted suicide. Baltimore, Md.: Penguin Books, 1966.

16. Malden LT, Sutherland C, Tattersall MHN, et al. Dying of cancer: factors influencing the place of death of patients. Med J Aust 1984; 141:147-50.

17. Angell M. Respecting the autonomy of competent patients. N Engl J Med 1984; 310:1115-6.

18. Sacred congregation for the doctrine of the faith: declaration on euthanasia. Ottawa, Ont.: Publications Service, Canadian Conference of Catholic Bishops, 1980.

19. Social principles—socal community. In: Discipline of the United Methodist Church. Nashville, Tenn.: United Methodist, 1980:91.

20. Health, life and death . . . a christian perspective. Minneapolis: American Lutheran Church, 1977.

21. Jacobs L. What does Judaism say about . . . ? Jerusalem: Keter, 1973: 128-9.

22. Man dies after court lets him halt treatment. Minneapolis Star and Tribune. October 23, 1982:4A.

23. Rust M. Key ruling awaited on terminating treatment. Am Med News 1984; 27(45):1, 29-30.

24. Suber DG, Tabor WJ. Withholding of life-sustaining treatment from the terminally ill, incompetent patient: who decides? I. JAMA 1982; 248:2250-1.

25. Paris JJ. The New York Court of Appeals rules on the rights of incompetent dying patients: the conclusion of the Brother Fox case. N Engl J Med 1981; 304:1424-5.

26. Suber DG, Tabor WJ. Withholding of life-sustaining treatment from the terminally ill, incompetent patient: who decides? II. JAMA 1982; 248:2431-2.

27. Pearlman RA, Inui TS, Carter WB. Variability in physician bioethical decision-making: a case study of euthanasia. Ann Intern Med 1982; 97:420-5.

28. Epstein FH. Responsibility of the physician in the preservation of life. Arch Intern Med 1979; 139:919-20.

29. Petty TL. Mechanical last 'rights.' Arch Intern Med 1982; 142:1442-3.

30. Hilfiker D. Allowing the debilitated to die: facing our ethical choices. N Engl J Med 1983; 308:716-9.

31. Stenn F. A plea for voluntary euthanasia. N Engl J Med 1980; 303:891.

32. Wanzer SH, Adelstein SJ, Cranford RE, et al. The physician's responsibility toward hopelessly ill patients. N Engl J Med 1984; 310:955-9.

Death and Dying / Further Reading

Annas, George J. "Law and the Life Sciences: The Incompetent's Right to Die: The Case of Joseph Saikewicz." *Hastings Center Report* 8 (February 1978), 21–23.

Aries, Philippe. *Western Attitudes toward Death: From the Middle Ages to the Present.* Translated by Patricia M. Ranum. Baltimore: Johns Hopkins University Press, 1974.

Callahan, Daniel. "On Defining a 'Natural Death.'" *Hastings Center Report* 7 (June 1977), 32–37.

Cantor, Norman L. "A Patient's Decision to Decline Life-Saving Medical Treatment: Bodily Integrity vs. the Preservation of Life." *Rutgers Law Review* 26 (Winter, 1972), 228–64.

Imbus, Sharon H., and Zawacki, Bruce E. "Autonomy for Burned Patients When Survival is Unprecedented." *New England Journal of Medicine* 297 (August 11, 1977), 038–11.

Mack, Arien, Editor. *Death in the American Experience.* New York: Schocken Books, 1973.

Maguire, Daniel C. *Death by Choice.* New York: Doubleday, 1974.

Vanderpool, Harold Y. "The Ethics of Terminal Care." *Journal of the American Medical Association* 239 (February 27, 1978), 850–52.

Veatch, Robert M. *Death, Dying, and the Biological Revolution.* New Haven: Yale University Press, 1976.

Weir, Robert F., Editor. *Ethical Issues in Death and Dying.* New York: Columbia University Press, 1977.

PART FOUR

RESEARCH AND HUMAN EXPERIMENTATION

Hans Jonas
David D. Rutstein
Robert J. Levine
Diana Baumrind

15 *Philosophical Reflections on Experimenting with Human Subjects*

HANS JONAS, PH.D.

Jonas' article provides us with a comprehensive review of fundamental ethical issues in human experimentation. Part of the value of the article is his discussion of this topic within the context of the polarity between the individual and society. This fundamental theme is at the heart of the experimentation debate, and Jonas provides a basic description of the major issues. From this perspective, he also examines the motives either for participation in experiments or those used in the recruitment of volunteers. Jonas concludes by presenting basic rules for experimentation. The article points out general themes within the debate as well as providing specific resolutions of some of the important dilemmas.

Dr. Hans Jonas, Ph.D., is the Alvin Johnson Professor of Philosophy in the Graduate Faculty of The New School for Social Research, New York City

When I was first asked to comment "philosophically" on the subject of human experimentation, I had all the hesitation natural to a layman in the face of matters on which experts of the highest competence have had their say and still carry on their dialogue. As I familiarized myself with the material,[1] any initial feeling of moral rectitude that might have facilitated my task quickly dissipated before the awesome complexity of the problem, and a state of great humility took its place. Nevertheless, because the subject is obscure by its nature and involves fundamental, transtechnical issues, any attempt at clarification can be of use, even without novelty. Even if the philosophical reflection should in the end achieve no more than the realization that in the dialectics of this area we must sin and fall into guilt, this insight may not be without its own gains.

The Peculiarity of Human Experimentation

Experimentation was originally sanctioned by natural science. There it is performed on inanimate objects, and this raises no moral problems. But as soon as animate, feeling beings become the subjects of experiment, as they do in the life sciences and especially in medical research, this innocence of the search for knowledge is lost and questions of conscience arise. The depth to which moral and religious sensibilities can become aroused is shown by the vivisection issue. Human experimentation must sharpen the issue as it involves ultimate questions of personal dignity and sacrosanctity. One difference between the human experiments and the physical is this: The physical experiment employs small-scale, artificially devised substitutes for that about which knowledge is to be obtained, and the experimenter extrapolates from these models and simulated conditions to nature at large. Something deputizes for the "real thing"—balls rolling down an inclined plane for sun and planets, electric discharges from a condenser for real lightning, and so on. For the most part, no such substitution is possible in the biologial sphere. We must operate on the original itself, the real thing in the fullest sense, and perhaps affect it irreversibly. No simulacrum can take its place. Especially in the human sphere, experimentation loses entirely the advantage of the clear division between vicarious model and true object. Up to a point, animals may fulfill the proxy role of the classical physical experiment. But in the end man himself must furnish knowledge about himself, and the comfortable separation of noncommittal experiment and definitive action vanishes. An experiment in education affects the lives of its subjects, perhaps a whole generation of schoolchildren. Human experimentation for whatever purpose is always *also* a responsible, nonexperimental, definitive dealing with the subject himself. And not even the noblest purpose abrogates the obligations this involves.

Can both that purpose and this obligation be satisfied? If not, what would be a just compromise? Which side should give way to the other? The question is inherently philosophical as it concerns not merely pragmatic difficulties and their arbitration, but a genuine conflict of values involving principles of a high order. On principle, it is felt, human beings *ought not* to be dealt with in that way (the "guinea pig" protest); on the other hand, such dealings are increasingly urged on us by considerations, in turn appealing to principle, that claim to override those objections. Such a claim must be carefully assessed, especially when it is swept along by a mighty tide. Putting the matter thus, we have already made one important assumption rooted in our "Western" culture tradition: The prohibitive rule is, to that way of thinking, the primary and axiomatic one; the permissive counter-rule, as qualifying the first, is secondary and stands in need of justification. We must justify the infringement of a primary inviolability, which needs no justification itself; and the justification of its infringement must be by values and needs of a dignity commensurate with those to be sacrificed.

"Individual Versus Society" as the Conceptual Framework

The setting for the conflict most consistently invoked in the literature is the polarity of individual versus society—the possible tension between the individual good and the common good, between private and public welfare. Thus, W. Wolfensberger speaks of "the tension between the long-range interests of society, science, and progress, on one hand, and the rights of the individual on the other."[2] Walsh McDermott says: "In essence, this is a problem of the rights of the individual versus the rights of society."[3] Somewhere I found the "social contract" invoked in support of claims that science may make on individuals in the matter of experimentation. I have grave doubts about the adequacy of this frame of reference, but I will go along with it part of the way. It does apply to some extent, and it has the advantage of being familiar. We concede, as a matter of course, to the common good some pragmatically determined measure of precedence over the individual good. In terms of rights, we let some of the basic rights of the individual be overruled by the acknowledged rights of society—as a matter of right and moral justness and not of mere force or dire necessity (much as such necessity may be adduced in defense of that right). But in making that concession, we require a careful clarification of what the needs, interests, and rights of society are, for society—as distinct from any plurality of individuals—is an abstract and as such is subject to our definition, while the individual is the primary concrete, prior to all definition, and his basic good is more or less known. Thus, the unknown in our problem is the so-called common or public good and its potentially superior claims, to which the individual good must or might sometimes be sacrificed, in circumstances that in turn must also be counted among the unknowns of our questions. Note that in putting the matter in this way—that is, in asking about the right of society to individual sacrifice—the consent of the sacrificial subject is no necessary part of the *basic* question.

"Consent," however, is the other most consistently emphasized and examined concept in discussions of this issue. This attention betrays a feeling that the "social" angle is not fully satisfactory. If society has a right, its exercise is not contingent on volunteering. On the other hand, if volunteering is fully genuine, no public right to the volunteered act need be construed. There is a difference between the moral or emotional appeal of a cause that elicits volunteering and a right that demands compliance—for example, with particular reference to the social sphere, between the *moral claim* of a common good and society's *right* to that good and to the means of its realization. A moral claim cannot be met without consent; a right can do without it. Where consent is present anyway, the distinction may become immaterial. But the awareness of the many ambiguities besetting the "consent" actually available and used in medical research prompts recourse to the idea of a public right conceived independently of (and valid prior to) consent; and, vice versa, the awareness of the problematic nature of such a right makes even its advocates still insist on the idea of consent with all its ambiguities: An uneasy situation exists for both sides.

Nor does it help much to replace the language of "rights" by that of "interests" and then argue the sheer cumulative weight of the interests of the many over against those of the few or the single individual. "Interests" range all the way from the most marginal and optional to the most vital and imperative, and only those sanctioned by particular importance and merit will be admitted to count in such a calculus— which simply brings us back to the question of right or moral claim. Moreover, the appeal to numbers is dangerous. Is the number of those afflicted with a particular disease great enough to warrant violating the interests of the nonafflicted? Since the number of the latter is usually so much greater, the argument can actually turn around to the contention that the cumulative weight of interest is on *their* side. Finally, it may well be the case that the individual's interest in his own inviolability is itself a public interest such that its publicly condoned violation, irrespective of numbers, violates the interest of all. In that case, its protection in *each* instance would be a paramount interest, and the comparison of numbers will not avail.

These are some of the difficulties hidden in the conceptual framework indicated by the terms "society-individual," "interest," and "rights." But we also spoke of a moral call, and this points to another dimension—not indeed divorced from the societal sphere, but transcending it. And there is something even beyond that: true sacrifice from highest devotion, for which there are no laws or rules except that it must be absolutely free. "No one has the right to choose martyrs for science" was a statement repeatedly quoted in the November, 1967, *Daedalus* conference. But no scientist can be prevented from making himself a martyr for his science. At all times, dedicated explorers, thinkers, and artists have immolated themselves on the altar of their vocation, and creative genius most often pays the price of happiness, health, and life for its own consummation. But no one, not even society, has the shred of a right to expect and ask these things. They come to the rest of us as a *gratia gratis data.*

The Sacrificial Theme

Yet we must face the somber truth that the *ultima ratio* of communal life is and has always been the compulsory, vicarious sacrifice of individual lives. The primordial sacrificial situation is that of outright human sacrifices in early communities. These were not acts of blood-lust or gleeful savagery; they were the solemn execution of a supreme, sacral necessity. One of the fellowship of men had to die so that all could live, the earth be fertile, the cycle of nature renewed. The victim often was not a captured enemy, but a select member of the group: "The king must die." If there was cruelty here, it was not that of men, but that of the gods, or rather of the stern order of things, which was believed to exact that price for the bounty of life. To assure it for the community, and to assure it ever again, the awesome *quid pro quo* had to be paid ever again.

Far be it from me, and far should it be from us, to belittle from the height of our enlightened knowledge the majesty of the underlying conception. The particular *causal* views that prompted our ancestors have long since been relegated to the realm of superstition. But in moments of national danger we still send the flower of our young manhood to offer their lives for the continued life of the community, and if it is a just war, we see them go forth as consecrated and strangely ennobled by a sacrificial role. Nor do we make their going forth depend on their own will and consent, much as we may desire and foster these: We conscript them according to law. We conscript the best and feel morally disturbed if the draft, either by design or in effect, works so that mainly the disadvantaged, socially less useful, more expendable, make up those whose lives are to buy ours. No rational persuasion of the pragmatic necessity here at work can do away with the feeling, mixed of gratitude and guilt, that the sphere of the sacred is touched with the vicarious offering of life for life. Quite apart from these dramatic occasions, there is, it appears, a persistent and constitutive aspect of human immolation to the very being and prospering of human society—an immolation in terms of life and happiness, imposed or voluntary, of few for many. What Goethe has said of the rise of Christianity may well apply to the nature of civilization in general: *"Opfer fallen hier, / Weder Lamm noch Stier, / Aber Menschenopfer unerhoert."*[4] We can never rest comfortably in the belief that the soil from which our satisfactions sprout is not watered with the blood of martyrs. But a troubled conscience compels us, the undeserving beneficiaries, to ask: Who is to be martyred? in the service of what cause? and by whose choice?

Not for a moment do I wish to suggest that medical experimentation on human subjects, sick or healthy, is to be likened to primeval human sacrifices. Yet something sacrificial is involved in the selective abrogation of personal inviolability and the ritualized exposure to gratuitous risk of health and life, justified by a presumed greater, social good. My examples from the sphere of stark sacrifice were intended to sharpen the issues implied in that context and to set them off clearly from the kinds of obligations and constraints imposed on the citizen in the normal course of things or generally demanded of the individual in exchange for the advantages of civil society.

The "Social Contract" Theme

The first thing to say in such a setting-off is that the sacrificial area is not covered by what is called the "social contract." This fiction of political theory, premised on the primacy of the individual, was designed to supply a rationale for the *limitation* of individual freedom and power required for the existence of the body politic, whose existence in turn is for the benefit of the individuals. The principle of these limitations is that their *general* observance profits all, and that therefore the individual observer, assuring this general observance for his part, profits by it himself. I observe property rights because their general observance assures my own; I observe traffic rules because their general observance assures my own safety; and so on. The obligations here are mutual and general; no one is singled out for special sacrifice. For the most part, *qua* limitations of my liberty, the laws thus deducible from the hypothetical "social contract" enjoin me from certain actions rather than obligate me to positive actions (as did the laws of feudal society). Even where the latter is the case, as in the duty to pay taxes, the rationale is that I am myself a beneficiary of the services financed through these payments. Even the contributions levied by the welfare state, though not originally contemplated in the liberal version of the social contract theory, can be interpreted as a personal insurance policy of one sort or another—be it against the contingency of my own indigence, the dangers of disaffection from the laws in consequence of widespread unrelieved destitution, or the disadvantages of a diminished consumer market. Thus, by some stretch, such contributions can still be subsumed under the principle of enlightened self-interest. But no complete abrogation of self-interest at any time is in the terms of the social contract, and so pure sacrifice falls outside it. Under the putative terms of the contract alone, I cannot be required to die for the public good. (Thomas Hobbes made this forcibly clear.) Even short of this extreme, we like to think that nobody is entirely and one-sidedly the victim in any of the renunciations exacted under normal circumstances by society "in the general interest"—that is, for the benefit of others. "Under normal circumstances," as we shall see, is a necessary qualification. Moreover, the "contract" can legitimize claims only on our overt public actions and not on our invisible private being. Our powers, not our persons, are beholden to the commonweal. In one important respect, it is true, public interest and control do extend to the private sphere by general consent: in the compulsory education of our children. Even there, the assumption is that the learning and what is learned, apart from all future social usefulness, are also for the benefit of the individual in his own being. We would not tolerate education to degenerate into the conditioning of useful robots for the social machine.

Both restrictions of public claim in behalf of the "common good" —that concerning one-sided sacrifice and that concerning the private sphere—are valid only, let us remember, on the premise of the primacy of the individual, upon which the whole idea of the "social contract" rests. This primacy is itself a metaphysical axiom or option peculiar to our Western tradition, and the whittling away of this axiom would threaten the tradition's whole foundation. In passing, I may remark that systems adopting the alternative primacy of the community as their axiom are naturally less bound by the restrictions we postulate. Whereas we reject the idea of "expendables" and regard those not useful or even recalcitrant to the social purpose as a burden that society must carry (since their individual claim to existence is as absolute as that of the most useful), a truly totalitarian regime, Communist or other, may deem it right for the collective to rid itself of such encumbrances or to make them forcibly serve some social end by conscripting their persons (and there are effective combinations of both). We do not normally—that is, in nonemergency conditions—give the state the right to conscript labor, while we do give it the right to "conscript" money, for money is detachable from the person as labor is not. Even less than forced labor do we countenance forced risk, injury, and indignity.

But in time of war our society itself supersedes the nice balance of the social contract with an almost absolute precedence of public necessities over individual rights. In this and similar emergencies, the sacrosanctity of the individual is abrogated, and what for all practical purposes amounts to a near-totalitarian, quasi-Communist state of affairs is *temporarily* permitted to prevail. In such situations, the community is conceded the right to make calls on its members, or certain of its members, entirely different in magnitude and kind from the calls normally allowed. It is deemed right that a part of the population bears a disproportionate burden of risk of a disproportionate gravity; and it is deemed right that the rest of the community accepts this sacrifice, whether voluntary or enforced, and reaps its benefits—difficult as we find it to justify this acceptance and thus benefit by any normal ethical categories. We justify it transethically, as it were, by the supreme collective emergency, formalized, for example, by the declaration of a state of war.

Medical experimentation on human subjects falls somewhere between this overpowering case and the normal transactions of the social contract. On the one hand, no comparable extreme issue of social survival is (by and large) at stake. And no comparable extreme sacrifice or forseeable risk is (by and large) asked. On the other hand, what is asked goes decidedly beyond, even runs counter to, what it is otherwise deemed fair to let the individual sign over of his person to the benefit of the "common good." Indeed, our sensitivity to the kind of intrusion and use involved is such that only an end of transcendent value or overriding urgency can make it arguable and possibly acceptable in our eyes.

Health as a Public Good

The cause invoked is health and, in its more critical aspect, life itself—clearly superlative goods that the physician serves directly by curing and the researcher indirectly by the knowledge gained through his experiments. There is no question about the good served nor about the evil fought—disease and premature death. But a good to whom and an evil to whom? Here the issue tends to become somewhat clouded. In the attempt to give experimentation the proper dignity (on the problematic view that a value becomes greater by being "social" instead of merely individual), the health in question or the disease in question is somehow predicated of the social whole, as if it were society that, in the persons of its members, enjoyed the one and suffered the other. For the purposes of our problem, public interest can then be pitted against private interest, the common good against the individual good. Indeed, I have found health called a national resource, which of course it is, but surely not in the first place.

In trying to resolve some of the complexities and ambiguities lurking in these conceptualizations, I have pondered a particular statement, made in the form of a question, which I found in the *Proceedings* of the November *Dædalus* conference: "Can society afford to discard the tissues and organs of the hopelessly unconscious patient when they could be used to restore the otherwise hopelessly ill, but still salvageable individual?" And somewhat later: "A strong case can be made that society can ill afford to discard the tissues and organs of the hopelessly unconscious patient; they are greatly needed for study and experimental trial to help those who can be salvaged."[5] I hasten to add that any suspicion of callousness that the "commodity" language of these statements may suggest is immediately dispelled by the name of the speaker, Dr. Henry K. Beecher, for whose humanity and moral sensibility there can be nothing but admiration. But the use, in all innocence, of this language gives food for thought. Let me, for a moment, take the question literally. "Discarding" implies proprietary rights—nobody can discard what does not belong to him in the first place. Does society then own my body? "Salvaging" implies the same and, moreover, a use-value to the owner. Is the life-extension of certain individuals then a public interest? "Affording" implies a critically vital level of such an interest—that is, of the loss or gain involved. And "society" itself—what is it? When does a need, an aim, an obligation become social? Let us reflect on some of these terms.

What Society Can Afford

"Can Society afford . . .?" Afford what? To let people die intact, thereby withholding something from other people who desperately need it, who in consequence will have to die too? These other, unfortunate people indeed cannot afford not to have a kidney, heart, or other organ of the dying patient, on which they depend for an extension of their lease on life; but does that give them a right to it? Does it oblige society to procure it for them? What is it that *society* can or cannot afford—leaving aside for the moment the question of what it has a *right* to? It surely can afford to lose members through death; more than that, it is built on the balance of death and birth decreed by the order of life. This is too general, of course, for our question, but perhaps it is well to remember. The specific question seems to be whether society can afford to let some people die whose death might be deferred by particular means if these were authorized by society. Again, if it is merely a question of what society can or cannot afford, rather than of what it ought or ought not to do, the answer must be: Of course, it can. If cancer, heart disease, and other organic, noncontagious ills, especially those tending to strike the old more than the young, continue to exact their toll at the normal rate of incidence (including the toll of private anguish and misery), society can go on flourishing in every way.

Here, by contrast, are some examples of what, in sober truth, so-

ciety cannot afford. It cannot afford to let an epidemic rage unchecked; a persistent excess of deaths over births, but neither too
great an excess of births over deaths; too low an average life-expectancy even if demographically balanced by fertility, but neither too
great a longevity with the necessitated correlative dearth of youth in
the social body; a debilitating state of general health; and things of
this kind. These are plain cases where the whole condition of society is
critically affected, and the public interest can make its imperative
claims. The Black Death of the Middle Ages was a *public* calamity of
the acute kind; the life-sapping ravages of endemic malaria or sleeping
sickness in certain areas are a public calamity of the chronic kind. A
society as a whole can truly not "afford" such situations, and they
may call for extraordinary remedies, including, perhaps, the invasion
of private sacrosanctities.

This is not entirely a matter of numbers and numerical ratios. Society, in a subtler sense, cannot "afford" a single miscarriage of justice, a single inequity in the dispensation of its laws, the violation of
the rights of even the tiniest minority, because these undermine the
moral basis on which society's existence rests. Nor can it, for a similar
reason, afford the absence or atrophy in its midst of compassion and
of the effort to alleviate suffering—be it widespread or rare—one form
of which is the effort to conquer disease of any kind, whether "socially" significant (by reason of number) or not. And in short, society
cannot afford the absence among its members of *virtue* with its readi-
ness to sacrifice beyond defined duty. Since its presence—that is to
say, that of personal idealism—is a matter of grace and not of decree,
we have the paradox that society depends for its existence on intangi-
bles of nothing less than a religious order, for which it can hope, but
which it cannot enforce. All the more must it protect this most precious capital from abuse.

For what objectives connected with the medico-biological sphere
should this reserve be drawn upon—for example, in the form of accepting, soliciting, perhaps even imposing the submission of human
subjects to experimentation? We postulate that this must be not just
a worthy cause, as any promotion of the health of anybody doubtless-
ly is, but a cause qualifying for transcendent social sanction. Here one
thinks first of those cases critically affecting the whole condition,
present and future, of the community. Something equivalent to what
in the political sphere is called "clear and present danger" may be invoked and a state of emergency proclaimed, thereby suspending certain otherwise inviolable prohibitions and taboos. We may observe
that averting a disaster always carries greater weight than promoting a

good. Extraordinary danger excuses extraordinary means. This covers human experimentation, which we would like to count, as far as possible, among the extraordinary rather than the ordinary means of serving the common good under public auspices. Naturally, since foresight and responsibility for the future are of the essence of institutional society, averting disaster extends into long-term prevention, although the lesser urgency will warrant less sweeping licenses.

Society and the Cause of Progress

Much weaker is the case where it is a matter not of saving but of improving society. Much of medical research falls into this category. A permanent death rate from heart failure or cancer does not threaten society. So long as certain statistical ratios are maintained, the incidence of disease and of disease-induced mortality is not (in the strict sense) a "social" misfortune. I hasten to add that it is not therefore less of a human misfortune, and the call for relief issuing with silent eloquence from each victim and all potential victims is of no lesser dignity. But it is misleading to equate the fundamentally human response to it with what is owed to society: It is owed by man to man—and it is thereby owed by society to the individuals as soon as the adequate ministering to these concerns outgrows (as it progressively does) the scope of private spontaneity and is made a public mandate. It is thus that society assumes responsibility for medical care, research, old age, and innumerable other things not originally of the public realm (in the original "social contract"), and they become duties toward "society" (rather than directly toward one's fellow man) by the fact that they are socially operated.

Indeed, we expect from organized society no longer mere protection against harm and the securing of the conditions of our preservation, but active and constant improvement in all the domains of life: the waging of the battle against nature, the enhancement of the human estate—in short, the promotion of progress. This is an expansive goal, one far surpassing the disaster norm of our previous reflections. It lacks the urgency of the latter, but has the nobility of the free, forward thrust. It surely is worth sacrifices. It is not at all a question of what society can afford, but of what it is committed to, beyond all necessity, by our mandate. Its trusteeship has become an established, ongoing, institutionalized business of the body politic. As eager beneficiaries of its gains, we now owe to "society," as its chief agent, our individual contribution toward its *continued pursuit.* Maintaining the existing level requires no more than the orthodox means of taxation and enforcement of professional standards that raise no problems. The more optional goal of pushing forward is also more exacting. We have this syndrome: Progress is by our choosing an acknowledged interest of society, in which we have a stake in various degrees; science is a necessary instrument of progress; research is a necessary instrument of science; and in medical science experimentation on human subjects is a necessary instrument of research: Therefore, human experimentation has come to be a societal interest.

The destination of research is essentially melioristic. It does not serve the preservation of the existing good from which I profit myself and to which I am obligated. Unless the present state is intolerable, the melioristic goal is in a sense gratuitous, and not only from the vantage point of the present. Our descendants have a right to be left an unplundered planet; they do not have a right to new miracle cures. We have sinned against them if by our doing we have destroyed their inheritance—which we are doing at full blast; we have not sinned against them if by the time they come around arthritis has not yet been conquered (unless by sheer neglect). And generally, in the matter of progress, as humanity had no claim on a Newton, a Michelangelo, or a St. Francis to appear, and no right to the blessings of their unscheduled deeds, so progress, with all our methodical labor for it, cannot be budgeted in advance and its fruits received as a due. Its coming-about at all and its turning out for good (of which we can never be sure) must rather be regarded as something akin to grace.

The Melioristic Goal, Medical Research, and Individual Duty

Nowhere is the melioristic goal more inherent than in medicine. To the physician, it is not gratuitous. He is committed to curing and thus to improving the power to cure. Gratuitous we called it (outside disaster conditions) as a *social* goal, but noble at the same time. Both the nobility and the gratuitousness must influence the manner in which self-sacrifice for it is elicited and even its free offer accepted. Freedom is certainly the first condition to be observed here. The surrender of one's body to medical experimentation is entirely outside the enforceable "social contract."

Or can it be construed to fall within its terms—namely, as repayment for benefits from past experimentation that I have enjoyed myself? But I am indebted for these benefits not to society, but to the past "martyrs," to whom society is indebted itself, and society has no right to call in my personal debt by way of adding new to its own. Moreover, gratitude is not an enforceable social obligation; it anyway does not mean that I must emulate the deed. Most of all, if it was wrong to exact such sacrifice in the first place, it does not become right to exact it again with the plea of the profit it has brought me. If, however, it was not exacted, but entirely free, as it ought to have been, then it should remain so, and its precedence must not be used as a social pressure on others for doing the same under the sign of duty.

Indeed, we must look outside the sphere of the social contract, outside the whole realm of public rights and duties, for the motivations and norms by which we can expect ever again the upwelling of a will to give what nobody—neither society, nor fellow man, nor posterity—is entitled to. There are such dimensions in man with transsocial wellsprings of conduct, and I have already pointed to the paradox, or mystery, that society cannot prosper without them, that it must draw on them, but cannot command them.

What about the moral law as such a transcendent motivation of conduct? It goes considerably beyond the public law of the social contract. The latter, we saw, is founded on the rule of enlightened self-interest: *Do ut des*—I give so that I be given to. The law of individual conscience asks more. Under the Golden Rule, for example, I am required to give as I wish to be given to under like circumstances, but not in order that I be given to and not in expectation of return. Reciprocity, essential to the social law, is not a condition of the moral law. One subtle "expectation" and "self-interest," but of the moral order itself, may even then be in my mind: I prefer the environment of a moral society and can expect to contribute to the general morality by my own example. But even if I should always be the dupe, the Golden Rule holds. (If the social law breaks faith with me, I am released from its claim.)

Moral Law and Transmoral Dedication

Can I, then, be called upon to offer myself for medical experimentation in the name of the moral law? *Prima facie*, the Golden Rule seems to apply. I should wish, were I dying of a disease, that enough volunteers in the past had provided enough knowledge through the gift of their bodies that I could now be saved. I should wish, were I desperately in need of a transplant, that the dying patient next door had agreed to a definition of death by which his organs would become available to me in the freshest possible condition. I surely should also wish, were I drowning, that somebody would risk his life, even sacrifice his life, for mine.

But the last example reminds us that only the negative form of the Golden Rule ("Do not do unto others what you do not want done unto yourself") is fully prescriptive. The positive form ("Do unto others as you would wish them to do unto you"), in whose compass our issue falls, points into an infinite, open horizon where prescriptive force soon ceases. We may well say of somebody that he ought to have come to the succor of B, to have shared with him in his need, and the like. But we may not say that he ought to have given his life for him. To have done so would be praiseworthy; not to have done so is not blameworthy. It cannot be asked of him; if he fails to do so, he reneges on no duty. But *he* may say of himself, and only he, that he ought to have given his life. *This* "ought" is strictly between him and himself, or between him and God; no outside party—fellow man or society—can appropriate its voice. It can humbly receive the supererogatory gifts from the free enactment of it.

We must, in other words, distinguish between moral obligation and the much larger sphere of moral value. (This, incidentally, shows up the error in the widely held view of value theory that the higher a value, the stronger its claim and the greater the duty to realize it. The highest are in a region beyond duty and claim.) The ethical dimension far exceeds that of the moral law and reaches into the sublime solitude of dedication and ultimate commitment, away from all reckoning and rule—in short, into the sphere of the *holy*. From there alone can the offer of self-sacrifice genuinely spring, and this—its source—must be honored religiously. How? The first duty here falling on the research community, when it enlists and uses this source, is the safeguarding of true authenticity and spontaneity.

The "Conscription" of Consent

But here we must realize that the mere issuing of the appeal, the calling for volunteers, with the moral and social pressures it inevitably generates, amounts even under the most meticulous rules of consent to a sort of *conscripting*. And some soliciting is necessarily involved. This was in part meant by the earlier remark that in this area sin and guilt can perhaps not be wholly avoided. And this is why "consent," surely a non-negotiable minimum requirement, is not the full answer to the problem. Granting then that soliciting and therefore some degree of conscripting are part of the situation, who may conscript and who may be conscripted? Or less harshly expressed: Who should issue appeals and to whom?

The naturally qualified issuer of the appeal is the research scientist himself, collectively the main carrier of the impulse and the only one with the technical competence to judge. But his being very much an interested party (with vested interests, indeed, not purely in the public good, but in the scientific enterprise as such, in "his" project, and even in his career) makes him also suspect. The ineradicable dialectic of this situation—a delicate incompatibility problem—calls for particular controls by the research community and by public authority that we need not discuss. They can mitigate, but not eliminate the problem. We have to live with the ambiguity, the treacherous impurity of everything human.

Self-Recruitment of the Research Community

To whom should the appeal be addressed? The natural issuer of the call is also the first natural addressee; the physician-researcher himself and the scientific confraternity at large. With such a coincidence—indeed, the noble tradition with which the whole business of human experimentation started—almost all of the associated legal, ethical, and metaphysical problems vanish. If it is full, autonomous identification of the subject with the purpose that is required for the dignifying of his serving as a subject—here it is; if strongest motivation—here it is; if fullest understanding—here it is; if freest decision—here it is; if greatest integration with the person's total, chosen pursuit—here it is. With self-solicitation, the issue of consent in all its insoluble equivocality is bypassed *per se*. Not even the condition that the particular purpose be truly important and the project reasonably promising, which must hold in any solicitation of others, need be satisfied here. By himself, the scientist is free to obey his obsession, to play his hunch, to wager on chance, to follow the lure of ambition. It is all part of the "divine madness" that somehow animates the ceaseless pressing against frontiers. For the rest of society, which has a deep-seated disposition to look with reverence and awe upon the guardians of the mysteries of life, the profession assumes with this proof of its devotion the role of a self-chosen, consecrated fraternity, not unlike the monastic orders of the past; and this would come nearest to the actual, religious origins of the art of healing.

It would be the ideal, but not a real solution to keep the issue of human experimentation within the research community itself. Neither in numbers nor in variety of material would its potential suffice for the many-pronged, systematic, continual attack on disease into which the lonely exploits of the early investigators have grown. Statistical requirements alone make their voracious demands; were it not for what I have called the essentially "gratuitous" nature of the whole enterprise of progress, as against the mandatory respect for invasion-proof selfhood, the simplest answer would be to keep the whole population enrolled, and let the lot, or an equivalent of draft boards, decide which of each category will at any one time be called up for "service." It is not difficult to picture societies with whose philosophy this would be consonant. We are agreed that ours is not one such and should not become one. The specter of it is indeed among the threatening utopias on our own horizon from which we should recoil, and of whose advent by imperceptible steps we must beware. How then can our mandatory faith be honored when the recruitment for experimentation goes outside the scientific community, as it must in honoring another commitment of no mean dignity? We simply repeat the former question: To whom should the call be addressed?

"Identification" as the Principle of Recruitment in General

If the properties we adduced as the particular qualifications of the members of the scientific fraternity itself are taken as general criteria of selection, then one should look for additional subjects where a maximum of identification, understanding, and spontaneity can be expected—that is, among the most highly motivated, the most highly educated, and the least "captive" members of the community. From this naturally scarce resource, a descending order of permissibility leads to greater abundance and ease of supply, whose use should become proportionately more hesitant as the exculpating criteria are relaxed. An inversion of normal "market" behavior is demanded here —namely, to accept the lowest quotation last (and excused only by the greatest pressure of need), to pay the highest price first.

As such a rule of selection is bound to be rather hard on the number-hungry research industry, it will be asked: Why all the fuss? At this point we had better spell out some of the things we have been tacitly presupposing all the time. What is wrong with making a person an experimental subject is not so much that we make him thereby a means (which happens in social contexts of all kinds), as that we make him a thing—a passive thing merely to be acted on, and passive not even for real action, but for token action whose token object he is. His being is reduced to that of a mere token or "sample." This is different from even the most exploitative situations of social life; there the business is real, not fictitious. The subject, however much abused, remains an agent and thus a "subject" in the other sense of the word. The soldier's case, referred to earlier, is instructive: Subject to most unilateral discipline, forced to risk mutilation and death, conscripted without, perhaps against, his will—he is still conscripted with his capacities to act, to hold his own or fail in situations, to meet real challenges for real stakes. Though a mere "number" to the High Command, he is not a token and not a thing. (Imagine what he would say if it turned out that the war was a game staged to sample observations on his endurance, courage, or cowardice.)

These compensations of personhood are denied to the subject of experimentation, who is acted upon for an extraneous end without being engaged in a real relation where he would be the counterpoint to the other or to circumstance. Mere "consent" (mostly amounting to no more than permission) does not right this reification. The "wrong" of it can only be made "right" by such authentic identification with the cause that it is the subject's as well as the researcher's cause—whereby his role in its service is not just permitted by him, but *willed*. That sovereign will of his which embraces the end as his own restores his personhood to the otherwise depersonalizing context. To be valid it must be autonomous and informed. The latter condition can, outside the research community, only be fulfilled by degrees; but the higher the degree of the understanding regarding the purpose and the technique, the more valid becomes the endorsement of the will. A margin of mere trust inevitably remains. Ultimately, the appeal for volunteers should seek this free and generous endorsement, the appropriation of the research purpose into the person's own scheme of ends. Thus, the appeal is in truth addressed to the one, mysterious, and sacred source of any such generosity of the will—"devotion," whose forms and objects of commitment are various and may invest different motivations in different individuals. The following, for instance, may be responsive to the "call" we are discussing: compassion with human suffering, zeal for humanity, reverence for the Golden Rule, enthusiasm for progress, homage to the cause of knowledge, even longing for sacrificial justification (do not call that "masochism," please). On all these, I say, it is defensible and right to draw when the research objective is worthy enough: and it is a prime duty of the research community (especially in view of what we called the "margin of trust") to see that this sacred source is never abused for frivolous ends. For a less than adequate cause, not even the freest, unsolicited offer should be accepted.

The Rule of the "Descending Order" and Its Counter-Utility Sense

We have laid down what must seem to be a forbidding rule. Having faith in the transcendent potential of man, I do not fear that the "source" will ever fail a society that does not destroy it—and only such a one is worthy of the blessings of progress. But "elitistic" the rule is (as is the enterprise of progress itself), and elites are by nature small. The combined attribute of motivation and information, plus the absence of external pressures, tends to be socially so circumscribed that strict adherence to the rule might numerically starve the research process. This is why I spoke of a descending order of permissibility, which is itself permissive, but where the realization that it is a *descending* order is not without pragmatic import. Departing from the august norm, the appeal must needs shift from idealism to docility, from high-mindedness to compliance, from judgment to trust. Consent spreads over the whole spectrum. I will not go into the casuistics of this penumbral area. I merely indicate the principle of the order of preference: The poorer in knowledge, motivation, and freedom of decision (and that, alas, means the more readily available in terms of numbers and possible manipulation), the more sparingly and indeed reluctantly should the reservoir be used, and the more compelling must therefore become the countervailing justification.

Let us note that this is the opposite of a social utility standard, the reverse of the order by "availability and expendability": The most valuable and scarcest, the least expendable elements of the social organism, are to be the first candidates for risk and sacrifice. It is the standard of *noblesse oblige*; and with all its counter-utility and seeming "wastefulness," we feel a rightness about it and perhaps even a higher "utility," for the soul of the community lives by this spirit.[6] It is also the opposite of what the day-to-day interests of research clamor for, and for the scientific community to honor it will mean that it will have to fight a strong temptation to go by routine to the readiest sources of supply—the suggestible, the ignorant, the dependent, the "captive" in various senses.[7] I do not believe that heightened resistance here must cripple research, which cannot be permitted; but it may slow it down by the smaller numbers fed into experimentation in consequence. This price—a possibly slower rate of progress—may have to be paid for the preservation of the most precious capital of higher communal life.

Experimentation on Patients

So far we have been speaking on the tacit assumption that the subjects of experimentation are recruited from among the healthy. To the question "Who is conscriptable?" the spontaneous answer is: Least and last of all the sick—the most available source as they are under treatment and observation anyway. That the afflicted should not be called upon to bear additional burden and risk, that they are society's special trust and the physician's particular trust—these are elementary responses of our moral sense. Yet the very destination of medical research, the conquest of disease, requires at the crucial stage trial and verification on precisely the sufferers from the disease, and their total exemption would defeat the purpose itself. In acknowledging this inescapable necessity, we enter the most sensitive area of the whole complex, the one most keenly felt and most searchingly discussed by the practitioners themselves. This issue touches the heart of the doctor-patient relation, putting its most solemn obligations to the test. Some of the oldest verities of this area should be recalled.

The Fundamental Privilege of the Sick

In the course of treatment, the physician is obligated to the patient and to no one else. He is not the agent of society, nor of the interests of medical science, the patient's family, the patient's co-sufferers, or future sufferers from the same disease. The patient alone counts when he is under the physician's care. By the simple law of bilateral contract (analogous, for example, to the relation of lawyer to client and its "conflict of interest" rule), he is bound not to let any other interest interfere with that of the patient in being cured. But manifestly more sublime norms than contractual ones are involved. We may speak of a sacred trust; strictly by its terms, the doctor is, as it were, alone with his patient and God.

There is one normal exception to this—that is, to the doctor's not being the agent of society vis-à-vis the patient, but the trustee of his interests alone—the quarantining of the contagious sick. This is plainly not for the patient's interest, but for that of others threatened by him. (In vaccination, we have a combination of both: protection of the individual and others.) But preventing the patient from causing harm to others is not the same as exploiting him for the advantage of others. And there is, of course, the abnormal exception of collective catastrophe, the analogue to a state of war. The physician who desperately battles a raging epidemic is under a unique dispensation that suspends in a nonspecifiable way some of the strictures of normal practice, including possibly those against experimental liberties with his patients. No rules can be devised for the waiving of rules in extremities. And as with the famous shipwreck examples of ethical theory, the less said about it the better. But what is allowable there and may later be passed over in forgiving silence cannot serve as a precedent. We are concerned with non-extreme, non-emergency conditions where the voice of principle can be heard and claims can be adjudicated free from duress. We have conceded that there are such claims, and that if there is to be medical advance at all, not even the superlative privilege of the suffering and the sick can be kept wholly intact from the intrusion of its needs. About this least palatable, most disquieting part of our subject, I have to offer only groping, inconclusive remarks.

The Principle of "Identification" Applied to Patients

On the whole, the same principles would seem to hold here as are found to hold with "normal subjects": motivation, identification, understanding on the part of the subject. But it is clear that these conditions are peculiarly difficult to satisfy with regard to a patient. His physical state, psychic preoccupation, dependent relation to the doctor, the submissive attitude induced by treatment—everything connected with his condition and situation makes the sick person inherently less of a sovereign person than the healthy one. Spontaneity of self-offering has almost to be ruled out; consent is marred by lower resistance or captive circumstance, and so on. In fact, all the factors that make the patient, as a category, particularly accessible and welcome for experimentation at the same time compromise the quality of the responding affirmation that must morally redeem the making use of them. This, in addition to the primacy of the physician's duty, puts a heightened onus on the physician-researcher to limit his undue power to the most important and defensible research objectives and, of course, to keep persuasion at a minimum.

Still, with all the disabilities noted, there is scope among patients for observing the rule of the "descending order of permissibility" that we have laid down for normal subjects, in vexing inversion of the utility order of quantitative abundance and qualitative "expendability." By the principle of this order, those patients who most identify with and are cognizant of the cause of research—members of the medical profession (who after all are sometimes patients themselves)—come first; the highly motivated and educated, also least dependent, among the lay patients come next; and so on down the line. An added consideration here is seriousness of condition, which again operates in inverse proportion. Here the profession must fight the tempting sophistry that the hopeless case is expendable (because in prospect already expended) and therefore especially usable; and generally the attitude that the poorer the chances of the patient the more justifiable his recruitment for experimentation (other than for his own benefit). The opposite is true.

Nondisclosure as a Borderline Case

Then there is the case where ignorance of the subject, sometimes even of the experimenter, is of the essence of the experiment (the "double blind"-control group-placebo syndrome). It is said to be a necessary element of the scientific process. Whatever may be said about its ethics in regard to normal subjects, especially volunteers, it is an outright betrayal of trust in regard to the patient who believes that he is receiving treatment. Only supreme importance of the objective can exonerate it, without making it less of a transgression. The patient is definitely wronged even when not harmed. And ethics apart, the practice of such deception holds the danger of undermining the faith in the bona fides of treatment, the beneficial intent of the physician—the very basis of the doctor-patient relationship. In every respect, it follows that concealed experiment on patients—that is, experiment under the guise of treatment—should be the rarest exception, at best, if it cannot be wholly avoided.

This has still the merit of a borderline problem. This is not true of the other case of necessary ignorance of the subject—that of the unconscious patient. Drafting him for nontherapeutic experiments is simply and unqualifiedly impermissible; progress or not, he must never be used, on the inflexible principle that utter helplessness demands utter protection.

When preparing this paper, I filled pages with a casuistics of this harrowing field, but then scratched out most of it, realizing my dilettante status. The shadings are endless, and only the physician-researcher can discern them properly as the cases arise. Into his lap the decision is thrown. The philosophical rule, once it has admitted into itself the idea of a sliding scale, cannot really specify its own application. It can only impress on the practitioner a general maxim or attitude for the exercise of his judgment and conscience in the concrete occasions of his work. In our case, I am afraid, it means making life more difficult for him.

It will also be noted that, somewhat at variance with the emphasis in the literature, I have not dwelt on the elements of "risk" and very little on that of "consent." Discussion of the first is beyond the layman's competence; the emphasis on the second has been lessened because of its equivocal character. It is a truism to say that one should strive to minimize the risk and to maximize the consent. The more demanding concept of "identification," which I have used, includes "consent" in its maximal or authentic form, and the assumption of risk is its privilege.

No Experiments on Patients Unrelated to Their Own Disease

Although my ponderings have, on the whole, yielded points of view rather than definite prescriptions, premises rather than conclusions, they have led me to a few unequivocal yeses and noes. The first is the emphatic rule that patients should be experimented upon, if at all, *only* with reference to *their* disease. Never should there be added to the gratuitousness of the experiment as such the gratuitousness of service to an unrelated cause. This follows simply from what we have found to be the *only* excuse for infracting the special exemptions of the sick at all—namely, that the scientific war on disease cannot accomplish its goal without drawing the sufferers from disease into the investigative process. If under this excuse they become subjects of experiment, they do so *because*, and only because, of *their* disease.

This is the fundamental and self-sufficient consideration. That the patient cannot possibly benefit from the unrelated experiment therapeutically, while he might from experiments related to his condition, is also true, but lies beyond the problem area of pure experiment. Anyway, I am discussing nontherapeutic experimentation only, where *ex hypothesi* the patient does not benefit. Experiment as part of therapy—that is, directed toward helping the subject himself—is a different matter altogether and raises its own problems, but hardly philosophical ones. As long as a doctor can say, even if only in his own thought: "There is no known cure for your condition (or: You have responded to none); but there is promise in a new treatment still under investigation, not quite tested yet as to effectiveness and safety; you will be taking a chance, but all things considered, I judge it in your best interest to let me try it on you"—as long as he can speak thus, he speaks as the patient's physician and may err, but does not transform the patient into a subject of experimentation. Introduction of an untried therapy into the treatment where the tried ones have failed is not "experimentation on the patient."

Generally, there is something "experimental" (because tentative) about every individual treatment, beginning with the diagnosis itself; and he would be a poor doctor who would not learn from every case for the benefit of future cases, and a poor member of the profession who would not make any new insights gained from his treatments available to the profession at large. Thus, knowledge may be advanced in the treatment of any patient, and the interest of the medical art and all sufferers from the same affliction as well as the patient may be served if something happens to be learned from his case. But this gain to knowledge and future therapy is incidental to the *bona fide* service to the present patient. He has the right to expect that the doctor does nothing to him just in order to learn.

In that case, the doctor's imaginary speech would run, for instance, like this: "There is nothing more I can do for you. But you can do something for me. Speaking no longer as your physician but on behalf of medical science, we could learn a great deal about future cases of this kind if you would permit me to perform certain experiments on you. It is understood that you yourself would not benefit from any knowledge we might gain; but future patients would." This statement would express the purely experimental situation, assumedly here with the subject's concurrence and with all cards on the table. In Alexander Bickel's words: "It is a different situation when the doctor is no longer trying to make [the patient] well, but is trying to find out how to make others well in the future."[8]

But even in the second case of the nontherapeutic experiment where the patient does not benefit, the patient's own disease is enlisted in the cause of fighting that disease, even if only in others. It is yet another thing to say or think: "Since you are here—in the hospital with its facilities—under our care and observation, away from your job (or, perhaps, doomed), we wish to profit from your being available for some other research of great interest we are presently engaged in." From the standpoint of merely medical ethics, which has only to consider risk, consent, and the worth of the objective, there may be no cardinal difference between this case and the last one. I hope that my medical audience will not think I am making too fine a point when I say that from the standpoint of the subject and his dignity there is a cardinal difference that crosses the line between the permissible and the impermissible, and this by the same principle of "identification" I have been invoking all along. Whatever the rights and wrongs of any experimentation on any patient—in the one case, at least that residue of identification is left him that it is his own affliction by which he can contribute to the conquest of that affliction his own kind of suffering which he helps to alleviate in others; and so in a sense it is his own cause. It is totally indefensible to rob the unfortunate of this intimacy with the purpose and make his misfortune a convenience for the furtherance of alien concerns. The observance of this rule is essential, I think, to attenuate at least the wrong that nontherapeutic experimenting on patients commits in any case.

On the Redefinition of Death

My other emphatic verdict concerns the question of the redefinition of death—acknowledging "irreversible coma as a new definition for death."[9] I wish not to be misunderstood. As long as it is merely a question of when it is permitted to cease the artificial prolongation of certain functions (like heartbeat) traditionally regarded as signs of life, I do not see anything ominous in the notion of "brain death." Indeed, a new definition of death is not even necessary to legitimize the same result if one adopts the position of the Roman Catholic Church, which here for once is eminently reasonable—namely that "when deep unconsciousness is judged to be permanent, extraordinary means to maintain life are not obligatory. They can be terminated and the patient allowed to die."[10] Given a clearly defined negative condition of the brain, the physician is allowed to allow the patient to die his own death by any definition, which of itself will lead through the gamut of all possible definitions. But a disquietingly contradictory purpose is combined with this purpose in the quest for a new definition of death, in the will to advance the moment of declaring him dead: Permission not to turn off the respirator, but, on the contrary, to keep it on and thereby maintain the body in a state of what would have been "life" by the older definition (but is only a "simulacrum" of life by the new) —so as to get at his organs and tissues under the ideal conditions of what would previously have been "vivisection."[11]

Now this, whether done for research or transplant purposes,

seems to me to overstep what the definition can warrant. Surely it is one thing when to cease delaying death, but another when to start doing violence to the body; one thing when to desist from protracting the process of dying, but another when to regard that process as complete and thereby the body as a cadaver free for inflicting on it what would be torture and death to any living body. For the first purpose, we need not know the exact borderline with absolute certainty between life and death—we leave it to nature to cross it wherever it is, or to traverse the whole spectrum if there is not just one line. All we need to know is that coma is irreversible. For the second purpose we must know the borderline; and to use any definition short of the maximal for perpetrating on a *possibly* penultimate state what only the ultimate state can permit is to arrogate a knowledge which, I think, we cannot possibly have. *Since we do not know the exact borderline between life and death,* nothing less than the maximum definition of death will do—brain death plus heart death plus any other indication that may be pertinent—before final violence is allowed to be done.

It would follow then, for this layman at least, that the use of the definition should itself be defined, and this in a restrictive sense. When only permanent coma can be gained with the artificial sustaining of functions, by all means turn off the respirator, the stimulator, any sustaining artifice, and let the patient die; but let him die all the way. Do not, instead, arrest the process and start using him as a mine while, with your own help and cunning, he is still kept this side of what may in truth be the final line. Who is to say that a shock, a final trauma, is not administered to a sensitivity diffusely situated elsewhere than in the brain and still vulnerable to suffering? a sensitivity that we ourselves have been keeping alive? No fiat of definition can settle this question.[12] But I wish to emphasize that the question of possible suffering (easily brushed aside by a sufficient show of reassuring expert consensus) is merely a subsidiary and not the real point of my argument; this, to reiterate, turns on the indeterminacy of the boundaries between *life and death,* not between sensitivity and insensitivity, and bids us to lean toward a maximal rather than a minimal determination of death in an area of basic uncertainty.

There is also this to consider: The patient must be absolutely sure that his doctor does not become his executioner, and that no definition authorizes him ever to become one. His right to this certainty is absolute, and so is his right to his own body with all its organs. Absolute respect for these rights violates no one else's rights, for no one has a right to another's body. Speaking in still another, religious vein: The expiring moments should be watched over with piety and be safe from exploitation.

I strongly feel, therefore, that it should be made quite clear that the proposed new definition of death is to authorize *only* the one and *not* the other of the two opposing things: only to break off a sustaining intervention and let things take their course, not to keep up the sustaining intervention for a final intervention of the most destructive kind.

There would now have to be said something about nonmedical experiments on human subjects, notably psychological and genetic, of which I have not lost sight. But having overextended my limits of space by the most generous interpretation, I must leave this for another occasion. Let me only say in conclusion that if some of the practical implications of my reasonings are felt to work out toward a slower rate of progress, this should not cause too great dismay. Let us not forget that progress is an optional goal, not an unconditional commitment, and that its tempo in particular, compulsive as it may become, has nothing sacred about it. Let us also remember that a slower progress in the conquest of disease would not threaten society, grievous as it is to those who have to deplore that their particular disease be not yet conquered, but that society would indeed be threatened by the erosion of those moral values whose loss, possibly caused by too ruthless a pursuit of scientific progress, would make its most dazzling triumphs not worth having. Let us finally remember that it cannot be the aim of progress to abolish the lot of mortality. Of some ill or other, each of us will die. Our mortal condition is upon us with its harshness but also its wisdom—because without it there would not be the eternally renewed promise of the freshness, immediacy, and eagerness of youth; nor, without it, would there be for any of us the incentive to number our days and make them count. With all our striving to wrest from our mortality what we can, we should bear its burden with patience and dignity.

REFERENCES

1. G. E. W. Wolstenholme and Maeve O'Connor (eds.), *CIBA Foundation Symposium, Ethics in Medical Progress: With Special Reference to Transplantation* (Boston, 1966); "The Changing Mores of Biomedical Research," *Annals of Internal Medicine* (Supplement 7), Vol. 67, No. 3 (Philadelphia, September, 1967); *Proceedings of the Conference on the Ethical Aspects of Experimentation on Human Subjects,* November 3-4, 1967 (Boston, Massachusetts; hereafter called *Proceedings*); H. K. Beecher, "Some Guiding Principles for Clinical Investigation," *Journal of the American Medical Association,* Vol. 195 (March 28, 1966), pp. 1135-36. H. K. Beecher, "Consent in Clinical Experimentation: Myth and Reality," *Journal of the American Medical Association,* Vol. 195 (January 3, 1966), pp. 34-35; P. A.

Freund, "Ethical Problems in Human Experimentation," *New England Journal of Medicine*, Vol. 273 (September 23, 1965), pp. 687-92; P. A. Freund, "Is the Law Ready for Human Experimentation?", *American Psychologist*, Vol. 22 (1967), pp. 394-99; W. Wolfensberger, "Ethical Issues in Research with Human Subjects," *World Science*, Vol. 155 (January 6, 1967), pp. 47-51; See also a series of five articles by Drs. Schoen, McGrath, and Kennedy, "Principles of Medical Ethics," which appeared from August to December in Volume 23 of *Arizona Medicine*. The most recent entry in the growing literature is E. Fuller Torrey (ed.), *Ethical Issues in Medicine* (New York, 1968), in which the chapter "Ethical Problems in Human Experimentation" by Otto E. Guttentag should be especially noted.

2. Wolfensberger, "Ethical Issues in Research with Human Subjects," p. 48.

3. *Proceedings*, p. 29.

4. *Die Braut von Korinth:* "Victims do fall here,/Neither lamb nor steer,/Nay, but human offerings untold."

5. *Proceedings*, pp. 50-51.

6. Socially, everyone is expendable relatively—that is, in different degrees; religiously, no one is expendable absolutely: The "image of God" is in all. If it can be enhanced, then not by any one being expended, but by someone expending himself.

7. This refers to captives of circumstance, not of justice. Prison inmates are with respect to our problem in a special class. If we hold to some idea of guilt, and to the supposition that our judicial system is not entirely at fault, they may be held to stand in a special debt to society, and their offer to serve—from whatever motive—may be accepted with a minimum of qualms as a means of reparation.

8. *Proceedings*, p. 33. To spell out the difference between the two cases: In the first case, the patient himself is meant to be the beneficiary of the experiment, and directly so; the "subject" of the experiment is at the same time its object, its end. It is performed not for gaining knowledge, but for helping him—and helping him in the *act* of performing it, even if by its results it also contributes to a broader testing process currently under way. It is in fact part of the treatment itself and an "experiment" only in the loose sense of being untried and highly tentative. But whatever the degree of uncertainty, the motivating anticipation (the wager, if you like) is for success, and success here means the subject's own good. To a pure experiment, by contrast, undertaken to gain knowledge, the difference of success and failure is not germane, only that of conclusiveness and inconclusiveness. The "negative" result has as much to teach as the "positive." Also, the true experiment is an act distinct from the uses later made of the findings. And, most important, the subject experimented on is distinct from the eventual beneficiaries of those findings: He lets himself be used as a means toward an end external to himself (even if he should at some later time happen to be among the beneficiaries himself). With respect to his own present needs and his own good, the act is gratuitous.

9. "A Definition of Irreversible Coma," Report of the *Ad Hoc* Committee of Harvard Medical School to Examine the Definition of Brain Death, *Journal of the American Medical Association*, Vol. 205, No. 6 (August 5, 1968), pp. 337-40.

10. As rendered by Dr. Beecher in *Proceedings*, p. 50.

11. The Report of the *Ad Hoc* Committee no more than indicates this possibility with the second of the "two reasons why there is need for a definition": "(2) Obsolete criteria for the definition of death can lead to controversy in obtaining organs for

transplantation." The first reason is relief from the burden of indefinitely drawn out coma. The report wisely confines its recommendations on application to what falls under this first reason—namely, turning off the respirator—and remains silent on the possible use of the definition under the second reason. But when "the patient is declared dead on the basis of these criteria," the road to the other use has theoretically been opened and will be taken (if I remember rightly, it has even been taken once, in a much debated case in England), unless it is blocked by a special barrier in good time. The above is my feeble attempt to help doing so.

12. Only a Cartesian view of the "animal machine," which I somehow see lingering here, could set the mind at rest, as in historical fact it did at its time in the matter of vivisection: But its truth is surely not established by definition.

16 *The Ethical Design of Human Experiments*

DAVID D. RUTSTEIN, M.D.

Beginning with the premise that it is ethical to experiment on humans in carefully controlled conditions, Rutstein goes on to the specific problem of how to design scientific experiments that will both produce the information needed and yet be ethical. This focus helps us to think our way through the many dilemmas inherent in this situation. The presentation is enhanced by its balanced blending of both ethical reasoning and scientific analysis. Rutstein clearly states his premise and arguments and thus provides the opportunity to engage in a genuine ethical and scientific dialogue.

Dr. David D. Rutstein, M.D., is Ridly Watts Professor of Preventive Medicine at Harvard Medical School

This analysis of the ethical considerations governing human experiments is based on the assumption that it is ethical under carefully controlled conditions to study on human beings mechanisms of health and disease and to test new drugs, biological products, procedures, methods, and instruments that give promise of improving the health of human beings, of preventing or treating their diseases, or postponing their untimely deaths. Without such an assumption, there can be no systematic method of medical advance. Progress would have to depend on the surreptitious, illegal, or unsupervised research and testing of new modes of prevention and treatment of disease. The ethical standards of such irregular activities would certainly be at a far lower level than can be guaranteed when the testing of new methods of treatment is openly practiced.

Proceeding on that assumption, how can one design experiments upon human beings that will yield the desired scientific information and yet avoid or keep ethical contraindications to a minimum? This question is asked in the belief that in the design of the experiment itself many ethical dilemmas may be resolved. Attention must be given to the ways an experiment can be designed to maintain its scientific validity, meet ethical requirements, and yet yield the necessary new knowledge.

Let us concentrate on laying out new guidelines that might lead to the solution of ethical problems rather than on focusing our attention on the difficulties that these problems present. The ethical requirements that have created the most difficulty are obtaining informed consent from the potential subject; the need for the subject to derive a health benefit from the experiment; and keeping the risk to the subject as small as possible. Such questions are important and relevant because ethical considerations are paramount when experiments are to be performed on human subjects. It is the thesis of this essay that in the design of a human experiment it is mandatory to select those experimental conditions, subjects, and methods of measurement that impose the fewest ethical constraints. Such an approach will not cause the ethical problems of human experiments to disappear. If a definitive attempt is made, during the planning stages of an experiment on human beings, to keep the ethical as well as scientific criteria in mind, it is possible often to perform the necessary research to yield the desired information.

Scientifically Unsound Studies Are Unethical

It may be accepted as a *maxim that a poorly or improperly designed study involving human subjects*—one that could not possibly yield scientific facts (that is, reproducible observations) relevant to the question under study—*is by definition unethical.* Moreover, when a study is in itself scientifically invalid, all other ethical considerations become irrelevant. There is no point in obtaining "informed consent" to perform a useless study. A worthless study cannot possibly benefit anyone, least of all the experimental subject himself. Any risk to the patient, however small, cannot be justified. In essence, the scientific validity of a study on human beings is in itself an ethical principle.

How, then, can the experimental human subject be protected from incompetent investigators so that he will not become a victim in feckless studies? There are *two lines of* defense. The research committee of a medical school, institution, or hospital must be concerned with the ethical principles as well as the scientific validity of the proposals placed before them. To perform this task effectively, every committee must have among its membership a biostatistician to insure scientific validity and an expert (for whom there is as yet no name) who is concerned with the ethical aspects of human experimentation. The biostatistician can assist the committee in evaluating the scientific quality of the proposed investigation and make recommendations for improvement of the scientific aspects of the study design. *Experiments on human beings must not be performed without a carefully drawn protocol, which in turn can best be prepared in consultation with experts in study design.* In the same way, experts in the ethical aspects of human experimentation should assist the committee in passing on the ethical issues of proposed studies and in recommending modifications that might make the studies ethically acceptable.

The second line of defense can be provided by editors and editorial boards of journals that publish scientific reports of human experiments. If higher scientific standards of publication were established and adhered to, it would soon become clear to investigators that there would be small likelihood that improperly designed studies would be published. Automatically, many human subjects would be protected against participation in unsound and unethical medical research. When there has been a clear-cut violation of ethical principles, scientific reports of human studies should be refused publication. The reason for such refusal should be clearly stated.

For appropriate evaluation of manuscripts, therefore, the membership of editorial boards should include biostatisticians and experts in the ethical aspects of human experimentation to provide advice to the board and to the editor in their respective fields.

Anticipating Ethical Problems

Whenever possible, it is necessary to anticipate serious ethical problems in human experimentation in order to explore ways in which they can be avoided or kept to a minimum in the design of the experiment. The experiments in human heart transplantation are a case in point, particularly in the selection of the heart donor.

Death is not a simultaneous, instantaneous event for all of the organs of the body. Some organs die earlier than others—the brain being the most vulnerable. It is evident that the heart must be "alive" and free of disease at the time of transplantation if it is to be useful to the recipient. The selection of the heart donor, therefore, cannot be based on his "total death" in the usual sense—that is, a lack of any spontaneous activity and the complete absence of cerebral, cardiac, and pulmonary activity and of spinal reflex function.

As experience with this operation is accumulating, everyone concerned is becoming increasingly aware that to comply with both the scientific and ethical constraints, donor selection must be the responsibility of a specially constituted committee in hospitals where transplantation is performed and must not have among its members any member of the transplantation team. Within such a protective structure, the eligibility of the donor will in effect depend primarily on his having complete and irreversible cessation of cerebral function while the heart remains as normal as possible. Indeed, there may be clinical or electrocardiographic evidence at the time of donor selection that the heart continues to beat.

These criteria of eligibility represent a revolution in our cultural concept of death—and it has occurred by default. The dramatic nature of the heart transplant operation has obscured the underlying change in our ethical concept of deciding when an individual is dead—that is, when a physician may act as if there is no longer any need for treating the patient "to save his life." Until recently, if the heart were still beating, treatment would continue. It is remarkable that this major ethical change has occurred right before our eyes, and that this change is more and more widely accepted with little public discussion of its significance.

This new definition of heart donor eligibility that substitutes "irreversible brain damage" for "total death" raises more questions than it answers. Does acceptance of this concept mean that it is no longer necessary to treat, for example, the senile patient who would meet such criteria? How do eligible donors differ in principle from totally feeble-minded individuals? What are the implications for the inheritance of property if the heart of an intestate donor is kept beating with a pacemaker while the search for a recipient goes on and the donor's wife dies during the interval? Does this new definition of death for the heart donor open up new channels of criminal activity that will lead to the burking of patients to increase the supply of eligible donors?

Let us examine the nature of this revolutionary change in our ethics and pursue its implications to their logical conclusion. Substituting "irreversible brain damage" for "complete absence of any living manifestations in any organ" as essential in the diagnosis of "death" forces us to examine the meaning of the phrase "irreversible brain damage." The presently recommended definition of "irreversible brain damage" demands a complete absence of all manifestations of brain function, all the way from the higher levels of cortical activity down through the centers governing the emotions, sensations, automatic functions, and muscular control and including the spinal reflexes with, however, two special exceptions—the centers controlling respiration and circulation. These centers are excluded for practical and not for ethical reasons. In severely ill patients, the function of these centers can be taken over by machines that may not be stopped until the diagnosis of death is made on other counts. Moreover, for successful heart transplantation, the heart must be "alive" if it is to benefit the recipient.

Why do we insist on the absence of all activity of all of the other subcortical centers if we are willing in our diagnosis of irreversible brain damage to disregard these two centers of essentially automatic function? Again the reason is a practical one. We do not yet know how to make a firm diagnosis of irreversible brain damage limited to the higher cortical centers. We therefore turn in our ignorance to the requirement that all nervous activity be absent (with the exceptions noted) as the basis for the new diagnosis of "death." Again we are confronted with a practical and not a conceptual or ethical reason.

It is clear that in accepting the new definition of "irreversible brain damage" as equivalent to death in man, we are really concerned only with irreversible damage of higher cortical centers. We are saying that in man "life" exists only when he is aware of and can respond to his environment or, if he cannot, that he may recover to a point where he will react consciously within his environment. It remains then for intensive research to be conducted so that physicians will be able to identify specifically the irreversible loss of activity of higher cortical centers and distiguish it from lower reflex function. If, as a result, a reliable diagnosis of irreversible damage of higher cortical centers could be made and this concept generally accepted, the new diagnosis of death would be concerned only with the permanent loss of those functions that distinguish man from other animals. Eventually, many of the great problems imposed on society with its growing senile population might be overcome. In the meantime, however, it should be clear to all of us that such a concept has already been accepted in principle by those who would replace "irreversible brain damage" for "total absence of the functions of all organs" as satisfactory for the diagnosis of death in man.

It would have been better if some of these questions had been explored before the first heart transplantation was performed. Heart donor eligibility is becoming so complex that in the present stage of diagnosis the ethical problem of donor eligibility might best be avoided by the development of a suitable mechanical heart.

Asking the Right Question

The design of an experiment depends at first on the question asked by the investigator. Some questions are in themselves unethical. One cannot ask whether plague bacilli are more virulent in human beings when injected into the bloodstream than when they are sprayed into the throat. One may obtain hints as to the answer to such a question by epidemiologic comparison of the spread of pneumonic plague (spread from the lungs into the air) and bubonic plague (spread by insect bite). Anecdotal information on the spread of plague can also be obtained through the study of laboratory accidents. But a deliberate experiment to answer this question cannot be performed.

The human experiments performed by the Nazis during World

War II horrified the world because they were designed to answer unethical questions. "How long can a human being survive in ice cold water?" will, it is to be hoped, never again be a question to be answered by a scientific experiment. Thus, as a first step in the design of any human experiment, we must first be sure that the question itself is an ethical one.

Moreover, an unethical experiment can sometimes be converted into an ethical one by rephrasing the question. In drug testing, for example, it is not ethical to design an experiment to answer the question: "Is treatment of the disease with the new drug more effective than no treatment at all?" In answering such a question, the patients in the control group would literally have to receive "no treatment" and that is completely unacceptable. Instead, if the patients in the control group are given the best possible current treatment of the disease, we may now ask an ethical question: "Is treatment with the new drug more effective than the generally accepted treatment for this particular disease?"

We faced this problem in the design of the United States-United Kingdom Cooperative Rheumatic Fever Study, which was concerned with measuring the relative effectiveness of cortisone and ACTH in the treatment of that disease.[1] We could not give rheumatic fever patients in the control group "no treatment." We would have had to go so far as to prohibit bed rest, which in itself may be helpful to rheumatic fever patients, because patients in bed have a slower heart rate. Instead, we asked the question: "Is treatment with ACTH or cortisone better, worse, or the same as the best generally accepted drug treatment for this disease?"

Our control group, in addition to all the other non-specific treatments which the treated groups also received, were given large doses of aspirin—the generally accepted drug treatment of the time. A question that compares the new treatment with the most effective treatment of the time is not only ethical, but it is also the most practical question. If the new treatment is to replace the generally accepted treatment is must be demonstrated clearly to be better.

With a question framed in that way, one may obtain consent from the patient by explaining that he will receive either the best treatment of the time or the new drug. It is made clear that, although promising in animal and other experiments, the new drug has not yet been shown in human experiments to be better, worse, or the same as the generally accepted treatment. Most patients will accept these alternatives. The investigator himself would be reassured that he has done the best for his patient's health and safety, while evaluating a more promising remedy for his disease.

When designing a human experiment, the question under study

must not be so trivial as not to justify any risk to the human subject. One may not ask whether large doses of a cortico-steroid agent would remove freckles. Nor may there be an excessive risk when compared with the possible benefit of a successful experiment. One may not test in humans a "sure cure" for the common cold which causes paralysis in experimental animals. Thus, in selecting a question for human experimentation, the expectation of benefit to the subject and to mankind must clearly far exceed the risk to the human subject.

Ethical considerations that prohibit certain human experiments are similar in their effects as are scientific constraints on the design of experiments. At the moment, much research on infectious hepatitis, a serious human disease, is impossible because there is no method for isolating infectious hepatitis virus. No laboratory animal has been found which is susceptible to it and no other procedure for its isolation has been developed. This scientific constraint is serious because without isolation of the virus a vaccine cannot be made for the protection of susceptible human beings. Human beings are susceptible and theoretically could be used for the growth of large quantities of virus needed for vaccine manufacture, but now we face the ethical constraint. It is not ethical to use human subjects for the growth of a virus for any purpose. Here, then, we have an example of a scientific constraint that in turn creates an ethical constraint, both of which interfere with the conduct of experiments important to life and health. When asking a question that might be answered by human experimentation, both the scientific and ethical demands must carefully be taken into account. Unless both are satisfied, the experiment cannot be performed.

The Ethics of Controlled Human Experimentation

Controls are essential in such human experiments as the testing of a drug or a surgical procedure. In order to evaluate new therapy, it is necessary to identify those additional benefits of the new remedy which exceed the improvement that might be expected in the course of the natural history of the disease. To be sure, in a disease such as human rabies, which is practically 100 per cent fatal, controlled observations are not needed because any recovery of treated patients is an obvious benefit. Acute leukemia and virulent tumors such as reticulum-cell sarcoma are other examples of diseases whose natural history is one of immutable progression to death and where benefit can be identified without a controlled experiment.

Most diseases do not fall into such a clear-cut category. Even diseases such as cancer of the breast have such a variable course that one is not certain to this moment if surgery prolongs the life of the patient suffering from this disease. The variability of the disease from patient to patient makes it difficult, if not impossible, to evaluate the additional effectiveness of the surgical remedy without a controlled study.

Controlled studies also keep the investigator from leaving the world of reality. The enthusiastic research worker often concentrates on whether the new treatment seems to work. Psychologically, he is apt to pay less attention to possible harmful effects of the new treatment. The result of this attitude is documented repeatedly by the myriad of treatments that make the headlines and promise miraculous cures on the front pages of our best newspapers, only to be completely discarded a few years later. This phenomenon is not without its harmful effects. The definite, albeit limited, benefits of established treatments are often cast aside in favor of the dramatic new, but as yet unproven method of treatment for a human disease. For example, before the advent of the sulfa drugs and antibiotics, there were fairly effective procedures that alleviated and at times cured urinary-tract infection. When these new therapeutic agents became available, some physicians concentrated on intensive therapy with one of the new agents and often felt that it was no longer necessary to practice many of the important details of treatment that had been given in the past. Now, after several decades, there is a gradual return to a more balanced regimen of treatment that places each of the antibiotics in proper perspective in the total treatment of urinary-tract infection. In such situations, a controlled study that is properly performed permits a clean comparison of the helpful and harmful effects of the new treatment and of the older established method of therapy. If, in addition, circumstances permit the ethical use of a placebo control, information can also be obtained about the natural history of the disease.

One might ask whether it is unethical not to perform a controlled human experiment. The Pasteur experiment with rabies vaccine is classic. Controlled human experimentation was completely unknown when Pasteur first tested his new vaccine on those Russian *muzhiks* who were bitten by rabid wolves. All were given the vaccine and all recovered. The result was so dramatic and so electrifying that further experimentation seemed unnecessary. When it was later learned, however, that the chances were relatively low of developing this uniformly fatal disease—human rabies—even after a bite from a known rabid animal, and that the vaccine itself causes paralysis which is not infrequently fatal, it became important to determine whether the vaccine really does more good than harm.

But it became impossible to do a controlled experiment on rabies vaccine. After the general acceptance of the treatment, if a controlled experiment were to be performed, and if a subject in the control group developed rabies, the experimenter might not only be sued for malpractice, but might even be deemed criminally culpable for not having given the patient the "accepted treatment of the time." This same situation is now developing in the estimation of the benefits of heart transplantation and in measuring the value of intensive-care units in the treatment of heart attacks from coronary disease.

In hospitals where heart transplantation is performed, there are many more eligible recipients than donors. It would be relatively easy to randomize the procedure and measure the effectiveness of this new operation. Whenever a heart from a human donor became available, a random selection could be made among all of the eligible recipients. Those not selected would then comprise a control group whose course and outcome could be compared with those of the recipients of a transplanted heart.

The same situation obtains in the treatment of heart attacks from coronary disease in intensive-care units. There is as yet no published control study demonstrating the effectiveness of intensive care in the treatment of acute myocardial infarction. Once again, a control study is possible because in any one center the numbers eligible for care may far exceed the available facilities. A randomly allocated control study would provide the precise information that is needed to estimate the value of this procedure.[2] Instead, we are already beginning to hear ex-cathedra statements of the effectiveness of intensive-care units that are unsupported by the required scientific evidence.

Even up to the present moment, many patients suffer severe discomfort or are permanently harmed from treatments whose validity has been based on uncontrolled observations. Thousands of hypertensive patients in the 1930's and '40's were subjected to extensive surgery for the removal of their thoracolumbar sympathetic nervous system in the belief that the progress of the disease would be arrested. The treatment is no longer used.

Would this problem have been resolved had controlled studies been performed by means of random allocation in which half of the patients would have had sham operations? In an analogous situation when uncontrolled evidence suggested that the internal mammary artery operation might be helpful in the treatment of angina pectoris, Dr. Henry Beecher recommended a study in which the patients in the control groups would be given a sham operation.[3] He indicated that a far smaller total number of human subjects would have been needed and a definitive answer could be obtained by such a procedure. Although scientifically sound, I do not believe that it is ethical to perform sham operations on human subjects because of the operative risk and the lack of potential benefit to the patient. Instead, controlled studies could have been performed with the randomly allocated control patients being given the best medical treatment of the time together with a period of bed rest similar to that of the surgical convalescent.

The history of diseases of unknown etiology is replete with serially accepted and discarded fads of treatment. Peptic ulcer is an example. The Sippy rigid alkali and milk diet became the Meulengracht meat diet and in time became a bland diet with enough alkali to relieve the patient's symptoms. The short-circuiting surgical operation of gastro-enterostomy changed to one for removal of a large portion of the acid-secreting part of the stomach—partial gastrectomy—and then to the less traumatic procedure of removing the nerve supply to the stomach and upper intestine—vagotomy. Along the way, a procedure for freezing the stomach was introduced, then discarded, not because the fad had worn itself out, but because it was obviously harmful. All these treatments might or might not have been accompanied with psychiatric therapy. To this day, the treatment of peptic ulcer, as is the case of many diseases of unknown etiology, is an art with little solid scientific support.

In essence, a new treatment of a disease may be better, worse, or the same as the generally accepted one. The controlled clinical trial has not only been effective in rejecting useless treatments, but perhaps even more helpful in recognizing a harmful therapy, such as the anticoagulant treatment of cerebral thrombosis. That treatment was earning growing acceptance until, in a controlled clinical trial, it was recognized that cerebral hemorrhage was a more frequent complication in the group treated with anticoagulants than among the patients in the control group.[4] The trial was terminated.

One may conclude that if the question under study is an ethical one, and if the design of the study is sound, taking both the scientific and the ethical constraints into consideration, controlled studies when indicated impose fewer ethical problems than uncontrolled human experiments.

"Benefiting" the Subject

Years ago, after I had administered the first dose of streptomycin to a human patient, there was a need to obtain "normal" values for the absorption and excretion of this new antibiotic.[5] Because of the toxicity (subsequently eliminated) of the early lots of the antibiotics, it did not seem ethical to test normal subjects who could not conceivably benefit from the procedure.

A satisfactory compromise was reached. Streptomycin in early laboratory experiments gave promise of being effective in the treatment of infections due to gram-negative enteric bacilli—one of which is the typhoid bacillus. A typhoid carrier—that is, an individual who has recovered from typhoid fever, but continues to carry this pathogenic bacillus in his gall bladder, intestine, or genito-urinary tract—is relatively "normal" so far as the aims of our experiment were concerned. Moreover, he could have conceivably benefited from the experiment by elimination of his carrier state.

As a result of strict public health controls, the typhoid carrier is the pariah or leper of modern society. Everyone who knows him avoids him. Invited guests will not enter his home, and he will not be invited elsewhere. Indeed, the entire family suffers. Because of the great desire to be relieved of this burden, many typhoid carriers willingly volunteered, and the experiment on the absorption and excretion of streptomycin was performed on them. Unfortunately, the eradication of their carrier state was temporary, and it returned after drug therapy was stopped. But there was a possible benefit to the subject that could only be ascertained by experiment. The necessary human data on the absorption and excretion of streptomycin were collected.

A Proposed Design for Testing New Drugs

We will explore the hypothesis that a system of drug testing can be developed that will satisfy scientific requirements, meet a higher standard of ethical principles than now obtains, and yet release a new drug for general use more rapidly than is now feasible.

Now that the Federal Food and Drug Administration has imposed and implemented rigorous scientific standards for drug testing, there are frequent complaints that the procedure itself may be unethical in that it is so costly, time-consuming, and demanding of highly qualified investigators that the benefit to the public of the new therapeutic agent is unnecessarily delayed. And, yet, the critics are properly loath to recommend a return to a system that might permit a toxic drug, such as Thalidomide, to be sold in the open market. The horns of the dilemma are clearly visible—potential benefit on the one hand, and potential harm, on the other.

In outlining a plan to resolve this dilemma, let us first explore the existing process of rigorous testing through which a new drug becomes available for widespread use. From time to time, evidence is presented that a new medicament may be useful in the prevention or treatment of a particular disease. At that point, it is tested in animals for toxicity and for therapeutic efficacy in an appropriate model (for example, an animal disease or a laboratory test for inhibiting the growth of or eradicating a pathogenic micro-organism). If such efforts are successful—that is, if the drug continues to demonstrate therapeutic usefulness without serious toxicity—a decision finally is made to explore the use of the new drug in a few carefully selected patients.

Ideally, this next stage is carried out by a few investigators who have had great experience with the disease under study and who are most likely to detect in relatively few patients variations produced by the drug from fluctuations in the natural history of the illness. Let us assume that this hurdle has been surmounted and that the drug is deemed apparently effective, relatively safe, and ready for a large controlled clinical test. Assume also that an estimate has been made of the number of patients needed for a precise evaluation of the drug were its effectiveness to continue to be the same.

A controlled clinical trial is then instituted. An appropriate question is asked and a protocol of experiment is developed to satisfy scientific and ethical requirements. Patients are randomly admitted to treatment and control groups. Measurements of effectiveness and toxicity are made, recorded, and analyzed sequentially. If the results are satisfactory, a final decision is reached concerning the widespread availability of the new therapeutic agent. The drug may then be released and then monitored for continued effectiveness and for rare manifestations of severe toxicity.

At the present time, this process—performed in accordance with an ethical and scientifically precise plan—postpones the widespread use of an effective drug, involves too many competent investigators for too long a period of time, and through repetition in many countries throughout the world imposes the hazards of testing the same drug on an unnecessarily large number of human subjects. The process raises ethical questions because it is unethical to expose to unnecessary risk more human subjects than are needed to ascertain the scientific fact. Fortunately, when the situation is carefully analyzed, many of these difficulties may be overcome without sacrificing scientific standards or ethical principles.

The time required for testing can be reduced, and there can be an earlier release of the drug, if the trial is performed collaboratively, instead of haphazardly, by a group of investigators in different hospitals using a common protocol of experiment. In a coordinating center, the data are analyzed sequentially to be sure that the dose is maximal, the method of administration effective, and toxicity minimal. When satisfactory results are obtained, the drug could be released immediately for general use.

The collaborative clinical trial avoids one of the great ethical problems of drug testing. In any one hospital, when evidence that a new drug may be effective begins to become manifest, there are increasing pressures on the investigator to release it for general use before a statistically significant sample of patients has been studied.

At that point, in a collaborative study, the number of cases in all of the centers in the study is usually large enough to provide a solid estimate of the efficacy of the agent as well as of the nature and the degree of its toxicity.

A collaborative program by itself in any one country will not necessarily reduce the number of human subjects who are exposed to the risk of testing a particular drug. The number of human subjects can be reduced, however, by international agreements among developed countries that adhere to drug testing standards similar to our own.[6] A well-designed international collaborative and cooperative study in which the new drug could be tested on a specified but much smaller number of human subjects could suffice for all. At present, in many advanced countries a valid sample of treated and control patients is collected, and with relatively little exchange of information, the same experiments are repeated in many countries. The present process wastes professional skills and medical resources, unnecessarily exposes too many human subjects to the risk of drug testing, and is thereby unethical.

Experience in the United States-United Kingdom Cooperative Rheumatic Fever Study has demonstrated that international cooperation in drug testing can be successful.[7] From that experience, it is urged that an international agency, such as the World Health Organization, or an international pharmaceutical manufacturers' association explore the possibility of rapid, efficient international drug testing.

There are, of course, political and economic objections, including conflicts in patent policy, protection of trade secrets, and disturbance of international drug marketing agreements. These should be faced squarely to see whether or not a solution can be found so that the benefits of international testing might be reaped. One obvious benefit is much earlier marketability of the drug.

Another benefit for pharmaceutical companies adhering to the agreement is protection against damage suits resulting from relatively uncommon toxicity of the drug. For example, if it is determined by the international agency that to assure effectiveness and lack of serious toxicity a drug should be tested on a specific number of cases and the requirement is met by the manufacturer, it should be *prima facie* evidence that he cannot be responsible for severe drug reactions that occur less frequently than the number of cases treated. Thus, if it is estimated from preliminary testing that five hundred cases should be included in the clinical trial, and this requirement is satisfied and the drug released, a manufacturer could not reasonably be expected to be responsible for a rare, severe reaction that might occur in only one of two thousand patients.

In summary, then, an international drug testing program, including a monitoring system for following the continued effectiveness and the rare manifestations of toxicity of the drug, would decrease the number of human subjects at risk and bring the benefits of the new agent to the world in a shorter period of time.

Modern Design of Human Experiments

The advent of the electronic computer has increased the efficiency of biomedical research and, in turn, has had its ethical implications. In the days of collecting laboratory measurements on the smoked drum, it was easier to collect data than to analyze them. Indeed, final interpretation of experiments was often delayed for months as data were collated and analyzed by hand tabulations, often made by the investigator himself in odd moments between the pressing needs of laboratory duties and teaching. Rarely was the analysis of data given priority over his other activities. At the top of the list was the next experiment, the gross results of which were eagerly anticipated while the detailed analysis was again postponed.

As a result of these traditional limitations on data handling and processing, and with the increasing complexity of our understanding of biological systems, there has been a growing tendency to design experiments in simplified systems where at any one time a few variables can be measured with great precision. This method of research has yielded a great deal of generally applicable biological knowledge. But because the systems of the human body are so complex and the new simplified approach to research so remote from them, the research results have become less and less applicable to the solution of problems of human health and disease. Indeed, the clinical problem that may have originally inspired the research program may often be forgotten as the scientist concentrates on further and further detailed study of his simplified system. As a corollary, when such clinical investigations became more remote from human subjects, fewer ethical problems were created.

With the advent of the electronic computer, the underlying situation was completely reversed. The revolution in data handling and processing has now made it much easier to analyze and interpret than to collect scientific data. The analysis of scientific data, if the experiment's design is sound, should now take relatively little time and effort. Indeed, the immediate availability of an analysis of the data of an experiment should permit the scientist to concentrate on the significance of the experimental results. The scientist now has the time to take into consideration the results of this last experiment so as to plan better the next one.

More importantly, clinical experimentation no longer need be limited to the study of a few variables at any one time in simplified systems. Experiments can presently be designed to study the complex interrelationships of many variables at the same time. For example, instead of studying the salt and water metabolism of the kidney as if it were completely independent of all the other functions of this organ, it is now possible to study total organ function. Indeed, computer handling of data makes it feasible to study total body functions. Furthermore, with on-line data collection and analysis in real time, it is feasible, for example, to build into a physiologic experiment many contingent measurements depending upon what happens in the earlier stages of the experiment. With such study design, medical research can deal more directly with complex systems in the human subject. Moreover, because the research system is closer to that of the human being, the experimental results should be more easily applicable to the improvement of health and the prevention and treatment of human disease.

This modern method of research—with its more complicated design and more intensive and thorough study of each human subject— is uncovering new ethical questions: How long can one safely run a particular experiment on a patient with a certain disease? How much blood may be collected for research purposes over a specified period of time and how frequently may the experiment be repeated? Will a particularly long continued intensive experiment interfere with the best treatment of the patient? It is clear that more comprehensive clinical experiments requiring more intensive scientific planning will also demand more careful attention to the protection of the human subject. Moreover, now that more complete experiments can be performed, human subjects must not be "wasted" in trivial experiments. This is not to say that simple but complete and penetrating experiments should not be performed. It is a plea for more meticulous planning based on modern technology, computer facilities, and biostatistical consultation to yield more applicable experimental results without increasing the risk to the human subject. It will force us to ask the question: "Is it ethical to perform *limited experiments* if, with more careful planning and with no increased risk to the patient, much more valuable information could be collected of more immediate applicability to patients, including the subject himself?"

The design of medical experiments may also under certain circumstances help to surmount existing ethical problems. It is often difficult to justify ethically a human experiment concerned with the study of normal metabolism or physiology or with the changes produced by a particular illness, because benefits to the subject are likely to be limited. To be sure, the more profound study of the patient's condition implicit in the research measurements may yield information that permits better treatment of his disease. But we can do better than that. A properly designed experiment with on-line computer analysis of properly programmed data makes feasible the study of a physiologic, metabolic, or pathologic mechanism and simultaneously the evaluation of a therapeutic agent. For example, in the study of the mechanism of circulatory collapse in severe infections not amenable to antibiotic therapy, the testing of a drug or, perhaps in the future, the trial of a mechanical heart booster could be interwoven and both studies completed at the same time. Such design assures the experimenter that he could benefit the human subjects of his experiments.

Modern design of human experiments opens up new vistas in the understanding of complex biological systems with immediate promise of human benefit. Experiments so designed should yield more knowledge at the same risk to the human subject—and this is an ethical benefit. But these more complex experiments also uncover new ethical problems demanding increasing vigilance in the protection of the human subject.

The Role of Mathematical Theory

When it is impossible for ethical reasons to perform a given experiment to test a particular hypothesis, it may be useful to turn to the mathematician for the deduction of an alternative hypothesis which could be tested by experiment. As W. G. Cochran has pointed out:

A fruitful mathematical theory will predict the results of experiments not yet carried out—in some cases impossible to carry out. In the intensive studies of the Rhesus factor during the 1940's, Mendelian analysis predicted the existence of two genes not then discovered and the seriologic properties of two new antibodies. Epidemic theory can indicate by how much the probability of a major epidemic will be reduced by immunization of any given proportion of the susceptible population in a public-health program. In evolution and the study of inbreeding, the consequences of forces acting over many generations can be worked out.[8]

The increasing role of mathematics in the medical sciences should make this approach more and more feasible.

If we can agree that scientific medical research can continue to serve ethically as the basis for medical progress, there is an immediate need to re-examine the design of human experiments from both the scientific and ethical points of view; to reshape the design of human experiments and take advantage of new technology; to increase, improve, make more relevant the data collected in human experiments, and yet, at the same time, strengthen the ethical principles of medical research.

REFERENCES

1. Rheumatic Fever Working Party of the Medical Research Council of Great Britain and the Sub-committee of Principal Investigators of the American Council on Rheumatic Fever and Congenital Heart Disease, American Heart Association, "A Joint Report: The Treatment of Acute Rheumatic Fever in Children. A Cooperative Clinical Trial of ACTH, Cortisone, and Aspirin," *Circulation*, Vol. 11 (1955), pp. 343-77; *British Medical Journal*, Vol. 1 (1955), pp. 555-74.

2. Since this manuscript was presented and submitted, it has been learned that two control studies are now under way in the United Kingdom.

3. H. K. Beecher, "Surgery as Placebo—A Quantitative Study of Bias," *Journal of the American Medical Association*, Vol. 176 (1961), pp. 1102-1107.

4. A. B. Hill, J. Marshall, and D. A. Shaw, "A Controlled Clinical Trial of Long-Term Anticoagulant Therapy in Cerebrovascular Disease," *Quarterly Journal of Medicine*, Vol. 29, New Series (1960), pp. 597-609.

5. D. D. Rutstein, R. B. Stebbins, R. T. Cathcart, and R. M. Harvey, "The Absorption and Excretion of the Streptomycin in Human Chronic Typhoid Carriers, *Journal of Clinical Investigation*, Vol. 24 (1945), pp. 898-909.

6. Such an agreement should not be confused with the rumored surreptitious drug testing said to be conducted at times by a few United States drug manufacturers in countries not having standards so rigid as those of the Food and Drug Administration in the United States.

7. Rheumatic Fever Working Party of the Medical Research Council of Great Britain and the Sub-committee of Principal Investigators of the American Council on Rheumatic Fever and Congenital Heart Disease, American Heart Association, A Joint Report Prepared by D. D. Rutstein and E. Densen, "The Natural History of Rheumatic Fever and Rheumatic Heart Disease: Ten-Year Report of a Cooperative Clinical Trial of ACTH, Cortisone, and Aspirin," *Circulation*, Vol. 32, pp. 457-76; *British Medical Journal*, Vol. 2, pp. 607-615; *Canadian Medical Association Journal*, Vol. 93 (1965), pp. 519-31.

8. W. G. Cochran, "The Role of Mathematics in the Medical Sciences," *New England Journal of Medicine*, Vol. 265 (1961), p. 176.

17 Clarifying the Concepts of Research Ethics

ROBERT J. LEVINE

The way in which words are used by different groups of people has always caused a variety of problems; this is particularly true in ethics where a different understanding of a word can give a completely different outcome to an argument. One of the major contributions that the National Commission for the Protection of Human Subjects has made is the clarification of a variety of terms that are routinely used in discussing ethical issues in the conducting of research on human subjects. In this article, Levine discusses the Commission's definition of research and practice, its abandoning of the distinction between therapeutic and nontherapeutic research, the clarification of the concept of risk and the different purposes of obtaining informed consent and its relationship to a consent form.

Robert J. Levine, M.D., is Professor of Medicine at the Yale University School of Medicine

One of the most important achievements of the National Commission for the Protection of Human Subjects of Biomedical and Behavioral Research (the Commission) was to begin the process of correcting the conceptual and semantic errors that had undermined virtually all previous attempts to develop rational public policy on research involving human subjects. The fruits of this achievement are seen most clearly in the later reports of the Commission—on children,[1] on those institutionalized as mentally infirm,[2] and on Institutional Review Boards (IRBs).[3] Earlier reports, for example, on the fetus,[4] were flawed in several respects[5] because they were prepared before the Commission had completed its conceptual clarifications. Four of these clarifications are especially important. The Commission (1) developed satisfactory definitions of research and practice; (2) abandoned the distinction between therapeutic and nontherapeutic research; (3) clarified the concept of risk; and (4) identified the different purposes of informed consent and the consent form.

DISTINCTIONS BETWEEN RESEARCH AND PRACTICE

Distinguishing research from practice might not seem to present any problems. Yet, the legislative history of the Act that created the Commission reflects the fact that some physicians regarded this as a very important and exceedingly difficult task.[6] Jay Katz identified "drawing the line between research and accepted practice . . . (as) the most difficult and complex problem facing the Commission." And Thomas Chalmers asserted: "It is extremely hard to distinguish between clinical research and the practice of good medicine. Because episodes of illness and individual people are so variable, every physician is carrying out a small research project when he diagnoses and treats a patient."

Chalmers, of course, was only echoing the views of many distinguished physicians who had spoken to this issue earlier. For example, in *Experimentation with Human Subjects,* Hermann Blumgart stated: "Every time a physician administers a drug to a patient, he is in a sense performing an experiment."[7] To this Francis Moore added: "Every (surgical) operation of any type contains certain aspects of experimental work."[8] While these statements are true, they tend to cloud the real issues and make it more difficult to distinguish research from practice.

Bewildered by these statements, Congress directed the Commission to "consider . . . the boundaries between biomedical or behavioral research involving human subjects and the accepted and routine practice of medicine."[9] The Commission, after its deliberations, concluded in *The Belmont Report* that there were no overlapping boundaries. Rather, when used correctly, the terms "practice" and "research" describe mutually exclusive sets of activities.[10]

> For the most part, the term "practice" refers to interventions that are designed solely to enhance the well-being of an individual patient or client and that have a reasonable expectation of success. The purpose of medical or behavioral practice is to provide diagnosis, preventive treatment or therapy to particular individuals. By contrast, the term "research" designates an activity designed to test a hypothesis, permit conclusions to be drawn and thereby to develop or contribute to generalizable

knowledge (expressed, for example, in theories, principles and statements of relationships) (pp. 2–3).

The Commission further observed:

The distinction between research and practice is blurred partly because both often occur together (as in research designed to evaluate a therapy) and partly because notable departures from standard practice are often called "experimental" when the terms "experimental" and "research" are not carefully defined (p. 2).

In order to state its views clearly, the Commission avoided such terms as "experimentation" and "experimental"[11] unless it carefully defined the intended sense of the word.[11a] Further, it identified two classes of practices that are commonly confused with research and provided advice as to how to deal with them.

Nonvalidated practices. A class of procedures performed by physicians conforms to the definition of "practice" to the extent that these procedures are "designed solely to enhance the well-being of an individual patient or client." However, they may not have been tested sufficiently often or sufficiently well to meet the standard of having "a reasonable expectation of success." The Commission uses various terms to describe these procedures: "innovative therapies,"[12] "nonvalidated practices,"[13] and, most commonly, "interventions that hold out the prospect of direct benefit for the individual subjects."[14] The regulations of the Food and Drug Administration refer to "investigational" drugs or devices. In my opinion, the best designation for this class of procedures is "nonvalidated practices."[15] Novelty is not the attribute that defines this class of practices; rather it is the lack of suitable validation of the safety or efficacy of the practice.

In *The Belmont Report,* the Commission focuses upon innovations:

When a clinician departs in a significant way from standard or accepted practice, the innovation does not, in and of itself, constitute research. The fact that a procedure is "experimental," in the sense of new, untested or different, does not automatically place it in the category of research. Radically new procedures of this description *should,* however, be made the object of formal research at an early stage in order to determine whether they are safe and effective (emphasis supplied). Thus, it is the responsibility of medical practice committees, for example, to insist that a major innovation be incorporated into a formal research project (p. 3).

Thus, performing a procedure that is innovative, or, for some other reason, nonvalidated is not research; rather, it is a form of practice that ought to be made the object of formal research. The Commission concludes that when research is designed to evaluate a practice, the entire activity—research and practice components—should be reviewed by an IRB.[16] However, the harm-benefit analysis of the nonvalidated practice component should be conducted according to the standards of practice, not research, a point to which I shall return in the section on therapeutic versus nontherapeutic research.

Practice for the benefit of others. The Commission recognizes still another class of activities that conforms to its definition of practice in that it has "a reasonable expectation of success"; however, it is not designed *solely* to enhance the well-being of an individual patient. This class includes some interventions that are applied to one individual in order to enhance the well-being of another (for example, blood donation and organ transplants), and some others that have the dual purpose of enhancing the well-being of a particular individual and, at the same time, providing some benefit to others (for example, vaccination). While these activities often raise harm-benefit questions similar to those presented by research,[17] the Commission concluded that they need not be reviewed by an IRB.[18]

THERAPEUTIC VERSUS NONTHERAPEUTIC RESEARCH

It is not clear when the distinction between therapeutic and nontherapeutic research began to be made in discussions of the ethics and regulation of research. The Nuremberg Code (1947) draws no such distinction. The Declaration of Helsinki (1964) distinguishes nontherapeutic clinical research from clinical research combined with professional care. In the 1975 revision of this Declaration, "medical research combined with professional care" is designated "clinical research," while "nontherapeutic biomedical research involving human subjects" is designated "non-clinical biomedical research."

One major problem with this dichotomy is illustrated by placing one principle of the Helsinki Declaration developed for clinical research (II.6) in immediate proximity to one developed for nonclinical research (III.2):

II.6 The doctor can combine medical research with professional care, the objective being the acquisition of new medical knowledge only to the extent that medical research is justified by its potential diagnostic or therapeutic value for the patient. III.2 The subjects should be volunteers—either healthy persons or patients for whom the experimental design is not related to the patient's illness.

This classification has several unfortunate (and unintended) consequences, two of which are:

1. Many types of research cannot be defined as either therapeutic or nontherapeutic. Consider, for example, the placebo-controlled, "double-blind," drug trial, in which neither patient nor physician knows whether the drug or the placebo is being administered. Certainly, the administration of a placebo for research purposes is not "justified by its potential diagnostic or therapeutic value for the patient." Therefore, according to the principles, this is nontherapeutic, and those who receive the placebo must be "either healthy persons or patients for whom the experimental design is not related to the patient's illness." This, of couse, makes no sense.

2. A strict interpretation of the Declaration of Helsinki would lead to the conclusion that all rational research designed to explore the pathogenesis of a disease is to be forbidden. Since it cannot be justified as prescribed in principle II.6., it must be considered nontherapeutic and therefore done only on healthy persons or patients not having the disease one wishes to investigate. Again, this makes no sense.

By 1974, when the Commission was first convened, the distinction between therapeutic and nontherapeutic research had assumed a central position in most discussions of the ethics and regulation of research involving human subjects. These discussions generally reflected the assumption that there was a class of activities that could be defined as "therapeutic research" and that this was always done—at least in part—for the benefit of the subject. They further reflected the assumption that "nontherapeutic research," because it was not done for the benefit of the subject, was somehow more ethically suspect; that it required stronger justification to proceed; and that it required more stringent mechanisms designed to safeguard the rights and welfare of the subjects. In fact, there were some DHEW proposals to foreclose entire categories of "non-beneficial research" without regard to considerations of whether any risk was involved.[19]

The Commission's first report, *Research on the Fetus,* did not show much promise of correcting these problems; it presented the following definitions:

Research refers to a systematic collection of data or observations in accordance with a designed protocol.

Therapeutic research refers to research designed to improve the health condition of the research subject by prophylactic, diagnostic or treatment methods that depart from standard medical practice but hold out a reasonable expectation of success.

Nontherapeutic research refers to research not designed to improve the health condition of the ... subject (p. 6).

Of course, there is no such thing as a "systematic collection of data or observations ... designed to improve the health condition of a research subject ... that departs from standard medical practice." Thus, the Commission developed recommendations for the conduct of a null set of activities.[20]

After its report on the fetus was completed, the Commission began the process of systematically addressing the general conceptual charges in its mandate. As it developed its definitions of research and medical practice, it identified a distinct class of activities called "nonvalidated practices." It is these practices that are "designed to improve the health condition of the research subject by prophylactic, diagnostic or treatment methods that depart from standard medical practice." These practices are therapeutic but they are not research. As the Commission concluded, research should be done to validate these practices—that is, by establishing their safety and efficacy.

In all subsequent reports, the Commission completely abandoned the language of therapeutic and nontherapeutic research and used instead the concept of nonvalidated practice, for example: "Research on practices, both innovative and accepted, which have the intent and reasonable probability of improving the health or well-being of the individual prisoner ..."[21] The same concept is reflected in Recommendation 4 on children[22] and Recommendation 3 on those institutionalized as mentally infirm;[23] these Recommendations make it clear that the risks and benefits of therapeutic maneuvers are to be analyzed similarly, notwithstanding the status of a maneuver as either nonvalidated or standard (accepted): "The relation of anticipated benefit to such risk ... (should be) at least as favorable to the subjects as that presented by available alternative approaches." The risks of research maneuvers (designed to benefit the collective) are perceived differently. If they are more than minimal, special justifications and procedural protections are required.

THE CONCEPT OF RISK

It is widely believed that being a research subject is a highly risky undertaking. This assumption is clearly reflected in the legislative history of the Act that established the Commission; it is further reflected in some of the Commission's early deliberations. For example, because the Commission considered the role of research subject a hazardous occupation, it called upon the philospher Marx Wartofsky to analyze the distinctions between this and other hazardous occupations.[24]

Biomedical researchers have contributed to this incorrect belief.[25] For example, it is often stated that accepting the role of subject nearly always entails the assumption of some risk without specifying the nature of the risk. To many members of the public and to many analysts who are not themselves researchers, the word "risk" seems to carry the implication of some possibly dreadful consequence; this is made to seem even more terrifying when it is acknowledged that, in some cases, the very nature of this dreadful consequence cannot be anticipated. And yet, when biomedical researchers discuss risk, they more commonly mean a possibility that something like a bruise might be observed after a venipuncture.[26]

Some recent data indicate that, in general, it is not especially hazardous to be a research subject. For example, John D. Arnold estimates the risks of physical or psychological harm to subjects in Phase I drug testing[27] are slightly greater than those of being an office secretary, one-seventh those of window washers, and one-ninth those of miners. Chris J. D. Zarafonetis and his coworkers found that, in Phase I drug testing among prisoners, a "clinically significant medical event" occurred once every 26.3 years of individual subject exposure.[28] In 805 protocols involving 29,162 prisoner volunteers over 614,534 days, there were 58 adverse drug reactions, none of which produced death or permanent disability. The only subject who died did so while receiving a placebo. Philippe Cardon and his colleagues, in a large-scale survey of investigators designed to determine the incidence of injuries to research subjects, found that in "nontherapeutic" research, the risk of being disabled either temporarily or permanently was substantially less than that of being similarly harmed in an accident.[29] None of the nearly 100,000 subjects of "nontherapeutic research" died. The apparent hazards of being a subject in "therapeutic research" were substantially greater. This reflects the fact that the subjects of "therapeutic research" tend to have diseases that produce disability or death. Although no direct comparisons were made, it appears that the frequency of either death or disability in subjects of "therapeutic research" was substantially lower than similar unfortunate outcomes in comparable medical settings involving no research.

Mere inconvenience and minimal risk. In considering the burdens imposed upon the human research subject, risk of physical or psychological injury ought to be distinguished from various phenomena that are more appropriately referred to as inconvenience, discomfort, and embarrassment; "mere inconvenience" is a general term for these phenomena.[30] Research presenting the burden of mere inconvenience is characterized as presenting no greater risk of consequential injury to the subject than that inherent in his or her particular life situation.

This class of research is by far the most common. In general, what researchers ask is that a prospective subject give up some time (for example, to reside in a clinical research center, to be observed in a physiology laboratory, or to fill out a questionnaire). Often there is a request to draw some blood or to collect urine or feces.

The term "mere inconvenience" is used in Recommendation 1 in the Commission's report on prisoners.[31] Other reports attempt to reflect a similar conceptualization by using the term "minimal risk."[32] For example:

> Minimal risk[33] is the probability and magnitude of physical or psychological harm that is normally encountered in the daily lives, or in the routine medical or psychological examination, of healthy children.[33a]

Incorporation of this concept into the Commission's recommendations has had a very important effect. Like HEW, the Commission has recognized that stringent procedures—such as review at the national level by an Ethics Advisory Board (EAB)—may be necessary to protect subjects from harm. However, because HEW viewed virtually all research subjects as being "at risk," without distinguishing harm from inconvenience, it proposed bureaucratic procedural protections for all research on certain classes of persons. The favorable effect of the Commission's conceptual clarification is to bring the benefit of these procedural protections to the small minority of research proposals in which some meaningful purpose might be served. For example, proposals to do research involving children must be reviewed by the EAB only if more than minor increments above minimal risk are presented by interventions that do not "hold out the prospect of direct benefit for the individual subjects."[34]

INFORMED CONSENT

HEW regulations require that for all grants and contracts supporting research, development, and related activities in which human subjects are involved, an IRB must determine whether these subjects will be placed at risk. If risk is involved the IRB must assure that "legally effective informed consent will be obtained by adequate and appropriate methods." HEW interpretations of the meaning of "at risk" create a requirement for informed consent in virtually all of these activities. A careful reading of HEW regulations indicates that informed consent must always be documented on a consent form.[35]

Various critics have argued that these requirements are not merely a waste of time, but they also cause many investigators to disregard significant aspects of obtaining informed consent and its documenta-tion.[36] In addition, prospective "subjects" are commonly burdened by the necessity of making decisions that are made to seem more conse-quential than they really are.[37]

The Commission has recommended changes in the regulations that respond to these criticisms. These recommendations not only re-flect the conceptual clarifications I have discussed but also elucidate the function of informed consent and the very different purposes of its documentation on a consent form. Informed consent is designed to show respect for the research subjects' right to self-determination—that is, to make free choices. Researchers tell the subjects what they wish to do and the subjects decide whether they wish to become in-volved. For example, by telling prospective subjects of the risks in-volved in procedures, researchers provide them with an opportunity to protect themselves by deciding whether the potential benefits are worth the risks.

The purpose of documenting consent on a consent form is entire-ly different. It is designed to protect the investigator and the institu-tion against legal liability.[38] The retention of a signed consent form tends to give the advantage to the investigator in any adversary pro-ceeding. In fact, signed consent forms may be detrimental to subjects' interests even in the absence of litigation; their availability in institu-tional records may lead to violations of privacy and confidentiality.[39]

Recognizing these facts, the Commission recommends that there need be no written documentation of consent if the IRB determines either: "(1) The existence of signed consent forms would place sub-jects at risk, or (2) the research presents no more than minimal risk and involves no procedures for which written consent is normally re-quired" (p. 21).

The Commission goes even further by pointing out some circum-stances in which informed consent itself is unnecessary. These in-clude research activities in which:

(1) The subjects' interests are determined to be adequately pro-tected in studies of documents, records or pathological speci-mens and the importance of the research justifies such invasion of the subjects' privacy, or (2) in studies of public behavior where the research presents no more than minimal risk, is unlikely to cause embarrassment, and has scientific merit (p. 21).

Finally, it should be noted that the Commission has abandoned the use of the word "consent," except in situations in which an indi-vidual can provide "legally effective consent" on his or her own behalf. Respect for persons such as children or others who have either immature or impaired capacities for rational self-determination is manifested by negotiating for "assent" or, at least, by recognizing and respecting a "deliberate objection." As a corollary to this decision, the Commission does not use such terms as "proxy consent" or "consent of a legally authorized representative"; the parent or guardian of such a person is asked to give "permission." This terminology was introduced in the Commission's recommendations on children and on those institutionalized as mentally infirm; it is tentatively adopted in HEW proposed regulations on these two classes of subjects.

CONCLUSIONS

In its later reports the Commission recommended policies that are far more rational than those developed by any of its predecessors. To illustrate this I have compared these recommendations with earlier HEW final and proposed regulations, the Declaration of Helsinki, and an early report of the Commission. The Commission's achievement can be partially attributed to the identification and correction of several conceptual and semantic errors that had undermined previous attempts to develop suitable standards for the ethical conduct of research involving human subjects.

Still, many authors continue to use these incorrect concepts in their current writings in this field. For example, several commentators have used the language of therapeutic and nontherapeutic research in their analyses of the Commission's reports on prisoners, children, and those institutionalized as mentally infirm. This indicates that they do not understand the recommendations that they are analyzing. Such analyses, if taken seriously, could contribute to the development of a regressive public policy. As Confucius said:[40]

> If language is not used rightly,
> then what is said is not what is meant.
> If what is said is not what is meant,
> then that which ought to be done is left undone;
> if it remains undone, morals and art will be corrupted;
> if morals and art are corrupted, justice will go awry;
> and if justice goes awry, the people will stand about
> in helpless confusion.

REFERENCES

1. Commission, *Report and Recommendations: Research Involving Children.* DHEW Publication No. (OS) 77-0004, Washington, 1977.

2. Commission, *Report and Recommendations: Research Involving Those Institutionalized as Mentally Infirm.* DHEW Publication No. (OS) 78-0006, Washington, 1978.

3. Commission, *Report and Recommendations: Institutional Review Boards.* DHEW Publication No. (OS) 78-0008, Washington, 1978.

4. Commission, *Report and Recommendations: Research on the Fetus.* DHEW Publication No. (OS) 76-127, Washington, 1975.

5. Robert J. Levine, "The Impact on Fetal Research of the Report of the National Commission for the Protection of Human Subjects of Biomedical and Behavioral Research," *Villanova Law Review* 22 (1977), 367–82.

6. E. M. Kay, "Legislative History of Title II—Protection of Human Subjects of Biomedical and Behavioral Research—of the National Research Act: P.L. 93–348." Prepared for the National Commission, 1975, pp. 16–18.

7. Hermann L. Blumgart, "The Medical Framework for Viewing the Problems of Human Experimentation," in *Experimentation with Human Subjects,* Paul A. Freund, ed. (New York: George Braziller, 1970), pp. 39–65.

8. Francis D. Moore: "Therapeutic Innovation: Ethical Boundaries in the Initial Clinical Trials of New Drugs and Surgical Procedures," in *Experimentation with Human Subjects,* pp. 358–78.

9. Public Law 93–348: The National Research Act.

10. Commission, *The Belmont Report: Ethical Principles and Guidelines for the Protection of Human Subjects of Research.* DHEW Publication No. (OS) 78-0012, Washington, 1978.

11. To experiment means to test something or to try something out. In another sense, an experiment is a tentative procedure, especially one adopted in uncertainty as to whether it will bring about the desired purposes or results. Much of the practice of diagnosis and therapy is experimental in nature. For example, a physician tries out a drug to see if it brings about the desired result in the patient. If it does not, the physician either increases the dose, changes to another therapy, or adds a new therapeutic modality to the first drug. All of this "experimentation" is done in the interests of enhancing the well-being of the patient.

When experimentation is conducted for purposes of developing generalizable knowledge, it is regarded as research. One of the problems presented by much research designed to test the safety or efficacy of drugs is that this activity is much less experimental than the practice of medicine. It must, in general, conform to the specifications of a protocol. Thus, the individualized dosage adjustments and changes in therapeutic modalities are less likely to occur in the context of a clinical trial than they are in the practice of medicine. This deprivation of the "experimentation" ordinarily done to enhance the well-being of a patient is one of the burdens imposed on the patient-subject in a randomized clinical trial.

11a. Robert J. Levine and Karen Lebacqz: "Some Ethical Considerations in Clinical Trials," *Clinical Pharmacology and Therapeutics* 25 (1979), 728–41.

12. Early drafts of *The Belmont Report.*

13. Commission, *Report and Recommendations: Research Involving Prisoners.* DHEW Publication No. (OS) 76–131, Washington, 1976.

14. Commission, *Report and Recommendations: Research Involving Children* and *Report and Recommendations: Research Involving Those Institutionalized as Mentally Infirm.*

15. See Levine, "The Impact on Fetal Research of the Report of the National Commission. . . . ," pp. 380–82.

16. Commission, *The Belmont Report,* p. 4.

17. Robert J. Levine: "On the Relevance of Ethical Principles and Guidelines Developed for Research to Health Services Conducted or Supported by the Secretary, DHEW" in: *Appendix to the Commission's Report: Ethical Guidelines for the Delivery of Health Services by DHEW.* DHEW Publication No. (OS) 78-0011, Washington, 1978, pp. 2.14–2.16.

18. While the concept of "practice for the benefit of others" is reflected in *The Belmont Report* (p. 3), the term is not used. A more complete description of this class of practices and the problems it presents may be found in Levine, "On the Relevance of Ethical Principles. . . . ," pp. 2.11–2.13.

19. DHEW: Proposed Policy, Federal Register 39 (No. 165) (August 23, 1974), 30648–57.

20. I do not wish to be excessively critical of the Commission's first report. The Commission was required by Congress to place fetal research first on its agenda. Considering the time constraints imposed by Congress, the report is remarkably good.

21. Commission, *Report and Recommendations: Research Involving Prisoners,* p. 15.

22. Commission, *Report and Recommendations: Research Involving Children,* pp. 5–6.

23. Commission, *Report and Recommendations Involving Those Institutionalized as Mentally Infirm,* pp. 11–13.

24. Marx W. Wartofsky: "On Doing It for Money," in *Appendix to Reference No. 13.* DHEW Publication No. (OS) 76-132, Washington, 1976, pp. 3.1–3.24.

25. Robert J. Levine: "Nondevelopmental Research on Human Subjects: The Impact of the Recommendations of the National Commission for the Protection of Human Subjects of Biomedical and Behavioral Research," *Federation Proceedings* 36 (1977) 2359–64; and Robert J. Levine, "Commentary: Terminological Inexactitude," in *Legal and Ethical Issues in Human Research and Treatment: Psychopharmacologic Considerations,* Donald M. Gallant and Robert Force, eds. (New York: Spectrum Publications, 1978), pp. 85–98.

26. A comprehensive discussion of the origins and consequences of this belief is beyond the scope of this essay. Further details may be found in the articles cited in reference 25.

27. J. D. Arnold: "Alternatives to the Use of Prisoners in Research in the United States," in *Appendix to reference 13,* pp. 8.1–8.18.

28. C. J. D. Zarafonetis et al, "Clinically Significant Adverse Effects in a Phase 1 Testing Program," *Clinical Pharmacology and Therapeutics* 24 (1978) 127–32.

29. Philippe V. Cardon, F. William Dommel, and Robert R. Trumble: "Injuries to Research Subjects: A Survey of Investigators," *New England Journal of Medicine* 295 (1976) 650–54.

30. Robert J. Levine, "Appropriate Guidelines for the Selection of Human Subjects for Participation in Biomedical and Behavioral Research," in *Appendix I to reference 10,* DHEW Publication No. (OS) 78-0013, pp. 4.8–4.10.

31. Commission, *Report and Recommendations: Research Involving Prisoners*, p. 14.

32. Commission, *Report and Recommendations: Research Involving Children*, p. xx.

33. The Commission's choice of the term "minimal risk" troubles me. It is one of the unusual instances that the Commission decided to stipulate a definition for words in common usage. The use of stipulated definitions in regulations commonly creates confusion. Citations of regulations using this term will be misinterpreted by the unsophisticated reader, unless the full stipulated definition is reproduced in each citation.

    The unsophisticated reader might think that the intended meaning is that presented in standard dictionaries; "minimal" means least possible. The term "risk" is even more problematic. For examples: could minimal risk mean an infinitesimal chance of a substantial harm? A substantial chance of an infinitesimal harm? In this case the confusion will be compounded by the fact that the term is used in the report on children (p. xx) with one stipulated definition, in the report on those institutionalized as mentally infirm with a different definition (p. 8), and in the report on the fetus (p. 73) with no definition.

33a. Robert J. Levine: "The Role of Assessment of Risk-Benefit Criteria in the Determination of the Appropriateness of Research Involving Human Subjects," in *Appendix I to reference No. 10*, pp. 2.1–2.59.

34. Commission: *Report and Recommendations: Research Involving Children*, p. 10.

35. Robert J. Levine: "The Nature and Definition of Informed Consent in Various Research Settings," in *Appendix I to reference No. 10*, pp. 3.1–3.91.

36. Franz J. Ingelfinger, "The Unethical in Medical Ethics," *Annals of Internal Medicine*, 83 (1975), 264–69.

37. Angela R. Holder and Robert J. Levine: "Informed Consent for Research on Specimens Obtained at Autopsy or Surgery: A Case Study in the Overprotection of Human Subjects," *Clinical Research* 24 (1976), 68–77.

38. Levine, "On the Relevance of Ethical Principles, . . . ," pp. 2.17–2.19.

39. Karen Lebacqz and Robert J. Levine, "Respect for Persons and Informed Consent to Participate in Research," *Clinical Research* 254 (1977), 101–07.

40. Lois DeBakey, "Literacy: Mirror of Society," *Journal of Technical Writing and Communication* 8 (1978), 297–319.

18 *Research Using Intentional Deception*

DIANA BAUMRIND

This article continues Baumrind's development of arguments against the use of deception in research. Here she presents three ethical rules which proscribe deceptive practices and examines the costs of such deception to subjects, the professions, and society. This evaluation is set within the context of social psychological experimentation, and Baumrind concludes by presenting ethically acceptable research strategies.

Diana Baumrind is a Research Psychologist at the University of California, Berkeley

Abstract: Ethical issues concerning the use of intentional deception in research with human participants are revisited 10 years after the publication of the 1973 APA guidelines on the conduct of research with human subjects. Intentional deception is defined. The present status of guidelines concerning intentional deception and the incidence and extremity of deception being used are reviewed, leading to the conclusion that the former has not decreased the latter. My position proscribing intentionally deceptive research is grounded in rule-utilitarian metaethics by contrast to act-utilitarian and deontological metaethics; three ethical rules proscribing intentional deception in the research setting are presented. The costs to subjects, the profession, and society are reviewed, and arguments are brought to bear against the scientific benefits claimed for deceptive instructions. In this context, the scientific problems with social psychological experimentation are discussed. Finally, certain recommendations for research strategies in lieu of deception paradigms, and for appropriate debriefing, are offered.

In a series of articles (Baumrind, 1964, 1971, 1972, 1975a, 1975b, 1978, 1979), beginning with a critique of the Milgram (1964) paradigm, I argue that the use of intentional deception in the research setting is unethical, imprudent, and unwarranted scientifically. In response to my latest article (Baumrind, 1979), Baron (1981) offered "an openly optimistic rejoinder." He claimed that deception research is necessary to accomplish beneficial scientific ends and that as a result of the guidelines researchers now use informed consent and thorough debriefing. Two respondents took exception to Baron's optimistic rejoinder. Dresser (1981) pointed out that in distorting a study's true purpose the investigator necessarily grounds participants' willingness to cooperate on misinformed consent. Goldstein (1981) argued that participants' rights to autonomy, dignity, and privacy are necessarily violated by deceptive research practices and rejected Baron's assurance that experimenters were now sensitized to ethical issues. Surveys of the major social psychological journals suggest that Goldstein is correct and Baron's optimism is unwarranted. Ten years after publication of the *Ethical Principles in the Conduct of Research With Human Participants* (American Psychological Association, 1973), I was invited to revisit these issues in the context of a symposium on ethics of deception research delivered to the International Society for Research on Aggression.

By intentional deception I mean withholding information in order to obtain participation that the participant might otherwise decline, using deceptive instructions and confederate manipulations in laboratory research, and employing concealment and staged manipulations in field settings. Because perfect communication between human beings is impossible to achieve, there will always be some degree of misunderstanding in the contract between researcher and subject. Full disclosure of everything that could possibly affect a given subject's decision to participate is not possible, and therefore cannot be ethically required. Provided that participants agree to postponement of full disclosure of the purposes of the research, absence of full disclosure does not constitute intentional deception. The investigator whose purpose is "to take the person unaware by trickery" or to "cause the person to believe the false" in order to minimize ambiguity about causal inference is intentionally deceiving subject–participants to further the investigator's scientific ends or career goals.

Investigators continue to use intentional deception and to justify its use. Epistemological superiority is accorded to deceptive methods as a means of controlling the demand characteristics of the setting by assuring that all subjects believe the situation to be realistic and perceive it in the same way. If intentional deception does not accomplish this objective, its epistemological superiority is doubtful, which in turn casts doubt on the benefits of intentional deception and thus on the justification for its use. Although the examples I offer are drawn largely from aggression research, the justification for deceptive practices arises from the research paradigm that guides experimental social psychology as a whole. It is necessary, therefore, to examine that paradigm.

PRESENT STATUS OF DECEPTION RESEARCH

If deceit is used to obtain consent, by definition it cannot be informed. Deceptive instructions logically contradict the informed consent provision contained in all federal and professional ethical guidelines. Yet these guidelines do permit each of the provisions guaranteeing informed consent to be waived provided that some or all considerations such as the following pertain:

(a) The research objective is of great importance and cannot be achieved without the use of deception; (b) on being fully informed later (Principle E), participants are expected to find the procedures reasonable and to suffer no loss of confidence in the integrity of the investigator or of others involved; (c) research participants are allowed to withdraw from the study at any time (Principle F), and are free to withdraw their data when the concealment or misrepresentation is revealed (Principle H); and (d) investigators take full responsibility for detecting and removing stressful aftereffects of the experience (Principle I). (American Psychological Association, 1982, p. 41)

No strategic guidelines are included to assure that these considerations pertain. Institutional review boards (IRBs), as well as investigators, are at liberty to set their own.

Neither the incidence nor the magnitude of deception reported in social psychological research appears to have decreased since 1973. Thus, the APA guidelines appear to serve an expressive rather than a deterrent function. McNamara and Woods (1977) reported a rise to 57% in a survey covering the years 1971 to 1974. In the most recent study (Smith & Richardson, 1983), approximately half of the 464 psychology undergraduates surveyed reported that the experiment in which they had participated used deception. Both figures exceed Seeman's (1969) figures of 18% in 1948 and 37% in 1963. The maximum magnitude of reported deception has not decreased as four exemplars published since the 1973 APA guidelines will illustrate: (a) Milgram's paradigm was duplicated by Shanab and Yahya (1977) with children as young as six; graphic reports of the children's reactions document trembling, lip biting, and nervous laughter; (b) White (1979) used a typical aggression paradigm in which a confederate angered real subjects by evaluating them personally in a highly negative and insulting manner; subjects were then asked to administer shocks to the confederate, after being given a false cover story as to the purpose of the experiment; (c) Zimbardo, Andersen, and Kabat (1981) induced partial deafness through posthypnotic suggestion to study the effect of unrecognized hearing deficit on the development of paranoia; Zimbardo et al. then misinformed subjects as to the purpose of the experiment and what experiences they would undergo and recruited subjects with the promise that they would continue to play a part in his research, a promise that was not kept; and (d) Marshall and Zimbardo (1979) used multiple high-magnitude deceptions to study the affective consequences of inadequately explained physiological arousal; they misinformed subjects about the purpose of the experiment; they manipulated physiological arousal via injection of epinephrine or placebo after telling subjects that they would receive a vitamin injection; and they misled subjects into thinking their responses were not being monitored when they were. They then postponed debriefing for six weeks until all subjects had been tested. The IRB permitted all of the above manipulations, balking only at a planned "angry" condition on the basis that it was unethical to induce anger in unsuspecting subjects.

Rule-Utilitarian Objections
to Deception Research

The cost-benefit analysis arising from the metaethical justification called *act-utilitarianism* (Frankena, 1963) is used to justify these exceptions. By contrast, *deontological* or *rule-utilitarian* metaethical positions do not lend themselves to justification of the use of deceptive research practices. From both these more stringent metaethical positions, if informed consent is a right of participants and intentional deception a necessary violation of that right, then intentional deception is to be avoided in the research setting.

The thesis of act-utilitarianism is that a particular act is right if, and only if, no other act the agent could perform at the time would have, on the agent's evidence, better consequences. From an act-utilitarian stance, if in the opinion of the investigator, the requirements of the research demand that the participants be kept unaware that they are being studied or deception must be used to create a psychological reality in order to permit valid inference, then failure to obtain informed consent, concealment, and deception could be justified. The decision would be made by the investigator applying a cost-benefit calculus to the specific situation. Act-utilitarianism, by comparison with rule-utilitarianism, falls short as a metaethical system of justification because (a) it fails to consider the substantive rights of the minority, (b) it fails to take long-range costs into account, and (c) it is subjective and not generalizable. It takes little to convince a researcher or a review board of his or her peers that the long-range benefits of a clever bit of deceptive manipulation outweigh the short-range costs to participants of being deceived. The long-range costs to subjects and society are unknown and therefore are easy for investigators and review boards to dismiss. It is difficult to imagine more extreme instances of deception than those provided by Zimbardo's experiments, and yet both were approved by the Stanford IRB, subsequent to 1973, just as Milgram's experiments had been reviewed favorably at Yale prior to 1973.

Deontological moralists (e.g., Wallwork, 1975) claim that the basic judgments of obligation are perceived as being given intuitively without recourse to consideration of what serves as the common good. For deontologists such as Kant, the principle of justice or truth or the value of life stands by itself without regard to any balance of good over evil for self, society, or the universe. By contrast, I hold, with Waddington (1960), that the function of ethical beliefs is to mediate human evolution so that there can be no principles, including preservation of life, distributive justice, and trustworthiness that are absolutely inviolable.

I ground my judgment that intentional deception in the research setting is morally wrong not in act-utilitarianism (which is too relativistic) or in a deontological categorical imperative (which is too dogmatic), but rather in rule-utilitarianism, the view that an act is right if, and only if, it would be as beneficial to the common good in a particular social context to have a moral code permitting that act as to operate under a rule that would prohibit that act. In Western society, as a result of innate or learned behaviors associated with optimum survival for our community, most of us elevate rules of social living that maximize the opportunity for self-determination so that we may hold each other accountable for our actions. Also, we share strong aversions to certain types of actions. We are averse to hurting others, killing others, and telling lies, and so we feel that we must *justify* these acts if we intentionally commit them. Those of us who are rule-utilitarians grant that even actions to which we have strong moral aversions are justifiable in certain contexts. Thus, retaliative aggression may be justifiable provided that it is proportionate to the grievance; killing may be justifiable if our victim is an enemy or a murderer or a fetus under three months; telling lies may be justifiable if intended to benefit the recipient and not the liar; hurting others may be justifiable if we are dentists or surgeons. However, by justifying morally aversive acts we legitimate them, and this, too, has social consequences, because harm inflicted self-righteously may appear to demand no reparation and is not self-correcting.

Why is intentional deception in the context of the research endeavor so wrong from a rule-utilitarian perspective? At least three ethical rules generally accepted in Western society proscribe deceitful research practices: (a) the right of self-determination within the law, which translates in the research setting to the right of informed consent; (b) the obligation of a fiduciary (in this case, the researcher) to protect the welfare of the beneficiary (in this case, the subject); and (c) the obligation, particularly of a fiduciary, to be trustworthy in order to provide sufficent social stability to facilitate self-determined agentic behavior. Consistent wtih a rule-utilitarian position, I propose to ground these rules teleologically by arguing that their adoption benefits modern Anglo-American society more than contradictory rules, thus explaining their general acceptance.

The principle of *informed consent* is a manifestation of the basic right granted each individual in Anglo-American political philosophy and tradition to be self-determining and let alone so long as the individual is not interfering with the rights of other individuals or the public. According to Sir William Blackstone (1765–1769/1941), individuals surrender to society many rights and privileges that they would be free to exercise in a state of nature, in exchange for benefits that each receives as a member of society. Each citizen retains, however, certain rights and privileges that the public may not abrogate without the citizen's consent. Thus, subjects have the right to judge for themselves whether being lied to or learning something painful about themselves constitutes psychological harm for them. A violation of an individual's right of informed consent is a breach of the social contract and thus legitimates retaliative lawlessness because only in a rule-following environment may we be held fully accountable for the consequences of our actions. Therefore, social scientists must exercise their right to seek knowledge within the constraints imposed by the right to informed consent of those persons from whom they would obtain that knowledge.

Further, the basic rules of fiduciary law apply to the researcher-subject and the teacher–student relationships (Holder, 1982). A fiduciary obligation pertains when a person, called the *fiduciary*, is dealing with another under circumstances involving the placing of a special confidence. The overriding duty of the fiduciary is loyalty and trustworthiness by contrast to the principle of "caveat emptor," which may apply to some sales relations. If challenged, the burden of proof is on the fiduciary to show loyalty and trustworthiness. It is illogical for an investigator to justify the use of deceit by appealing to the special quality of the investigator–subject relationship when it is just that special quality that enables the investigator to recruit participants and establishes the fiduciary obligations of the investigator to be trustworthy in relations with them. If the rule that justifies scientific experimentation is "You shall know the truth, and the truth shall set you free," then that rule applies also in the conduct of science.

Finally, violation of trust is generally held to be immoral, and even more so in a fiduciary relationship, especially when the subject is also a student for whom the experimenter serves as a model. If the student is beguiled, his or her trust has been misplaced. If the student is not beguiled, then deceptive instructions do not undermine trust. Psychology undergraduates in heavily experimental departments expect rigged lotteries, deceptive instructions, and the use of confederates. Those who adopt a gameset are not likely to be disillusioned because they do not assume that the experimenter is trustworthy. Under those conditions, subjects may be beguiled, but they are not betrayed. The wrong done as well as the harm done is trivial. But to the extent that students routinely suspend belief, then experimental control has not been achieved by deceptive instructions, and there are no benefits to weigh against the costs. The costs include encouraging students to lie in the interests of science and career advancement.

Even from the permissive stance of an act-utilitarian cost-benefit analysis, it is the responsibility of investigators who wish to use deceptive practices that fail to conform to the informed consent provision of the ethical guidelines to demonstrate first, that the social and scientific benefits of their proposed research objectives are indeed sufficiently significant to offset the costs to participants, the profession, and society; second, that the research paradigm will effectively accomplish those objectives; and third, that those objectives cannot be accomplished equally well by using nondeceptive research paradigms. We proceed now to reexamine the costs and benefits of deception research.

Costs of Deception Research

The costs of deceptive research practices accrue to the participants, to the scientific enterprise, and to society.

Harm Done to the Subject

A brief excerpt from an autobiographical account of a former secretary who typed my earlier articles illustrates the subtle but serious harm that can be done to subjects by undermining their trust in their own judgment and in fiduciaries as well as the reluctance many have to admit, even to themselves, that they have been duped.

This experiment [involving deceptive feedback about quality of performance relative to peers] confirmed my conviction that standards were completely arbitrary . . . because the devastating blow was struck by a psychologist, whose competence to judge behavior I had never doubted before. . . . It is not a matter of "belief" but of fact that I found the experience devastating.

I was harmed in an area of my thinking which was central to my personal development at that time. Many of us who volunteered for the experiment were hoping to learn something about ourselves that would help us to gauge our own strengths and weaknesses, and formulate rules for living that took them into account. When, instead, I learned that I did not have any trustworthy way of knowing myself—or anything else—and hence could have no confidence in any lifestyle I formed on the basis of my knowledge, I was not only disappointed, but felt that I had somehow been cheated into learning, not what I needed to learn, but something which stymied my very efforts to learn. I told literally no one about it for eight years because of a vague feeling of shame over having let myself be tricked and duped. It was only when I realized that I was not peculiar but had, on the contrary, had a *typical* experience that I first recounted it publicly. (Baumrind, 1978, pp. 22–23)

Anecdotal evidence such as this has been challenged as heresay. A number of studies have been undertaken to establish whether subjects are harmed by deception experiments. The results are equivocal. However, most of these studies rely on self-report rather than behavioral evidence. About 80% of subjects, when asked, say that they were glad to have participated in the experiment. This is used illogically to establish that subjects suffered no harm. Thus, Milgram (1974, p. 195) justified his shocking procedure by citing results of a follow-up questionnaire in which 84% of subjects said they were glad to have participated in the experiment. However, as Patten (1977) pointed out, it is logically inconsistent for Milgram to use the self-reported judgments of overly acquiescent ("destructively obedient") subjects to establish the ethical propriety of his experiments. Similarly, Marshall and Zimbardo's (1979) subjects were chosen for their hypnotic suggestibility and would be expected to defer compliantly to the experimenter's expertise. After all, if self-reports could be regarded as accurate measures of the impact of experimental conditions, we could dispense entirely with experimental manipulation and behavioral measures, substituting instead vivid descriptions of environmental stimuli to which subjects would be instructed to report how they would act.

Self-report questionnaires used to assess participants' reactions are tacked on as an afterthought and generally lack psychometric sophistication. Subjects' self-reported gladness to be stressed and deceived may be explained by a variety of psychological mechanisms in addition to deferential compliance discussed above. These mechanisms include reduction of cognitive dissonance, identification with the aggressor, and masochistic obedience. It takes well-trained clinical interviewers to uncover true feelings of anger, shame, or altered self-image in participants who believe that what they say should conform with their image of a "good subject." Ring, Wallston, and Corey (1970), in their follow-up interview exploring subjective reactions to a Milgram-type obedience experiment, reported that many subjects stated that they were experiencing difficulty in trusting adult authorities. In a recently reported study of the effects of debriefing (Smith & Richardson, 1983), about 20% of 464 introductory psychology undergraduates reported experiencing harm. In the harm group, 61% had participated in a deception experiment as compared to 38% in the no-harm group. Students who had participated in deception experiments tended to perceive psychologists as less trustworthy than did nondeceived participants. Even subjects who deny other harmful effects do report decreased trust in social scientists following deception research. For example, citing instances of experimental deception:

> Fillenbaum (1966) found that deception led to increased suspiciousness (even though subjects tended not to act on their suspicions), and Keisner (1971) found that deceived and debriefed subjects were "less inclined to trust experimenters to tell the truth" (p. 7). Other authors (Silverman, Shulman, & Wiesenthal, 1970; Fine & Lindskold, 1971) have noted that deception decreases compliance with demand characteristics and increases negativistic behavior. (In Wahl, 1972, p. 12)

Decreased trust in fiduciaries then is a generally acknowledged cost of deception itself. Even if we choose to accept self-report data as veridical, 20% of subjects report such harm and the proportion is highest for deception research. From an ethical and legal perspective, harm is done to *each* individual. The harm the minority of subjects report they have suffered is not nullified by the majority of subjects who claim to have escaped unscathed, any more than the harm done victims of drunk drivers can be excused by the disproportionate number of pedestrians with sufficient alacrity to avoid being run over by them.

From a rule-utilitarian perspective, the procedural issue concerns where the locus of control should rightly reside. The generally accepted principle of respect for self-determination dictates that the locus of control should reside with each participant. The subject, like the investigator, retains the right to decide whether the likely benefits to self and society outweigh the likely costs to self and society. The investigator is not privileged to weigh the costs to the subjects against the benefits to society. The principle of informed consent allows the subject to decide how to dispose of his or her person. The subject acting as sovereign agent may freely agree to incur risk, inconvenience, or pain. But a subject whose consent has been obtained by deceitful and fraudulent means has become an object for the investigator to manipulate. A subject can only regain sovereignty by claiming to have been a subject all along and not an object. Not surprisingly, subjects tend to affirm their agency by denying that they have allowed themselves to be treated as objects, and when queried by an experimenter, most will say that they were glad to have been subjects.

Harm Done to the Profession

The harm done by deception researchers accrues to the profession and to the larger society as well as to the individual. The scientific costs of deception in research are considerable. These costs include (a) exhausting the pool of naive subjects, (b) jeopardizing community support for the research enterprise, and (c) undermining the commitment to truth of the researchers themselves.

The power of the scientific community is conferred by the larger community. Social support for behavioral science research is jeopardized when investigators promote parochial values that conflict with more universal principles of moral judgment and moral conduct. The use of the pursuit of truth to justify deceit risks the probable effect of undermining confidence in the scientific enterprise and in the credibility of those who engage in it. As a result of widespread use of deception, psychologists are suspected of being tricksters. Suspicious subjects may respond by role-playing the part they think the investigator expects, doing what they think the investigator wants them to do (Orne, 1962), or pretending to be naive. The *practice* of deceiving participants and of justifying such deception undermines the investigators' own integrity and commitment to truth. Short-term gains are traded for the cumulative costs of long-term deterioration of investigators' ethical sensibilities and integrity and damage to their credibility.

Harm Done to Society

The moral norm of reciprocity proscribing deceitful social relations both acknowledges and places a positive value on the fact that the elements of social reality are reciprocally determined. The inherent cost of behaving deceitfully in the research setting is to undermine trust in expert authorities. If conduct in the laboratory or natural setting cannot be isolated from conduct in daily life, the implications are far-reaching. In a popular article entitled "Snoopology," John Jung (1975) discussed some probable effects of experimentation in real-life situations with persons who did not know they were serving as experimental subjects. These included increased self-consciousness in public places, broadening of the aura of mistrust and suspicion that pervades daily life, inconveniencing and irritating persons by contrived situations, and desensitizing individuals to the needs of others by "boy-who-cried-wolf" effects so that unusual public events are suspected of being part of a research project.

Truth telling and promise keeping serve the function in social relations that physical laws do in the natural world; these practices promote order and regularity in social relations, without which intentional actions would be very nearly impossible. By acting in accord with agreed-upon rules, keeping promises, acting honorably, and following the rules of the game, human beings construct for themselves a coherent consistent environment in which purposive behavior becomes possible.

BENEFITS OF DECEPTION

Even if a simple cost-benefit calculus consistent with act-utilitarianism is adopted and we agree to weigh the costs to subjects against the benefits to humankind, we must still inquire as to what these benefits might be. Consideration of the benefits of a proposed investigation within the context of a cost-benefit ethical analysis requires more stringent standards for what constitutes scientifically and socially valid research than in a purely empirical context. I will argue that the scientific and social benefits of deception research cannot be established with sufficient certitude to tip the scale in favor of procedures that wrong subjects. The deception paradigms employed by experimental social psychologists do not and cannot deliver the reduction in ambiguity that could justify what would otherwise be regarded as ethically unacceptable research practices. Deceptive practices do not succeed in accomplishing the scientific objectives that are used to justify such deception, any better than methods that do not require deception. If the phenomenon being studied is socially important it can be studied in natural or clinical contexts that do not require laboratory manipulation to produce. If laboratory controls are required to create a counterfactual condition that exists nowhere, then in order to claim benefits, it must first be shown that the counterfactual conditions are possible to create in situ and that the common good would be enhanced by doing so.

The claim is made that deceptive manipulations are required to create a psychological reality under experimental conditions that permit valid inference. This claim is based on two assumptions: (a) deceptive instructions create a uniform psychological reality; and (b) causal inference in the social sciences can be achieved with a high level of certitude. But neither of these assumptions has gone unchallenged by critics of experimental social psychological methods.

Deception does not create a uniform psychological reality when subjects in an experiment differ in their level of naiveté or in their responses to the possibility of experimental manipulation. It is now common knowledge among many kinds of prospective subjects that deception is employed routinely in social psychological experiments. The tendency of some subjects to assign idiosyncratic meaning rather than to buy the experimenter's cover story, even when it is true, defeats the purpose of deceptive instructions, which is to control subject set. There is evidence that investigators untrained in phenomenological assessment methodology will fail to detect subject suspiciousness. Page (1973) has shown that asking subjects fewer than four questions will classify only 5% of subjects as suspicious, whereas extended questionnaires will yield about 40% suspicious subjects, and the behaviors of suspicious subjects in the experimental situation are generally found to differ from those who are not. Referring to laboratory research, Seeman (1969) concluded, "In view of the frequency with which deception is used in research we may soon be reaching a point where we no longer have naive subjects, but only naive experimenters" (p. 1026).

The traditional experimental social psychologist justifies deception research on the logical positivist presupposition that laboratory observations *could* provide unassailable knowledge if only we were able to produce a uniform psychological reality and do away with error variance. The objective of the traditional social psychology experiment is to enable the experimenter to infer unambiguously the existence and direction of causal relations by ruling out alternative causal explanations. Controls requiring deceptive instructions are introduced with the implicit expectation that their use can provide such unassailable knowledge. But the claim that observations can provide value-free, objective knowledge has been challenged by philosophers and scientists at least since Heisenberg's (1958) principle was enunciated. From the perspective of their critics, experimental controls distort by controlling the phenomena the investigator is attempting to explain. The meaning subjects assign to a situation depends upon the characteristics of that situation, as well as upon subject characteristics. A psychological mechanism observed to operate under one set of experimental conditions often fails to replicate under a somewhat different set of experimental conditions because the meaning persons give a situation is contextual and purposive and dependent upon factors that the experimenter may not even be aware of, such as the strangeness of the situation from the perspective of the subject. Typically the conjunction of events in a laboratory situation is atypical, and the effect of constraining the options a subject has is itself a factor that distorts the responses given and the behavior observed. Whereas laboratory methods construct situations and contexts for persons and then assess how they respond to these extrinsicially constructed situations, persons in their natural settings typically construct or select their own social worlds among the options available. Bronfenbrenner (1977) called for an ecological perspective in developmental and social research precisely because he disputed the possibility that subjects *could* assign the same meaning to their behavior in the natural setting as they did in the highly artificial laboratory setting.

Thus, it can be argued that laboratory conditions create the very ambiguity they are intended to dispel. For example, Gardner (1978) could not replicate Glass and Singer's (1972) findings of negative aftereffects of noise when subjects knew that they had the option of discontinuing participation. Assurance of freedom to withdraw removed the effect of the noise stressor. If Glass and Singer intended to study the negative aftereffects of noise per se, their experimental manipulation was inappropriate. If, on the other hand, they intended to study the effects of *inescapable* noise, their experimental situation was highly relevant, but clearly violated participants' right to withdraw. Similarly, the experimental condition created by Milgram in his studies of "destructive obedience" exemplifies a highly ambiguous control that seriously compromises the generalizability of his findings. Because subjects were paid for their participation and recruited on that basis, obedience in Milgram's setting for some subjects might have reflected a sense of fair play and employee loyalty rather than, as for other subjects, shocking obedience. Moreover, Milgram's experimental directives were incongruous and bizarrre, thus confusing and distressing the subject. Furthermore, the experimenter's orders were legitimized by the laboratory setting, thus permitting subjects to resolve their sense of incongruity by trusting the good will of the investigator toward both subject and confederate. Far from illuminating real life, as he claimed, Milgram in fact appeared to have constructed a set of conditions so internally inconsistent that they could not occur in real life. His application of his results to destructive obedience in military settings or Nazi Germany (Milgram, 1974) is metaphoric rather than scientific.

Not only was the situation artificial in Milgram's experiment, but all the necessary data were provided by the graduate student confederates who demonstrated conclusively by obeying Milgram's instructions to inflict suffering upon the subjects that normal, well-intentioned people will hurt others who are innocent. The confederates justified their actions on the same bases as the subjects justified theirs, that they were inflicting no real harm. Because subjects' motives could not unambiguously be called destructive obedience and the behavior of his graduate student confederates could, Milgram's deceitful manipulation was neither necessary nor could it permit valid inference to the real-life situations to which Milgram generalized his results.

Defenders of laboratory manipulations have attempted to rebut the criticism that laboratory experiments lack external validity and therefore do not produce knowledge of benefit to society that could justify misinforming subjects. Berkowitz and Donnerstein (1982) argued that laboratory experiments are oriented mainly toward testing causal hypotheses concerning mediational processes and are not carried out to determine the probability that a certain event will occur in a particular population. They claimed that, in theoretically oriented investigations, the specific manipulations and measures are merely arbitrary operational definitions of general theoretical constructs and the subject sample is merely an arbitrary group from the general universe of all humans to which the hypothesis is assumed to apply.

> We now have come to our central thesis: The meaning the subjects assign to the situation they are in and the behavior they are carrying out plays a greater part in determining the generalizability of an experiment's outcome than does the sample's demographic representativeness or the setting's surface realism. (Berkowitz & Donnerstein, 1982, p. 249)

But if the specific operations were interchangeable as Berkowitz and Donnerstein claimed, the context and subject populations could be altered without changing the results. However, failure to replicate social psychological findings when probed by a critical investigator is more the rule than the exception in social psychology, and the failure to replicate can seldom be attributed unambiguously to a controlled change in experimental conditions. Results do not survive even minor changes in the experimental conditions, such as notifying subjects that they may withdraw from an experiment. Therefore, Berkowitz and Donnerstein were incorrect in claiming that the specific operations typically employed in social psychological experiments are interchangeable. In the event that the variables that are untied and independently manipulated in the laboratory setting are necessarily or typically confounded in the natural setting, conditions in the laboratory cannot or will not be replicable. Psychological processes do not occur in a psychosocial vacuum. When the task, variables, and setting can have no real-world counterparts, the processes dissected in the laboratory also cannot operate in the real world. In that case, deceptive research practices cannot be justified by their benefits to science and society.

Furthermore, deceptive practices cannot be justified unless they result in findings that are controversial because the benefit to society of noncontroversial, that is, trivial, findings is minimal. Berkowitz and Donnerstein markedly attenuated the importance of causal hypotheses by claiming that experimenters ask only, *can* "alterations in Variable X lead to changes in Variable Y?" This is generally a trivial question because we almost always know prior to conducting the experiment that the answer is yes. Generally, the phenomenon has already been shown to occur in real life. For example, did Zimbardo and his colleagues (1981) really need to induce partial deafness through posthypnotic suggestion to confirm what is a generally acknowledged clinical observation that unexplained deafness in older people induces suspiciousness?

The mechanistic model of development implied by experimental social psychological procedures is not really applicable to social psychological phenomena. If the Cartesian, mechanistic world view is insufficient to explain the physical world, then it is certainly not adequate to explain biosocial and psychosocial phenomena. If physical reality is subject to indeterminacy introduced by the observer, as Heisenberg (1958) assured us it is, how much more true is this of human behavior? The level of complexity of social phenomena and the implausibility of treating human beings as interchangeable or even as identical with themselves over time sharply limit the level of certitude that can accompany any empirical generalization in the sociobehavioral sciences.

A little ingenuity may well yield fruitful alternatives to deception (see Geller, 1982, for a systematic review of such alternatives). If a phenomenon is socially significant it can frequently be observed in situ, making experimental manipulation unnecessary. Alternatively, experimenters could act as subjects in their own experiments and employ introspection. Aggression can certainly be studied in situ. Aggression researchers can study acts intended to harm others in such naturalistic situations as organized sports, which vary along relevant parameters such as rules and normative expectations. Investigators interested in studying how people justify intentionally causing others to suffer in real life have the option of introspective examination of their own behavior as participants in the research process. Thus, in lieu of the familiar teacher–learner aggression paradigm (Berkowitz & Geen, 1966) in which a confederate makes a series of preplanned errors on a word-association task and subjects deliver shocks to the confederate, investigators and their confederates could introspect. It turns out that subjects believe that they are benefiting the learner and therefore are not behaving aggressively in the sense of intending to inflict harm (Kane, Joseph, & Tedeschi, 1976). Experimenters and their confederates argue just as research subjects do that their motives in inflicting emotionally painful discomfort are altruistic or justified by role expectations, even though an objective observer might regard the behavior of confederates and subjects as equally aggressive. For example, Milgram justified his deceptive procedure by suggesting that many subjects were grateful for the insight into their own destructively obedient tendencies that the experiment and debriefing afforded. Investigators could also study retaliative aggression without using deception by introducing certain non-deceptive experimental conditions in which they acted as real, rather than confederate, subjects. Immediately after the usual perfunctory debriefing in deception research, subjects would be instructed to demonstrate behaviorally how they feel about their participation by delivering 0 to 20 mild but genuine electric shocks to the forearm of the experimenter who designed the research. In addition to providing data on subjects' response to deception and some data on retaliative aggression, this aversive reinforcement coda might have the added advantage of rendering superfluous any need for extrinsically imposed codes mandating ethical practices in the conduct of research with human participants.

The suggestion that psychologists serve as their own subjects and introspect was made before me by the investigators whose work Marshall and Zimbardo (1979) failed to replicate:

> In these days of ethical guidelines and human subjects committees, this may very well be the end of the matter, for it is unlikely that anyone will do experiments such as ours or Marshall and Zimbardo's for quite a while, if ever again. On the particular issue at stake, however, this is probably of little moment, for this is one issue on which the readers can serve as their own subjects. If they will do a thorough introspective job after convincing a physician to inject them with .5 cc of a 1:1000 solution of epinephrine, they can decide which of us is right. (Schachter & Singer, 1979, p. 995)

Debriefing

Effective debriefing does not nullify the wrong done participants by deceiving them and may not even repair their damaged self-image or ability to trust adult authorities. Subjects did, after all, commit acts that they believed at the time could be harmful to others, and they were in fact, entrapped into committing those acts by an authority whom they had reason to trust. And if the participants (subjects and confederates) are students, they have, in fact, been provided with a model of behavior in which scientific ends are used to justify deceitful means.

However, if an investigator does elect to use deception, he or she must include an effective debriefing procedure in order to reduce the long-range costs of deception and offer partial reparation to subjects. Sieber (1983) offered carefully considered recommendations for debriefing when deception is used. She argued convincingly that deceptive debriefing is especially unethical and that debriefing in deception research should be undertaken only by a skilled and sympathetic professional, or it may do more harm than good. For example, Mills (1976) presented in detail a debriefing scenario that he developed over 20 years of debriefing, and that provides the participant with an educational experience as well as a truthful account of the experiment's actual nature. The experiment is explained very gradually and every point reviewed until the subject understands. Subjects are given time to reorganize their perceptions of the experiment and their responses to it, from possible humiliation and discomfort to self-acceptance and, it is to be hoped, sympathetic understanding of the researcher's perspective. Subjects are offered a genuine opportunity to withdraw their data after having received a full explanation of the purposes of the experiment. Moreover, by adding to the investigators' emotional and fiscal costs, painstaking and effective debriefing procedures introduce a noncoercive but persuasive deterrent to investigators who are contemplating deception research.

REFERENCES

American Psychological Association, Committee for the Protection of Human Participants in Research. (1973). *Ethical principles in the conduct of research with human participants.* Washington, DC: Author.

American Psychological Association, Committee for the Protection of Human Participants in Research. (1982). *Ethical principles in the conduct of research with human participants* (2nd ed.). Washington, DC: Author.

Baron, R. A. (1981). The "Costs of deception" revisited: An openly optimistic rejoinder. *IRB: A Review of Human Subjects Research, 3*(1), 8–10.

Baumrind, D. (1964). Some thoughts on ethics of research: After reading Milgram's "Behavioral study of obedience." *American Psychologist, 19*, 421–423.

Baumrind, D. (1971). Principles of ethical conduct in the treatment of subjects: Reaction to the draft report of the Committee on Ethical Standards in Psychological Research. *American Psychologist, 26*, 887–896.

Baumrind, D. (1972). Reactions to the May 1972 draft report of the Ad Hoc Committee on Ethical Standards in Psychological Research. *American Psychologist, 27*, 1082–1086.

Baumrind, D. (1975a). It neither is nor ought to be: A reply to Wallwork. In E. C. Kennedy (Ed.), *Human rights and psychological research: A debate on psychology and ethics* (pp. 83–102). New York: Thomas Y. Crowell.

Baumrind, D. (1975b). Metaethical and normative considerations governing the treatment of human subjects in the behavioral sciences. In E. C. Kennedy (Ed.), *Human rights and psychological research: A debate on psychology and ethics* (pp. 37–68). New York: Thomas Y. Crowell.

Baumrind, D. (1978). Nature and definition of informed consent in research involving deception. In *The Belmont Report: Ethical principles and guidelines for the protection of human subjects of research* (DHEW Publication No. (OS) 78-0014, 23-1-23-71). Washington, DC: The National Commission for the Protection of Human Subjects of Biomedical and Behavioral Research.

Baumrind, D. (1979). IRBs and social science research: The costs of deception. *IRB: A Review of Human Subjects Research, 1*(6), 1–4.

Berkowitz, L., & Donnerstein, E. (1982). External validity is more than skin deep: Some answers to criticisms of laboratory experiments. *American Psychologist, 37*, 245–257.

Berkowitz, L., & Geen, R. G. (1966). Film violence and the cue properties of available targets. *Journal of Personality and Social Psychology, 3*, 525–530.

Blackstone, W. (1941). *Commentaries on the laws of England.* Washington, DC: The Washington Law Book Co. (Original work published 1765–1769)

Bronfenbrenner, U. (1977). Toward an experimental ecology of human development. *American Psychologist, 32*, 513–531.

Dresser, R. S. (1981). Deception research and the HHS final regulations. *IRB: A Review of Human Subjects Research, 3*(4), 3–4.

Fillenbaum, S. (1966). Prior deception and subsequent experimental performance: The "faithful" subject. *Journal of Personality and Social Psychology, 4*, 532–537.

Fine, R. H., & Lindskold, S. (1971). Subject's experimental history and subject-based artifact. *Proceedings of the Annual Convention of the American Psychological Association, 6*, 289–290.

Frankena, W. (1963). *Ethics.* Englewood Cliffs, NJ: Prentice-Hall.

Gardner, G. T. (1978). Effects of federal human subjects regulations on data obtained in environmental stressor research. *Journal of Personality and Social Psychology, 36*, 628–634.

Geller, D. M. (1982). Alternatives to deception: Why, what, and how? In J. E. Sieber (Ed.), *The ethics of social research: Surveys and experiments* (pp. 40–55). New York: Springer-Verlag.

Glass, D. C., & Singer, J. E. (1972). *Urban stress: Experiments on noise and social stressors.* New York: Academic Press.

Goldstein, R. (1981). On deceptive rejoinders about deceptive research: A reply to Baron. *IRB: A Review of Human Subjects Research, 3*(8), 5–6.

Heisenberg, W. K. (1958). *Physics and philosophy:* New York: Harper & Row.

Holder, A. R. (1982). Do researchers and subjects have a fiduciary relationship? *IRB: A Review of Human Subjects Research, 4*(1), 6–7.

Jung, J. (1975). Snoopology. *Human behavior, 4*(10), 56–59.

Kane, T. R., Joseph, J. M., & Tedeschi, J. T. (1976). Person perception and the Berkowitz paradigm for the study of aggression. *Journal of Personality and Social Psychology, 33,* 663–673.

Keisner, R. (1971). *Debriefing and responsiveness to overt experimenter expectancy cues.* Unpublished manuscript, Long Island University, Long Island, NY.

Marshall, G. D., & Zimbardo, P. G. (1979). Affective consequences of inadequately explained physiological arousal. *Journal of Personality and Social Psychology, 37,* 970–988.

McNamara, J. R., & Woods, K. M. (1977). Ethical considerations in psychological research: A comparative review. *Behavior Therapy, 8,* 703–708.

Milgram, S. (1964). Issues in the study of obedience: a reply to Baumrind. *American Psychologist, 19,* 848–952.

Milgram, S. (1974). *Obedience to authority.* New York: Harper & Row.

Mills, J. (1976). A proecedure explaining experiments involving deception. *Personality and Social Psychology Bulletin, 2,* 3–13.

Orne, M. T. (1962). On the social psychology of the psychological experiment: With particular reference to demand characteristics and their implications. *American Psychologist, 17,* 776–783.

Page, M. M. (1973). On detecting demand awareness by post-experimental questionnaire. *Journal of Social Psychology, 91,* 305–323.

Patten, S. C. (1977). Milgram's shocking experiments. *Philosophy, 52,* 425–440.

Ring, K., Wallston, K., & Corey, M. (1970). Mode of debriefing as a factor affecting subjective reaction to a Milgram-type obedience experiment: An ethical inquiry. *Representative Research in Social Psychology, 1,* 67–88.

Schachter, S. & Singer J. (1979). Comments on the Maslach and Marshall-Zimbardo experiments. *American Psychologist, 37,* 989–995.

Seeman, J. (1969). Deception in psychological research. *American Psychologist, 24,* 1025–1028.

Shanab, M. E., & Yahya, K. A. (1977). A behavioral study of obedience in children. *Journal of Personality and Social Psychology, 35,* 530–536.

Sieber, J. E. (1983). Deception in social research III: The nature and limits of debriefing. *IRB: A Review of Human Subjects Research, 5*(3), 1–4.

Silverman, I., Shulman, A. D., & Wiesenthal, D. L. (1970). Effects of deceiving and debriefing psychological subjects on performance in later experiments. *Journal of Personality and Social Psychology, 14,* 203–212.

Smith, S. S., & Richardson, D. (1983). Amelioration of deception and harm in psychological research: The important role of debriefing. *Journal of Personality and Social Psychology, 44,* 1075–1082.

Waddington, C. H. (1960). *The ethical animal.* Chicago: University of Chicago Press.

Wahl, J. M. (1972, April). The utility of deception: An empirical analysis. In *Symposium on Ethical Issues in the Experimental Manipulation of Human Beings,* Western Psychological Association, Portland, Oregon.

Wallwork, E. (1975). In defense of substantive rights: A reply to Baumrind. In E. C. Kennedy (Ed.), *Human rights and psychological research* (pp. 103–125). New York: Thomas Y. Crowell.

White, L. A. (1979). Erotica and aggression: The influence of sexual arousal, positive affect, and negative affect on aggressive behavior. *Journal of Personality and Social Psychology, 37,* 591–601.

Zimbardo, P. G., Andersen, S. M., & Kabat, L. G. (1981, June). Induced hearing deficit generates experimental paranoia. *Science, 212,* 1529–1531.

Research and
Human Experimentation/Further Reading

Barber, Bernard, et al. *Research on Human Subjects: Problems of Social Control In Medical Experimentation.* New York: Russell Sage Foundation, 1973.

Capron, Alexander Morgan. "Informed Consent in Catastrophic Disease Research and Treatment." *University of Pennsylvania Law Review* 123 (December, 1974), 340–438.

Childress, James F. "Compensating Injured Research Subjects: I. The Moral Argument." *Hastings Center Report* 6 (December, 1976), 21–27.

Eisenberg, Leon. "The Social Imperatives of Medical Research." *Science* 198 (December, 1977), 1105–10.

"The Freedom of Inquiry and Subjects." *American Journal of Psychiatry* 134 (August, 1977), 891–913.

Fried, Charles. *Medical Experimentation: Personal Integrity and Social Policy. Volume 5 of Clinical Studies.* Edited by A. G. Bearn, D. A. K. Black, and H. H. Hiatt. New York: Elsevier, 1974.

Katz, Jay, Edited with Alexander A. Capron and Eleanor Swift Glass. *Experimentation With Human Beings.* New York: Russell Sage Foundation, 1972.

Rivlin, Alice M., and Timpane, P. Michael, Editors. *Ethical and Legal Issues of Social Experimentation.* Washington, D.C.: The Brookings Institution, 1975.

Roth, Loren H., et al. "Tests of Competency to Consent to Treatment." *American Journal of Psychiatry* 134 (March 1977), 279–84.

Walters, LeRoy. "Some Ethical Issues in Research Involving Human Subjects." *Perspectives in Biology and Medicine.* 20 (Winter, 1977), 193–211.

PART FIVE

ETHICAL DILEMMAS IN OBTAINING INFORMED CONSENT

Karen Lebacqz
Robert J. Levine
Benjamin Freedman
Alan Soble
Sissela Bok

19 Respect for Persons and Informed Consent to Participate in Research

KAREN LEBACQZ AND ROBERT J. LEVINE

This article investigates the foundations of and requirements for informed consent. Basing the requirement on the ethical principle of respect for persons, the authors argue that major disagreements over the requirement come from two different interpretations of the principle: 1) it requires that we protect another from harm and 2) it requires that we respect another's right to self-determination.

Karen Lebacqz is an Associate Professor of Ethics at the Pacific School of Religion
Robert J. Levine is Professor of Medicine at the Yale University School of Medicine

The first sentence of the Nuremberg Code (1947), "The voluntary consent of the human subject is absolutely essential," signals the centrality of the consent requirement in research using human subjects. Prior to Nuremberg, statements of medical and other professional organizations made no mention of the necessity for consent. Subsequently, the tendency to focus on "informed consent" has been reinforced by public outcry over the inadequacy of consent in certain landmark cases: *eg*, Willowbrook,[1, at p. 1007] Jewish Chronic Disease Hospital,[1, at p. 9] Tea Room Trade,[1, at p. 325] and most recently, Tuskegee.[2] Indeed, the issue of informed consent has so dominated recent discussion of the ethics of research that one might be led to think erroneously that other issues (*eg*, research design, selection of subjects) are either less important or more satisfactorily resolved.

The purpose of this essay is to explore the foundations of and requirements for informed consent. The requirement is best derived from the ethical principle of *respect for persons;* we contend that the major disagreements over the requirement arise from two conflicting interpretations of the principle: (1) it requires that we protect another from harm, and (2) it requires that we respect another's right to self-determination—ie, to be left alone or to make free choices. We shall provide examples of how these differing views have been expressed in the development of the legal requirements for informed consent to biomedical research.[a]

RESPECT FOR PERSONS

The principle of respect for persons was stated formally by Immanuel Kant: "So act as to treat humanity, whether in thine own person or in that of any other, in every case as an end withal, never as a means only."[5, at p. 441] However, what it means to treat a person as an *end* and not only as a *means* to another's end may be variously interpreted.

One interpretation of respect for persons is that it requires that we protect others from harm. This interpretation would be in accord with the Hippocratic admonition ". . . to help, or at least, to do no harm." The consent requirement can be justified as a form of helping, or at least not harming, the patient: seeking consent provides a mechanism for ascertaining what the patient might consider a "benefit" and whether the patient considers the anticipated benefits worth the taking of the risks.

However, a focus on benefits and harms does not establish a strict requirement for informed consent; physicians could avoid seeking consent in any situation in which they consider that informing the patient would be more harmful than beneficial. Such reasoning is commonly used to legitimate incomplete disclosure (*infra*).

Another interpretation of respect for persons is that it requires us to leave them alone—even to the point of allowing them to choose activities that might be harmful (*eg*, parachuting). Authors who share this interpretation speak of respecting a person's autonomy, self-determination, liberty, and so on. As stated by Justice Cardozo[1, at p. 526]: ". . . Every human being of adult years and sound mind has a right to determine what shall be done with his (*sic*) own body. . . ." In this interpretation of the principle, the purpose of informed consent is to assure the person's right to choose; the requirement for it cannot be overridden by concern for the possible harm that might be done by informing the person.[b]

AUTONOMY VERSUS PROTECTION

The tensions between protecting persons from harm and respecting their autonomy are reflected in two rather distinct approaches to interpret respect for persons to require the fostering of a covenantal relationship in which subjects are protected by giving truly *informed* consent. Benjamin Freedman,[8] on the other hand, construes the principle as requiring primarily and almost exclusively a respect for the individual's *freedom* to choose, regardless of whether the choice is informed.

For Jonas and Ramsey, the use of persons as means to another's end, as in research, is justified only if they so identify with the purposes of research that they *will* them as their own. Only such absolute identification rectifies the "sacrifice" of the individual for the collective good. Researcher and subject become "co-adventurers." The consent requirement affirms a basic covenantal bond between subject and researcher, and ensures that the person is not used simply as a means to an end.

While the focus on the will of persons suggests a primary interest in their freedom of choice, Jonas and Ramsey also argue that in order to establish a proper covenant (to become truly "co-adventurers"), the subject's consent must be *informed:* it must reflect a genuine appreciation of the purposes and especially of the risks of the research. The less one understands the risks and identifies with the purposes of research, the less valid is one's consent and the less desirable one's participation. Hence, for Jonas and Ramsey respect for the individual's autonomy is always strongly tempered by a concern to protect subjects from harm through ensuring that their consent is informed.

Therefore, the ideal subjects are those maximally able to identify with the goals of research and to understand the risk—namely, researchers themselves![6, at p. 17] Recognizing the need for a larger subject population than this ideal would permit, Jonas proposes a "descending order of permissibility" for the recruitment ("conscription") of volunteers. Therefore, he would be reluctant to allow the use of such vulnerable subjects as the sick.

While neither Jonas nor Ramsey focuses exclusively on patients as subjects, their treatment of informed consent appears to be influenced largely by the medical practice model. The stress on covenantal bonds and on the duty to do no harm is analogous to traditional assumptions about the physician-patient relationship. Research is seen as a violation of covenant because the physician-researcher no longer has the good of the patient-subject at heart and the subject is asked to sacrifice for the good of others.

This interpretation reflects certain assumptions which can be challenged:

1. The medical practice model may not be appropriate for many types of research: *eg,* social and behavioral research.[9, at p. 17]

Even in biomedical research—particularly basic research—there is often no physician-patient relationship between investigator and subject; thus one may question the relevance of discussing either the creation or the violation of these particular covenantal bonds.[c]

2. Research is not generally so risky (so much of a "sacrifice") as Jonas and Ramsey assume.[d]

3. This "ideal" model is probably impracticable.[15]

The most important challenge to the Jonas-Ramsey construction of the requirements for informed consent lies in an alternative interpretation of the principle of respect for persons. Freedman[8] interprets the principle to include a respect for the validity of an expression of will that is not "informed," even if the price of not being "informed" is not being able to "protect" oneself. Overprotection is seen as a form of dehumanization and lack of respect. For example, to classify persons as incompetent in order to "protect" them from their own judgments is the worst form of abuse.

In this interpretation, respect for persons means primarily to let persons alone and respect their expressions of autonomy. Protecting the welfare of persons must not ʰe bought at the price of repudiating their autonomy. "Fully informɛ ɪ consent" is not only unattainable, but in most cases undesirable! Rather, contends Freedman, we should strive for "valid" consent, which entails ". . . only the imparting of that information which the patient/subject requires in order to make a responsible decision." The two fundamental requirements are that the choice be responsible[e] and that it be voluntary. A person may *choose* not to be fully informed, and a decision based on less information (or different information) than another person might consider essential is not to be regarded as a sign of irresponsibility. Thus Freedman opens up the possibility of a "valid yet ignorant consent." Information and protection must not be forced upon potential subjects.

REQUIREMENTS FOR INFORMED CONSENT

According to the Nuremberg Code, to consent to participate in research one must: (a) have the "legal capacity" to give consent, (b) be "so situated as to be able to exercise free power of choice," (c) have "sufficient knowledge" on which to decide, and (d) have "sufficient . . . comprehension" to make an "enlightened" decision. Most commentators agree that compromise of any one of these conditions jeopardizes the ethical acceptability of research. However, they differ on what constitutes a compromise, in part owing to different interpretations of what is required by the underlying principle of respect for persons.

"Free Power of Choice"

The Nuremberg Code proscribes ". . . any element of force . . . or other ulterior form of constraint or coercion . . ." in obtaining consent. Any flagrant coercion—*eg*, as when competent, comprehending persons are forced to submit to research against their expressed wills—clearly renders consent invalid.

Yet, more subtle or indirect "constraints" or "coercions" may obtain when prospective subjects are highly dependent, impoverished, or needy, as exemplified by persons who are confined involuntarily in institutions. Some commentators argue that consent to participate in research is not sufficiently voluntary when it is given (a) to procure financial reward in situations offering few alternatives for remuneration; (b) to seek release from an institution either by evidencing "good behavior" or by ameliorating the condition for which one was confined; or (c) to please physicians or authorities upon whom one's continued welfare depends.[16]

In contrast, Cornell West[17] argues that such indirect constraints (or inner motivations) do not invalidate consent by making it involuntary. True coercion, he asserts, consists in a *threat*—*eg*, a threat to put prisoners in "the hole" unless they cooperate. Consent given under such circumstances would not be voluntary. But offers of reward—*eg*, better living conditions or financial remuneration—are not, strictly speaking, "coercion" and do not render consent involuntary. While West agrees with other commentators that rewards should not be so high as to constitute "undue" or "unfair" inducement and that advantage should not be taken of the confined circumstances of prisoners, mental patients, and other institutionalized persons, his argument nonetheless provides grounds for rejecting an overprotection of confined persons on the basis that they cannot give valid consent. Parenthetically, we note that many prisoners protest such overprotection and do not consider it an appropriate expression of respect for them as persons.

Competence and Comprehension

The Nuremberg Code requires both "legal capacity" to consent and "sufficient understanding" to reach an "enlightened" decision, without specifying what is meant by either. Contemporary interpretations tend to link the two, defining competence in terms of comprehension—*eg*, the ability to evaluate relevant information,[18, at p. 55] to understand the consequences of action,[19, at p. 183] or to reach a decision for rational reasons.[3, at p. 203; 5, at p. 445] However, Joseph Goldstein[20, at p. 15] charges that this link is "pernicious," since refusal to participate in research might be judged "irrational" and used as grounds for declaring a person incompetent. He argues that the purpose of the consent requirement is to guarantee the exercise of free choice, not to judge the rationality of the choice. Here again we see the tension between the desire to protect the individual (by ensuring the "rationality" of choice) and the requirement to respect that individual's freedom of choice.

This tension is further highlighted in debates about the validity of "proxy consent" to do research on subjects who lack the legal capacity to consent. Arguing strictly from the interpretation that respect for persons requires that we let them alone, Ramsey claims that the use of a nonconsenting subject (*eg*, a child) is wrong whether or not there is risk, simply because it involves an "unconsented touching." "Wrongful touching" is rectified only when it is for the good of the individual, because then the person is treated as an end as well as a means. Hence, proxy consent may be given for nonconsenting subjects only when the research includes therapeutic[f] interventions related to the subject's own recovery.[7, at p. 11]

But in a strict interpretation of leaving alone, the unconsented touching of a competent adult is wrong even if it benefits that person. Why, then, should benefit justify such touching for a child (or other subject unable to give consent)? Richard McCormick proposes that the validity of such interventions rests on the presumption that the person, if capable, *would* consent to therapy. This presumption in turn derives from a person's obligation to seek therapy—an obligation which people possess simply as human beings.[18, at p. 9] Because people have an obligation to seek their own well-being, we presume they *would* consent if they *could* and thus presume also that "proxy consent" for therapeutic interventions will not violate respect for them as persons.

By analogy, people have other obligations, as members of a moral community, to which one would presume their consent; this presumption justifies "proxy consent." One such obligation is to contribute to the general welfare when to do so requires little or no sacrifice. Hence, McCormick concludes that nonconsenting subjects may be used in research not directly related to their own benefit so long as the research fulfills an important social need and involves no discernible risk. In McCormick's view, respecting persons includes recognizing that they are members of a moral community with attendant obligations.

To this, Ramsey counters that children, at least, are not adults with a full range of duties and obligations. Therefore, they have no obligation to contribute to the general welfare and respect for them requires that they be protected from harm and from unconsented touching.

While Freedman[8] adopts Ramsey's premise that a child is not a moral being in the same sense as an adult, his analysis yields a different conclusion. Precisely because children are *not* autonomous they have no right to be let alone. Instead they have a right to custody. Thus the only relevant moral issue is the risk involved in research; the child must be protected from harm. Freedman, therefore, agrees with McCormick that children may be used in research unrelated to their therapy provided it presents them no discernible risk.

The inevitable conflict between the goals of promoting autonomy and providing protection are thus demonstrated in disagreements over both the standards of competence and the use of incompetent subjects.

Disclosure of Information

The Nuremberg Code requires that the subject be told "the nature, duration, and purpose of the experiment; the method and means by which it is to be conducted; all inconveniences and hazards reasonably to be expected; and the effects upon his (*sic*) health or person which may possibly come. . . ." There is no universal agreement on what constitutes "sufficient knowledge" to give an "informed" consent. Many commentators disagree over what sorts of information should be provided.[8] Those who agree on the need for disclosure of information of a particular sort—*eg*, the risks—often disagree on the extent of the information that must be provided. The Nuremberg Code requires explication of hazards "reasonably" to be expected. Does this include an infinitesimal chance of a substantial harm? A substantial chance of an infinitesimal harm?

Disagreements over particulars arise in part from disagreements about underlying standards: is disclosure to be determined by (1) general medical practice or opinion, (2) the requirements of a "reasonable person," or (3) the idiosyncratic judgment of the individual? While the legal trend may be shifting from the first to the second,[24, at p. 25] it may be argued that only the third is truly compatible with the requirement of respect for the autonomy of the individual person.[3, at pp. 31-37;23, at pp. 25-28]

Yet even those who adopt the third standard disagree as to its implications. As noted earlier, Freedman holds that the idiosyncratic judgment of the individual is overriding—to the point that the prospective subject can choose to have less information than a "reasonable" person might require. Veatch, however, argues that anyone refusing to accept as much information as would be expected of a "reasonable person" should not be accepted as a subject.[23, at p. 29]

Professional codes (eg, AMA code) and federal regulations[22] reflect the traditional medical maximum of "do no harm" and the legal doctrine of *therapeutic privilege* according to which a physician may withhold information when in his/her judgment disclosure is either infeasible or potentially harmful.[3, at p. 35] Recent critics have argued that invoking the doctrine of therapeutic privilege to justify withholding of information from a prospective subject in order to assure cooperation in a research project is almost never appropriate; it gives the investigator entirely too much license to serve vested interests by withholding information[h] that might be material to the decision of a prospective subject.[3, at p. 36]

The Consent Form

Considerations of informed consent in federal regulations and by members of Institutional Review Boards tend to focus on the composition and disposition of consent forms—ie, the *documentation* of the negotiations for informed consent.[11, at pp. 52-65] While the purpose of the *negotiations* for consent is to make operational the requirements of the principle of respect for persons, the purposes of the documentation are different. The most important function of meticulous and formal documentation of informed consent is to protect the interests of the investigator and the institution.[26, at p. 18] The net effect of the documentation may, in fact, be harmful to the interests of the subject: The retention of a signed consent form tends to give the advantage to the investigator in any adversary proceeding; moreover, the availability of such documents in institutional records may lead to violations of privacy and confidentiality.[27, at pp. 74-86] Indeed, Albert Reiss suggests that a change in the current system of documentation might better serve the interests of subjects: Where investigators now retain consent forms signed by subjects, Reiss would prefer that subjects retain statements of responsibility signed by investigators.[27]

Conclusions and Implications

The consent requirement is derived from the ethical principle of respect for persons. Most major disagreements over the requirements arise from two conflicting interpretations of the principle: (1) it requires that we protect another from harm, and (2) it requires that we respect another's right to self-determination—ie, to be left alone or to make free choices. Tensions between these conflicting interpretations are reflected in debates over who is sufficiently free to give valid consent, whether subjects must make rational decisions, whether consent is valid if it is not informed, and so on.

The recent trend in the evolution of federal regulation of research reflects an emphasis on the protection interpretation of the principle. This is manifest by, among other things, increasing requirements for formal and meticulous documentation of the negotiations for informed consent (mistakenly thought to provide protection for subjects) as well as proposals to establish consent committees and to assign monitoring functions to Institutional Review Boards. The development of excessive or inappropriate mechanisms for the protection of subjects is contrary to the interpretation that the principle of respect for persons requires that we respect another's right to self-determination.

It will be necessary to clarify further the principle of respect for persons and its interpretation in the requirement to give consent to participate in research. Because we see overprotection as a form of disrespect for persons, we favor an approach to consent that emphasizes the autonomy of prospective subjects.

REFERENCES AND NOTES

1. Katz J: Experimentation with Human Beings, New York, Russell Sage Foundation, 1972.

2. Final Report of the Tuskegee Syphilis Study, Ad Hoc Advisory Panel, Washington, DC, DHEW, Apr 1973.

3. Annas GJ, Glantz LH, Katz BF: The law of informed consent to human experimentation. Prepared for The National Commission for the Protection of Human Subjects of Biomedical and Behavioral Research, Jun 1976.

4. Fried C: Medical Experimentation, Personal Integrity and Social Policy. Amsterdam, North-Holland Publishing Company, 1974.

5. Macklin R, Sherwin S: Experimenting on human subjects, philosophical perspectives. Case Western Reserve Law Rev 25:434–471, 1975.

6. Jonas H: Philosophical reflections on experimenting with human subjects. In Freund PA (ed): Experimentation with Human Subjects. New York, George Braziller, 1970, pp. 1–31.

7. Ramsey P: The Patient as Person. New Haven, Yale University Press, 1970.

8. Freedman B: A moral theory of informed consent. Hastings Center Rep 5 (No. 4):32–39, 1975.

9. Baumrind D: Nature and definition of informed consent in research involving deception. Prepared for The National Commission for the Protection of Human Subjects of Biomedical and Behavioral Research, Jan, 1976.

10. Feinstein AR: Medical ethics and the architecture of clinical research. Clin Pharmacol Therapeut 15:316–334, 1974.

11. Levine RJ: The nature and definition of informed consent in various research settings. Prepared for The National Commission for the Protection of Human Subjects of Biomedical and Behavioral Research, Dec, 1975.

12. Levine RJ: Appropriate guidelines for the selection of human subjects for participation in biomedical and behavioral research. Prepared for The National Commission for the Protection of Human Subjects of Biomedical and Behavioral Research, Feb, 1976.

13. Arnold JD: Alternatives to the use of prisoners in research in the United States. Prepared for The National Commission for the Protection of Human Subjects of Biomedical and Behavioral Research, Mar, 1976.

14. Cardon PV, Dommel FW, Trumble RR: Injuries to research subjects. N Eng J Med 295:650–654, 1976.

15. Ingelfinger FJ: Informed (but uneducated) consent. N Eng J Med 287:465–466, 1972.

16. Branson R: Philosophical perspectives on experimentation with prisoners. Prepared for The National Commission for the Protection of Human Subjects of Biomedical and Behavioral Research, Feb, 1976.

17. West CR: Philosophical perspective on the participation of prisoners in experimental research. Prepared for The National Commission for the Protection of Human Subjects of Biomedical and Behavioral Research, Jan, 1976.

18. Shuman SI: The emotional, medical and legal reasons for the special concern about psychosurgery. In Ayd FJ Jr (ed): Medical, Moral and Legal Issues in Mental Health Care. Baltimore, Williams and Wilkins, 1974.

19. Katz J: Human rights and human experimentation. In Protection of Human Rights in the Light of Scientific and Technological Progress in Biology and Medicine (Proc 8th Round Table of Council for International Organizations of Medical Sciences, 1973), Geneva, World Health Organization, 1974.

20. Goldstein J: On the right of the institutionalized mentally infirm to consent to or refuse to participate as subjects in biomedical and behavioral research. Prepared for The National Commission for the Protection of Human Subjects of Biomedical and Behavioral Research, Feb, 1976.

21. McCormick RA: Proxy consent in the experimentation situation. Perspect Biol Med 18:2–20, 1974.

22. DHEW: Protection of human subjects: technical amendments. Fed Reg 40(50): 11854–11858, Mar 13, 1975.

23. Veatch RM: Three theories of informed consent: philosophical foundations and policy implications. Prepared for The National Commission for the Protection of Human Subjects of Biomedical and Behavioral Research, Feb, 1976.

24. Curran WJ: Ethical issues in short term and long term psychiatric research. In Ayd FJ Jr (ed): Medical, Moral and Legal Issues in Mental Health Care. Baltimore, William and Wilkins, 1974.

25. Ashley BM: Ethics of experimenting with persons. In Schoolar JC, Gaitz CM (eds): Research and the Psychiatric Patient. New York, Brunner and Mazel, 1975.

26. Levine RJ: On the relevance of ethical principles and guidelines developed for research to health services conducted or supported by the Secretary, DHEW. Prepared for The National Commission for the Protection of Human Subjects of Biomedical and Behavioral Research, May, 1976.

27. Reiss AJ: Selected issues in informed consent and confidentiality with special reference to behavioral-social science research-inquiry. Prepared for the National Commission for the Protection of Human Subjects of Biomedical and Behavioral Research, Feb, 1976.

a. It should be recognized that the legal grounding for the requirement for consent to research[3, at pp. 29-37; 4, at p. 18-25] is based on the outcome of litigation of disputes arising almost exclusively in the context of the practice of medicine. There is very nearly no case law upon which legal standards for consent to research, as distinguished from practice, might be defined (there is one Canadian case: *Halushka v. University of Saskatchewan*).

b. The law defines, in general, the circumstances under which a patient, or by extension, a research subject, may recover damages for having been wronged or harmed as a consequence of failure to negotiate adequate consent.[3, at p. 29-37] Traditionally, failure to negotiate adequate consent was treated as a *battery* action. In accord with the view that respect for persons requires us to leave them alone, the law of battery makes it wrong *a priori* to touch, treat, or do research upon a person without the person's consent. Whether or not harm befalls the person is irrelevant; it is the "unconsented-to touching" that is wrong.

The modern trend in malpractice litigation is to treat cases based upon failure to obtain proper consent as *negligence* rather than battery actions. The negligence doctrine combines elements of patient benefit and self-determination. To bring a negligence action, a patient/subject must prove: that the physician had a *duty* toward the patient; that the duty was *breached;* that *damage* occurred to the patient; and that the damage was *caused* by the breach. In contrast to battery actions, negligence actions remove as a basis for the requirement for consent the simple notion that "unconsented-to touching" is a wrong—rather, such touching is wrong (actionable) only if it is negligent and results in harm; otherwise, the patient/subject cannot recover damages.

Under both battery and negligence doctrines, consent is invalid if any information is withheld that might be considered material to the decision to give consent.

c. Whether or not negotiations for informed consent to research should be conducted according to different standards than consent to practice is a controversial matter. Feinstein[10] has observed that it is our custom to adhere to a "double standard": "An act that receives no special concern when performed as part of clinical practice may become a major ethical or legal issue if done as part of a formally designed investigation." In his view there is less need for formality in the negotiations for informed consent to a relationship where the interests of research and practice are conjoined—*eg,* as in research conducted by a physician-investigator having the aim of demonstrating the safety and/or efficacy of a non-validated therapeutic maneuver—than when the only purpose of the investigator-subject relationship is to perform research. Capron,[1, at p. 574] on the other hand, has asserted: "Higher requirements for informed consent should be imposed in therapy than in investigation, particularly when an element of honest experimentation is joined with therapy." Levine[11, at pp. 41-42] concluded that patients are entitled to the same degree of thoroughness of negotiations for informed consent as are subjects. However, patients may be offered the opportunity to delegate decision-making authority to a physician while subjects should rarely be offered this option. The most important distinction is that the prospective subject should be informed that in research, as contrasted with practice, the subject will be at least in part a means and perhaps only a means to another's end.

d. Most research does not present risk of physical or psychological harm; rather, it calls upon the subject to assume a burden that might more appropriately be named inconvenience.[12, at p. 8-11] The researcher calls upon subjects to give of their time, to perform tasks that might be tedious or embarrassing, or to experience transitory pains or other discomfort. The risk of physical or psychological harm from Phase I drug testing, for example, has been estimated as slightly greater than that of being an office secretary, $\frac{1}{7}$ that of window washers and $\frac{1}{9}$ that of miners.[13, at p. 18] For biomedical research generally, the following estimates have been reported[14]: In basic research (called "nontherapeutic" by the authors) the risk of being disabled either temporarily or permanently is substantially less than that of being similarly harmed by an accident. The risks of dying or becoming disabled in what the authors call "therapeutic research" are much higher; however, they seem much less than the risks of similar unfortunate outcomes for comparable patients in other medical settings involving no research.

e. A full elaboration of Freedman's use of the word *responsible* is beyond the scope of this essay. Interested readers are referred to his paper.[8]

f. This argument is based on the erroneous assumption—which Ramsey shares with many other authors—that research can be dichotomized into two distinct sets: "therapeutic" and "nontherapeutic." Authors using this classification usually argue that, since the purpose of "therapeutic research" is to benefit the subject, it is more easily justified than "nontherapeutic research." These arguments fail because they do not recognize that activities commonly referred to as "therapeutic research" generally include maneuvers designed to benefit persons other than the subject—*eg,* randomization is designed to develop generalizable knowledge about the safety and efficacy of therapies. The many problems that have been created by the categorization of research as "therapeutic" and "nontherapeutic" are elaborated in two essays in a forthcoming issue of the *Villanova Law Review:* (1) Lebacqz, K.: Some reflections on *Report and Recommendations: Research on the Fetus;* (2) Levine, R.J.: The impact on fetal research of the report of The National Commission for the Protection of Human Subjects of Biomedical and Behavioral Research.

g. Codes developed subsequent to Nuremberg have modified its requirements in various ways: disclosure of the purpose of research is often ignored, and other stipulations such as disclosure of the availability of alternative modes of treatment are added. Federal regulations[22] require (1) a fair explanation of procedures; (2) disclosure of risks; (3) explanation of benefits; (4) description of alternatives; (5) an offer to answer questions; and (6) a statement that the subject may withdraw at any time.

While these requirements have the force of law, they are by no means exhaustive of possible standards for disclosure. To them one might add: a statement of overall purpose; a clear invitation to participate in research, distinguishing maneuvers required for research purposes from those necessary for therapy; an explanation of why the particular person is invited (selected); a suggestion that the prospective subject might wish to discuss the research with another person; and an explanation (when appropriate) of the fact that the risks are unknown (much biomedical research is designated to determine the nature, probability and magnitude of harms that might be produced by a therapeutic maneuver).[11] Veatch[23] would add the names of members of any review boards that had approved the research, an explanation of who is responsible for harm done, and an explanation of the right, if any, to continue receiving treatments found useful.

h. Similarly, in research activities contingent upon subjects' lack of awareness of purposes or procedures it has been thought permissible to either withhold information or practice deliberate deception provided harms are minimized and subjects "debriefed" (given a full explanation) afterwards. Baumrind[9] opposes deceptive practices arguing not only that they violate the principle of respect for persons but also that eventually they will invalidate research on scientific grounds. Various proposals have been made to minimize the need for and harmful effects of deceptive practices: subjects might be invited to consent to incomplete disclosure with a promise of full disclosure at the termination of the research[11, at pp. 30-31]; subjects might be told as much as possible and asked to consent for specified limits of time and risk[25, at p. 19]; and consent based on full disclosure might be negotiated with mock or "surrogate" populations.[12, at pp. 26-29]

20 The Validity of Ignorant Consent to Medical Research

BENJAMIN FREEDMAN

This article examines the issues and implications connected with the critical question: "Can a consent obtained from a free and competent adult under conditions of ignorance be valid?" If such is not the case, many medical practices may be jeopardized. But, on the other hand, if this is the case, have we not lost the value of autonomy? This essay provides a thorough examination, from a theoretical and practical dimension, of the major ethical difficulties associated with attempts to inform the subject and obtain a genuinely informed consent.

Benjamin Freedman is Associate for Bioethics at the Westminster Institute for Ethics and Human Values, Westminster College, London, Ontario, Canada

C an a consent obtained from a free and competent adult under conditions of ignorance be valid? Would it make any difference if the consent obtained were to a nontherapeutic rather than a therapeutic procedure? If it were offered to an investigator rather than to a clinician? Is it possible that the subject's right to grant informed consent to all proposed procedures is one that he or she cannot waive? Can we say that a patient is acting responsibly in agreeing to participate in a research program under conditions of ignorance? And, if we believe that such ignorant consent is the very model of irresponsibility, does the investigator have the right to refuse to deal with willfully ignorant subjects?

The requirement of informed consent to medical therapy and research is today more than a principle; it is a cliché. An earlier discussion of mine on the doctrine, a major point of which was to provide reasons for thinking a consent could be valid in spite of ignorance, appeared, despite my best efforts and those of the editors, under the title "A Moral Theory of Informed Consent."[1] It seems that one can no more separate the "informed" from the "consent" than one can buy a pant from a tailor. Yet one useful way of discussing an ethical principle is by means of the extreme case, and ignorant consent surely qualifies. In addition, the problems raised by the recognition of an ignorant consent are quite commonly present (in an unrecognized form) in research generally.

I am not concerned, except incidentally, in the status of ignorant consent under the present law and regulation of research. The position taken by law and regulation should follow upon, though it need not be identical with, ethical analysis. Those moral investigations collected as the Appendix to the National Commission's Belmont Report would more realistically have been dubbed the prologue to that report.

IGNORANT CONSENT: DEFINITIONS AND PREVALENCE

Saying that ignorant consent is the obverse of informed consent does not seem to get us very far. It does, however, point out that the concept of ignorance is parasitic upon that of information, so that each of the various theories of informed consent generates a different view of what constitutes ignorant consent.

Consider an individual, Brown, undergoing invasive electrophysiological studies for clinical reasons. He is a candidate for concurrent noninvasive research; e.g., his body-surface will be "mapped" electrocardiographically to ascertain correlations between the clinically induced phenomena and the map tracings. The mapping is, from the subject's point of view, entirely nontherapeutic. Upon being invited to participate in a study described to him as posing some discomfort but no intrinsic risk (i.e., no risk over and above that accompanying the clinical investigations he has agreed to), the subject consents. The investigator indicates that further information is generally provided before the subject makes up his mind: the nature of the experiment, its potential benefits, and so on; but the subject declines to be further informed. We will assume here (as we generally assume, in the absence of contrary indications) that the subject is competent and is not acting under duress. Leaving aside for the moment the question of its validity, has the subject offered an ignorant consent?

In defining informal consent for research one major position has been to a large extent abandoned. That is the "professional standard," the idea that an investigator has only the obligation to disclose those elements that would commonly be disclosed by other investigators conducting similar research. This leaves us with two different approaches to the problem of describing an adequate amount of information.

The first of these is procedure-based. Robert Levine, for example, lists eleven elements that informed consent should satisfy.[2] These include such things as the purpose of the research, the reason for selecting this individual as a subject, the procedures to be followed and the discomforts that the subject will suffer as a result of them, and so on. Other elements may be added; for example, Robert Veatch[3,p.34] would include the need for "a specific disclosure of the presence of a control group within the research design" and an explanation of who is to be held responsible should the subject be harmed in the course of the research (in anticipated and unanticipated ways).

By the procedure-based understanding of informed consent, Brown has clearly consented under conditions of ignorance. Far from being cognizant of such esoterica as the presence of a control group, or the names of the members of the institutional review board (IRB) that had approved the protocol, he does not even know the nature and purpose of the research. The only element of which he is aware is that of risk, and even here he is not fully informed. By this standard, Brown is ignorant; and so for those adopting that standard, the question arises as to whether he can serve as a subject.

Yet although many investigators concentrate their attention upon satisfying the procedure-based understanding, most commentators believe it to be a derivative of some more general principle, that of fitting the information provided to the informational requirements of reasonable people. How much information, and what kinds, would be used by a reasonable individual in deciding whether to agree to participate as a subject in this research? For both Levine and Veatch, and indeed for many others who discuss the "elements" of informed consent, these items do not stand alone, but are generated by reference to the needs of ordinary people.

On the face of it, though, this particular subject-centered standard of information would agree that Brown's consent was an ignorant one. The average reasonable person is likely to require much more information than was supplied in this case before agreeing to participate.

There is one further complication, however. Rather than focusing upon that information desired by the average reasonable person, we might maintain that this standard is also a mere derivative. More fundamental is the requirement that this subject be given information that allows him to decide about participation. And by this individualized standard, Brown, it would be said, is fully informed: all that he feels he needs to know is that he will undergo some added discomfort, with no attendant risk, to an already uncomfortable, therapeutically indicated procedure.

This theory, however, would be solving what is a difficult moral question by mere verbal fiat. Saying that Brown is informed is analogous to saying that an anorectic is sated before the table has been set for dinner. There is another way, however, of construing the theory, which leaves the moral problem intact. Let us take this as a tentative construct of a theory of *valid* consent, rather than informed consent. Ordinarily, people require a certain amount of information to make up their minds. A fully individualized standard, though, when applied to competent eccentrics (or the competent harried) suggests that the informational component can be waived. The question remains, however, as to whether such a waiver ought morally to be respected by the investigator, in the sense that he will be prepared to proceed without supplying the standard elements of information. For all theories, then, we may say that there is a moral question of ignorant consent. An ignorant consent is offered when an individual consents in violation of the common informational components required by reasonable people.

Defined in this way, it turns out that people often rely on ignorant consent, most obviously in the case of placebo administration, blind or double-blind. The average reasonable person would surely want to know, prior to ingesting a little pink pill, whether it is composed of sugar or of some substance that is presumed or suspected to be pharmacologically active. In allowing research involving placebos, we rely upon the idea that a subject may morally choose to remain ignorant of information that is ordinarily crucial to reasonable decision making. Knowledge that one may receive a placebo, if one is informed of being in a clinical trial, does not satisfy ordinary informational requirements. If placebo-controlled drug trials are licit, as most maintain, it is because it is felt that an ignorant consent may be valid.

In the (somewhat paradoxical) context of the desire to rectify ethically troubling situations, a more radical scheme has been proposed along the same lines. In the search to reconcile deceptive research strategies, social-psychological or otherwise, with the doctrine of consent, some have proposed that a prior consent to be deceived be obtained from an entire prospective subject population (e.g., all first-year psychology students).[4] They could be told that any experiment of which they would be the subject will pose no (physical) risk, and will have been approved by an IRB, which is concerned to safeguard their rights; but they would not be told when, or whether, or how they will be studied. Upon consenting in that fashion, the students would in effect know that they will either be the subjects of an experiment or not, which gives them no significant advantage over the first-year students in logic, who have blissfully wiped their minds clean of all mundane knowledge.

There is a further situation, undocumented but surely common, in which ignorant consent is relied upon. Alter Brown's situation to correspond with a more common pattern of informing subjects. He has just been handed an informed consent sheet, describing the research in the moderate detail to which we are accustomed. He glances at it, lays it aside, asks the research nurse if the study poses any risk, and is told that it will involve some discomfort but no risk. Thereupon, he signs the consent sheet.

Is this situation different in any morally relevant way from the earlier? It is hard to see how. He has been told exactly the same things. In each case, he had readily at hand the opportunity to be further informed: in the first case, through the researcher's offer; in the second case, through reading the sheet. Those who would be inclined to accept Brown's participation are tacitly admitting the validity of an ignorant consent; and are likely to reconstrue the requirement of informing the subject to one of offering the subject the opportunity to be informed.

To recapitulate: insistence upon the subject's prior informed consent, taken to include those things that the average reasonable person would want to know before participating in research, would eliminate one common pattern of clinical research, one favored technique of justification for psychological research, and one plausible pattern of agreement to all research. Given these results, it is surprising to find considerable resistance to the concept of ignorant consent in the ethical literature.

These three results, taken together, provide us with a sort of argument for the validity of ignorant consent, or at least with a distasteful alternative: for it seems that one must either accept its validity, or eschew these practices. One could respond that all they have demonstrated is that in cases such as these the value of the progress of science overrides that of consent. But this response fails on three grounds. First, consent itself, as opposed to information, does not seem to be dispensable in all these cases; surely not for the first case, of placebo administration; nor for the third. Advance knowledge that a subject is unwilling to trouble himself to be informed supplies no exemption for experimentation without due notice and consent. As for the second case, that of deceptive experimentation, those who have proposed prior ignorant consent have done so precisely in the belief that consent ought never be discarded.

Second, the value of scientific progress does not seem to be much at stake in the last instance, unless it is felt that the prevalent attitude among prospective subjects is one of indifference toward information. Most tellingly, though, there is a third reason. The presumption that the objection has made is that scientific progress is a value that can stand alone against autonomy. Why should ignorance in the service of science be admitted, while a free choice of ignorance is to be resisted?

Yet it must be admitted that ignorance is not among the nobler objectives of mankind. Perhaps respect for autonomy need not embrace autonomous foolishness. Perhaps the physician/investigator should not let his or her protocol be used as a new setting for irresponsibility. Even if a prima facie case has been made for validity of some ignorant consents, Brown's case need not be considered settled.

Against Ignorant Consent

The Kantian idea of summing up morality in the principle that you must never treat others as a means to your end alone has a reverse side as well: a duty to never allow yourself to be treated as a means either. Charles Fried has applied this idea to the physician-patient relationship:[5,p.100]

> It might be, after all, that a patient will treat his doctor like some kind of medicine, like a more or less inanimate object used to arrive at an end. And a doctor might connive in such an instrumental relationship. But I take it to be the goal of a fully human life that important relationships be lived significantly and as human relationships.

The respecting of humanity is, then, a two-way street and must be done in one's own person as well as toward others. As a physician must not connive with a patient who wishes to contract for a service and pretend that its provision is impersonal, so it could be argued that an investigator must not connive with a subject in narrowing the focus of their interaction. Paul Ramsey may be suggesting a similar point in his characterization of informed consent to research as constituting a "covenant" between the parties as representing a "canon of loyalty."[6]

There is, however, another aspect. In therapy, the willingness to consent upon the physician's recommendation, in the absence of information, may be representative of trust and faith in another. Indeed, apart from the deranged, some functional equivalent of trust is undoubtedly present whenever one person is prepared to act (or be acted upon) in response to another's say-so. To exclude trust from the repertoire of human relationships would be an extreme application of the Kantian dictum, whose intellectual freight is too heavy to be borne in the run-of-the-mill research situation. We manage to make purchases at the grocery store without treating the cashier (or being treated by the cashier) as an end-in-oneself. Fried himself is not prepared to go quite that far. "It may well be," he says, "that no human relationship should ever assume this willfully truncated, merely instrumental aspect," but—significantly—that is a matter about which he does not "care to argue."

It is worth carrying a similar trend of thought a little farther. We commonly speak of the "right to informed consent," which is possessed by the subject. Is it possible that this is a right that the subject may not waive (by rejecting the opportunity to be informed)? Typically, the exercise of rights is a personal option; one may have the right to unemployment compensation, and choose not to apply. Might there be another sort of right, which one could be forced to exercise; and, if so might informed consent be such a right?

One example is that of public education: there is a right to be educated, one possessed by the resident and enforceable against the government. But education (or at least occupancy of a classroom chair during school hours) is not an option. Put another way, there is a right to education but no right to truancy. Informed consent could be said to be a kind of education.

The example is not apposite, however, for the very quality whose presence is presupposed by informed consent is supposed to be absent in reference to education. That quality is competency. We presume that children are incompetent to make the irrevocable decision to absent themselves from grade school; once this presumption of incompetency is defeated by mature years, education becomes an option-right. Yet if we did not believe the subject to be competent, informed consent would not be required, or would serve at best as an ancillary, perhaps in the form of a veto, to decisions made by another.

Another analogy is the right to a fair trial, as defined by whatever judicial norms may have been established in the jurisdiction in question. A person may not waive the right to a fair trial, in the interests of getting on with it, and submit to a kangaroo court. (For a while, it appeared from media accounts that this was just the situation in which convicted Utah murderer Gary Gilmore found himself, as appeals were entered on his behalf to stay a sentence which he wished consummated.[7]) The reason that this right should not be waivable, it may be said, is that what is at stake is not just one person's fate, but the public perception of the integrity of a social institution. Justice should not lend itself, or be thought to be lending itself, to procedures that are less than fair (less than just).

This analogy is quite compelling, for in the same way ignorant consent causes the institution of research to fall into public disrepute. Research may in fact be much more vulnerable to such a result than is the judiciary. But this factor cannot be said to be in itself determinative. For one thing, it presupposes a point that is at issue: whether there is anything wrong in proceeding with a subject who has chosen ignorance. There are criteria for establishing fair procedures that are independent of a defendant's preferences (so that his or her wishes may conflict with the procedures). It is less clear that informed consent procedures are intended to do anything more than to institutionalize practices that will enable prospective subjects to make a free choice. In addition, the need to protect the institution against harmful public perceptions is relative to the seriousness of the matter at issue. A defendent is given latitude to choose expedited proceedings in inverse proportion to the seriousness of the charge. A similar principle could be applied to research. Extreme care should be taken with nontherapeutic procedures that pose extreme risk. Ignorant consent remains plausible in a case like that of Brown.

A curious reversal of this Kantian position results in yet another objection to the validity of ignorant consent to research. In contrast to Fried's Kantian position in which ignorant consent to therapy is more suspect than is that to (most) research, a number of sources suggest that the positions should be reversed. This may be the case, for example, in current Canadian law, although doctrine has not matured sufficiently to be certain. In a recent case from the Supreme Court of Canada[8,p.13] appears the only judicial acknowledgment that I am acquainted with of the validity of ignorant consent to therapy: "It is, of course, possible that a particular patient may waive aside any question of risks and be quite prepared to submit to the surgery or treatment, whatever they be. Such a situation presents no difficulties." By way of possible contrast, the leading Canadian case on consent to research, *Halushka* v. *University of Saskatchewan*,[9] adopted a firm standard of full disclosure:

> There can be no exceptions to the ordinary requirements of disclosure in the case of research as there may well be in ordinary medical practice. The researcher does not have to balance the probable effect of lack of treatment against the risk involved in the treatment itself. . . . The subject of medical experimentation is entitled to a full and frank disclosure of all the facts, probabilities and opinions which a reasonable man might be expected to consider before giving his consent.

Veatch and Levine state clearly that ignorant consent to therapy should be handled differently from such a consent to research. Veatch's approval of ignorant consent to therapy is, in any event, given grudgingly. He feels that "it can be seriously questioned at the ethical level whether one is justified in waiving information necessary to make a consent informed." Justified or not, he feels it may be followed in "cases of routine patient care." In cases of research, however, there is a "preferable course": "The investigator can turn to other subjects."[3,p.33]

While Veatch explains what is wrong with ignorant consent—it represents an abdication of responsibility to determine one's medical future—he gives no basis for distinguishing between therapy and research. Indeed, as we saw with Fried, any distinction would seem to work the other way; one's medical care is likely to be more important, not to mention more risky, than is the case for participation in most research. But a plausible argument is given by Levine,[10,p.3] who similarly believes that "patients may be offered the opportunity to delegate decision-making authority to a physician while subjects (of any experiment bearing any consequential possibility of harm) should rarely be offered this option." The difference is that "the patient may ordinarily assume that the health care professional will be acting in his (or her) best interests. . . . The subject, on the other hand, should feel very [much] less secure in delegating decision-making authority to the investigator."

There are two issues here: whether it is clever (or moral, or responsible) to participate as a subject under conditions of ignorance, and what response ought the investigator make to such a subject. Levine's remarks are directed toward the first question,[11] while Veatch is speaking of the second.

As to the first, the answer must surely be that it all depends: most obviously, on the state of the individual and on the truncated information delivered. Any IRB member will be acquainted with many protocols that, in retrospect, hardly called for the amount of ethical reflection that was (by standard procedures) brought to bear. Investigators, if not subjects, will know this; some discrimination is called for. When a research protocol warrants considerable examination, a subject may be told that the matter calls for more consideration than an off-hand agreement.

Only in case the subject wishes to proceed, after such a warning, is it relevant to consider Veatch's proposal, that the investigator look elsewhere for subjects. A fairly serious judgment is after all being imposed when we find that someone has acted irresponsibly and in a sense impose our judgment upon him or her. In an important sense, by the way—for, lacking that judgment of irresponsibility, the subject would, presumably, have been accepted.

There is a third question, however, which requires consideration. At the level of establishing regulations, should provision be made for accepting ignorant consents? Given the imaginative ways in which any regulations or guidelines established will be (predictably) circumvented, is it not safer to foreclose this kind of loophole?

If we recall the kind of ignorant consent under discussion, however, this point loses a good deal of its force. Ignorant consent is that offered under less information than that used by the reasonable person in arriving at a decision. Both Veatch and Levine specify the kinds of things reasonable people want to know. Veatch includes the names of those who reviewed the protocol from an ethical viewpoint, and the individual who will be held liable should some harm accrue to the subject. Levine includes a statement of the overall purpose of the research.

Plainly, these are not matters that are of common concern to reasonable people. The fact that one might reasonably want to know the details of these matters served as sufficient reason for this inclusion; else, an investigator (or IRB) might be led to claim that such matters are none of the subject's business. They patently might be the subject's business; it is not unreasonable to want to know about these things; but it is not unreasonable to fail to have the slightest interest in them (prior to body-mapping through electrocardiography, for example).

The lists of those elements that constitute information for the reasonable person in fact represent a compendium of maximal information, rather than a minimum norm. It is quite possible that the disinterest shown by a subject in the details of what will happen could be of such a magnitude as to give the researcher pause. He or she may even consider that he or she would rather not bother with such a subject. If he or she is that unreasonable now, what might he or she be like later on—during the research, or afterwards? But most frequently, it will not be the case that "ignorant consent" will be as troubling as this. Even reasonable people are not necessarily troubled with a burning curiosity about technical and bureaucratic details. Researchers and IRBs are not charged with the mission of infecting subjects with such obsessions.

What Is To Be Done?

The conclusions that I draw relate more to our own attitudes than to recommendations that the practice of research be altered substantially. In contrast to some of the writers that have been discussed, I don't believe that *any* general perspective on ignorant consent can be justified. A subject may or may not be acting responsibly in offering an ignorant consent. A researcher might or might not be justified in refusing to deal with such a subject. An IRB might or might not wish, in the context of a particular protocol, to grant latitude regarding the amount of information that must be imparted.

It may seem that there is not a great deal at stake in recognizing (or failing to recognize) the validity of ignorant consent, but it is a problem worthy of consideration.

It is worthwhile being clear about our crucial terms: e.g., recognizing the difference between what a reasonable person might want to know, and what he or she ought to know. And as we have noted ignorant consent is relied upon quite commonly. Beyond these, however, how we handle this problem says something about our evaluation of freedom. People's decisions are not being respected as such if no allowance is made for the uncommon, the idiosyncratic response.

A general problem is, I think, expressed in this narrow one: the relationship between the norms governing ordinary life and those applied to medical practice and research. What has no doubt been often said by harried clinicians and investigators bears reflection: Is it wise to hold medicine—staff, patients, subjects—to standards of rationality and conduct in excess of those applied when they leave the clinic?

ACKNOWLEDGMENTS

The author wishes to acknowledge Deborah Thornton, research assistant at Westminster Institute, for her very substantial contribution to my thinking on this subject.

REFERENCES

1. Freedman, B.: A moral theory of informed consent, *Hastings Center Report* 5 (No. 4): 32-39, August 1975.

2. Levine, R.J.: The nature and definition of informed consent in various research settings. In National Commission for the Protection of Human Subjects of Biomedical and Behavioral Research, *Appendix to the Belmont Report*, Vol. I. U.S. Government Printing Office, DHEW publication no. (OS)78-0013, pp. 3-1 to 3-91.

3. Veatch, R.M.: Three theories of informed consent: philosophical foundations and policy implications. In *Appendix to the Belmont Report*, Vol. II, DHEW publication no (OS)78-0014, pp. 26-1 to 26-66.

4. Diener, E. and Crandall, R. *Ethics in social and behavioral research*. Chicago: University of Chicago Press, 1978, pp. 95-96. Bok, S. *Lying: Moral Choice in public and private life*. New York: Pantheon, 1978, pp. 194-195. Milgram, S.: Subject reaction: The neglected factor in the ethics of experimentation. *Hastings Center Report* 7 (No. 5): 19-23, October, 1977, at 23.

5. Fried, C. *Medical experimentation: Personal integrity and social policy*. New York: American Elsevier, 1974.

6. Ramsey, P. *The patient as person*. New Haven: Yale University Press, 1970 (esp. Chapter I).

7. For an account, see Norman Mailer, *The Executioner's Song.* Boston: Little, Brown and Co., 1979.

8. *Reibl v. Hughes* (1980), 114 D.L.R. (3d) 1, 14 C.C.L.T. 1, 33 N.R. 361 (S.C.C.).

9. (Sask. 1965), 52 W.W.R. 608. In Katz, J., Capron, A.M. and Glass, E.S. *Experimentation with human beings.* New York: Russell Sage Foundation, 1972, pp. 569-573 at 572.

10. Levine, R.J.: The boundaries between biomedical or behavioral research and the accepted and routine practice of medicine. In *Appendix to the Belmont Report,* Vol. I., pp. 1-1 to 1-44.

11. Levine should be exempted from any implication that the amount of information that reasonable people may desire *must* be imparted to all prospective subjects. He had stated in "The Nature and Definition . . ." (see ref. 2) that the negotiations regarding informed consent "should be determined on a protocol by protocol basis" by the local IRB (p. 75). More recently, he has clarified his view still further: the reasonable person standard serves as a minimum baseline. *At least* that much information must be *offered* to prospective subjects, who "may reject a fact by either ignoring or forgetting it," but who "may not do so without having been made aware, however transiently, of its existence." *Ethics and Regulation of Clinical Research.* Baltimore: Urban and Schwarzenberg, 1981, p. 78.

21 Deception and Informed Consent in Research

ALAN SOBLE

The practice of deceiving some subjects in a social science or other research protocol seems to contradict one of the very core elements of the concept of informed consent: informing the subject. In this article, Soble surveys a variety of approaches which argue either for not obtaining consent prior to participation in a protocol involving deception or provides strategies by which some form of consent can be obtained by the subject prior to participation in the experiment. This survey article provides a good guide for thinking one's way through the many problematic issues surrounding deception in research.

Alan Soble, Ph.D., is with the Department of Philosophy, University of New Orleans

The principle of informed consent generally includes two necessary conditions for the proper treatment of human subjects in experimentation. The first condition, which has been widely discussed, is that the consent be obtained from subjects who agree to participate *voluntarily,* where voluntarism is understood negatively as the absence of coercion. The second condition, which is less often discussed, is that the consent must be *informed.* The Articles of the Nuremberg Tribunal and The Declaration of Helsinki both state that the subjects must be told the duration, methods, possible risks, and the purpose or aim of the experiment. The most recent HEW regulations agree: informed consent has not been obtained if there has been any element of deceit or fraud. These guidelines reflect our ordinary moral view that deception is morally unacceptable.

During the past quarter-century the size of the scientific research establishment has vastly increased. Medical, sociological, and psychological research is being carried out at our universities and other institutions at a rapid rate. The success of this effort, measured in terms of the amount of knowledge gained, has been well documented. In some of this research, however, the human beings serving as subjects are deceived as to the purpose of the experiment. In social psychology, for example, the incidence of the use of deceptive research designs has been estimated to be as high as 38 percent,[1] and even though deception is less common in medical research, many examples are available.[2] One immediate response is to say that "the experiment ought not to be performed and the desired knowledge should be sought by means of a different research design."[3] But this response overlooks the crucial point that certain bits of knowledge cannot, for logical reasons alone, be obtained without the use of deception. The testing of some hypotheses, within both psychology and medicine, requires that the subjects not be informed of the purpose or aim of the experiment being conducted.

We are faced then with a moral dilemma. Since the search for knowledge is at least morally permissible (if not, to a certain extent, morally obligatory), and since the use of deception is morally unacceptable (at least on a *prima facie* basis), in some situations both moral desiderata cannot be satisfied. And it is not clear which moral value ought to be sacrificed for the sake of the other.

I am aware of a handful of proposed solutions for this dilemma. First, we can maintain that subjects ought to be told the full purpose of an experiment for which they have volunteered. In this view no experiments logically requiring deception are permissible. Second, we can say that the subject's knowing the purpose of an experiment is not a central element of informed consent and therefore that experiments using deception are always permissible, as long as they satisfy the other conditions of the principle of informed consent. These are the two extreme solutions.[4]

The other positions are more complicated. According to one proposal, ineliminable deception is permissible *only* when there are substantial paternalistic reasons for withholding the purpose of the experiment from the subjects. According to another proposal, deception is permissible *only* when there are firm utilitarian reasons for doing so. This view, the standard argument for the use of deception, claims that the knowledge to be gained from deceptive experiments is so valuable to society that it is only a minor defect that persons must be deceived in the process. Finally, a number of strategies have been recently proposed to resolve the dilemma. These include the method of *ex post facto* consent (getting approval of the subjects retroactively), the method of presumptive consent (getting approval from a group of mock subjects and inferring that the real subjects would have consented), the method of prior general consent (in effect, getting consent to deceptive procedures well before the experiment is actually conducted), and a method that combines prior general consent and proxy consent. Before I discuss each of these ways of resolving the dilemma, let me examine briefly the major presupposition that underlies the dilemma.

Are Deceptive Designs Necessary?

Many types of experiments seem to require that the subjects not be told the purpose of the study, and in some cases that they be induced to hold false beliefs about the nature of the experiment during the experiment itself. Experiments, for example, that are designed to yield information about the influence of expectation or other psychological factors on the psychoactivity of drugs or on physiological processes would be ruined if subjects were told that what was being studied was their "mental" contribution to drug effects. Often subjects are not merely ignorant as to whether they have received the drug being tested or a placebo, but rather are told that they will receive one of these but in fact receive the other. Similarly, experiments designed to test for the existence of psychological phenomena such as obedience and trustworthiness seem necessarily to involve the use of deception.[5] Telling subjects that what is being studied is, for example, the extent to which they conform with the judgments of persons who are really cohorts of the experimenter, will destroy the attempt to discover the extent of conformity.

But how does one go about proving that deception is required in order to obtain certain bits of knowledge? In some cases, of course, it is quite easy. If what we want to know is something like "the effect of LSD-25 on the behavior of a group of unsuspecting enlisted men," it is quite obvious that the subjects must be deceived in order to assure that they are unsuspecting. This is an easy case because the statement of the relevant hypothesis being tested will include reference to deceived persons. But the hypothesis that persons will tend to judge in conformity with the judgments of persons in their immediate vicinity does not contain a reference to deceived subjects. It *seems* obvious that knowledge about conformity requires that we deceive subjects, but how can this intuition be supported?

Certainly, there is a way of proving that a given case of the use of deception was *not* required: all we need to do is to construct an experiment that is designed to yield the same information but that does not involve any deception. But the failure to find such an alternative nondeceptive research design does not prove that the deception *was* required by the nature of the knowledge being sought. The failure may only show how unimaginative we are in constructing research designs. (This is very ironic. Some deceptive research designs are extraordinarily ingenious.[6]) At least for this reason we ought not to take lightly the claim that deceptive research is ultimately justifiable because deceptive designs are necessary.

Knowledge that can be obtained only by using a deceptive research design must be contrasted with knowledge that can be obtained without deception but that can be obtained more efficiently by employing deception. Deception that is motivated out of a need to secure enough subjects, or deception that is pragmatically useful in terms of conserving time, effort, and expense, is not generally deception that is required purely on account of the nature of the knowledge being sought.[7] In these cases, of course, the dilemma I outlined earlier does not arise. But we have to be careful, for there is the danger that if we do allow deception because it is logically necessary for the testing of specific hypotheses, then it becomes slightly more plausible to argue that deception that saves the experimenter (and society) time, effort, and money also should be permitted. One major fault of the paternalistic and utilitarian solutions to the dilemma is that they also tend to justify deception that is only pragmatically, and not logically, required.

Before discussing the various proposals, I would like to comment on two related issues. First, the dilemma as I have stated it involves the acceptability of deceiving subjects who know, at least, that they are subjects in an experiment. What they do not know is precisely what experiment they are subjects in. Experiments done especially within sociology, however, involve deception in which the subjects do not even know that they are subjects in the experiment (covert observation, for example).[8] I will not discuss the issue of the morality of this practice here, for in covert observation there is apparently not simply a violation of the "informed" condition of the principle of informed consent, but also a violation of the "voluntary" condition. Discussion of this issue would take us too far from the resolution of the dilemma.

Second, my discussion is meant only to examine the acceptability of deception in thoroughly experimental situations, and is not meant to bear upon the use of deception by physicians and others in situations that are purely therapeutic. Therefore, my conclusion on the acceptability of deceptive techniques in experimentation does not necessarily apply to the morality of placebo therapy and the practice of lying to patients in the course of treating disease or disability.

The Paternalistic Defense of Deception

A defender of research employing ineliminable deception might try to justify the deception by relying on an argument like this: the deceptive procedures employed in these experiments can be viewed as being therapeutic for the subjects, and since there are many contexts in which the principle of informed consent is temporarily abandoned for the sake of persons who need therapy (for example, unconscious adults requiring emergency treatment), it ought to be acceptable temporarily to ignore the principle in these experiments.[9]

The argument, however, does not provide an adequate way of resolving the dilemma. First, it is not a global justification of the use of ineliminable deception, for it would only justify a small percentage of the experiments in question, those in which some real benefit to the subjects could be demonstrated. But there are more serious problems with the argument. It assumes much too quickly that the experimenter who plans to deceive subjects can know that the subjects will agree that the deception is in fact beneficial for them. Even if it is true, however, that the subjects do agree that the deception is beneficial for them (by, for example, exposing to them certain psychological traits they have but would rather not have), this does not mean that the deception was also therapeutic. Possessing certain psychological traits may not be beneficial for a person, but possessing these traits does not constitute being unhealthy, and therefore procedures that tend to expose and to remove these traits cannot be called "therapeutic." But even if it makes some sense to say that the removal of certain psychological traits is therapeutic, whether a procedure that removes these traits is therapeutic will depend on the context in which the procedure is carried out. Persons presenting themselves at a physician's office or at a clinic acknowledge that the context is a therapeutic one, but this acknowledgement is absent when persons volunteer for experiments.

Finally, the paternalistic argument carries the danger of justifying not only ineliminable deception but also deception motivated out of a concern to conserve time, effort, and expense. The paternalistic argument can be extended to something like this: deception that conserves the experimenter's time and effort, which enables the experimenter to carry out the research less expensively, ultimately is beneficial for each of the *individual* subjects, who are of course taxpayers. (The paternalistic argument might also say that the money saved could be reallocated and used in, for example, cancer research. The deception then can be tied to a therapeutic intent.) But an argument like this would justify more deception than we would find comfortable.

THE UTILITARIAN DEFENSE OF DECEPTION

A utilitarian justification of the use of ineliminable deception is far superior to a paternalistic one because it does not have to blur the distinction between therapy and experiments. It is also more plausible because it argues that the deception is acceptable because it promises to benefit in many cases the whole of society and not merely the individuals who participate as subjects. Simply put, the utilitarian argues that experiments utilizing ineliminable deception and that do *not* cause any other harm to subjects are acceptable because the knowledge gained from them is socially valuable. When balancing the needs of society and a desire of individual subjects not to be deceived, experiments that do contribute substantially to our knowledge are justified.

Like the paternalistic argument, the utilitarian argument does not provide a global justification of experiments employing ineliminable deception. If the deceptive procedure is accompanied by the possibility of grave harm to the subjects, then the needs of society no longer overshadow the needs of the subjects. Or if the deceptive procedure is part of an experiment that is designed to yield only trivial knowledge, there is no longer a justification for the experiment. Even so, the utilitarian argument has the potential for justifying most of the experiments recently carried out that employ deception. But I do not find the argument to be a convincing one.

One weakness of the utilitarian argument can be seen by examining what the argument has to prove. Certainly we can agree that the scientific research establishment as a whole is to be justified on utilitarian grounds. The reason we spend so much time, effort, and money on research is that the research as a whole is bound to have beneficial results for society and the individuals who make up society. But the utilitarian argument has to prove that because the research establishment itself is justified on utilitarian grounds, anything else done within that establishment is also justified by utilitarian considerations. In particular, the utilitarian argument has the burden of showing that not only the principle of informed consent is ultimately based on utilitarian considerations, but also that exceptions to the principle (for example, the use of ineliminable deception) are also grounded in utilitarian considerations.

This argument may be very difficult to prove. For example, one who relied on a notion of "rules" developed by John Rawls[10] might say that, yes, the principle of informed consent can be justified on utilitarian grounds, and yes, the research establishment can be similarly justified. But this Rawlsian would go on to claim that a system of experimentation on human subjects that publicly included a rule

permitting violations of the principle of informed consent (by allowing ineliminable deception) would not be justified on utilitarian
grounds, given certain sociological, psychological, economic, and
ideological properties of this society. For example, public outrage at
the use of deception could undermine the status of the experimental
scientists and eventually result in a curtailment of research and a subsequent decrease in the knowledge that the research establishment
provides. The use of deception then from a utilitarian point of view
would be counterproductive. The heavy burden of the utilitarian is
thus to show that it is unreasonable to believe that the proposed
modification of the principle of informed consent would be counterproductive in this way.

Alternatively, the utilitarian can drop the requirement that a rule
permitting violations of the principle of informed consent must be
public. This modification might eliminate the possibility that deception is counterproductive. But I think that this alternative is inadequate, for at least three reasons. First, it relies on the assumption,
which is likely false, that this deception (the failure to make a rule
public) is especially immune from discovery. Indeed, it could turn out
that this deception, when exposed, is more counterproductive than
the deception permitted by the public rule in certain experiments.
Second, it solves the dilemma about the use of deception in experiments by introducing deception at another level, and therefore in a
sense just begs the question. Third, in allowing rules to be nonpublic,
it seems to violate one of the so-called logical or conceptual requirements of morality.

The utilitarian argument is also not convincing because it ignores
the history or the genesis of the principle of informed consent.[11] The
whole point of the principle (including its prohibition of deception) is
precisely to protect individual rights against exactly these sorts of
claims of social need or benefit. Those who designed and those who
now support the principle freely admit that there might be utilitarian
reasons for not always obeying the principle, but they announce that
the individual has a sphere of autonomy that cannot be sacrificed or
invaded for the good of society. To try to justify experiments employing ineliminable deception on utilitarian grounds would be to
deny the intent and significance of a principle that has only recently
appeared in our history, that took much effort to develop and apply,
and that represents one of the major advances of modern society. In a
word, the utilitarian argument proposes that we undo the moral progress we have made in this century.

Finally, like the paternalistic argument, the utilitarian argument
would justify too much deception. If experiments employing ineli-

minable deception are acceptable for utilitarian reasons, then what about deception motivated by pragmatic considerations? Indeed, the utilitarian justification of merely pragmatic deception seems stronger than the corresponding paternalistic justification of pragmatic deception. Again we end up allowing more deception than we find comfortable, and the utilitarian argument therefore does not provide a safe way of resolving the dilemma.[12]

Ex Post Facto Consent: Another Defense

Stanley Milgram has tried to justify the ineliminable deception used in his obedience experiments this way:

> Misinformation . . . [and] illusion . . . are justified for one reason only; they are, in the end, accepted and endorsed by those who are exposed to them. . . . *The central moral justification for allowing a procedure of the sort used in my experiments is that it is judged acceptable by those who have taken part in it.*[13]

The thrust of this argument is that the principle of informed consent can be modified to allow for consent being obtained after a procedure has been carried out on subjects, rather than before, in order to permit the successful execution of deceptive techniques vital to the knowledge being sought. I want to argue that such a modification is not acceptable.

Consider first the possibility that after the experiment is over, some of the subjects do not agree that they should have been deceived. We already know that violations of the principle of informed consent, when the principle is understood in its usual way as requiring consent prior to an experiment, have been increasingly met by claims of subjects that they deserve compensation and that punitive measures be directed at the experimenters. But an experimenter who wants to rely on *ex post facto* consent is in a rather shaky position. If any subject withholds consent afterwards, this subject was a participant in an experimental procedure to which he or she *never* consented. Their failure to agree means that such subjects never should have been exposed to the experimental procedures. They would have, I think, a good argument for compensation. The experimenter who relies on *ex post facto* consent therefore faces practical problems that endanger the continuance of the research, professional standing, and perhaps financial status.[14] But even if compensation is exacted, this does not mean that it was morally correct that the procedures were carried out. The 1.3 percent of Milgram's subjects who expressed disapproval afterwards were morally wronged, and it is no defense to say that 98.7 percent found the deception acceptable.

Consider now the situation in which all the subjects do approve afterwards. Is it safe to say that this postexperimental approval counts as *bona fide* consent? Steven Patten has argued that the approval of Milgram's subjects was not really consent.[15] We know, says Patten, from Milgram's study that persons are submissive to authority; this gives us reason to think that when the subjects approved afterwards they were merely obeying (once again) and not really consenting. Although Patten has a point here, I think his argument is too strong. If the subjects in Milgram's experiments are representative of people in general, then *no* experiments at all on human subjects would be permissible. For if we take Patten's point seriously, it means that we ought not to believe any subject who shows up for an experiment; the subject's showing up is just an act of obedience and real consent cannot be obtained. From Patten's argument, then, we can only draw the conclusion that Milgram's study is only as objectionable as any other study. It does not provide a way of singling out deceptive experiments as especially objectionable.

The approval given by the subjects afterwards might not really be consent because the experimental procedures themselves elicit the approval of the subjects or make it difficult for them not to agree afterwards. Consent, whether it be prior or retroactive, ought to be *independent* approval of the experimental procedures. (One might want to interpret the requirement of independence simply as the requirement that consent be given voluntarily.) I don't want to argue that *ex post facto* consent is always nonindependent, but rather that many experimental procedures do contain ingredients that elicit the subsequent approval of the subjects. Because obtaining consent prior to an experiment is the best way to ensure that consent is independent, we ought not to allow deceptive procedures that can be given approval only, if at all, in retrospect.

In the case of Milgram's studies, it is plausible that persons who have been exposed (to themselves and, quasi-publicly, to the experimenters) as obedient and as unfaithful to their own moral beliefs will be embarrassed and shamed by this exposure and will attempt to alleviate their unpleasant position by agreeing afterwards that the experimenters were correct to have used deception. Even those subjects who were not obedient during the course of the experiment have good reasons for giving approval afterwards. To disapprove of the deception would be to undermine their fine performance. Thus for both obedient and defiant subjects the nature of the experiment provides powerful psychological reasons (self-respect, exculpation, self-righteousness) for giving approval afterwards.[16]

What is astounding is that Milgram recognizes the influence of just these kinds of psychological factors on other features of his experiment but not on the credibility of retrospective approval. Commenting on the fact that 3.8 percent of the obedient subjects *later* said that they were certain that the learner was not receiving real shocks, Milgram writes:

> Even now I am not willing to dismiss those subjects because it is not clear that their rejection of the technical illusion was a cause of their obedience or a consequence of it. Cognitive processes may serve to rationalize behavior. . . . [S]ome subjects may have come to this position as a post facto explanation. It cost them nothing and would go a long way toward preserving their positive self-conception.[17]

If the doctrine of *ex post facto* consent is to be taken seriously, surely the burden of proof is on the one who wants to justify the use of deception in research to demonstrate convincingly that retrospective approval has in no way been manufactured by the experimental procedures. It is necessary to eliminate the possibility that the procedures for which consent is requested do not themselves elicit that consent.[18]

PRESUMPTIVE CONSENT: A PROPOSAL

Robert Veatch has proposed a method for resolving the dilemma and thereby for permitting ineliminable deception:

> In those rare, special cases where knowledge of the purpose would destroy the experiment . . . it might be acceptable to ask a group of mock subjects drawn from the same experimental population if they would consent to participate in the experiment knowing its purpose. If there is substantial agreement (say, 95 percent), then it seems reasonable to conclude that most real subjects would have agreed to participate even if they had had the information that would destroy the experiment's validity.[19]

It seems to me that Veatch's proposal is just as controversial as the dilemma it was intended to resolve. His method relies on our assuming that real subjects *would* consent on the basis of what other persons *do* consent to. Although in some cases (for example, when a person in need of treatment is temporarily unconscious) we allow that the next-of-kin consent to therapy assuming that the patient would consent, the experimental situation is too far removed from these emergency cases for this kind of hypothetical reasoning to be compelling.

An objection that was raised to the doctrine of *ex post facto* consent can be raised in this context also. Why does Veatch settle for only 95 percent agreement from the mock subjects? This figure suggests that

Veatch is willing to expose 5 percent of the subject population to procedures to which they would not have consented, had they known the information that they in fact do not know. If we were to use his method, we ought to set the level of mock subject agreement at 100 percent. In a typical nondeceptive experiment, there are some persons who, having heard the terms of the experiment, decide not to participate. This percentage can be weeded out at the start. But in an experiment involving ineliminable deception and governed by presumptive consent, if the agreement of the mock subjects is only 95 percent, then those persons who would have been weeded out are not going to be weeded out. (A side thought: regarding the "voluntary" element of the principle of informed consent, would we allow an experiment in which we have evidence that only 95 percent of the subjects *would* have consented?)

Of course, if the criterion of mock subject agreement is set as high as 100 percent then perhaps in practice Veatch's proposal will mean that very few deceptive experiments will be carried out. This possibility does not fit very well with Veatch's apparent sympathy with the attempt to gain knowledge with deceptive and otherwise nonharmful experiments. Furthermore, even if all the mock subjects give approval, this in no way guarantees that all the real subjects would have consented had they known the purpose of the experiment. Even when the criterion is set as high as it can be, there is still a possibility that some subjects will be exposed to procedures to which they would not have consented.

Note also that Veatch's proposal has a loose tie with Milgram's suggestion of *ex post facto* consent. If we were to use a group of real subjects in a deceptive experiment on the grounds that mock subjects have given their approval, we are using real subjects on the strength of a claim that is somewhat testable. It would be nice to know, afterwards, whether the percentage of mock subjects who agreed was a reliable indicator of the percentage of real subjects who would have agreed. In order to obtain this information we must seek the approval of the real subjects *ex post facto*. But it is possible that this check on the accuracy of the prediction, however, may very well be contaminated by the influence of the experimental procedures themselves.[20]

PRIOR GENERAL CONSENT: STILL ANOTHER METHOD

Milgram has proposed another method designed to satisfy the principle of informed consent and at the same time make deceptive experiments possible:

[Prior general consent] is a form of consent that would be based on subjects' knowing the general types of procedures used in psychological investigations, but without their knowing what specific manipulations would be employed in the particular experiment in which they would take part. The first step would be to create a pool of volunteers to serve in psychology experiments. Before volunteering to join the pool people would be told explicitly that sometimes subjects are misinformed about the purposes of an experiment. . . . Only persons who had indicated a willingness to participate in experiments involving deception . . . would, in the course of the year, be recruited for experiments that involved [deception].[21]

This proposal fails to resolve the dilemma because it creates a new dilemma: experiments based upon this proposal *either* will yield no useful information at all *or* will require that additional experiments be performed which do violate the principle of informed consent (see fn. 20). If an experiment relying on this technique for recruitment yields no useful information, then the technique has not preserved one of the original goals we had: to secure valuable information. And if experiments relying on this technique require (for their validity, as I argue below) that further experiments be done which do involve violations of the principle of informed consent, then the technique has not preserved our other goal.

The first question is whether we could have reason to believe that any deception eventually carried out on this subject pool really worked and really provided us with the information we were seeking. At first glance, if people know or think that the procedures to which they have consented involve deception, then they will be more suspicious of the experimental protocol and may very well not be "tricked" in the necessary way. Even when subjects are *not* told in advance that the experiment involves deception, there is always some doubt as to whether the illusion was successful and whether the experiment has generated any useful knowledge. But if the technique of prior general consent is used, the subjects know in advance that they might be exposed to deception, and this knowledge makes the success of the illusion even more problematic. In order to show that the knowledge gained in experiments relying on prior general consent is useful, experimenters will have to demonstrate that subjects' foreknowledge of the deception did not interfere with the success of the illusion. And, as far as I can tell, to establish this kind of fact one must resort to deceptive procedures.[22] If this is so, prior general consent does not solve the dilemma. One might say here that even though it is true that only those subjects who generally consented to deception are used in deceptive experiments, this pool of subjects does not have to know this fact about itself. Withholding *this* information from the subjects would certainly bypass the problems I just mentioned but at the cost of replacing one act of deception with another.

The second question is whether the information gained in an experiment relying on this technique is useful because the only subjects who are exposed to deceptive procedures are those who express a willingness to be exposed to deception. Application of this technique, that is, restricts the nature of the subject pool and may possibly insert a bias into the characteristics of the research population. This complaint is raised often in the context of sex research; the information obtained by studying only those who volunteer for sex experiments may be misleading because the research population is lacking other kinds of persons. If deceptive procedures are carried out only upon those who are willing to undergo deception, then psychological studies may be misleading because they have excluded from the research population those people who were not willing to undergo deception and who may have different personality structures or profiles than willing subjects. Again, in order to show that such a bias is not present, it is quite likely that deceptive experiments *not* relying on prior general consent will have to be carried out. At the very least, the burden of proof is on the experimenter who relies on prior general consent to establish that the knowledge is not contaminated by either of the two factors I mentioned. And in establishing this, the experimenter must not conduct experiments that violate the principle of informed consent.

Prior General Consent and Proxy Consent

I have so far rejected all but one of the more complicated ways of resolving the dilemma. In addition to the method that I am about to describe, then, the only positions left are the two extreme views. According to one, no experiments involving ineliminable deception are permissible; according to the other, all such experiments are permissible. This latter alternative wants to decrease substantially the significance of the "informed" condition of the principle of informed consent. But there is very little that can be said in favor of doing so. I have already suggested that paternalistic and utilitarian arguments for exceptions to the prohibition on the use of deception are inadequate. But paternalistic and utilitarian reasons are the only ones we could have for decreasing the significance of the "informed" condition. The second extreme solution, then, is in practice no different from the solutions proposed by the paternalist or by the utilitarian. There are simply no other arguments to use in defending the second extreme solution.

There are of course perfectly good reasons for accepting the first extreme solution. Experiments without deception respect those individuals who have already volunteered to be subjects at least in part for the sake of other people. Conversely, experiments with deception show disrespect for these persons who have willingly undertaken the risks of an experiment so that other persons might benefit. Deceiving an experimental subject who has volunteered is an acute expression of ingratitude. And it deserves the scorn that we ordinarily give to the person who passes through the cafeteria line twice but pays only once. There is, however one final method that seems to satisfy our requirements; it allows some ineliminable deception, and so preserves the search for knowledge, without (1) expressing ingratitude to the subjects and (2) undermining the epistemological status of the data collected during the experiment. In this method prior general consent is combined with proxy consent.[23]

I suggest that we make the method of prior general consent applicable to the whole realm of experimental science employing human subjects. If the method of prior general consent is employed for any and every subject pool, the likelihood that forewarning of deception will disrupt the experimental illusion is greatly decreased. In this method, furthermore, the experimental bias introduced in Milgram's proposal (only those subjects who consented in general to deception would be used in deceptive experiments) is overcome in the following way. Subjects are *not* told that only those who approve of deception will be used in experiments utilizing deception; rather, all subjects are candidates for participating in deceptive experiments. But the usual objection to doing this is vitiated by the use of an additional procedure: proxy consent. Each subject in the pool designates some relative or friend as one who will inspect the experiment in which the subject might participate. This relative or friend is empowered by the subject to reject or accept experiments on the basis of whether they posed too much risk, employed deception that was too devious, or was aimed at providing knowledge that might be misused. The proxy makes these judgments from the point of view of the subject who has empowered him or her to do so. It is important to note that combining the method of prior general consent with that of proxy consent combines what is acceptable from both Milgram's and Veatch's proposals. From Milgram's it takes the idea that consent to deception is compatible with the principle of informed consent; from Veatch's proposal it takes the idea that we can resolve the dilemma by consulting persons other than the subjects themselves. But the method of proxy consent used as a conjunct to prior general consent has an obvious advantage to Veatch's proposal: the necessity of having to argue from the approval of mock subjects to the hypothetical approval of real subjects is eliminated by consulting persons empowered by the real subjects to give consent for them.

A procedure employing both prior general consent (as standard for all subject pools) and proxy consent is very far removed from what exists at the present: the use of deception in experiments without the protection for subjects of either prior general consent or proxy consent. For this reason many changes will have to be made in the structure of experimental science using human subjects; so many changes, in fact, that I suspect that the initial reaction of experimental scientists will be that the proposal is impractical, that it will create too many bureaucratic impediments to the conduct of research. Indeed, the experimental scientist could argue that the method, in solving the original dilemma, gives rise to a new dilemma. Either we employ the method of prior general/proxy consent (and abandon a large part of the research enterprise because the method is too costly in terms of time, effort, and money), or we retain the large bulk of the research enterprise (but employ a less ethically satisfying method of obtaining the approval of the subjects). My response to this argument would be to say that as long as we reject the paternalistic and utilitarian arguments for the use of ineliminable deception because those justifications could very well justify deception required only for pragmatic reasons, then we must also be prepared to embrace the relative inefficiency of the method of general/proxy consent. Pragmatic considerations, we had decided, are not compelling enough to warrant the less-than-full satisfaction of the principle of informed consent.

REFERENCES

1. See Donald Warwick, "Social Scientists Ought to Stop Lying," *Psychology Today* (February 1975), p. 105; and Jay Katz, *Experimentation with Human Beings* (New York: Russell Sage Foundation, 1972), pp. 323–433, esp. p. 358. A very recent example is the experiment done by Diane Ruble, "Premenstrual Symptoms: A Reinterpretation," *Science* 197 (1977), 291–292.

2. Three recent examples are: Robert Heaton, "Subject Expectancy and Environmental Factors as Determinants of Psychedelic Flashback Experience," *Journal of Nervous and Mental Disease* 161 (1975), 157–65; Monte S. Buchsbaum, Robert D. Coursey, and Dennis L. Murphy, "The Biochemical High-Risk Paradigm: Behavioral and Familial Correlates of Low Platelet Monoamine Oxidase Activity," *Science* 194 (1976), 339–41; and C. P. O'Brien, Thomas Testa, T. J. O'Brien, J. P. Brady, and Barbara Wells, "Conditioned Narcotic Withdrawal in Humans," *Science* 195 (1977), pp. 1000–02.

3. Sissela Bok, "The Ethics of Giving Placebos," *Scientific American* 231 (November 1974), 17–23.

4. Perry London says that "neither extreme position will do for those of us who are equally concerned with the need for valid scientific information and for the protection of human subjects" (*Psychology Today* [November 1977], p. 23), and he laments the fact that the current HEW guidelines "offer no clues as to when some amount of deception may be necessary and proper." The guidelines however do seem to be rather explicit in prohibiting "any element of force, fraud, deceit, duress . . ." (*Federal Register, 39,* No. 105, at section 46.3c).

5. For example: Seymour Feshbach and Robert Singer, *Television and Aggression* (San Francisco: Jossey-Bass, 1971); C. K. Hofling, E. Brotzman, S. Dalrymple, N. Graves, and C. M. Pierce, "An Experimental Study in Nurse-Physician Relationships," *Journal of Nervous and Mental Disease* 143 (1966), 171–80; Stanley Milgram, *Obedience to Authority* (New York: Harper & Row, 1974); L. Paige, "The Effects of Oral Contraceptives on Affective Fluctuations Associated With the Menstrual Cycle," *Psychosomatic Medicine* 33 (1971), 515–37. An interesting discussion and a number of references can be found in S. Wolf, "The Pharmacology of Placebos," *Pharmacological Review,* 11 (1959), 689-704.

6. For an experiment involving extensive deception of different types, see Stuart Valins, "Cognitive Effects of False Heart-Rate Feedback," *Journal of Personality and Social Psychology* 4 (1966) 400–08. Incidentally, Valin's comment on p. 401 is noteworthy. "Male introductory psychology students, whose course *requirements* included 6 hours of participation in experiments, *volunteered* for a psychophysiological experiment" (italics added).

7. One might want to interpret the San Antonio oral contraceptive study in this way. For discussion, see Robert Veatch, "Medical Ethics: Professional or Universal?" *Harvard Theological Review* 65 (1972), 550, and his " 'Experimental' Pregnancy," *Hastings Center Report,* 1 (1971), 2–3, and the editors' note in Robert Hunt and John Arras, eds., *Ethical Issues in Modern Medicine* (Encino, Cal.: Mayfield, 1977), p. 266. Some deception in personality studies is carried out because the investigators fear, ironically, that the subjects would otherwise lie when answering questionnaires. Is this deception logically required by the knowledge being sought, or is it only pragmatically useful in obtaining that knowledge?

8. For example: D. Rosenhan, "On Being Sane in Insane Places," *Science* 179 (1973) 250–59; and Laud Humphreys, *Tearoom Trade. Impersonal Sex in Public Places* (Chicago: Aldine, 1975), enlarged edition. A general critique of Humphreys is presented by Donald Warwick, "Tearoom Trade: Means and Ends in Social Research," *Hastings Center Studies* 1 (1973), 27–38; and Murray Wax has recently discussed problems of consent in sociology, in "Fieldworkers and Research Subjects: Who Needs Protection?" *Hastings Center Report* 7, No. 4 (August 1977), 29–32.

9. See the remarks of some of Milgram's subjects after they had been debriefed, in *Obedience to Authority,* pp. 196 and 200, and the "Foreword" to *Tearoom Trade* by Lee Rainwater, pp. xiv–xv.

10. John Rawls, "Two Concepts of Rules," *Philosophical Review* 64 (1955), 3–32. For a similar position see H. L. A. Hart, "Prolegomenon to the Principles of Punishment," in *Punishment and Responsibility* (New York: Oxford University Press, 1968), pp. 1–27.

11. A concise history can be found in Alan Donagan, "Informed Consent in Therapy and Experimentation," *Journal of Medicine and Philosophy* 2 (1977), 307–29.

12. It might be argued that some studies employing ineliminable deception are permissible or even mandatory because they are designed to expose or produce facts

about the occurrence of harmful or immoral activities (for example, the studies done by Rosenhan and Hofling). But this utilitarian argument justifies only a very small percentage of the experiments involving ineliminable deception. Furthermore, there are dangers in this rationale, in that the argument not only comes close to justifying police entrapment but also suggests that policework is a legitimate activity for scientists.

13. *Obedience to Authority*, pp. 198–99. Milgram's position is repeated in his "Subject Reaction: The Neglected Factor in the Ethics of Experimentation," *Hastings Center Report* 7, No. 5 (August 1977). 21.

14. Murray Wax (in "Fieldworkers and Research Subjects," p. 32) does not mention compensation to subjects when *ex post facto* consent is not obtained, but only punitive measures taken against the experimenter by professional peers.

15. "The Case That Milgram Makes," *Philosophical Review* 86 (1977), 350–64.

16. The fact that Milgram's subjects were given supportive debriefing may also have influenced their retroactive approval. See A. K. Ring, et al., "Mode of Debriefing as a Factor Affecting Subjective Reaction to a Milgram-type Experiment—An Ethical Inquiry," in Katz, *Experimentation on Human Beings*, pp. 395–99.

17. *Obedience to Authority*, pp. 173–74. See also *ibid.*, p. 204.

18. An example from ordinary life will help explain my point. Consider a man who persists with amorous advances, as in attempted seduction, in spite of the fact that the woman is verbally and physically resisting. If later, having finally given in, she expresses approval, we cannot take her approval at face value because it has been induced by the procedure she has approved of. Her approval is not independent of the procedure being judged.

19. "Ethical Principles in Medical Experimentation," in *Ethical and Legal Issues of Social Experimentation*, A. M. Rivlin and P. M. Timpane, eds. (Washington: The Brookings Institution, 1975), p. 52. Milgram also makes this suggestion, in "Subject Reaction," p. 23.

20. This last objection to Veatch's proposal is similar to an objection raised by Milgram to the technique known as "role-playing." In role-playing, the subject is fully informed but is asked to go through the experimental protocol *as if* he or she didn't know the relevant information. Clearly, role-playing does not involve any violation of the principle of informed consent. But, as Milgram points out, "we must still perform the crucial experiment [with deception] to determine whether role-played behavior corresponds to nonrole-played behavior" ("Subject Reaction," p. 23). What the experimental scientist needs to do, then, is to show *without* the use of deception that role-played and nonrole-played behavior closely correspond, and this may be impossible to do.

21. "Subject Reaction," p. 23.

22. See, for example, L. J. Stricker, S. Messick, and D. N. Jackson, "Suspicion of Deception: Implications for Conformity Research," *Journal of Personality and Social Psychology* 5 (1967), pp. 379–89; and Z. Rubin and J. C. Moore, Jr., "Assessment of Subjects' Suspicions," *Journal of Personality and Social Psychology* 17 (1971) 163–70.

23. This method was suggested to me by Professor Richard T. Hull, Department of Philosophy, SUNY/Buffalo.

22 *The Ethics of Giving Placebos*

SISSELA BOK

This article explores one specific ethical dilemma in experimentation: placebos and their use in blind or double-blind studies. The ethical focus is on the meaning and role of informed consent in such experiments which necessarily imply a withholding of important knowledge from the subject. Bok carefully leads us through a variety of problems and draws up specific conclusions on the use of the placebo. This article provides an excellent test case for an examination of the scientific and ethical principles that are inherent in this type of human experimentation.

Dr. Sissela Bok, Ph.D., teaches at Brandeis University, Waltham, MA.

In 1971 a number of Mexican-American women applied to a family-planning clinic for contraceptives. Some of them were given oral contraceptives and other were given placebos, or dummy pills that looked like the real thing. Without knowing it the women were involved in an investigation of the side effects of various contraceptive pills. Those who were given placebos suffered from a predictable side effect: 10 of them became pregnant. Needless to say, the physician in charge did not assume financial responsibility for the babies. Nor did he indicate any concern about having bypassed the "informed consent" that is required in ethical experiments with human beings. He contented himself with the observation that if only the law had permitted it, he could have aborted the pregnant women!

The physician was not unusually thoughtless or hardhearted. The fact is that placebos are so widely prescribed for therapeutic reasons or administered to control groups in experiments, and are considered so harmless, that the fundamental issues they raise are seldom confronted. It appears to me, however, that physicians prescribing placebos cannot consider only the presumed benefit to an individual patient or to an experiment at a particular time. They must also take into account the potential risks, both to the patient or the experimental subject and to the medical profession. And the ethical dilemmas that are inherent in the various uses of placebos are central to such an estimate of possible benefits and risks.

The derivation of "placebo," from the Latin for "I shall please," gives the word a benevolent ring, somehow placing placebos beyond moral criticism and conjuring up images of hypochondriacs whose vague ailments are dispelled through adroit prescriptions of beneficent sugar pills. Physicians often give a humorous tinge to instructions for prescribing these substances, which helps to remove them from serious ethical concern. One authority wrote in a pharmacological journal that the placebo should be given a name previously unknown to the patient and preferably Latin and polysyllabic, and "it is wise if it be prescribed with some assurance and emphasis for psycho-therapeutic effect. The older physicians each had his favorite placebic prescriptions—one chose tincture of Condurango, another the Fluid-extract of *Cimicifuga nigra*." After all, are not placebos far less dangerous than some genuine drugs? As another physician asked in a letter to *The Lancet*: "Whenever pain can be relieved with two milliliters of saline, why should we inject an opiate? Do anxieties or discomforts that are allayed with starch capsules require administration of a barbiturate, diazepam or propoxyphene?"

Before the 1960's placebos were commonly defined as just such pharmacologically inactive medications as salt water or starch, given primarily to satisfy patients that something is being done for them. It has only gradually become clear that any medical procedure has an implicit placebo effect and, whether it is active or inactive, can serve as a placebo whenever it has no specific effect on the condition for which it is prescribed. Nowadays fewer sugar pills are prescribed, but X rays, vitamin preparations, antibiotics and even surgery can function as placebos. Arthur K. Shapiro defines a placebo as "any therapy (or component of therapy) that is deliberately or knowingly used for its nonspecific, psychologic or psycho-physiologic effect, or that. . ., unknown to the patient or therapist, is without specific activity for the condition being treated."

Clearly the prescription of placebos is intentionally deceptive only when the physician himself knows they are without specific effect but keeps the patient in the dark. In considering the ethical issues attending deception with placebos I shall exclude the many procedures in which physicians have had—or still have—misplaced faith; that includes most of the treatments prescribed until this century and a great many still in use but of unproved or even disproved value.

Considering that in the past most therapies had little or no specific effect (yet sometimes succeeded thanks to faith on the part of healers and sufferers) and that we now have more effective remedies, it might be thought that the need to resort to placebos would have decreased. Improved treatment and diagnosis, however, have raised the expectations of patients and health professionals alike and consequently the incidence of reliance on placebos has risen. This is true of placebos given both in experiments and for therapeutic effect.

Modern techniques of experimentation with humans have vastly expanded the role of placebos as controls. New drugs, for example, are compared with placebos in order to distinguish the effects of the drug from chance events or effects associated with the mere administration of the drug. They can be tested in "blind" studies, in which the subjects do not know whether they are receiving the experimental drug or the placebo, and in "double-blind" studies, in which neither the subjects nor the investigators know.

Experiments involving humans are now subjected to increasingly careful safeguards for the people at risk, but it will be a long time before the practice of deceiving experimental subjects with respect to placebos is eradicated. In all the studies of the placebo effect that I surveyed in a study initiated as a fellow of the Interfaculty Program in Medical Ethics at Harvard University, only one indicated that those subjected to the experiment were informed that they would receive placebos; indeed, there was frequent mention of intentional deception. For example, a study titled "An Analysis of the Placebo Effect in Hospitalized Hypertensive Patients" reports that "six patients . . . were asked to accept hospitalization for approximately six weeks . . . to have their hypertension evaluated and to undertake a treatment with a new blood pressure drug. . . . No medication was given for the first five to seven days in the hospital. Placebo was then started."

As for therapeutic administration, there is no doubt that studies conducted in recent decades show placebos can be effective. Henry K. Beecher studied the effects of placebos on patients suffering from conditions including postoperative pain, angina pectoris and the common cold. He estimated that placebos achieved satisfactory relief for about 35 percent of the patients surveyed. Alan Leslie points out, moreover, that "some people are temperamentally impatient and demand results before they normally would be forthcoming. Occasionally, during a period of diagnostic observation or testing, a placebo will provide a gentle sop to their impatience and keep them under control while the important business is being conducted.

A number of other reasons are advanced to explain the continued practice of prescribing placebos. Physicians are acutely aware of the uncertainties of their profession and of how hard it is to give meaningful and correct answers to patients. They also know that disclosing uncertainty or a pessimistic prognosis can diminish benefits that depend on faith and the placebo effect. They dislike being the bearers of uncertain or bad news as much as anyone else. Sitting down to discuss an illness with a patient truthfully and sensitively may take much-needed time away from other patients. Finally, the patient who demands unneeded medication or operations may threaten to go to a more cooperative doctor or to resort to self-medication; such patient pressure is one of the most potent forces perpetuating and increasing the resort to placebos.

There are no conclusive figures for the extent to which placebos are prescribed, but clearly their use is widespread. Thorough studies have estimated that as many as 35 to 45 percent of all prescriptions are for substances that are incapable of having an effect on the condition for which they are prescribed. Kenneth L. Melmon and Howard F. Morrelli, in their textbook *Clinical Pharmacology*, cite a study of treatment for the common cold as indicating that 31 percent of the patients received a prescription for a broad-spectrum or medium-spectrum antibiotic, 22 percent received penicillin and 6 percent received sulfonamides—"none of which could possibly have any beneficial specific pharmacological effect on the viral infection per se." They point out further that thousands of doses of vitamin B-12 are administered every year "at considerable expense to patients without pernicious anemia," the only condition for which the vitamin is specifically indicated.

In view of all of this it is remarkable that medical textbooks provide little analysis of placebo treatment. In a sample of 19 popular recent textbooks in medicine, pediatrics, surgery, anesthesia, obstetrics and gynecology only three even mention placebos, and none of them deal with either the medical or the ethical dilemmas placebos present. Four out of six textbooks on pharmacology consider placebos, but with the exception of the book by Melmon and Morrelli they mention only the experimental role of placebos and are completely silent on ethical issues. Finally, four out of eight standard texts on psychiatry refer to placebos, again without ever mentioning ethical issues.

Yet little thought is required to see the dilemma placebos should pose for physicians. A placebo can provide a potent, although unreliable, weapon against suffering, but the very manner in which it can relieve suffering seems to depend on keeping the patient in the dark. The dilemma is an ethical one, reflecting contrary views about how human beings ought to deal with each other, an apparent conflict between helping patients and informing them about their condition.

This dilemma is pointed up by the concept of informed consent: the idea that the individual has the right to give prior consent to, and even to refuse, what is proposed to him in the way of medical care. The doctrine is recognized in proliferating "bills of rights" for patients. The one recommended by the American Hospital Association states, for example, that the patient has the right to complete, understandable information on his diagnosis, treatment and prognosis; the right to whatever information is needed so that he can give informed consent to any treatment; the right to refuse treatment to the extent permitted by law.

Few physicians appear to consider the implications of informed consent when they prescribe placebos, however. One reason is surely that the usefulness of a placebo may be destroyed if informed consent is sought, since its success is assumed to depend specifically on the patient's ignorance and suggestibility. Then too the substances employed as placebos have been considered so harmless, and at the same time so potentially beneficial, that it is easy to assume that the lack of consent cannot possibly matter. In any case health professionals in general have not considered the possibility that the prescription of a placebo is so intrinsically misleading as to make informed consent impossible.

Some authorities have argued that there need not be any deception at all. Placebos can be described in such a way that no outright verbal lie is required. For example: "I believe these pills may help you." Lawrence J. Henderson went so far as to maintain that "it is meaningless to speak of telling the truth, the whole truth and nothing but the truth to a patient . . . because it is . . . a sheer impossibility. . . . Since telling the truth is impossible, there can be no sharp distinction between what is false and what is true."

Can one really think of prescribing placebos as not being deceptive at all as long as the words were sufficiently vague? In order to answer this question it is necessary to consider the nature of deception. When someone intentionally deceives another person, he causes that person to believe what is false. Such deception may be verbal, in which case it is a lie, or it may be nonverbal, conveyed by gestures, false visual cues or the myriad other means human beings have devised for misleading one another. What is common to all intentional deception is the intent to deceive and the providing of misleading information, whether that information is verbal or nonverbal.

The statement that a placebo may help a patient is not a lie or even, in itself, deceitful. Yet the circumstances in which a placebo is prescribed introduce an element of deception. The setting in a doctor's office or hospital room, the impressive terminology, the mystique of the all-powerful physician prescribing a cure—all of these tend to give the patient faith in the remedy; they convey the impression that the treatment prescribed will have the ingredients necessary to improve the patient's condition. The actions of the physician are therefore deceptive even if the words are so general as not to be lies. Verbal deception may be more direct, but all kinds of deception can be equally misleading.

The view that merely withholding information is not deceptive is particularly inappropriate in the case of placebo prescriptions because information that is material and important is withheld. The crucial fact that the physician may not know what the patient's problems are is not communicated. Information concerning the prognosis is vague and information about the specific way in which the treatment may affect the condition is not provided. Henderson's view fails to make the distinction between such relevant information, which it is usually feasible to provide, and infinite details of decreasing importance, which to be sure can never be provided with any completeness. It also fails to distinguish between two ways in which the information reaching the patient may be altered: it may be withheld or it may be distorted. Often the two are mingled. Consider the intertwining of distortion, mystification and failure to inform in the following statement, made to unsuspecting recipients of placebos in an experiment performed in a psychiatric outpatient clinic: "You are to receive a test that all patients receive as part of their evaluation. The test medication is a nonspecific autonomous nervous system stimulant."

Even those who recognize that placebos are deceptive often dispel any misgivings with the thought that they involve no serious deception. Placebos are regarded as being analogous to the innocent white lies of everyday life, so trivial as to be quite outside the realm of ethical evaluation. Such liberties with language as telling someone that his necktie is beautiful or that a visit has been a pleasure, when neither statement reflects the speaker's honest opinion, are commonly accepted as being so trivial that to evaluate them morally would seem unduly fastidious and, from a utilitarian point of view, unjustified. Placebos are not trivial, however. Spending for them runs into millions of dollars. Patients incur greater risks of discomfort and harm than is commonly understood. Finally, any placebo uses that are in fact trivial and harmless in themselves may combine to form nontrivial practices, so that repeated reliance on placebos can do serious harm in the long run to the medical profession and the general public.

Consider first the cost to patients. A number of the procedures undertaken for their placebo effect are extremely costly in terms of available resources and of expense, discomfort and risk of harm to patients. Many temporarily successful new surgical procedures owe their success to the placebo effect alone. In such cases there is no intention to deceive the patient; physician and patient alike are deceived. On occasion, however, surgery is deliberately performed as a placebo measure. Children may undergo appendectomies or tonsillectomies that are known to be unnecessary simply to give the impression that powerful measures are being taken or because parents press for the operation. Hysterectomies and other operations may be performed on adults for analogous reasons. A great many diagnostic procedures that are known to be unnecessary are undertaken to give patients a sense that efforts are being made on their behalf. Some of these carry risks; many involve discomfort and the expenditure of time and money. The potential for damage by an active drug given as a placebo is similarly clear-cut. Calvin M. Kunin, T. Tupasi and W. Craig have described the ill effects—including death—suffered by hospital patients as a result of excessive prescription of antibiotics, more than half of which they found had been unneeded, inappropriately selected or given in incorrect dosages.

Even inactive placebos can have toxic effects in a substantial proportion of cases; nausea, dermatitis, hearing loss, headache, diarrhea and other symptoms have been cited. Stewart Wolf reported on a double-blind experiment to test the effects of the drug mephenesin and a placebo on disorders associated with anxiety and tension. Depending on the symptom studied, roughly 20 to 30 percent of the patients were better while taking the pills and 50 to 70 percent were unchanged, but 10 to 20 percent were worse—"whether the patient was taking mephenesin or placebo." A particularly serious possible side effect of even a harmless substance is dependency. In one case a psychotic patient was given placebo pills and told they were a "new major tranquilizer without any side effects." After four years she was taking 12 tablets a day and complaining of insomnia and anxiety. After the self-medication reached 25 pills a day and a crisis had occurred, the physician intervened, talked over the addictive problem (but not the deception) with the patient and succeeded in reducing the dose to two a day, a level that was still being maintained a year later. Other cases have been reported of patients' becoming addicted or habituated to these substances to the point of not being able to function without them, at times even requiring that they be stepped up to very high dosages.

Most obvious, of course, is the damage done when placebos are given in place of a well-established therapy that is clearly indicated for the patient's condition. The Mexican-American women I mentioned at the outset, for example, were actually harmed by being given placebo pills in the guise of contraceptive pills. In 1966 Beecher, in an article on the ethics of experiments with human subjects, documented a case in which 109 servicemen with streptococcal respiratory infections were given injections of a placebo instead of injections of penicillin, which was already known to prevent the development of rheumatic fever in such patients and which was being given to a larger group of patients. Two of the placebo subjects developed rheumatic fever and one developed an acute kidney infection, whereas such complications did not occur in the penicillin-treated group.

There have been a number of other experiments in which patients suffering from illnesses with known cures have been given placebos in order to study the course of the illness when it is untreated or to determine the precise effectiveness of the known therapy in another group of patients. Because of the very nature of their aims the investigators have failed to ask subjects for their informed consent. The subjects have tended to be those least able to object or defend themselves: members of minority groups, the poor, the institutionalized and the very young.

A final type of harm to patients given placebos stems not so much from the placebo itself as from the manipulation and deception that accompany its prescription. Inevitably some patients find out that they have been duped. They may then lose confidence in physicians and in bona fide medication, which they may need in the future. They may even resort on their own to more harmful drugs or other supposed cures. That is a danger associated with all deception: its discovery leads to a failure of trust when trust may be most needed. Alternatively, some people who do not discover the deception and are left believing that a placebic remedy works may continue to rely on it under the wrong circumstances. This is particularly true with respect to drugs, such as antibiotics, that are used sometimes for their specific action and sometimes as placebos. Many parents, for example, come to believe they must ask for the prescription of antibiotics every time their child has a fever.

The major costs associated with placebos may not be the costs to patients themselves that I have discussed up to this point. Rather they may be costs to new categories of patients in the future, to physicians who do not abuse placebo treatment and to society in general.

Deceptive practices, by their very nature, tend to escape the normal restraints of accountability and so can spread more easily. There are many instances in which an innocuous-seeming practice has grown to become a large-scale and more dangerous one; warnings against "the entering wedge" are often rhetorical devices but may sometimes be justified when there are great pressures to move along the undesirable path and when the safeguards against undesirable developments are insufficient. In this perspective there is reason for con-

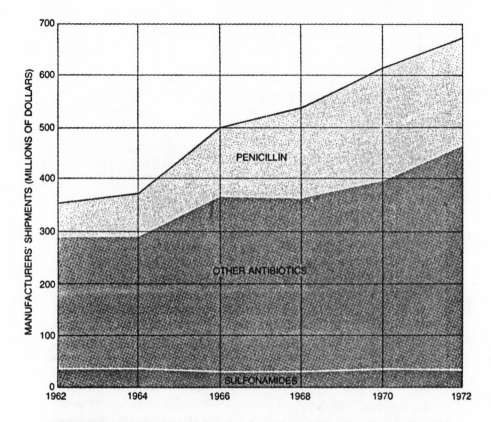

ANTIBIOTICS serve primarily as placebos when they are prescribed for minor virus diseases such as the common cold. Curves, based on Department of Commerce figures, show the value of manufacturers' shipments of systemic antibiotics and of sulfonamides, which are chemical anti-infective drugs. Among antibiotics, single penicillin preparations are shown separately. Antibiotic-sulfonamide combinations are included with other antibiotics.

cern about placebos. The safeguards are few or nonexistent against a practice that is secretive by its very nature. And there are ever stronger pressures—from drug companies, patients eager for cures and busy physicians—for more medication, whether it is needed or not. Given such pressures the use of placebos can spread along a number of dimensions.

The clearest danger lies in the gradual shift from pharmacologically inert placebos to more active ones. It is not always easy to distinguish completely inert substances from somewhat active ones and these in turn from more active ones. It may be hard to distinguish between a quantity of an active substance so low that it has little or no effect and quantities that have some effect. It is not always clear to physicians whether patients require an inert placebo or possibly a

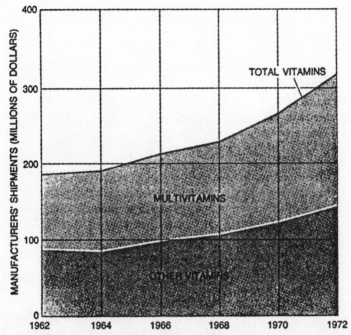

RISING SALES of vitamins (*left*) and of hematinics, or drugs that improve the quality of the blood (*right*), reflect their frequent prescription or purchase across the counter as placebos rather than for their specific effects. The Department of Commerce figures used here include proprietary preparations (sold across the counter) as well as "ethical" ones (sold only on a physician's prescription).

more active one, and there can be the temptation to resort to an active one just in case it might also have a specific effect. It is also much easier to deceive a patient with a medication that is known to be "real" and to have power. One recent textbook in medicine goes so far as to advocate the use of small doses of effective compounds as placebos rather than inert substances—because it is important for both the doctor and the patient to believe in the treatment! The fact that the dangers and side effects of active agents are not always known or considered important by the physician is yet another factor contributing to the shift from innocuous placebos to active ones.

Meanwhile the number of patients receiving placebos increases as more and more people seek and receive medical care and as their desire for instant, push-button alleviation of symptoms is stimulated by drug advertising and by rising expectations of what "science" can do. Reliance on placebic therapy in turn strengthens the belief that there really is a pill or some other kind of remedy for every ailment. As long ago as 1909 Richard C. Cabot wrote, in a perceptive paper on the subject of truth and deception in medicine: "The majority of placebos are given because we believe the patient . . . has learned to expect medi-

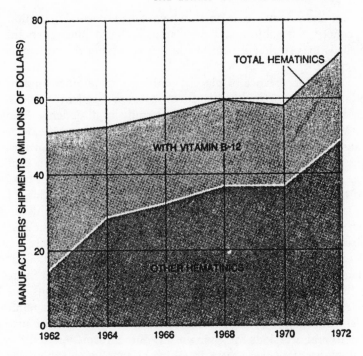

cine for every symptom, and without it he simply won't get well.
True, but who taught him to expect a medicine for every symptom?
He was not born with that expectation. . . . It is we physicians who
are responsible for perpetuating false ideas about disease and its cure.
. . . With every placebo that we give we do our part in perpetuating
error, and harmful error at that."

A particularly troubling aspect of the spread of placebos is that it
now affects so many children. Parents increasingly demand pills, such
as powerful stimulants, to modify their children's behavior with a
minimum of effort on their part; there are some children who may
need such medication but many receive it without proper diagnosis.
As I have mentioned, parents demand antibiotics even when told they
are unnecessary, and physicians may give in to the demands. In these
cases the very meaning of "placebo" has shifted subtly from "I shall
please the patient" to "I shall please the patient's parents."

Deception by placebo can also spread from therapy and diagnosis
to experimental applications. Although placebos can be given non-
deceptively in experimentation, someone who is accustomed to prescribing placebos therapeutically without consent may not take the
precaution of obtaining such consent when he undertakes an experiment on human subjects. Yet therapeutic deception is at least thought

to be for the patient's own good, whereas experimental deception may not benefit the subject and may actually harm him; even the paternalistic excuse that the investigator is deceiving the patient for his own good then becomes inapplicable.

Finally, acceptance of placebos can encourage other kinds of deception in medicine such as failure to reveal to a patient the risks connected with an operation, or lying to terminally ill patients. Medicine lends itself with particular ease to deception for benevolent reasons because physicians are so clearly more knowledgeable than their patients and the patients are so often in a weakened or even irrational state. As Melvin Levine has put it, "the medical profession has practiced as if the truth is, in fact, a kind of therapeutic instrument [that] . . . can be altered or given in small doses . . . [or] not used at all when deemed detrimental to the patients. . . . Many physicians have utilized truth distortion as a kind of anesthetic to promote comfort and ease treatment." Such practices are presumably for the good of patients. No matter how cogent and benevolent the reasons for resorting to deception may seem, when those reasons are considered in secret, without the consent of the doctored, they tend to be reinforced by less benevolent pressures, self-deception begins to blur nice distinctions and occasions for giving misleading information multiply.

Because of all these ways in which placebo usage can spread it is impossible to look at each incident of manipulation in isolation. There are no water-tight compartments in medicine. When the costs and benefits of any therapeutic, diagnostic or experimental procedure are weighed, not only the individual consequences but also the cumulative ones must be taken into account. Reports of deceptive practices inevitably filter out, and the resulting suspicion is heightened by the anxiety that threats to health always create. And so even the health professionals who do not mislead their patients are injured by those who do and the entire institution of medicine is threatened by practices lacking in candor, however harmless the results may appear to be in some individual cases.

What should be the profession's attitude with regard to placebos? In the case of most experimental applications there are ways of avoiding deception without abandoning placebo controls. Subjects can be informed of the nature of the experiment and of the fact that placebos will be administered; if they then consent to the experiment, the use of placebos cannot be considered surreptitious. Although the subjects in a blind or double-blind experiment will not know exactly when they are receiving placebos or even whether they are receiving them, the initial consent to the experimental design, including placebos, removes the ethical problems having to do with deception. If, on the other hand, there are experiments of such a nature that asking subjects for their informed consent to the use of placebos would invalidate the results or cause too many subjects to decline, then the experiment ought not to be performed and the desired knowledge should be sought by means of a different research design.

As for the diagnostic and therapeutic use of placebos, we must start with the presumption that it is undesirable. By and large, given the principle of informed consent as well as concern for human integrity, no measures that affect someone's health should be undertaken without explanation and permission. Placebos are not so trivial as to be unworthy of ethical evaluation; they carry a definite possibility of harm and discomfort to patients as well as high collective costs; as a result placebo prescriptions present a more serious inroad on patient decision making than has been appreciated up to now. Surreptitious diagnostic and therapeutic administration of placebos should therefore be ruled out whenever possible.

The prohibition should not be absolute, however. In some cases the balance of benefit over cost is so overwhelming that reasonable people would choose to be deceived. There is no clear formula that will quickly reveal in each case whether the benefits will greatly outweigh the possible harm. Much of the problem can be avoided if care is taken to avoid placebos if possible and to observe the following principles in the remaining cases: (1) Placebos should be used only after a careful diagnosis; (2) no active placebos should be employed, merely inert ones; (3) no outright lie should be told and questions should be answered honestly; (4) placebos should never be given to patients who have asked not to receive them; (5) placebos should never be used when other treatment is clearly called for or all possible alternatives have not been weighed.

If placebo medicine is to be thus limited, the information provided to both medical personnel and patients will have to change radically. Placebos, so often resorted to and yet so rarely mentioned, will have to be discussed from scientific as well as ethical points of view during medical training. Textbooks will have to confront the medical and ethical dilemmas analytically and exhaustively. Similarly, much education must be provided for the public. There must be greater stress on the autonomy of the patient and on his right to consent to treatment or to refuse treatment after being informed of its nature. Understanding of the normal courses of illnesses should be stressed, including the fact that most minor conditions clear up by themselves rather quickly. The great pressure patients exert for more medication must be countered by limitations on drug advertising and by information concerning the side effects and dangers of drugs.

I have tried to show that the benevolent deception exemplified by placebos is widespread, that it carries risks not usually taken into account, that it represents an inroad on informed consent, that it damages the institution of medicine and contributes to the erosion of confidence in medical personnel.

Honesty may not be the highest social value; at exceptional times, when survival is at stake, it may have to be set aside. To permit a widespread practice of deception, however, is to set the stage for abuses and growing mistrust. Augustine, considering the possibility of giving official sanction to white lies, pointed out that "little by little and bit by bit this will grow and by gradual accessions will slowly increase until it becomes such a mass of wicked lies that it will be utterly impossible to find any means of resisting such a plague grown to huge proportions through small additions."

Ethical Dilemmas In
Obtaining Informed Consent/Further Reading

Callan, Dennis E. "Patients' Rights and Informed Consent: An Emergency Case For Hospitals?" *California Western Law Review* 12 (Winter, 1976), 406–28.

Freedman, Benjamin. "A Moral Theory of Informed Consent." *Hastings Center Report.* 5 (August, 1975), 32–39.

Kelman, Herbert C. "The Rights of the Subject in Social Research: An Analysis in Terms of Relative Power and Legitimacy." *American Psychologist* 27 (November, 1972), 989–1016.

Macklin, Ruth. "Consent, Coercion, and Conflicts of Rights." *Perspectives in Biology and Medicine* 20 (Spring, 1977), 360–71.

Morris, R. Curtis, et al. "Guidelines for Accepting Volunteers: Consent, Ethical Implications, and The Function of Peerly View." *Clinical Pharmacology and Therapeutics* 13 (September, 1972), 782–802.

Patten, Stephen C. "The Case That Milgram Makes." *The Philosophical Review* (July, 1977), 350–63.

The following reports have all been issued by the National Commission for the Protection of Human Subjects Biomedical and Behavioral Research, and are available from the United States Printing Office.

1. Disclosure of Research Information Under the Freedom of Information Act. DHEW (OS) 77-003.

2. Report and Recommendations: Psychosurgery. DHEW (OS) 77-001.

3. Report and Recommendations: Research Involving Children. DHEW (OS) 77-004.

4. Report and Recommendations: Research Involving Prisoners. DHEW (OS) 76-131.

5. Report and Recommendations: Research Involving Those Institutionalized as Mentally Infirm. DHEW (OS) 78-006.

6. Report and Recommendations: Research On The Fetus. DHEW (OS) 76-127.

7. Report and Recommendations: Institutional Review Boards. DHEW (OS) 78-008.

8. Report and Recommendations: Ethical Guidelines for the Delivery of Health Services by DHEW. DHEW (OS) 78-0010.

PART SIX

GENETIC ENGINEERING AND GENETIC POLICY

The Presidential Commission
Tabitha M. Powledge
John Fletcher
James F. Childress
Kenneth Casebeer
Leon R. Kass
Clifford Grobstein
Michael Flower
John Mendeloff

23 *Social and Ethical Issues*

THE PRESIDENTIAL COMMISSION

This chapter presents an overview of several issues related to the potential for splicing genes. The Commission organized these issues under two major headings. First, the Commission addressed concerns about "playing God." This examined the religious dimension of the new genetics as well as possible limits on interventions into nature. Second, the consequences of gene splicing were evaluated. Here various applications were examined, the evolutionary impact discussed and harms and benefits compared. The Commission helpfully summarizes many of the major social and ethical issues related to the practice of genetics.

The Presidential Commission was formed to evaluate ethical dilemmas in medicine and behavioral research. Its Report, Splicing Life, *from which this chapter is taken, was published in 1983*

The preceding chapters have described the potential benefits of gene splicing, but they have also suggested the awesome and sometimes troubling implications that have shared this technology's spotlight. In this chapter, the Commission considers the social and ethical issues raised as society seeks ways to realize the benefits without incurring unacceptable risks. The Commission has found no ethical precepts that would preclude the initial clinical uses of gene splicing now being undertaken or planned or that would categorically prohibit the research procedures through which knowledge is currently being sought in this important field. But more distant possibilities—either in themselves or in conjunction with other scientific and social developments they may foster—could have less benign effects. Consequently, this Report recommends steps that can and should be taken to keep the social and ethical implications of gene splicing before the public and policymakers as these developments become feasible in the years ahead.

The Commission also believes, for several reasons, that balancing both present and future benefits and risks requires more than a simple arithmetical calculation. First, assessing this new technology through cost/benefit or risk/benefit analysis is complex because decisionmaking about gene splicing technology is characterized by several types and levels of uncertainty. The risks and benefits are poorly conceptualized and understood. Before they can be compared, they must be more clearly distinguished and articulated. Moreover, in many cases consensus—social or scientific—is lacking about whether a particular outcome is in fact a benefit or a detriment. For example, some people regard the prospect of eliminating a genetic disorder in future generations as laudable, while others worry about the unforeseeable consequences of making alterations in germ-line cells. Second, while some people focus on particular consequences of various applications of genetic engineering technology, others are concerned about the acceptability of genetic manipulation per se. In this context, balancing risks against benefits makes little sense because actions, not consequences, are at issue.

In the first part of this chapter, the Commission considers theological and secular attitudes toward the technology as such, rather than toward its possible consequences, and attempts to clarify the nature of these concerns. The Commission then turns to an examination of the types of risks at issue. Although the focus is on spelling out the meaning and significance of certain risks, the benefits being sought through genetic manipulations—and those foregone if progress is thwarted—are also part of the equation.

It should be emphasized that this discussion does not limit itself to concerns about gene splicing that the scientific community or the Commissioners view as valid. Moreover, this chapter is not a comprehensive survey of the social and ethical issues in genetic engineering. Since this Report addresses primarily the potential human uses of gene splicing, there is, for example, no detailed treatment of the subject of laboratory or industrial "biohazards" (that is, the danger of microorganisms to those involved in their creation or manufacture, or to the general public should they escape from a controlled environment). The problems of laboratory hazards and occupational safety have been scrutinized for almost a decade by the United States Congress (through hearings and through studies by the Office of Technology Assessment and the Library of Congress), by RAC [Recombinant Advisory Committee], by various bodies at the Federal, state, and local level, and by numerous scientific organizations.[1]

Some of the doubts about the new technology may appear on close examination to be overly speculative or even fanciful. Nonetheless, they have been forcefully expressed in the popular press, by religious writers, and by members of the general public, and they represent important concerns about the responsible exercise of what may prove to be the means by which people achieve freedom from some of the dictates of their genetic inheritance.

The Commission believes it is important for society to address these concerns head-on. If some of these fears prove groundless, the clearing away of spurious issues will make it easier to focus on any problems of real concern. Without necessarily resolving the problems, the Commission tries to go beyond clarification of the issues to recommend concrete steps for dealing with them.

Concerns About "Playing God"

Hardly a popular article has been written about the social and ethical implications of genetic engineering that does not suggest a link between "God-like powers" and the ability to manipulate the basic material of life. Indeed, a popular book about gene splicing is entitled *Who Should Play God?*[2], and in their June 1980 letter to the President, the three religious leaders sounded a tocsin against the lack of a governmental policy concerning "[t]hose who would play God" through genetic engineering.[3]

Religious Viewpoints

The Commission asked the General Secretaries of the three religious organizations to elaborate on any uniquely theological considerations underlying their concern about gene splicing in humans. The scholars appointed by the organizations to address this question were asked to draw specifically on their particular religious tradition to explain the basis of concerns about genetic engineering; further commentary was provided by other religious scholars.[4]

In the view of the theologians, contemporary developments in molecular biology raise issues of responsibility rather than being matters to be prohibited because they usurp powers that human beings should not possess. The Biblical religions teach that human beings are, in some sense, co-creators with the Supreme Creator.[5] Thus, as interpreted for the Commission by their representatives, these major religious faiths respect and encourage the enhancement of knowledge about nature, as well as responsible use of that knowledge.[6] Endorsement of genetic engineering, which is praised for its potential to improve the human estate, is linked with the recognition that the misuse of human freedom creates evil and that human knowledge and power can result in harm.

While religious leaders present theological bases for their concerns, essentially the same concerns have been raised—sometimes in slightly different words—by many thoughtful secular observers of contemporary science and technology. Concerns over unintended effects, over the morality of genetic manipulation in all its forms, and over the social and political consequences of new technologies are shared by religious and secular commentators. The examination of the various specific concerns need not be limited, therefore, to the religious format in which some of the issues have been raised.

Fully Understanding the Machinery of Life

Although it does not have a specific religious meaning, the objection to scientists "playing God" is assumed to be self-explanatory. On closer examination, however, it appears to the Commission that it conveys several rather different ideas, some describing the power of gene splicing itself and some relating merely to its consequences.

At its heart, the term represents a reaction to the realization that human beings are on the threshold of understanding how the fundamental machinery of life works.[7] A full understanding of what are now great mysteries, and the powers inherent in that understanding, would be so awesome as to justify the description "God-like." In this view,

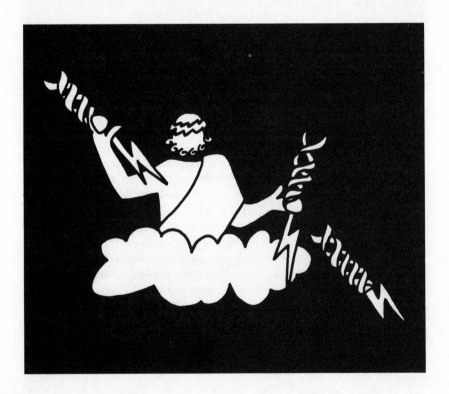

playing God is not actually an objection to the research but an expression of a sense of awe—and concern.

Since the Enlightenment, Western societies have exalted the search for greater knowledge, while recognizing its awesome implications. Some scientific discoveries reverberate with particular force because they not only open new avenues of research but also challenge people's entire understanding of the world and their place in it. Current discoveries in gene splicing—like the new knowledge associated with Copernicus and Darwin—further dethrone human beings as the unique center of the universe. By identifying DNA and learning how to manipulate it, science seems to have reduced people to a set of malleable molecules that can be interchanged with those of species that people regard as inferior. Yet unlike the earlier revolutionary discoveries, those in molecular biology are not merely descriptions; they give scientists vast powers for action.

Arrogant Interference with Nature

By what standards are people to guide the exercise of this awesome new freedom if they want to act responsibly? In this context, the charge that human beings are playing God can mean that in "creating new life forms" scientists are abusing their learning by interfering with nature.

But in one sense *all* human activity that produces changes that otherwise would not have occurred interferes with nature. Medical activities as routine as the prescription of eyeglasses for myopia or as dramatic as the repair or replacement of a damaged heart are in this sense "unnatural." In another sense, human activity cannot interfere with nature—in the sense of contravening it—since all human activities, including gene splicing, proceed according to the scientific laws that describe natural processes. Ironically, to believe that "playing God" in this sense is even possible would itself be hubris according to some religious thought, which maintains that only God can interfere with the descriptive laws of nature (that is, perform miracles).

If, instead, what is meant is that gene splicing technology interferes with nature in the sense that it violates God's prescriptive natural law or goes against God's purposes as they are manifested in the natural order, then some reason must be given for this judgment. None of the scholars appointed to report their views by the three religious bodies that urged the Commission to undertake this study suggested that either natural reason or revelation imply that gene splicing technology as such is "unnatural" in this prescriptive sense. Although each scholar expressed concern over particular applications of gene splicing technology, they all also emphasized that human beings have not merely the right but the duty to employ their God-given powers to harness nature for human benefit. To turn away from gene splicing, which may provide a means of curing hereditary diseases, would itself raise serious ethical problems.[8]

Creating New Life Forms

If "creating new life forms" is simply producing organisms with novel characteristics, then human beings create new life forms frequently and have done so since they first learned to cultivate new characteristics in plants and breed new traits in animals. Presumably the idea is that gene splicing creates new life forms, rather than merely modifying old ones, because it "breaches species barriers" by combining DNA from different species—groups of organisms that cannot mate to produce fertile offspring.

Genetic engineering is not the first exercise of humanity's ability to create new life forms through nonsexual reproduction. The creation of hybrid plants seems no more or no less natural than the development of a new strain of *E. coli* bacteria through gene splicing. Further, genetic engineering cannot accurately be called unique in that it involves the creation of new life forms through processes that do not occur in nature without human intervention. As described in Chapter Two [of *Splicing Life*] scientists have found that the transfer of DNA between organisms of different species occurs in nature without human intervention. Yet, as one eminent scientist in the field has pointed out, it would be unwarranted to assume that a dramatic increase in the frequency of such transfers through human intervention is not problematic simply because DNA transfer sometimes occurs naturally.[9]

In the absence of specific religious prohibitions, either revealed or derived by rational argument from religious premises, it is difficult to see why "breaching species barriers" as such is irreligious or otherwise objectionable. In fact, the very notion that there are barriers that must be breached prejudges the issue. The question is simply whether there is something intrinsically wrong with intentionally crossing species lines. Once the question is posed in this way the answer must be negative—unless one is willing to condemn the production of tangelos by hybridizing tangerines and grapefruits or the production of mules by the mating of asses with horses.

There may nonetheless be two distinct sources of concern about crossing species lines that deserve serious consideration. First, gene splicing affords the possibility of creating hybrids that can reproduce themselves (unlike mules, which are sterile). So the possibility of self-perpetuating "mistakes" adds a new dimension of concern, although here again, the point is not that crossing species lines is inherently wrong, but that it may have undesirable consequences and that these consequences may multiply beyond human control. As noted, the Commission's focus on the human applications of gene splicing has meant that it does not here address this important set of concerns, which lay behind the original self-imposed moratorium on certain categories of gene splicing research and which have been, and continue to be, addressed through various scientific and public mechanisms, such as RAC.[10]

Second, there is the issue of whether particular crossings of species—especially the mixing of human and nonhuman genes—might not be illicit. The moral revulsion at the creation of human-animal hybrids may be traced in part to the prohibition against sexual relations between human beings and lower animals. Sexual relations with lower animals are thought to degrade human beings and insult their God-given dignity as the highest of God's creatures. But unease at the prospect of human-animal hybrids goes beyond sexual prohibitions.

The possibility of creating such hybrids calls into question basic assumptions about the relationship of human beings to other living things. For example, those who believe that the current treatment of animals—in experimentation, food production, and sport—is morally suspect would not be alone in being troubled by the prospect of exploitive or insensitive treatment of creatures that possess even more human-like qualities than chimpanzees or porpoises do. Could genetic engineering be used to develop a group of virtual slaves—partly human, partly lower animal—to do people's bidding? Paradoxically, the very characteristics that would make such creatures more valuable than any existing animals (that is, their heightened cognitive powers and sensibilities) would also make the moral propriety of their subservient role more problematic. Dispassionate appraisal of the long history of gratuitous destruction and suffering that humanity has visited upon the other inhabitants of the earth indicates that such concerns should not be dismissed as fanciful.

Accordingly, the objection to the creation of new life forms by crossing species lines (whether through gene splicing or otherwise) reflects the concern that human beings lack the God-like knowledge and wisdom required for the exercise of these God-like powers. Specifically, people worry that interspecific hybrids that are partially human in their genetic makeup will be like Dr. Frankenstein's monster. A striking lesson of the Frankenstein story is the uncontrollability and uncertainty of the consequences of human interferences with the natural order. Like the tale of the Sorcerer's apprentice or the myth of the golem created from lifeless dust by the 16th century rabbi, Loew of Prague, the story of Dr. Frankenstein's monster serves as a reminder of the difficulty of restoring order if a creation intended to be helpful proves harmful instead. Indeed, each of these tales conveys a painful irony: in seeking to extend their control over the world, people may lessen it. The artifices they create to do their bidding may rebound destructively against them—the slave may become the master.

Suggesting that someone lacks sufficient knowledge or wisdom to engage in an activity the person knows how to perform thus means that the individual has insufficient knowledge of the consequences of that activity or insufficient wisdom to cope with those consequences. But if this is the rational kernel of the admonition against playing God, then the use of gene splicing technology is not claimed to be wrong as such but wrong because of its potential consequences. Understood in this way, the slogan that crossing species barriers is playing God does not end the debate, but it does make a point of fundamental importance.[11] It emphasizes that any realistic assessment of the potential consequences of the new technology must be founded upon a sober recognition of human fallibility and ignorance. At bottom, the warning not to play God is closely related to the Socratic injunction "know thyself": in this case, acknowledge the limits of understanding and prediction, rather than assuming that people can foresee all the consequences of their actions or plan adequately for every eventuality.[12]

Any further examination of the notion that the hybridization of species, at least when one of the species is human, is intrinsically wrong (and not merely wrong as a consequence of what is done with

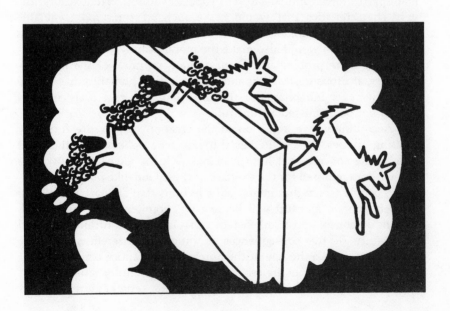

the hybrids) involves elaboration of two points. First, what characteristics are uniquely human, setting humanity apart from all other species? And second, does the wrong lie in bestowing some but not all of these characteristics on the new creation or does it stem from depriving the being that might otherwise have arisen from the human genetic material of the opportunity to have a totally human makeup? The Commission believes that these are important issues deserving of serious study.

It should be kept in mind, however, that the information available to the Commission suggests that the ability to create interspecific hybrids of the sort that would present intrinsic moral and religious concerns will not be available in the foreseeable future. The research currently being done on experimentation with recombinant DNA techniques through the use of single human genes (for example, the insertion of a particular human hemoglobin gene into mouse cells at the embryonic stage) or the study of cellular development through the combining of human genetic material with that of other species in a way that does not result in a mature organism (for example, *in vitro* fusion of human and mouse cells) does not, in the Commission's view, raise problems of an improper "breaching of the barriers."

CONCERNS ABOUT CONSEQUENCES

To appreciate the complexity of the problem of assessing potential consequences and the individual and societal ability to cope with them, the several types of uncertainty discussed in Chapter One [of *Splicing Life*] must be considered: the occurrence uncertainty that arises when it is not known whether a particular event will take place (or what sort of future it will take place in), the ethical uncertainty that follows from not knowing whether certain uses of a technology should be regarded as beneficial or harmful, and the conceptual uncertainty that attends new developments that challenge people's fundamental beliefs. The presence of any of these types of uncertainty complicates the task of estimating whether the potential benefits of genetic engineering outweigh the potential risks.

What Are the Likely Outcomes?

Medical applications. Two broad applications may be distinguished: the use of drugs produced by gene splicing (such as interferon or insulin) and the direct application of gene splicing to human beings through gene therapy or gene surgery.

The problems of personal safety involved in using drugs produced by gene splicing techniques do not appear to be radically different from those that accompany conventionally produced drugs. The basic scientific and ethical issues in this broad area are well known and need not be rehearsed here. The appropriate divisions within the Department of Health and Human Services (in particular, the relevant institutes of the NIH and the Office for Protection from Research Risks, regarding Federally supported research, and the Food and Drug Administration, regarding all drug and vaccine research) need to consider how to apply to genetically engineered drugs the existing mechanisms related to the margin of acceptable risk, the extent and type of animal and human studies required, the standards for manufacturers, and the decision to allow seriously ill patients to opt for more dangerous or less well tested experimental drugs.[13] According to the Department, appropriate steps are already being taken, especially by FDA, to resolve these issues, and the first product of gene splicing has already been approved.[14]

Some direct therapeutic applications of gene splicing technologies to human beings may present distinctive problems of uncertainty not ordinarily encountered in more conventional medical practice. Concern has been expressed that serious harm might result, for example, from a malfunctioning gene inserted by gene therapy. Yet even here the ethical and policy issues do not seem appreciably different from those involved in the development of any new diagnostic and therapeutic techniques. However, in the case of genetic interventions that involve alteration of germ cells, especially stringent animal testing and other precautions are appropriate, since any physical harms produced might extend to the subject's progeny.

Most experts agree there is a very small likelihood that inheritable changes in germ cells would inadvertently occur when the genetic material of somatic cells is being manipulated. However, the same animal tests and refinements of theoretical models that should precede the use of gene surgery in human beings may shed further light on whether such changes might produce inheritable changes in characteristic functions and whether they will influence germ cells. In both cases, the resolution of uncertainty depends upon increased understanding of how an inserted gene will perform its function.

Subjects of gene therapy or gene surgery might suffer psychological as well as physical harm. The revelation that a person has a genetic defect or is genetically predisposed to a disease may produce anxiety, fear or loss of self-esteem—feelings that may be intensified by the belief that the defect is a part of a person's constitution, rather than an outside influence. Similarly, patients might regard alterations of their genes as a more profound change than a surgical procedure or the ingestion of a drug. Experience with genetic screening and counseling suggests that the special significance of a genetic condition to the individual may be accompanied by social stigma based on ignorance, but that efforts to educate individual patients and their families as well as the general public can minimize this problem.[15]

Evolutionary impact on human beings. Some critics warn against the dangers of attempting to control or interfere with the "wisdom of evolution" in order to satisfy scientific curiosity.[16] Those who hold this view object in particular to crossing species lines by gene splicing because they believe that the pervasive inability of different species to produce fertile offspring by sexual reproduction must be an adapative feature, that is, it must confer some significant survival advantage. Thus they view species lines as natural protective barriers that human beings may circumvent only at their peril, although the harm such barriers are supposed to shield people from remains unspecified.

Most proponents of genetic engineering argue that the benefits it will bring are more tangible and important and will affect more people than those objecting suggest. Further, the notion of the "wisdom of evolution" that apparently underlies this consequentialist version of the objection to crossing species lines is not well founded. As the scientific theory of evolution does not postulate a plan that the process of evolution is to achieve, evolutionary changes cannot be said to promote such a plan, wisely or unwisely. Moreover, evolutionary theory recognizes (and natural history confirms) that a "wise" adaptation at one time or place can become a lethal flaw when circumstances change. So even if it could be shown that species barriers have thus far played an important adaptive role, it would not follow that this will continue. An evolutionary explanation of any inherited characteristic can at most show that having that characteristic gave an organism's ancestors some advantage in enabling them to live long enough to reproduce and that the characteristic has not yet proved maladaptive for the offspring.

Furthermore, as a philosopher concerned with assessing the risks of genetic engineering has recently noted, the ability to manipulate genes, both within and across species lines, may become a crucial asset for survival.

> There may . . . come a time when, because of natural or man-induced climatic change, the capacity to alter quickly the genetic composition of agricultural plants will be required to forestall catastrophic famine.[17]

The consequentialist version of the warning against crossing species lines seems, then, to be no more a conclusive argument against genetic engineering than the admonition that to cross species lines is wrong because it is playing God, But it does serve the vital purpose of urging that, so far as this is possible, the evolutionary effects of any interventions are taken into account.

One effect that is of particular concern to some observers is the loss of "heterozygote advantage"—the strength (in terms of individual health and species survival) engendered when members of a species have a variety of gene variants rather than all having the same gene. This advantage has two aspects. The first is the protection that varied genes offer for survival of a species in case of a radical change in environment or, more particularly, the occurrence of a novel pathogen. Of course, it would be virtually impossible to know which particular rare gene variant would prove to be valuable under such circumstances. This consideration would favor preserving as much genetic variation as possible, but it would be difficult to weigh this against the benefit to offspring of the variant gene in its homozygous form.

The second aspect is the advantage that may be conferred by a particular gene in past (and present) environments, perhaps accounting for its prevalence in a population. Although the existence of such an advantage could be construed as an argument against making inheritable gene changes, very little is actually known about the existence and nature of such advantages for most genes. The only instance that is widely acknowledged is the advantage, in terms of longevity and reproduction, possessed by sickle-cell carriers in tropical regions where malaria has been endemic.[18]

The possible beneficial effects of most gene variants are typically too small to be detected by current research methods—that is, other genetic and environmental effects on the health, longevity, and reproductive history of a population make it difficult to detect whether a particular gene confers any advantage on those who possess it. If it becomes feasible to remove an apparently deleterious gene from a population through routine use of gene surgery, the possible loss of heterozygote advantage will deserve careful evaluation.[19] Population geneticists tend to regard the loss of even minute advantages as serious, since such advantages can confer marked benefits on a species over a great many generations. Medical geneticists, on the other hand, are much less bothered by such losses because they believe that it should be possible to make up, through environmental manipulation (including medical treatment) for the loss of any advantage provided by a variant in any probable future environment.

Will Benefit or Harm Occur?

Parental rights and responsibilities. Current attitudes toward human reproductive activity are founded, in part, on several important assumptions, among them that becoming a parent requires a willingness, within very broad limits, to accept the child a woman gives birth to, that parents' basic duties to children are more or less clear and settled, and that reproduction and parenting are and should remain largely private and autonomous spheres of people's lives. The doors that genetic engineering can open challenge all three of these assumptions.

Genetic counseling and screening have already undercut the first assumption by enabling parents to make an informed decision to prevent the occurrence of some genetic defects by terminating pregnancy, by artificial insemination, or by avoiding conception. If gene therapy or gene surgery become available, parents could have more control over their children's characteristics. They will no longer face the stark alternatives of either playing the hand their child has been dealt by the "natural lottery" or avoiding birth or conception. Instead, they could prevent some genetic defects through gene surgery on the zygote and remedy others through gene therapy before the genetic defect produces irreversible changes in the child.

With this increased ability to act for the well-being of the child would come an expansion of parental responsibility. The boundaries of this responsibility—and hence people's conception of what it is to be a good parent—may shift rapidly. It seems safe to say that one important duty of a parent is to prevent or ameliorate serious defects (if it can be done safely) and that the duty to enhance favorable characteristics is less stringent and clear. Yet the new technological capabilities may change people's view of what counts as a defect. For example, if what is now regarded as the normal development of important cognitive skills could be significantly augmented by genetic engineering, then today's "normal" level might be considered deficient tomorrow. Thus ethical uncertainty about the scope of a parent's obligation is linked to conceptual uncertainty about what counts as a defect.

The problem of shifting conceptions of parental responsibility becomes even more complicated when the effects of parents' present actions on descendants beyond their immediate offspring are considered. Deciding whether to engineer a profound change in an expected or newborn child is difficult enough; if the change is inheritable, the burden of responsibility could be truly awesome.

Gene splicing technology may also change people's sense of family and kinship. On the one hand, the possibility of promoting significant inheritable changes through gene surgery may encourage people to think of their family as extending further into the future than they now do. On the other hand, knowing that future generations may employ an even more advanced technology to alter or replace the characteristics passed on to them may weaken people's sense of genetic continuity.

Traditional views of family and kinship associate reproduction with genetic contribution. If genetic engineering makes use of reproductive technologies such as artificial insemination and *in vitro* fertilization, it will increase the strains on this concept of lineage. Whether or not they are accurate, people's beliefs that they are linked to other members of their family by constitutional similarities may play an important role in a family's sense of solidarity and group identity. Knowledge that the genetic link between parents and children is only partial or nonexistent could attenuate these feelings of kinship and family and the sense of continuity and support that they foster. Experience with adoption illustrates successful integration of family members who are not biologically linked, but also demonstrates the importance some individuals place on an association with biological parents. Here, too, there may be as much uncertainty about whether such changes would be beneficial or harmful as there is about whether they are likely to occur.

Societal obligations. The concept of society's obligation to protect or enhance the health of children and future generations often rests on some notion of an adequate minimum of health care. This benchmark, in turn, depends upon assumptions about what counts as a serious defect or disability, on the one hand, and what constitutes normal functioning or adequate health, on the other. As technological capabilities grow, the boundary between these criteria will blur and shift, and with this will come changes in people's views about what society owes to children and to future generations.

As new technological capabilities raise the standard of normal functioning or adequate health, the scarcity of societal resources may raise anew a very difficult question that theorists of distributive justice have strongly disagreed about: where does justice to future generations end and generosity begin? This question is of vital practical import, for the demands of justice are characteristically thought of as valid claims or entitlements to be enforced by the coercive power of the state, while generosity is usually regarded as a private virtue.

Yet society has traditionally been reluctant to interfere with reproductive choice, at least in the case of competent adults. Even with the advent of genetic counseling and screening, social policy has for the most part scrupulously avoided restricting reproductive choice, either as a matter of justice or on any other grounds.[20] So long as the only alternatives are termination of pregnancy or avoidance of conception, any attempt to enforce a public policy designed to prevent genetic defects constitutes a severe infringement on freedom of reproductive choice. If genetic engineering and related reproductive technologies enable a marked reduction of genetic defects and the burden they impose on their victims and on societal resources, however, mandatory genetic treatments may be advocated. Involuntary blood transfusions of pregnant women have been ordered by courts when physicians conclude this is necessary to prevent serious harm to fetuses. Future developments in gene surgery or gene therapy may lead to further departures from the principle that a competent adult may always refuse medical procedures in nonemergency situations and from the assumption that parenting and reproduction are largely private and autonomous activities.

The commitment to equality of opportunity. Since the application of the burgeoning recombinant DNA technology will bring benefits as well as costs and since it will be funded at least in part by public resources, it is essential to ask several questions. Who will benefit from the new technology? And will the benefits be distributed equitably? Indeed, what sort of distribution would count as "fair" when the very thing that is being distributed (such as cognitive ability) is itself often the basis for distributing other things of value in society?[22]

The possibilities presented by gene therapy and gene surgery may in fact call into question the scope and limits of a central element of democratic political theory and practice: the commitment to equality of opportunity. One root idea behind the modern concept of equality of opportunity is the belief that because the social assets a person is born with are in no way earned or merited, it is unfair for someone's luck in the "social lottery" to determine that person's most basic prospects in life. Until recently, those who have sought to ground the commitment to equality of opportunity on this belief have only urged that social institutions be designed so as to minimize or compensate for the influence that the "social lottery" exerts on a person's opportunities.[23] Genetic engineering raises the question of whether equality of opportunity requires intervention in the "natural lottery" as well, for people's initial genetic assets, like their initial social assets, are unearned and yet exert a profound influence on opportunities in life. Even to ask this question challenges a fundamental assumption about the scope of principles of distributive justice, namely that they deal only with inequalities in social goods and play no role in regulating natural inequalities.

Genetic malleability and the sense of personal identity. The manipulation of genes that play an important role in regulating processes of growth and aging or that contribute significantly to personality or intelligence—if it ever becomes possible—could have considerable impact on the way people think of themselves. The current tendency is to think of a person as an individual of a certain character and personality that, following the normal stages of physical, social, and psychological development, is relatively fixed within certain parameters. But this concept—and the sense of predictability and stability in interpersonal relations that it confers—could quickly become outmoded if people use gene splicing to make basic changes in themselves over the course of a lifetime. People can already be changed profoundly through psychosurgery, behavior modification, or the therapeutic use of psychoactive drugs. But genetic engineering might possibly provide quicker, more selective, and easier means. Here again, uncertainty about possible shifts in some of people's most basic concepts brings with it evaluative and ethical uncertainty because the concepts in question are intimately tied to values and ethical assumptions. It is not likely that anything so profound as a change in the notion of personal identity or of normal stages of development over a lifetime is something to which people would have clear value responses in advance.

Changing the meaning of being human. Some geneticists have seen in their field the possibility of benefit through improving human traits.[24] Human beings have the chance to "rise above [their] nature" for "the first time in all time," as one leader in the field has observed:

> It has long been apparent that you and I do not enter this world as unformed clay compliant to any mold. Rather, we have in our beginnings some bent of mind, some shade of character. The origin of this structure—of the fiber in this clay—was for centuries mysterious. . . . Today . . . we know to look within. We seek not in the stars but in our genes for the herald of our fate.[25]

Will gene splicing actually make possible such changes in "human nature" for the first time? In some ways this question is unanswerable since there is great disagreement about which particular characteristics make up "human nature." For some people, the concept encompasses those characteristics that are uniquely human. Yet most human genes are actually found in other mammals as well; moreover, recent work by ethologists and other biologists on animal behavior and capacities is demonstrating that many characteristics once regarded as unique to human beings are actually shared by other animals, particularly by the higher primates, although an ability to record and study the past and to plan beyond the immediate future appears to be a singularly human trait.

Other people regard the critical qualities as those natural characteristics that are common to all human beings, or at least all who fall within a certain "normal range." "Natural" here means characteristics that people are born with as opposed to those that result from social convention, education, or acculturation.

To consider whether gene splicing would allow the changing of human nature thus breaks down into two questions. Which characteristics found in all human beings are inborn or have a large inborn basis? And will gene splicing techniques be able to alter or replace some of the genetic bases of those characteristics? As to the first, the history of religious, philosophical, and scientific thought abounds with fundamental disputes over human nature. Without a consensus on that issue the second question could only be answered affirmatively if it were clear that gene splicing will eventually allow the alteration of all natural characteristics of human beings.

As it is by no means certain that it will ever be possible to change the genetic basis of all natural characteristics, it seems premature to assume that gene splicing will enable changes in human nature. At most, it can perhaps be said that this technology may eventually allow some aspects of what it means to be human to be changed. Yet even that possibility rightly evokes profound concern and burdens everyone with an awesome and inescapable responsibility—either to develop and employ this capability for the good of humanity or to reject it in order to avoid potential undesirable consequences.

The possibility of changing human nature must, however, be kept in perspective. First, within the limits imposed by human beings' genetic endowment, there is already considerable scope by means other than gene splicing for changing some acquired characteristics that are distinctively human. For example, people's desires, values, and the way they live can be changed significantly through alterations in social and economic institutions and through mass education, indoctrination, and various forms of behavior control. Thus, even if gene splicing had the power that some people are concerned about, it would not be unique in its ability to produce major changes in what it means to be human— although it would be unusual in acting on the inheritable foundation of thoughts and actions. If the technology can ever be used in this way, the heritability of the changes ought probably to be regarded as significantly different from any changes now possible.[26]

Second, according to the theory of evolution, the genetic basis of what is distinctively human continually changes through the interplay of random mutation and natural selection. The concern, then, is that gene splicing will for the first time allow deliberate, selective, and rapid alterations to be made in the human genetic constitution.

Finally, concern about changing human nature may at bottom be still more narrowly focused upon those characteristics of human beings—whether unique to the species or not—that are especially valued or cherished. Here, too, there may be disagreement as to which characteristics are most valuable and the value of a given characteristic may depend upon the social or natural environment in which it is manifested.

In sum, the question of whether gene splicing will enable changes in human nature—and the ethical, social, and philosophical significance of such changes—cannot be determined until much more is known about human genetics, specifically the exact contribution of heredity to many human physical and, more important, behavioral traits. Indeed, one of the most important contributions genetic engineering could make to the science of behavioral genetics may be that it will help resolve the age-old controversy of nature versus nurture. If designed changes were possible, society would have to confront whether such changes should be made, and, if they should, which ones. The problems created by uncertainty are particularly notable here since any decision about what characteristics are "desirable" would depend on the world that people will be living in, which is itself unknowable in advance.

Unacceptable uses of gene splicing. A recent National Science Foundation survey indicates that though Americans are generally against restrictions on scientific research, "a notable exception was the opposition to scientists creating new life forms." The survey notes that

> Almost two thirds of the public believe that studies in this area should not be pursued. Fear of the unknown and of possible misuse of the discoveries by some malevolent dictator are among the reasons that could be given for opposition to such genetic engineering.[27]

Given the excesses of the eugenics movement in the United States and elsewhere in the early decades of this century and the role of eugenic theory in mass atrocities perpetrated by the Nazis, these fears cannot be dismissed as groundless. Some comfort may be drawn from the fact that although the possibility of directing human inheritance through simple breeding techniques has existed for centuries, it has not, with relatively minor exceptions, been attempted. Furthermore, the peculiar social and political circumstances that led to these attempts to control human reproduction through the coercive power of the state are not present in this country and are unlikely to occur in the foreseeable future.

Reassuring though they are, these answers are far from conclusive. Government control of sexual reproduction on a broad scale—through an enforced scheme for mating human beings—would require enormous repressive power and social control over individuals over an extended period of time. What might prove more tempting to a dictator or authoritarian ruling elite is the possibility of scientists rapidly making major changes in the genetic composition of a small group in the privacy of the laboratory.

Though there appears at present to be no evidence that the government of this or any other country is attempting to use gene splicing for unacceptable political purposes, the Commission believes that the appropriate posture for the public and the scientific community is one of vigilance. The best safeguards against such abuses are a continued support of democratic institutions and a commitment to individual rights combined with public education about the actual and potential uses of gene splicing technology. Of course, such efforts in this country would not avoid undesirable uses of genetic engineering by totalitarian governments, unless they led to effective international restrictions.[28]

A more subtle danger is that if genetically engineered changes ever become relatively easy to make, there may be a tendency to identify what are in fact social problems as genetic deficiencies of individuals or to assume that the appropriate solution to a given problem, whether social or individual, is genetic manipulation.[29] The relative ease of genetic methods (if gene therapy becomes an accepted medical technique) should most certainly not draw attention away from the underlying social causes of such problems.

Distributing the power to control gene splicing. Beyond any fear of the malevolent use of gene splicing, attention must be paid to a more basic question about the distribution of power: who should decide which lines of genetic engineering research ought to be pursued and which applications of the technology ought to be promoted?

This question is not ordinarily raised about medical technology in general. When it is, the assumption is that for the most part the key decisions are to be made by the relevant experts, the research community, and the medical profession, guided by the availability of research funds (which come predominately from Federal agencies) and by the dictates of medical malpractice law and of state and Federal regulatory agencies designed to protect the public from very tangible, unambiguous harms. Yet genetic engineering is more than a new medical technology. Its potential uses, as discussed, extend far beyond intervention to cure or prevent disease or to restore functioning. This more expansive nature makes it unlikely that decisions about the development of gene splicing technology can be made appropriately within institutions that have evolved to control medical technology and the practice of medicine.

Clearly, adequate institutional arrangements for decision-making about the further development of gene splicing technology must assign a substantial role to experts in the field. Yet it is important to understand the unavoidable limitations of technical expertise. On the one hand, there are the limitations of the experts' knowledge; on the other, there are the limitations of technical knowledge itself, no matter how thorough. Experts in genetic engineering can provide the most accurate available data, from which probability statements can be formulated. But neither geneticists nor scientists experienced in risk assessment have any special expertise about evaluative and conceptual uncertainties. An expert might conclude that there is a 5% probability that a certain harmful outcome will occur, but that knowledge is not sufficient for deciding whether such a probability is an acceptable degree of risk. Nor can scientific expertise answer the question of whether the burdens of risk would fall disproportionately upon some people, for this is a moral, not a scientific, question. This is not to say, of course, that scientific experts should not make moral judgments or that if they do they ought to be ignored. But the limitations of expertise must be clearly understood.

In general the public can reasonably rely on the judgments of experts in the field to the extent that at least three conditions are satisfied: (1) there is a strong consensus among the experts, (2) the process by which individuals come to be identified as experts is not unduly unfluenced by political factors or other forces unrelated to their qualifications as experts, and (3) the experts are not subject to serious conflicts of interest that are likely to distort their judgments or to make their advice unreliable.[30] Whether, or to what extent, these conditions are satisfied cannot be answered once and for all. Instead, they must be viewed as useful rules-of-thumb for assessing and reassessing the role of experts in the formation of responsible public policy.

Commercial-academic relations. Concern over the latter two points—unacceptable uses of the technology and the power to control it—have contributed to a growing public debate about the increased commercial involvement with university-based research on gene splic-

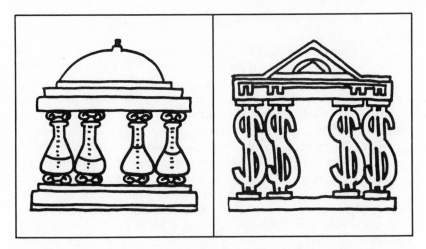

ing. Constraints on support for basic science research by the Federal government in the past decade have been compounded by economic problems that have reduced both state budgets for higher education and the grants of philanthropic foundations. Consequently, academic research scientists are turning increasingly to industry,[31] forming ties that have raised concern about how to accommodate the divergent goals and norms of science and industry.

Universities have historically been dedicated to increasing the general fund of knowledge through basic research, the open exchange of information and ideas, and the training of new researchers and scholars. These goals may run headlong into those of industry—the development of marketable products and techniques through applied research by maintaining a competitive posture, protecting trade secrets, and seeking patent protection.

The conflicts occasioned by these developments are not unique to genetic engineering; indeed, at the beginning of this century a number of expanding universities shifted their focus from the traditional arts and sciences as they became allied with the burgeoning electrical and chemical industries. Medicine, agriculture, econometrics, solid state physics, and computer science have all been advanced in part because of combined forces of industry and universities. Yet the recent similar developments in biotechnology present these issues in sharper relief for several reasons.

First, commercialization of biotechnology seems to be proceeding more rapidly than in chemistry and physics. And in gene splicing, the gap between theory and application—between a graduate student's work in the lab and a highly lucrative product—is often quite small.

Finally, the range of potential applications of the research is very broad.

Increased private funding for bioengineering research has therefore sparked questions about conflicts of interest and about the impact of commercialization on academe more generally.[32] Some see these issues as private concerns relating only to the particular universities and firms contracting with each other, a view reflected at a recent conference at Pajaro Dunes when university officials and industry representatives met in private to discuss concerns about commercialization. The participants at this privately funded conference of 5 leading universities and 11 corporations issued a statement intended to "get some general principles on the record" and "set an agenda for further discussion of the issues." The document raised questions of contract review and disclosure, exclusive licensure, and conflicts of interest encountered by university and faculty. It encouraged university faculties to continue examination of these issues over which commentators have noted that "[p]luralism and a certain measure of confusion prevail."[33]

Other issues are also at stake: Can professional virtue be maintained in the face of considerable financial temptations? How will private funding change professors' outlooks?[34] Will fewer be interested in teaching undergraduates? Will they encourage graduate students to focus on projects with maximum commercial potential, instead of those that would foster a more well rounded background? Will commercialization effect a shift from basic to applied research and, if so, with what consequences? Will the secrecy required by industry impede the free exchange of scientific information? What about conflicts of interest when the same academic department includes owners or employees of competitive bioengineering ventures? Will academic appointments and promotions be skewed to favor those who can attract private research funds to the university?

The Association of American Universities has recently suggested that it become a clearinghouse for information on commercialization.[35] These and related questions have also been the subject of debate in the press and before Congressional committees. Undoubtedly, such concerns spill over into the public arena when the question is whether the new agreements are "skimming off the cream produced by decades of taxpayer funded work," as Rep. Albert Gore, Jr., put it in opening Congressional hearings on the subject.[36] Only a continuing public debate over these as-yet-unresolved questions on the commercialization of biotechnology can ensure that the public's interests are being met—its interest in the integrity and credibility of scientific research, in a sound and balanced research agenda, and in the wise expenditure of Federal research dollars.

CONTINUING CONCERNS

A distinction has been drawn in this Report between two views: (1) that gene splicing technology is intrinsically wrong or contrary to important values and (2) that, while the technology is not inherently wrong, certain of its applications or consequences are undesirable. Regarding the latter, it has also been noted that genetic engineering involves an array of uncertainties beyond those usually found in technological developments. Not only is the occurrence of specific desirable or undesirable consequences impossible to predict but the application of gene splicing could have far-reaching consequences that could alter basic individual and social values.

The Commission could find no ground for concluding that any current or planned forms of genetic engineering, whether using human or nonhuman material, are intrinsically wrong or irreligious per se. The Commission does not see in the rapid development of gene splicing the "fundamental danger" to world safety or to human values that concerned the leaders of the three religious organizations.[37] Rather, the issue that deserves careful thought is: by what standards, and toward what objectives, should the great new powers of genetic engineering be guided?

Even though the many issues raised by gene splicing in human beings need to be considered one by one if their potential consequences are to be clearly assessed, it would be a mistake to compartmentalize the issues.[38] Although the Commission has not found any ethical, social, or legal barriers to continued research in this field, there remains an important concern expressed by the warning against "playing God." It not only reminds human beings that they are only human and will some day have to pay if they underestimate their own ignorance and fallibility; it also points to the weighty and unusual nature of this activity, which stirs elusive fears that are not easily calmed.

At this point in the development of genetic engineering no reasons have been found for abandoning the entire enterprise—indeed, it would probably be naive to assume that it could be. Given the great scientific, medical, and commercial interest in this technology, it is doubtful that efforts to foreclose important lines of investigation would succeed. If, for example, the United States were to attempt such a step, researchers and investment capital would probably shift to other countries where such prohibitions did not exist. To expect humanity to turn its back on what may be one of the greatest technological revolutions may itself betray a failure to recognize the limits of individual and social self-restraint. Even if important lines of research in this country or elsewhere could be halted, to do so would be to run a different sort of risk: that of depriving humanity of the great benefits genetic engineering may bring.

Assuming that research will continue somewhere, it seems more prudent to encourage its development and control under the sophisticated and responsive regulatory arrangements of this country, subject to the scrutiny of a free press and within the general framework of democratic institutions. In light of the potential benefits and risks—uncertain though they may be at this point—a responsible social policy on genetic engineering requires the cooperation of many institutions and organizations.

Efficient regulation and oversight will require considerable division of responsibility among different bodies and agencies. Legal controls will necessarily focus on the prevention of tangible harms to individuals and the environment. Nonetheless, the Commission believes it is crucial that those entrusted with such oversight and regulation do not lose sight of the more elusive, but equally important, concerns about the human significance of genetic engineering or neglect such concerns because they do not fit neatly into existing institutional jurisdictions. The continued development of gene splicing approved in this Report will require periodic reassessment as greater knowledge is gained about the ethical and social, as well as the technical, aspects of the subject.

REFERENCES

1. Office of Technology Assessment, U.S. Congress, IMPACTS OF APPLIED GENETICS—MICRO-ORGANISMS, PLANTS, AND ANIMALS, U.S. Government Printing Office, Washington (1981); Congressional Research Service, Library of Congress, GENETIC ENGINEERING, HUMAN GENETICS, AND CELL BIOLOGY—EVOLUTION OF TECHNOLOGICAL ISSUES, Report Prepared for the Subcomm. on Science, Research and Tech. of the House Comm. on Science and Tech., U.S. Government Printing Office, Washington (1976). [All cross-references in these notes refer to *Splicing Life*.]

2. Ted Howard and Jeremy Rifkin, WHO SHOULD PLAY GOD?, Dell Publishing Co., Inc., New York (1977).

3. *See* Appendix B, pp. 95-96 *infra*.

4. *See* Appendix D, pp. 107-10 *infra*, for a list of the religious commentators.

5. Seymour Siegel, *Genetic Engineering*, in PROC. OF THE RABBINICAL ASSEMBLY OF AMERICA, New York (1978) at 164.

6. In the Biblical tradition of the major Western religions, the universe and all that exists in it is God's creation. In pagan religion, the gods inhabit nature, which is thus seen as sacrosanct, but the Biblical God transcends nature. However, since God created the world, it has meaning and purpose. God has placed a special being on earth—humans—formed in the image of God and endowed with creative powers of intelligence and freedom. Human beings must accept responsibility for the effects brought about by the use of the great powers with which they have been endowed—for the betterment of the world—to uncover nature's secrets.

7. As science journalist Nicholas Wade has observed:

> We are about to enter an explosive phase of discovery in which we are going to reach close to the great goal of Western inquiry: the complete understanding of man as a physical-chemical system.

NOVA, LIFE: PATENT PENDING, WGBH Transcripts, Boston (1982) at 24.

8. Pope John Paul II, who had earlier been critical of genetic engineering, recently told a convocation on biological experimentation of the Pontifical Academy of Science of his approval and support for gene splicing when its aim is to "ameliorate the conditions of those who are affected by chromosomic diseases" because this offers "hope for the great number of people affected by those maladies."

> I have no reason to be apprehensive for those experiments in biology that are performed by scientists who, like you, have a profound respect for the human person, since I am sure that they will contribute to the integral well-being of man. On the other hand, I condemn, in the most explicit and formal way, experimental manipulations of the human embryo, since the human being, from conception to death, cannot be exploited for any purpose whatsoever. . . . I praise those who have endeavoured to establish, with full respect for man's dignity and freedom, guidelines and limits for experiments concerning man.

Pope John Paul II, *La sperimentozione in biologia deve contribuire al bene integrale dell'uomo,* L'OSSERVATORE ROMANO, Rome, Oct. 24, 1982, at 2.

9. Robert L. Sinsheimer, *Genetic Research: The Importance of Maximum Safety and Forethought* (Letter), N.Y. TIMES, May 30, 1977, at A-14.

10. Despite the great attention paid to the "biohazards" of the research with, and products of, gene splicing, the Environmental Impact Statement filed by NIH on its RAC guidelines focuses on the health effects on humans, plants, and animals and does not deal with ecosystems as entities. Subsequently, however, the Environmental Protection Agency has supported research on the effects of introducing recombinant organisms on the stability of various ecosystems.

> 11. [W]hat made the Gallilean and the other major scientific revolutions disturbing is the reductionism, that we become less than what we are. [T]hat is what is so uncertain about gene therapy, because it gets back to a very fundamental question. . . "Is there anything unique about humans?"

> And if there isn't anything unique about humans, there's nothing wrong with doing gene manipulation. But if there is something unique about humans, then it is wrong to pass over the barrier, wherever the barrier is—but we don't know where the barrier is.

> But as soon as you ask, "Where is the barrier?" you ask, "Is there a barrier?" And that's frightening. If there's nothing unique about humans—that's not a theological question but a very real one.

Testimony of Dr. French Anderson, transcript of 22nd meeting of the President's Commission (July 10, 1982) at 115-16.

12. As one physician-scientist has remarked, "We must all get used to the idea that biomedical technology makes possible many things we should never do." Leon Kass, *The New Biology: What Price Reducing Man's Estate?*, 174 SCIENCE 779 (1971). *See also, Ethical issues in experiments with hybrids of different species*, Appendix I, in Church and Society Office, MANIPULATING LIFE, World Council of Churches, Geneva (1982) at 28.

13. If there is any special concern in the evaluation of the products of gene splicing, it is only that in the initial stages of any new process there are uncertainties about some effects of the process. For example, bacterial contaminants are a unique by-product of gene splicing and in testing human insulin it was important to determine whether these contaminants induced deleterious antibodies in humans.

14. *See* note 10, Chapter Two *supra*, and accompanying text.

15. President's Commission for the Study of Ethical Problems in Medicine and Biomedical and Behavioral Research, SCREENING AND COUNSELING FOR GENETIC CONDITIONS, U.S. Government Printing Office, Washington (1983).

16. "Have we the right to counteract, irreversibly, the evolutionary wisdom of millions of years, in order to satisfy the curiosity of a few scientists? The future will curse us for it." Liebe F. Cavalieri, *New Strains of Life—Or Death*, N.Y. TIMES, Aug. 22, 1976 (Magazine), at 8, 68 (quoting Erwin Chargaff).

17. Stephen Stitch. *The Recombinant DNA Debate*, 7 PHIL. & PUB. AFF. 187 (1978).

18. *See* pp. 39-40 *supra*. Carriers of recessive diseases are people who possess one normal and one variant gene; they usually show no deleterious effects and may, as in the case of sickle-cell, have an advantage. The sickle-cell advantage is, however, dependent on time and place. In a temperate, nonmalarial area, or in a tropical climate from which the malaria parasite has been eliminated, carrying the sickle-cell gene would not confer an advantage.

19. A.M Capron, *The Law of Genetic Therapy*, in Michael P. Hamilton, ed., THE NEW GENETICS AND THE FUTURE OF MAN, William B. Eerdmans Pub. Co., Grand Rapids, Mich. (1972) at 133, 140 (raising question of a need for a living "genes savings bank").

20. SCREENING AND COUNSELING FOR GENETIC CONDITIONS, *supra* note 15, at second section of Chapter Two.

21. More specifically, it is important to ask whether the further development of gene splicing will reinforce or perhaps exacerbate existing social, cultural, and economic inequalities. This factor explains part of the concern that has been expressed about who will control this technology. Although objections have focused on corporations controlling access (through trade secrets and patents), Howard and Rifkin, *supra* note 2, at 189-207, the greatest abuses of genetics have involved governmental decisionmaking. Kenneth M. Ludmerer, GENETICS AND AMERICAN SOCIETY: A HISTORICAL APPRAISAL, Johns Hopkins Univ. Press, Baltimore (1972) at 121-34.

22. Suppose, for example, a society distributes certain scarce resources on the basis of merit—*e.g.*, intelligence, diligence, physical abilities. What if intelligence could be engineered upward? Who would merit this increase in merit? The very oddity of the inquiry calls into question the continued use of

intelligence as a basis for resolving competing claims—say, for admission to educational institutions or for access to the intelligence-raising technology itself. We could resort to the other coexisting merit attributes—unless they too were alterable by design. Under these conditions, how could we retain our system of merit distribution? If we could not, how would we then distribute the resources? By resort to a standard of efficiency? By leaving matters to a market? Or by designing a lottery?

Michael H. Shapiro, *Introduction to the Issue: Some Dilemmas of Biotechnology Research*, 51 S. Cal. L. Rev., 987, 1001-02 (1978) (citations omitted).

23. John Rawls, A Theory of Justice, Harvard Univ. Press, Cambridge, Mass. (1973) at 83.

24. Herman J. Muller is the scientist most associated with this view. In the mid-1960s he viewed selective breeding as a method for "a much greater, speedier, and more significant improvement of the population" than any direct rearrangement of genetic material possible in the 21st century. He advocated giving women "germinal choice" through artificial insemination of them with the genes for superior traits. Herman J. Muller, *Means and Aims in Human Genetic Betterment*, in T.M. Sonneborn, ed., Control of Human Heredity and Evolution, Macmillan Co., New York (1965) at 100. The list of the traits found desirable by Professor Muller changed dramatically over time, as did the types of individuals whose sperm should be used—Lenin appeared on the first list but disappeared during the Cold War. Garland E Allen, *Science and Society in the Eugenic Thought of H.J. Muller*, 20 BioScience 346 (1970).

25. Robert L. Sinsheimer, *The Prospect of Designed Genetic Change*, 32 Engineering and Science 8, 13 (April 1969). Prof. Sinsheimer took a different view from Prof. Muller. He contrasted the "older eugenics" of breeding, which would require a "massive social program," with the new eugenics that could permit "conversion of all the unfit to the highest genetic level" and "could, at least in principle, be implemented on a quite individual basis, in one generation, and subject to no existing social restrictions." *Id.* Prof. Sinsheimer subsequently became very doubtful about the wisdom of changing genes. *See* note 19, Chapter One *supra*.

26. If any one age really attains, by eugenics and scientific education, the power to make its descendants what it pleases, all men who live after it are patients of that power. They are weaker, not stronger: for though we may have put wonderful machines in their hands we have pre-ordained how they are to use them. . . . The real picture is that of one dominant age . . . which resists all previous ages most successfully and dominates all subsequent ages most irresistibly, and thus is the real master of the human species. But even within this master generation (itself an infinitesimal minority of the species) the power will be exercised by a minority smaller still. Man's conquest of Nature, if the dreams of the scientific planners are realized, means the rule of a few hundreds of men over billions upon billions of men.

C.S. Lewis, The Abolition of Man, Collier-Macmillan, New York (1965) at 70-71.

27. John Walsh, *Public Attitude Toward Science Is Yes, but-*, 215 Science 270 (1982) (quoting National Science Foundation. Science Indicators 1980).

28. Another misuse of gene splicing with international ramifications, described by the World Council of Churches as a "grave hazard," is "the deliberate production of pathogenic micro-organisms for biological warfare or terrorism." Paul Abrecht, ed., 2 Faith and Science in an Unjust World: Report of the World Council of Churches' Conference on Faith, Science and the Future, Fortress Press, Philadelphia (1980) at 53.

29. "In discussing the use of any science, including genetics, to solve social problems, it . . . becomes important to demarcate clearly the *limit* that scientific technique may be expected to contribute to an effective solution." Ludmerer, *supra* note 21, at 180. To take an extreme example, in a society in which gene surgery was widely used and accepted, it might be tempting to "solve" the problem of racial discrimination by making genetic changes to eliminate dark skin. A less fanciful example would be the decision to make genetic alterations in certain groups of workers who are exposed to dangerous chemicals in the workplace rather than to eliminate the dangers.

> Moreover, genetic research may denigrate the value that society has perceived in the moral and autonomous aspects of human conduct by forcing society to question the limits of free will and self-determination. Thus, genetic research has the power to reorder society's priorities and restructure its values; fundamentally, it can change the structures of human thought and the social construction of reality.

> Marc Lappé and Patricia Archbold Martin, *The Place of the Public in the Conduct of Science,* 52 S. Cal. L. Rev. 1535, 1537 (1978) (citations omitted).

30. *See* Stitch, *supra* note 17.

31. Estimates have put industry support of academic research at about $200 million per year. Although this represents only about 4% of what government contributes, it is a growing proportion. The formation in the past decade of about 200 new private ventures to pursue research and development in genetic engineering has been paralleled by increased interest on the part of existing industrial firms in universities that have strong programs in molecular biology. This interest has been capped by several well publicized multimillion dollar agreements.

> 32. That journey of discovery can only be undertaken once, and it would be better undertaken by people who have no interest in anything other than discovering the truth, whose hands are clean, whose motives can never be criticized. That's in the public's interest; that is in science's true interest. And if the commercialization, if this secondary goal of getting rich, ever starts to influence a scientist's primary goal, a university's primary goal of discovering the truth, then the scientists themselves, I hope, will have the sense to put a halt to it.

> Wade, *supra* note 7, at 24-25.

33. Barbara J. Culliton, *Pajaro Dunes: The Search for Consensus,* 216 Science 155 (1982); Draft Statement Pajaro Dunes Conference (March 25-27, 1982).

34. One physician-scientist who formerly held high budgetary and science advisory positions in the Federal government and who is presently the Dean of a school of public health has suggested that the financial agreements between universities and medical school faculty in the clinical departments could be "at least partially relevant" in finding a means of protecting the research and educational commitments of the basic-science faculties while generating added income. Gilbert S. Omenn, *Taking University Research into the Marketplace,* 307 New Eng. J. Med. 694, 699-700 (1982).

35. Letter from Robert M. Rosenzweig, chairman of the Association of American Universities Committee on University/Industry Relations, to Reps. Don Fuqua and Albert Gore, Jr. (Oct. 28, 1982) (on report of AAU study group).

36. *Commercialization of Academic Biomedical Research,* Hearings before the Subcomm. on Invest. and Oversight and the Subcomm. on Science, Research and Tech. of the House Comm. on Science and Tech., 97th Cong., 1st Sess., June 8, 1981, at 2.

37. *See* Appendix B, pp. 95-96 infra.

38. The predominant methodological strategy of biological research is reductionism: the isolation of the phenomenon under study from its usual circumstances, thereby reducing the number of variables that affect the analysis. This allows a clearer understanding of the "basic" processes, and has led to important discoveries.

The strength of reductionism is the principle of isolation. This principle, however, is also inherently limiting: the circumstances of the investigation are necessarily "unreal" in everyday terms. Of course, it may be that the isolated phenomena behave similarly under natural circumstances. This assumption, however, is often uncertain and may frequently be untrue. Moreover, the characteristics of those natural circumstances are rarely fully known. In some cases, knowledge of the multiple external influences upon biological processes could lead to a perception of those processes quite different from those obtained in the isolation of laboratory study. A critical understanding of present biological knowledge requires recognition of those methodological weaknesses. Public participation in science, by broadening the range of factors considered at each stage of investigation, provides a means of counteracting biases resulting from reductionist strategy.

Halsted R. Holman and Diana B. Dutton, *A Case for Public Participation in Science Policy Formation and Practice*, 51 S. CAL. L. REV. 1505, 1513-14 (1978) (citation omitted).

24 Guidelines for the Ethical, Social and Legal Issues in Prenatal Diagnosis

Tabitha M. Powledge and John Fletcher

This report from the Genetics Research Group of the Hastings Center proposes 18 guidelines which are relevant to ethical, social and legal issues in prenatal diagnosis. This interdisciplinary research group focused on nontechnical dimensions of technical and procedural problems, the use of the information after prenatal diagnosis has occurred, and problems of access to prenatal diagnosis.

John Fletcher is Director of Bioethics, National Institute of Health

Tabitha Powledge is an Associate for Genetics, Institute of Society, Ethics, and the Life Sciences

Medicine's ability to collect information about the fetus has increased dramatically in the last few years. A variety of technics—collectively known as prenatal diagnosis—have made it possible to learn much about a fetus's genetic and metabolic state, chromosomal constitution (including gender), bone structure and other information, and, moreover, to learn it earlier and earlier in gestation.

Many of the technics yield this information at a time that makes the selective abortion of a fetus legally possible. Selective abortion is morally unacceptable to many people. This report does not discuss this question in detail. It recognizes that selective abortion raises a variety of deeply troubling moral, social and legal questions that must always be kept in mind for the exercise of responsible decision making.

Since the release in the United States of a prospective study of mid-trimester amniocentesis in the fall of 1975 and its subsequent publication, the comparative safety and accuracy of this form of prenatal diagnosis has been widely accepted.[1] A study carried out in Canada and published shortly after the United States study disclosed similar findings.[2] As a result, it has been predicted that amniocentesis will soon become much more common, and ultimately part of standard obstetric practice, where indicated.

Rapid development of other forms of prenatal diagnosis is proceeding along several fronts. Ultrasound, often used as an adjunct of amniocentesis, is also used as a separate form of fetal diagnosis, not only for the detection of birth defects but also to establish gestational age, or to detect multiple pregnancy early.[3] This technic has been expanded to include real-time scanning, which yields a moving picture of the fetus.[4]

Another of the new procedures involves aspiration of blood from the placental vessels, making possible diagnosis of the hemoglobulinopathies and other blood and biochemical disorders.[5] In some centers this technic is accomplished by direct visualization of the fetus within the uterus by means of a tiny fiberoptic endoscope, also called the fetoscope.[6] This developing technology may also prove very helpful in the detection of a variety of other anomalies.

Early fetal assessment does not have to depend on methods that directly involve the uterus and its contents; the development of indirect diagnostic technics has also been proceeding rapidly. α-Fetoprotein levels in maternal serum can give information about birth defects, especially the neural-tube defects, on a mass basis.[7] This test is being widely used in the United Kingdom, where neural-tube defects are among the most common major malformations, and is also frequently employed in the United States and Canada. A pilot program in Nassau County, New York, has as its goal screening the serum of every pregnant woman in the county to identify those with high risk of fetal disease. Women with positive tests are then studied with more definitive diagnostic methods like ultrasonography and determination of α-fetoprotein concentrations in amniotic fluid.[8]

In short, various kinds of prenatal diagnoses are proliferating, and the array of technics is likely to expand even more in the future. None of them are without technical problems. Most are experimental and not yet standard practice. All of them also present other kinds of problems—moral, social, and legal as well—that, though often acknowledged, remain largely unresolved.

In early stages of the procedures' development, informal or ad hoc solutions to these problems must be attempted while experience is being acquired. But that is not a satisfactory long-term situation for society as a whole or for prenatal diagnosticians, many of whom are rightly uncomfortable cast in the unfamiliar and undesirable role of moral decision makers on behalf of society.

The Genetics Research Group of the Hastings Center, Institute of Society, Ethics and the Life Sciences, an interdisciplinary task force of people with academic training in law, medicine, philosophy, theology, biology, genetics and the social sciences, has been considering many of those questions for more than six years. Recently, this group decided to attempt a systematic exploration of them, with the intention of offering assistance to workers in this rapidly developing field. This document represents the result of that effort. Its purpose is to propose guidelines for the development and institutionalization of prenatal diagnostic programs and to help workers in this area provide the most favorable circumstances for thoughtful, informed, morally responsible decision making by parents.

Nontechnical Dimensions of Technical and Procedural Problems

The design, operation and validation of prenatal diagnostic technics, the organization and conduct of the programs themselves and the associated laboratory procedures involved have moral, social and legal dimensions often unrecognized or inadequately examined and discussed. This section considers these dimensions.

Prenatal diagnostic programs can be regarded as one type of screening program and should be organized in ways that are consonant with the principles of optimum screening programs. We emphasize "optimum" because most screening programs are conceded to be sometimes deficient in practice.[9] With the exception of prenatal diagnosis done for research purposes (dealt with in point 8, below), programs of prenatal diagnosis ought to meet at least the following criteria:

1. The programs should be designed to reach well defined groups of pregnant women known to be at risk.
2. Prenatal diagnosis should be undertaken only where high-quality laboratory work is available, even though, at the moment, lack of adequate laboratory services is an important barrier to the availability of amniocentesis. Though the current error rates are low, it is possible that frequency of error will increase as the technics become more widely applied by practitioners and laboratories new to the field, and by experienced workers burdened by a growing volume of tests. Laboratory tests must be standardized, and quality-control measures

implemented to assure accurate results. Inaccurate results have even heavier moral and legal consequences in prenatal diagnosis than in many screening procedures or other routine medical tests. To avoid the consequences, training programs for laboratory workers and a comprehensive prenatal-diagnosis laboratory monitoring and surveillance system should also be developed. Uncontrolled expansion of prenatal diagnosis and, particularly, inadequate laboratory work, would be a disastrous step for technics that can offer hope and reassurance to many families.

3. The lowest practical limits for false-positive and false-negative results should be established, and continuing attempts to improve test sensitivity should be made. In many other kinds of screening programs, a positive diagnosis is confirmed by additional tests, and a test that errs on the side of false-positive results is therefore acceptable. In most kinds of prenatal diagnosis, however, the test will be done only once, and a positive test result may lead to an abortion. False-negative results will lead to the undesired birth of an affected child. Error in either direction will cause pain and suffering in families, and may also open up the prenatal diagnostician to subsequent legal liability. Positive diagnoses should be confirmed, whether after abortion, stillbirth or live birth.

4. Efforts to follow up and evaluate all types of prenatal diagnosis procedures should be made and should be part of large programs from their outset, with the intention of determining the short-term and long-term safety for both mother and fetus. Reports of adverse psychologic responses by some parents when abortion is performed for a medical indication after prenatal diagnosis[10] raise troubling questions and need rapid validation or refutation, though care must also be taken to avoid unnecessary intrusion into family life. And though the short-term unfavorable health effects of amniocentesis and ultrasound appear to be minimal or nonexistent, we emphasize that very little is as yet known of their long-term consequences. Prudence dictates caution in the widespread application of any of these technics.

5. To assist prospective parents in the exercise of well informed and responsible decision making, they should be given adequate information about the procedure before prenatal diagnosis and adequate counseling after it. The professional should ascertain that the patient is aware of a number of extremely important factors relevant to a decision, such as the need for thoughtful consideration of the various options available, depending on the results of the diagnosis (abortion vs. possible al-

ternatives, taking into account the nature of the prenatally diagnosed condition and the present and future possibilities for prenatal and postnatal treatment); the possibility and meaning of inaccurate diagnoses ("falsely positive" or "falsely negative") and the consequences for the family in such an instance; the mechanics of the diagnostic intervention as well as the risks involved; the type of information that the procedure can and cannot provide; and the cost. Every effort should be made to include prospective fathers in the sessions.

6. The patient's privacy should be scrupulously protected ("patient" is here defined as the mother of the fetus, and, in most cases, the father as well). Great difficulties with this provision are to be expected, in view of the trend to genetic registries and similar medical-data banks, but those difficulties do not absolve the keepers of this information from their moral—and perhaps legal—obligation to protect patients. Central registries for epidemiologic data collection and needs assessment are justifiable, but individual patients should never be identifiable. Individual genetic disorders are, by definition, often found largely concentrated in particular racial and ethnic groups, but special care should be taken in the public presentation of these data not to perpetuate past instances of misinformation and stigmatization of particular groups.[11] It is desirable for physicians to follow their patients, but individually identifiable information should not be stored in centralized data banks. In the rare situation in which information obtained via prenatal diagnosis might be of direct benefit to collateral relatives, permission to disclose should be sought from the patients. If that permission is refused, professionals can face a conflict between their ethical and their legal obligations, and may need to justify disclosure from a legal standpoint.

7. The apparent trend toward performing amniocentesis in the office of the private physician, with the fluids sometimes being sent for assessment to commercial laboratories, should not be allowed to lead to a diminution of quality control in prenatal diagnosis. Nor does it relieve professionals of their obligation to maintain confidentiality, or to provide adequate counseling, information and follow-up study. Physicians should demonstrate competence in the technic—perhaps by way of special training—before applying it to their patients.

8. The distinction between attempts at prenatal diagnosis for research purposes and prenatal diagnosis as a relatively routine service for selected obstetric patients should be clear in the

minds of both the people performing the procedure and their patients. Research can be an important, rational and legitimate purpose of prenatal diagnosis, but researchers are under strong moral and legal obligation to make sure that their patients understand that, in these circumstances, they are experimental subjects as well as patients who may benefit from the procedure. The obligation to explain, so far as they are known, what the possible risks are, and to obtain the subject's comprehending consent to the procedure, is, if anything, greater for researchers than for ordinary physicians.

Use of Information after Prenatal Diagnosis

The desired and intended result of prenatal diagnosis is information about the presence or absence of a possible disease or defect in the fetus. In practice the test results are negative in more than 96 per cent of amniocentesis cases, thus providing these families with many months of relief from anxiety. In addition, pregnancies that would otherwise be terminated because the fetus is at a substantial risk of being abnormal can be carried to term. When diagnosis of the presence of disease or defect is made, parents and physicians use that information to make choices about subsequent action. The alternatives after such a diagnosis include abortion, treatment of the fetus in the rare cases in which prenatal therapy is or may be possible, bringing the pregnancy to term and providing the parents with whatever help is available for treating the condition after delivery, if possible, or bringing the pregnancy to term and arranging for the parents to give over their responsibilities by adoption, foster care or institutionalization. Each of these alternatives is intimately related to individual views on the ethics of abortion. Ethical considerations make it imperative to separate the fact of a positive diagnosis from the choice about the subsequent action. What parents and physicians should decide to do is not automatically dictated by the diagnosis, but ought to be shaped by their ethical and social views.

Most women who seek prenatal diagnosis want a child; prenatal diagnosis provides information that can enhance the freedom and responsibility of parents in reproductive decision making. Before development of prenatal diagnosis, parents and physicians were more at the mercy of outcomes unknown until delivery or after. However, the lack of a moral consensus on abortion also makes it inappropriate to suggest that women have a moral (or "medically indicated") obligation to undergo prenatal diagnosis.

One of the ultimate goals of prenatal diagnosis should be the treatment and eventual cure of disease in the fetus or infant. Many decades of work will be required to make substantial progress toward this goal, and, in the meantime, abortion in these cases is a limited and imperfect response when an effective therapy is lacking. Abortion is never therapeutic for the fetus, but we believe it can be morally justified for the relief of suffering and burden to family and society. These guidelines were developed in a moral framework favoring the protection of individual choice and the autonomy of parents, even when we disagree with their courses of action.

The profound conflict of values embodied in the abortion debate cannot be finally resolved in a set of guidelines that offer directions for choices that must always be made in the light of competing, and sometimes polar, claims. These guidelines cannot reconcile the views of those who believe that abortion is wrong virtually without exception with the views of those who exclude the welfare of the fetus completely from any argument about reproductive decisions. These guidelines attempt to respect the pluralism of values about abortion that exists in society, while offering concrete guidance in special cases that are cause for concern.

9. Prenatal diagnosis should not be denied to the woman who is at risk and desires the procedure, but has decided that she will not undergo an abortion no matter what the diagnosis. In the past, particularly before release of the collaborative studies, some researchers argued that such use of prenatal diagnosis offered possible risk to the unaffected fetus and was a waste of scarce resources; without abortion of an affected fetus, prenatal diagnosis was seen by them to have no purpose. By contrast, we regard the provision of information as an important and legitimate purpose of prenatal diagnosis. Depending on the disorder, certain families might find very useful a few months of planning and preparation for the birth of an affected child. In most cases, diagnosis of an unaffected fetus will provide months of relief from anxiety.

10. Counseling for the procedure should be noncoercive and respectful of parental views about abortion. Each family's life situation is special, and therefore, ideally, a counselor should have a tolerance for the moral ambiguities of abortion and the complexities of decision making.

11. In conditions for which both prenatal diagnosis and postnatal treatment are available, parents should be informed about both possibilities—including their relative disadvantages—and allowed to make their own decisions about what action to take. This is the situation that now prevails in the rare

metabolic disorder galactosemia. It has been argued that where treatment is available, the need for prenatal diagnosis vanishes. We believe that the medical profession should acknowledge that there are some families, particularly those who already have a child with a disorder, who will not want to bear another child who will need treatment, but who may wish to have additional, unaffected children. Prenatal diagnosis allows such families to have available wide choices about future childbearing, and it should not be denied them.

12. Prenatal ascertainment of sex in fetuses at risk for otherwise undiagnosable sex-linked disorders should be available to parents who want it. Since in such cases there will be at least a 50 per cent probability of aborting an unaffected fetus, which is an extremely unsatisfactory situation from both a moral and social perspective, the development of specific tests for the presence of such disorders should have a very high research priority.

13. Moral and legal strictures require that findings not be withheld from the parents, even when they are of disputed importance. This situation will become increasingly common as amniocentesis for Down's syndrome increases and chromosome anomalies of unknown or controversial consequence are discovered in the process. Prognosis for many children with these abnormalities is ambiguous, a well known example being the XYY condition.[12] We strongly recommend the development, perhaps under the auspices of an appropriate professional organization, of a series of fact sheets describing what is known about each of these conditions, to aid counselors who may have to give out this information. Counseling before prenatal diagnosis as part of the process of obtaining consent will alert couples to the possibility of such findings, giving them the choice of whether they want that information. Requests for both disclosure and nondisclosure should be honored.

14. Although we strongly oppose any movement aimed at making diagnosis of sex and selective abortion a part of ordinary medical practice and family planning, we recommend that no legal restrictions be placed on ascertainment of fetal sex. We think such restrictions would be ineffective and impossible to administer, would lead to subterfuge and, more important, would violate our objective of noninterference with parental choice, even when we disagree with that choice. Prenatal diagnosis is not now widely available for this purpose; indeed, amniocentesis is often refused to women who request it for that reason, largely on grounds that the procedure is expensive and possibly risky,

and should be reserved for grave medical conditions. Though we support the right of individual physicians to refuse to perform prenatal diagnosis for sex choice, we also recognize that in special situations, sex choice can appear to parents to be justifiable. We think most couples should not seek such information, however. Discouragement of this use of prenatal diagnosis, by pointing out that the risks and stresses of second-trimester abortions are not trivial, will mean that such cases will at least not be very great in number, though availability of earlier sex-ascertainment technics, now in development,[13] is likely to expand them considerably.

15. Standard medical practice on resuscitation, maintenance and treatment of newborns with severe abnormalities should apply in the event of a live birth after attempted abortion for a medical indication. Such measures may occasionally need to be considered because a positive prenatal diagnosis in most of its current forms is usually followed by a second-trimester abortion, occasionally close to the limits of viability for the fetus. Such infants should be regarded as members of the general class of gravely ill newborns, and decisions about them should be made on the same basis.

16. The existence of prenatal diagnosis should never be used as a justification for the withholding of support and services for those who are born with prenatally diagnosable diseases and whose parents want such support and services.

ACCESS

In the United States, women who undergo prenatal diagnosis belong largely to higher economic and social groups.[14] There are large numbers of women who are appropriate candidates for it and who might reasonably decide to use these technics, but for whom they have not been available. The last guidelines address that issue.

17. We endorse third-party payments, including Medicaid, for most kinds of prenatal diagnosis now available. In view of the data on economic and educational level of the typical prenatal-diagnosis patient, we regard the availability of prenatal diagnosis to pregnant women of lower educational and income levels as a very high priority, and subsidy, in one form or another, is critical to that availability.

18. The government, the medical profession, major foundations and voluntary health agencies could all do more, at

relatively low cost, to make the existence of prenatal diagnosis more widely known. This communication effort should be aimed at both professionals and consumers, but at a pace that does not create greater demand than existing services can safely meet.

We are indebted for the suggestions of the following people, though this acknowledgment is not necessarily meant to imply their endorsement of this report: Sherry Arnstein, M.S., National Center for Health Services Research; Stanley Bergen, Jr., M.D., College of Medicine and Dentistry of New Jersey; Arthur Caplan, Ph.D., Hastings Center; Joseph Fletcher, S.T.D., University of Virginia School of Medicine; Paul Freund, LL.B., Harvard Law School; Ruth Hanft, M.A., Department of Health, Education and Welfare; Leonard Isaacs, Ph.D., Michigan State University; Paul Ramsey, Ph.D., Princeton University; Philip Reilly, J.D., Yale University School of Medicine; Margaret Steinfels, M.A., Hastings Center; and Robert M. Veatch, Ph.D., Hastings Center.

REFERENCES

1. The NICHD National Registry for Amniocentesis Study Group: Midtrimester amniocentesis for prenatal diagnosis: safety and accuracy. JAMA 236:1471–1476, 1976

2. Simpson NE, Dallaire L, Miller JR, et al: Prenatal diagnosis of genetic disease in Canada: report of a collaborative study. Can Med Assoc J 115:739–748, 1976

3. Leopold GR, Asher WM: Ultrasound in obstetrics and gynecology. Radiol Clin North Am 12:127–146, 1974

4. Platt LD, Manning FA, Lemay M: Real-time B-scan-directed amniocentesis. Am J. Obstet Gynecol 130:700–703, 1978

5. Alter BP, Modell CB, Fairweather D, et al: Prenatal diagnosis of hemoglobinopathies: a review of 15 cases. N Engl J Med 295:1437–1443, 1976

6. Hobbins JC, Mahoney MJ: Fetoscopy in continuing pregnancies. Am J Obstet Gynecol 129:440–442, 1977

7. Wald NJ, Cuckle H, Brock DJH, et al: Maternal serum-alpha-fetoprotein measurement in antenatal screening for anencephaly and spina bifida in early pregnancy. Lancet 1:1323–1332, 1977

8. Macri JN, Weiss RR, Tillitt R, et al: Prenatal diagnosis of neural tube defects. JAMA 236:1251–1254, 1976

9. Wilson JMG, Jungner G: Principles and Practice of Screening for Disease, Geneva, World Health Organization, 1968

10. Blumberg BD, Golbus MS, Hanson KH: The psychological sequelae of abortion performed for a genetic indication. Am J Obstet Gynecol 122:799–808, 1975

11. Lappé M, Gustafson JM, Roblin R: Ethical and social issues in screening for genetic disease. N Engl J Med 286:1129–1132, 1972

12. Hamerton JL: Human population cytogenetics: dilemmas and problems. Am J Hum Genet 28:107–122, 1976

13. Pirani BBK, Pairaudeau N, Doran TA, et al: Amniotic fluid testosterone in the prenatal determination of fetal sex. Am J Obstet Gynecol 129:518–520, 1977

14. Bannerman RM, Gillick D, Van Coevering R, et al: Amniocentesis and educational attainment. N Engl J Med 297:449, 1977

25 *Public Policy Issues in Genetic Counseling*

JAMES F. CHILDRESS
KENNETH CASEBEER

This chapter examines the relation between public policy about genetics and the tensions between procreational freedom and other interests that might justify coercive policies: the welfare of offspring, society and future generations. The authors also argue that public policies have an inherent morality in that particularly in the case of genetic counseling, one must examine how those values relate to the author's assumption of a *prima facie* presumption in favor of reproductive freedom.

James F. Childress is Professor of Religion at the University of Virginia, and Kenneth Casebeer is at the Law School of the University of Miami, Coral Gables, Florida

This chapter offers a framework for discussing issues in public policy relating to genetic counseling by considering the interaction of public policy and genetic counseling and the tensions between procreational freedom and other interests. It tries to identify and sort out some of the central arguments about whether and how genetic counseling should be made a matter of public policy, and to show that arguments that counseling should be a subject of public policy are not separate from arguments that a particular policy should be enacted. Our framework is also normative, for we hold that our society recognizes a rebuttable presumption in favor of procreational freedom.

PUBLIC POLICY AND GENETIC COUNSELING

"Public policy is whatever governments choose to do or not to do" [1]. An adequate definition would also stress that public policy is purposive action, and, indeed, a course or pattern of action or inaction by government officials [2]. As such, public policies typically involve one or more of the following actions: allocation and distribution of benefits (eg services and goods) and burdens (eg taxation); regulation (eg prohibition or control of an activity); expression (eg affirmation of values). By no means exhaustive, these categories are designed to suggest some of the main types of public policies. Other essays in this volume treat directly some of these factors in relation to genetic counseling. For example, Twiss considers allocation, while Reilly and Capron discuss some issues in regulation such as licensing and confidentiality.

In defining "public policy" on a particular subject at a given time, our scrutiny must take in more than officially promulgated rules and regulations. Since a formal governmental policy may be one of inaction or laissez faire, various other forces, such as public opinion, may develop an informal or de facto policy. While de facto policies are sometimes only recognized in retrospect, they often decisively influence the direction of technological developments, such as genetic intervention. Indeed, informal policies may be so strong that the scope of eventual formal licensing or regulation becomes a foregone conclusion.

It is not appropriate to view public policy as merely a dependent variable. We cannot assume that the subject matter—genetic counseling—is clear and determined so that public policy only responds to an independent technological reality. As other essays in this volume indicate, genetic counseling is not monolithic. Despite certain major trends, there are significant disagreements about the goals of counseling (eg whether it is primarily to facilitate individual decisions about risk-taking or to prevent risk-taking), about its loyalties (eg to the family or to the society), about the counselor's virtues (eg directive or nondirective), and about standards of effectiveness (eg understanding by the counselees of changes in reproductive patterns). The content of public policies toward genetic counseling will (or should) depend on an interpretation of trends within the activity and a judgment about its proper direction.

The current state of genetic counseling is in part the result of past public policies as well as private choices, many of which did not directly concern counseling or even genetics. First, the gene pool and the risks of defects have been influenced, even if only to a small degree, by mutagenic agents, social intercourse and mobility, consanguinity laws, and so forth. Second, public programs in other areas of genetic intervention (such as screening) place demands upon, sometimes complement, and sometimes compete with genetic counseling. Third, the tools (such as amniocentesis and abortion) available to a counselor depend on previous public policies and court decisions [3]. The policies which guide counseling in part reflect deliberate choices about genetics and in part are simply by-products of public or mixed public/private choices regarding genetics, reproduction, and numerous other matters.

It is possible to evaluate public policies from many different standpoints and by many different standards. Green, for instance, insists that the "correctness or ethical acceptability" of public policies in genetics is not "a really important element in the political framework" [4]. Yet we believe that an evaluation of policies must take account of principles which are moral, legal and constitutional as well as political but which are at a base implicitly ethical in nature. Our discussion focuses on the content of public policy rather than the many processes (such as legislation) through which governmental decisions are made; a complete analysis would include both the content and the processes.

Procreational Freedom as a Right, Value, and Interest

It would be unfortunate to conceive public policy debates about genetic counseling solely in terms of individual rights or interests against societal interest, for there is a collective interest in protecting individuals' freedom. Moreover, the view that society balances individual and collective interests may be misleading since it implies that society puts various and often incommensurable values and rights on a scale to determine the best policy. Such language does not recognize procreational freedom as a presumptive or prima facie right that society is willing to override only under certain circumstances. The specially protected nature of procreational freedom can be discerned in many laws, court decisions, and social practices. By now the Supreme Court cases that affirm a constitutional right to privacy in the area of procreational choice—Roe v Wade, Griswold v Connecticut, and Eisenstadt v Baird—are well known [5]. The First, Fourth, Ninth, and Fourteenth Amendments have been read to prohibit state control of or intervention into private reproductive relationships and medical advice or response in regard to them.

The Social Value of Free Choice

The interrelation of societal and individual interests can take a number of forms. First, the public policy of a society may display a commitment to the value of free procreational choice and not merely a recognition of the individual's right to be free of interference. Thus, the government might fund programs to increase freedom in procreational decisions. Freedom, according to this line of thought, is more than an arbitrary, capricious gamble. Real freedom to decide about reproduction requires sound information about the risks (both probability and severity) of genetic defects and about the options for avoiding and reducing these risks or for coping with untoward results. Policies to maximize freedom could stress formal rather than substantive rationality: the rationality of choices of means to ends regardless of the rationality of the ends. They could aim to remove barriers to free decision, not to ensure that the counselees make the "right" decisions. From this perspective, society could insist that counseling be noncoercive and nondirective, that its goal be full communication, and that its efficacy be judged in terms of the counselees' level of understanding (not the "correctness" of their attitudes or behavior).

While freedom in reproduction has a high value in our society, there is little evidence that public policies primarily designed to enhance that freedom by facilitating informed choices have been given high priority in allocation of resources. Although the National Genetic Diseases Act [6] stresses "voluntary" choices, its paramount interest is not the increase of autonomy but the promotion of public health. It restricts its programs to voluntary counseling, but voluntariness is a "side constraint" not a goal [7]. Freedom is a limit on the pursuit of other ends, not an end in itself.

Freedom in the Positive Sense

A second type of interaction appears if we inquire about the obligations placed on the collectivity by the individual's rights regarding procreation. The focus here is on freedom in the positive sense, that is, the enhancement of choice rather than nonintervention by the state. If procreational freedom is a right of this type, there arises a positive duty on the part of the society not only to refrain from interference but to facilitate the full exercise of choice as well. It is apparent that past public choices in a complex social system markedly affect people's ability or options to implement procreational choice. Consequently, real liberty might depend on socially recognized responsibility toward individuals facing procreational choices. For example, the incidence and degree of genetic risk as well as the potential to respond to risk depend on the social process, especially when publicly funded advances in medical technology increase the likelihood that genetically defective newborns will survive, when rising medical costs restrict access of some segments of society to treatment for defective offspring, and when past public allocations of research funds place certain defective genotypes at risk of less attention than those thoroughly studied at public expense.

Freedom in the Negative Sense

The final area of concern includes those cases in which policy options that limit freedom of choice confront an individual's asserted right to be free from state interference. While procreational rights are recognized as fundamental, they have not been held to be absolute, and a compelling state interest can justify public intervention to restrict personal conduct that would otherwise be protected.

Any limits placed on the use of genetic counseling depend on its having markedly adverse social consequences. Such consequences may not only be attributed to the activity of counseling itself but to various techniques, procedures, and means of realizing the counselor's and counselee's goals. For example, screening and amniocentesis are important diagnostic procedures for identifying potentially "defective" offspring. Depending on what state in reproduction that the counselees seek advice, a variety of options—nonmarriage, contraception, artificial insemination, abortion, allowing defective newborns to die, treatment, and so forth—may all be means of avoiding or coping with genetically defective offspring. Several adverse social consequences could follow from permitting some of these available means. For example, allowing defective newborns to die when they need medical intervention [8] appears to violate numerous laws; continuation of such practices may necessitate several legal changes for consistency and coherence or could lead to a policy of enforcing relevant laws because of prosecutors' view on the immorality of the practice and the danger of its creating a "slippery slope" [9].

Given the various court decisions and policies that recognize the legitimacy of abortion, it is difficult to argue for a restrictive policy regarding amniocentesis simply because it may lead to abortion. Yet many counselors are reluctant to offer amniocentesis to parents who merely want to determine the sex of the fetus. So long as amniocentesis is a limited resource it seems justifiable to give low priority to counselees who have only this interest. But if scarcity is not now or ceases to be a problem, a policy of withholding amniocentesis from families who only want to identify the sex of the fetus may lack compelling justification. In some cases, parents are merely curious, and there is no legitimate reason for the state to foreclose harmless curiosity. In other cases, the health of the family or particular members could be adversely affected by the birth of either a male or a female, consequences which society may have no reason to compel. Finally, in the remaining cases, parents may have personal reasons for wishing to abort a fetus of one sex or the other. Since no reasons are required for abortion at certain stages of fetal development, it would be awkward and inconsistent for the state to rule out abortion based on fetal sex. Unless there is a change in public policy toward abortion generally, the possibility of abortion on grounds of sex cannot appropriately be used to deny access to amniocentesis once scarcity ceases to be a problem. Nevertheless, such a practice many have other adverse social consequences (eg altering the ratio of males to females) that might justify state-imposed restrictions.

The fundamental right of free procreational choice not only limits societal interference with genetic counseling in the absence of adverse social consequences, but it also stands as a "side constraint" on governmental attempts to realize other ends through various mandatory and coercive programs. As C. Fried has remarked, a right that does not stick in the spokes of someone's wheels is no right at all. The National Genetic Diseases Act allocates funds to achieve several ends, including public health, but it adheres to the "side constraint" of free procreational choice. Observing that twelve million Americans are affected by genetic diseases that often are "severely handicapping and debilitating and result in tragic physical, emotional, and financial burden on the individuals, their families, and society," this bill holds that "reducing the burden of genetic diseases deserves a high priority in Federal health legislation and will be cost beneficial to the American public." Its rationale is "to preserve and protect the health and welfare of all citizens. . . ." Yet it supports only "voluntary genetic testing and counseling programs," holding that any individual's participation in the programs shall be "wholly voluntary and shall not be a prerequisite to eligibility for or receipt of any other service or assistance from, or to participation in, any other program."

Even when compelling public interests justify overriding fundamental rights, such as free procreational choice, those rights usually do not disappear without leaving some traces. Suppose for purposes of argument that public health considerations (such as protection of the gene pool) justify some form of mandatory genetic counseling. The state must first try to realize its compelling interest by the "least restrictive alternative" since a fundamental right is involved [10]. For instance, since only a few genetic defects can be detected and even fewer can be prevented or treated, the improvement in the overall quality of the gene pool may be problematic. Futhermore, we could possibly get the same improvement by identifying and reducing the mutagenic agents in the environment that cause the same defects. Although it is difficult to determine the causes of genetic change, such an approach would not necessarily be less effective than compulsory counseling programs especially if we assume that religious and moral convictions as well as simple resentment will result in significant noncooperation or noncompliance. Thus, the courts might require that policy-makers show that less restrictive alternatives including voluntary programs and attempts to control mutagenic agents or the environment are not available before allowing mandatory counseling. Yet ironically for public policy, while the constitutionality of a proposed compulsory program depends only on presently feasible technological alternatives, the need for such drastic means of compulsion may be determined in part by wholly independent past public choices. Policy decisions to fund research and development to determine and alter the causes of genetic defects decided on their own merits thus set the future feasibility of alternatives to compulsion, illustrating the dynamic and continuous nature of public decision-making.

State regulations which restrict liberty (as, for example mandatory amniocentesis) must also provide "procedural due process" in Constitutional terms. "Procedural due process" usually means that the person must be granted a hearing after notice of the proposed course of action, perhaps provided with counsel and given an opportunity to present and interrogate witnesses. Furthermore, compulsory counseling programs that aim only at specific genetic defects may also run afoul of the guarantee of equal protection of the laws. Laws that categorize compulsion by identifiable but inherent traits, whether ethnic, racial, national origin, or perhaps sex, are inherently suspect and demand strict scrutiny for a compelling interest in utilizing the suspect classification. Even if, for example, a sickle cell program does not use racial identification, but focuses on those "at risk of the disease," the classification may still be suspect if only one racial group is found to be "at risk." Indeed, genetic makeup itself (which after all determines race) may come to be recognized as an immutable characteristic that demands strict justification [11]. Thus, the means of classification as well as the state end must be justified, and a very heavy burden would be required for compelling a particular group to undergo compulsory genetic intervention. The dangers of manipulation aimed at subjugation of a particular group and the unavoidable danger of public stigma would make such a program extremely problematic.

Regulation of genetic counseling need not be limited to civil or constitutional remedies for violations of publicly sanctioned duties. Bad results can be prevented and counseling itself channeled and shaped by legislation under the traditional police powers of the states to protect the public health and welfare. The states may act indirectly through incentive or funding schemes or more directly by detailing the manner and form all counseling must take. All the standards incorporated into bases for liability could be reworked into direct regulations. Violations, rather than leading to private damage actions, could be policed by revocations of licenses or even criminal penalties.

Regulations that set limits and impose duties in counseling will form a significant part of public policy. By taking into account public desires as well as present practices, they may aim at remedying harms, preventing incompetence, or facilitating development and use, and each aim reinforces the others. The extent of regulation will depend upon the type and importance of the state interests involved.

STATE INTERESTS AS JUSTIFICATIONS FOR COERCION

Now, what are some of the state interests that might justify one or more coercive policies? One argument for coercive policies—and even for directive counseling—is paternalism, which can be seen as the collective interest in restricting a person's liberty for his or her own benefit. Examples of paternalistic legislation are laws that require motorcyclists to wear helmets, make attempting a suicide a criminal offense, or prohibit drugs that can harm their users. Since genetic counselors typically have a better understanding of the effects of particular genetic diseases and their probability than counselees, the argument runs, they should take necessary steps to ensure certain results, particularly since counselees may be swayed by numerous irrational factors such as religious beliefs that stress the positive effects of suffering or that restrict the means to be used to prevent the harm that will come to families from genetic defects.

Paternalism is in fact rarely offered as a suffcient justification. Stronger reasons for coercive interventions center around the prevention of harm to persons other than those whose freedom is restricted. (Sometimes paternalistic reasons may also be cited, to avoid the charge of unfairly imposing burdens on a person or group for society's benefit. Thus, it might be argued that a restriction on one's procreational choice benefits one's family as much as it does society.) The list of "others" includes the genetically defective offspring, society and future generations.

Offspring

Some commentators have claimed that there is a tort of "wrongful life" and that every child has a right to a minimum quality of genetic inheritance [12]. Glass, for instance, maintains that "in a not-distant future time, owing to the advances of human genetics, the right of individuals to procreate must give place to a new paramount right: the right of every child to enter life with an adequate physical and mental endowment." [13] An argument such as Glass' might well point in the direction of a legal enforcement of genetic responsibility, although Glass, himself, was proposing only a moral, not a legal right. While the probable quality of life of potential offspring is relevant to parental decisions about risk-taking, it does not provide a solid foundation for coercive public policies, especially mandatory amniocentesis and abortion. Rarely does it appear by itself in discourse about public policies; and it seems to be limited to an exhortation to parents to base their decisions on what will be in their offspring's best interests.

Society

The public health, which appears in the National Genetics Diseases Act to justify funding voluntary programs, has also been invoked to justify coercive interventions in procreative decisions. For instance, in Buck v Bell in 1927, Justice Holmes appealed to the public health, along with other considerations including paternalism and fairness, to uphold a Virginia statute authorizing compulsory sterilization of the institutionalized mentally retarded: "The principle that sustains compulsory vaccination is broad enough to cover cutting the Fallopian tubes. . ." [14]. Much of our moral and legal reasoning is analogical. This is to be expected, since one fundamental principle of morality in general and justice in particular is that similar cases be treated in a similar way. Although analogical reasoning is necessary, particular analogies may be problematic. For Holmes, since the public health rationale is sufficient to sustain compulsory vaccination which invades privacy and bodily integrity, it is sufficient to uphold compulsory sterilization. Holmes overlooked the point that sterilization irreversibly prevents procreation and that it depends on uncertain theories of mental retardation and heredity. It is not at all clear that the holding in Buck v Bell would now be upheld, but regardless of the Supreme Court's decision, policy-makers can draw different and narrower boundaries on interference with procreation. While the strongest case for compulsory programs invokes the public health [15], even it depends on establishing clear connections between the classification of persons and the end that is sought; and those connections obviously hinge on well-founded theories of causation and prevention of genetic defects.

Many arguments about effects on society include the economic costs of trying to treat or care for defective offspring. The National Genetic Diseases Act refers to the "financial burden on the individuals, their families, and society," and insists that reducing genetic diseases will be "cost beneficial to the American public." Justice Holmes in Buck v Bell held that "three generations of imbeciles are enough" in part because they "sap the strength of the state. . . ." The drain on society's resources is a legitimate concern, but "there have also been intimations that a statute which compelled sterilization because of the potential financial drain on society posed by impecunious wards violates the Equal Protection Clause. . ." [16].

While economic costs cannot be ignored from the standpoint of public policy, a cost-benefit analysis that incorporates only such considerations is hardly adequate even if it is more quantifiable and manageable because it excludes other values. Furthermore, it is difficult to determine at what point economic values should override liberty.

Future Generations

Society has an interest in the quality of the gene pool particularly as it will affect the well-being of future generations. Interventions could be aimed at preventing further deterioration of the gene pool and even at reducing the frequency of deleterious genes. Nevertheless, evidence on the effects of altered reproduction patterns on the gene pool is quite mixed. As long as the effects remain speculative, procreational freedom should be undisturbed.

Although these three rationales for state interest in "genetic decisions" do not appear to justify coercion, even this brief review has pointed in the direction of a "minimal ethic of genetic responsibility," [Twiss, in this volume, p 255] in which harm to others, including society, is a relevant moral consideration for families who are trying to decide what to do with genetic information. But while we may present these considerations to ourselves and others (even occasionally in our roles as counselors), they seldom justify forcibly overriding autonomy. Some fear that voluntary programs, such as the ones encompassed in the National Genetic Diseases Act, may evolve into coercive programs, mandating counseling and even dictating certain procreative decisions. Whether such an evolution could be morally justified depends on the weight of scientific and other evidence about the magnitude of harm of genetic defects to various individuals and groups and the available means of preventing such harm. Whether particular moral considerations should be legally enforced is a moral and political question since conflicting values are at stake. To avoid harm or certain costs to others and to society is surely a reason for considering whether to override liberty, but we start from a presumption in favor of liberty in procreative decisions and it is difficult to determine when avoiding harm or costs is a sufficient, decisive, or conclusive reason.

THE MORALITY INHERENT IN PUBLIC POLICIES

So far we have emphasized the choice of public policies in instrumental terms: which policies will enable us to realize or at least to respect certain values and rights including the reduction of genetic defects and the preservation of autonomy. But rarely are public policies merely instrumental. They also express certain values and convictions, and often have effects, sometimes unanticipated, on other values and convictions. We need to ask what policies toward genetic counseling express and what they may affect.

First, increased interest in genetic counseling and related procedures and techniques may well alter attitudes toward procreative decisions in far-reaching ways. While we have long been interested in healthy babies, evidence suggests that we are rapidly coming to think about optimal or perfect babies. We even seem to phrase the options in terms of optimal baby or no baby. As Kass has suggested, such attitudes bespeak a transformation in the process of procreation, away from the family and into the laboratory. What began as a procedure to increase voluntary decision-making cannot now easily exclude the demand for optimal babies [17]. The costs of such a shift should enter into the formulation of public policy even if these costs cannot be quantified as readily as the tangible costs of birth defects.

Second, with an emphasis on prevention of birth defects in conjunction with procedures and techniques to realize that aim, what will happen to efforts to treat such defects and to care for those who suffer from them? A shift from curative medicine to preventive medicine may be marked by a different attitude toward those who need cure and care, those who have slipped through the net of prevention. Such attitudinal shifts can be expected to be more pronounced where prevention is unsuccessful because the parents have religious or moral scruples against a method (such as abortion) and where the costs of care are exceedingly large. What will be the effects of such changes in attitude?

Third, faced with limited resources for health care, including both prevention and therapy, a society could decide to exclude whole classes of disease from treatment. As Outka has stressed, such a strategy need not violate the principle of formal justice (treat similar cases in a similar way). It might take the form of refusing to support particular diseases that are rare and noncommunicable, have little prospect for rehabilitation, and require extended and very expensive care [18]. If such a strategy were adopted, one would expect pressure to add another criterion: could the disease have been prevented or avoided? While this criterion seems to add retributive factors to distributive ones, few would deny the relevance of effort to distributive justice even if they dispute its weight and significance. At any rate, society might decide to exclude treatment of a genetic disease that could have been avoided through a different choice about marriage, conception and abortion if that disease requires expensive care without any prospect for rehabilitation. However formally just and rational such a policy may appear, it has its own symbolic and cultural costs. Justice does not exhaust our vision of society, and a society that is merely just may lack many elements of humane caring. That cost should not be overlooked or downplayed.

Finally, public policies reflect social notions of health and disease which may direct or limit genetic counseling. Appearing to encompass firm "harm" and "welfare" judgments, they may actually rest on other hidden moral principles and values. What is or should be a moral or political problem may be converted into a medical one. Thus, the putatively objective labels of health and disease may serve to legitimate restrictions of liberty when other justifications would fall short. The rather severe measures taken in the name of treating "mental disease" supply a harrowing catalogue of the potential pernicious effects when the supposed neutral observations of medical science are translated into law. We should constantly probe assertions of harm and welfare, disease and health, to discover the unarticulated moral and political values on which the asserted justifications actually rest so as to determine whether they are strong enough to override other values and principles such as liberty and equality.

REFERENCES

1. Dye TR: Understanding Public Policy. Second edition. Englewood Cliffs, NJ: Prentice Hall, Inc., 1975, p 1.

2. Anderson JE: Public Policy-Making. New York: Praeger Publishers, 1975, p 3.

3. For example, the increasing use of amniocentesis is controversial precisely because it may be utilized during the stage of fetal development when abortion is legally permissible, ie, prior to fetal viability. See Roe vs Wade, 410 US 113 (1973). Suppose that technological advances result in fetal viability at an earlier stage of development than amniocentesis can be effectively used. If the legal prohibitions of abortion remain wedded to viability, rather than genetic counseling techniques, we can expect a drop in the use of amniocentesis. Or at least the justification for its use would be limited to information—to identify sex or to alert parents to what defects they can expect their child to have. Similar effects on the use of amniocentesis might occur as de facto public policy following a shift in moral attitudes critical of abortion. Waltz JR and Thigpen CR: Genetic Screening and Counseling: The Legal and Ethical Issues. Northwestern University Law Review 68:738, note 215, 1974.

4. Green HP: Law and Genetic Control: Public-Policy Questions. Ann NY Acad Sci 265: 170–177, 1976.

5. Roe vs Wade 410 US 113 (1973); Griswold vs Connecticut 381 US 479 (1965); Eisenstadt vs Baird 405 US 438 (1972).

6. National Genetic Diseases Act, S 7801, 94th Congress, 2nd, 1975.

7. Nozick R: Anarchy, State, and Utopia. New York: Basic Books, 1974.

8. For a defense of the practice, see Duff RS and Campbell AGM: "Moral and Ethical Dilemmas in the Special-Care Nursery." N Engl J Med 289:890–894, 1973; and On Deciding the Care of Severely Handicapped or Dying Persons: With Particular Reference to Infants. Pediatrics 57:487–493, 1976.

9. See Robertson JA: "Involuntary Euthanasia of Defective Newborns: A Legal Analysis." Stanford Law Review 27:213–269, 1975.

10. CF, eg Skinner vs Oklahoma, 316 US 535 (1942); Shapiro vs Thompson, 394 US 618 (1969).

11. See eg McLauflin vs Florida, 379 US 184 (1964). In McLauflin, a statute making interracial marriages a crime was struck down because of the per se use of race to distinguish the legal from the illegal. Similarly, the per se use of a particular genotype for a compulsory health treatment raises questions of definitional circularity in the rationale for using this means of classification.

12. For a legal analysis, see generally, Capron AM: Informed Decisionmaking in Genetic Counseling: A Dissent to the Wrongful Life Debate. Indiana Law Journal 48:581–604, Summer 1973.

13. Birch C, Abrecht P (eds): "Genetics and the Quality of Life." Elmsford, NY: Pergamon, 1975, pp 56–57. Glass' conception is a positive right to have a minimum level of genetic quality. This is an odd right since if the conditions are not present for its realization, the child is presumed to want no life at all. Furthermore, it is a right to something that we cannot guarantee. It might be better to avoid the language of rights in this context.

14. Buck vs Bell 274 US 200 (1927). But see also Skinner vs Oklahoma 316 US 535 (1942).

15. For example, the public health interest in compulsory vaccinations upheld in Jacobsen vs Massachusetts 197 US 11 (1905).

16. Price ME, Burt RA: Sterilization, State Action, and the Concept of Consent. Law and Psychology Review (Spring 1975): 62. They refer to Cook vs State, 9 Ore App 224, 495 P 2d 768 (1972).

17. See Kass L: Comments. "Early Diagnosis of Human Genetic Defects." Edited by Harris M. Fogarty International Center Proceedings No. 6 HEW Publication No. (NIH) 72–75, p 202. See also Kass L: Implications of Prenatal Diagnosis for the Human Right to Life. Ethical Issues in Human Genetics. Edited by Hilton B, et al. New York: Plenum, 1973, p 185.

18. Outka G: Social Justice and Equal Access to Health Care. Journal of Religious Ethics. 2:24, 1974.

26 *"Making Babies" Revisited*

Leon R. Kass, M.D.

The birth of Louise Brown whose conception occurred in vitro and was then transferred to her mother's uterus raised a number of questions about genetic engineering. Questions were also raised about the appropriateness of conducting research on the human embryo. Kass reviews a number of the arguments pro and con and then sets forth his own argument against the use of in vitro fertilization and embryo transplantation. Although the Ethics Advisory Board has allowed some research into in vitro fertilization, Kass nonetheless presents an interesting review of all of the arguments concerning this particular technology.

Leon Kass is with the University of Chicago Medical School

And the man knew not Eve his wife; but she conceived without him and bore Cain, and said: I have gotten a man with the help of Dr. Steptoe.

Ectogenesis IV, 1

And Isaac entreated the NIH for his wife, because she was barren; and the NIH let Itself be entreated of him, and Rebekah his wife conceived.

Ectogenesis XXV, 21

Seven years ago in the pages of this journal, in an article entitled "Making Babies—the New Biology and the 'Old' Morality" (Number 26, Winter 1972), I explored some of the moral and political questions raised by projected new powers to intervene in the processes of human reproduction. I concluded that it would be foolish to acquire and use these powers. The questions have since been debated in "bioethical" circles and in college classrooms, and they have received intermittent attention in the popular press and in sensational novels and movies. This past year they have gained the media limelight with the Del Zio suit against Columbia University, and more especially with the birth last

453

summer in Britain of Louise Brown, the first identified human baby born following conception in the laboratory.

Back in 1975, after prolonged deliberations, the National Commission for the Protection of Human Subjects of Biomedical and Behavioral Research issued its report and recommendations for research on the human fetus. And in the *Federal Register* of August 8, 1975, the Secretary of Health, Education, and Welfare published regulations regarding research, development, and related activities involving fetuses, pregnant women, and *in vitro* fertilization. These provided that no Federal monies should be used for *in vitro* fertilization of human eggs until a special Ethics Advisory Board reviews the special ethical issues and offers advice about whether government should support any such proposed research. There has been an effective moratorium on Federal support for human *in vitro* fertilization research since that time. But now the whole matter has once again become the subject of an intensive policy debate, for such a board has been established by HEW to consider whether the United States Government should finance research on human *in vitro* fertilization and embryo transfer.

The question has been placed on the policy table by a research proposal submitted to the National Institute of Child Health and Human Development by Dr. Pierre Soupart of Vanderbilt University. Dr. Soupart requested $465,000, over three years, for a study to define in part the genetic risk involved in obtaining early human embryos by tissue-culture methods. He proposes to fertilize about 450 human ova, obtained from donors undergoing gynecological surgery (i.e., not from women whom the research could be expected to help), with donor sperm, to observe their development for five to six days, and to examine them microscopically for chromosomal and other abnormalities before discarding them. In addition, Dr. Soupart proposes to study whether such laboratory-grown embryos can be frozen and stored without producing abnormalities; it is thought that temporary cold storage of human embryos might improve the success rate in the embryo-transfer procedure used to produce a child. Though Dr. Soupart does not now propose to do embryo transfers to women seeking to become pregnant, his research is intended to serve that goal: He seeks to reassure us that baby-making with the help of *in vitro* fertilization is safe; and he seeks to perfect the techniques introduced by Drs. Edwards and Steptoe in England.

Dr. Soupart's application was approved for funding by the National Institutes of Health review process in October 1977, but because of the administrative regulations it could not be funded without review by an Ethics Advisory Board. The Secretary of HEW, Joseph Califano, has constituted the 13-member Board, and charged it, not only with a decision on the Soupart proposal, but with an inquiry into all the scientific, ethical, and legal issues involved, urging it "to provide recommendations on broad principles to guide the Department in future decision making." The Board, comprising a distinguished group of physicians, academics, and laymen, has invited expert and public testimony on the widest range of questions. By the end of the first phase of its work, it will have held at least 11 meetings and public hearings all over the United States, offering all interested citizens or groups the chance to express their opinions.

I was asked by the Board to discuss the ethical issues raised by the proposed research on human *in vitro* fertilization, laboratory cultures of—and experimentation with—human embryos, and the intrauterine transfer of such embryos for the purpose of assisting human generation. In addition, I was asked to comment on the appropriateness of Federal funding of such research and on the implications of this work for the provision of health care. The present article is based largely on testimony given before the Ethics Advisory Board, at its Boston meeting, October 13–14, 1978.

II

How should one think about the ethical issues, here and in general? There are many possible ways, and it is not altogether clear which way is best. For some people ethical issues are immediately matters of right and wrong, of purity and sin, of good and evil. For others, the critical terms are benefits and harms, risks and promises, gains and costs. Some will focus on so-called rights of individuals or groups, e.g., a right to life or childbirth; still others will emphasize so-called goods for society and its members, such as the advancement of knowledge and the prevention and cure of disease.

My own orientation here is somewhat different. I wish to suggest that before deciding what to do, one should try to understand the implications of doing or not doing. The first task, it seems to me, is not to ask "moral or immoral?" "right or wrong?" but to try to understand fully the meaning and significance of the proposed actions.

This concern with significance leads me to take a broad view of the matter. For we are concerned here not only with the proposed research of Dr. Soupart, and the narrow issues of safety and informed consent it immediately raises, but also with a whole range of implications including many that are tied to definitely foreseeable consequences of this research and its predictable extensions—and touching even our common conception of our own humanity. The very establishment of a special Ethics Advisory Board testifies that we are at least tacitly aware that more is at stake than in ordinary biomedical research, or in experimenting with human subjects at risk of bodily harm. At stake is the *idea* of the *humanness* of our human life and the meaning of our embodiment, our sexual being, and our relation to ancestors and descendants. In reaching the necessarily particular and immediate decision in the case at hand, we must be mindful of the larger picture and must avoid the great danger of trivializing this matter for the sake of rendering it manageable.

III

What is the status of a fertilized human egg (i.e., a human zygote) and the embryo that develops from it? How are we to regard its being? How are we to regard it morally, i.e., how are we to behave toward it? These are, alas, all-too-familiar questions. At least analogous, if not identical, questions are central to the abortion controversy and are also crucial in considering whether and what sort of experimentation is properly conducted on living but aborted fetuses. Would that it were possible to say that the matter is simple and obvious, and that it has been resolved to everyone's satisfaction!

But the controversy about the morality of abortion continues to rage and divide our nation. Moreover, many who favor or do not oppose abortion do so despite the fact that they regard the pre-viable fetus as a living human organism, even if less worthy of protection than a woman's desire not to give it birth. Almost everyone senses the importance of this matter for the decision about laboratory culture of, and experimentation with, human embryos. Thus, we are obliged to take up the question of the status of the embryos, in a search for the outlines of some common ground on which many of us can stand. To the best of my knowledge, the discussion which follows is not informed by any particular sectarian or religious teaching, though it may perhaps reveal that I am a person not devoid of reverence and the capacity for awe and wonder, said by some to be the core of the "religious" sentiment.

I begin by noting that the circumstances of laboratory-grown blastocysts (i.e., 3-to-6-day-old embryos) and embryos are not identical with those of the analogous cases of 1) living fetuses facing abortion and 2) living aborted fetuses used in research. First, the fetuses whose fates are at issue in abortion are unwanted, usually the result of "accidental" conception. Here, the embryos are wanted, and deliberately created, despite certain knowledge that many of them will be destroyed or discarded.[1] Moreover, the fate of these embryos is not in conflict with the wishes, interests, or alleged rights of the pregnant women. Second, though the HEW guidelines governing fetal research permit studies conducted on the not-at-all-viable aborted fetus, such research merely takes advantage of available "products" of abortions not themselves undertaken for the sake of the research. No one has proposed and no one would sanction the deliberate production of live fetuses to be aborted for the sake of research, even very beneficial research.[2] In contrast, we are here considering the deliberate production of embryos for the express purpose of experimentation.

The cases may also differ in other ways. Given the present state of the art, the largest embryo under discussion is the blastocyst, a spherical, relatively undifferentiated mass of cells, barely visible to the naked eye. In appearance it does not look human; indeed, only the most careful scrutiny by the most experienced scientist might distinguish it from similar blastocysts of other mammals. If the human zygote and blastocyst are more like the animal zygote and blastocyst than they are like the 12-week-old human fetus (which already has a humanoid appearance, differentiated organs, and electrical activity of the brain), then there would be a much-diminished ethical dilemma regarding their deliberate creation and experimental use. Needless to say, there are articulate and passionate defenders of all points of view. Let us try, however, to consider the matter afresh.

First of all, the zygote and early embryonic stages are clearly alive. They metabolize, respire, and respond to changes in the environment; they grow and divide. Second, though not yet organized into distinctive parts or organs, the blastocyst is an organic whole, self-developing, genetically unique and distinct from the egg and sperm whose union marked the beginning of its career as a discrete, unfolding being. While the egg and sperm are alive as cells, something new and alive *in a different sense* comes into being with fertilization. The truth of this is unaffected by the fact that fertilization takes time and is not an instantaneous event. For after fertilization is *complete,* there exists a new individual, with its unique genetic identity, fully potent for the self-initiated development into a mature human being, if circumstances are cooperative. Though there is some sense in which the lives of egg and sperm are continuous with the life of the new organism-to-be (or, in human terms, that the parents live on in the child or child-to-be), in the decisive sense there is a discontinuity, a new beginning, with fertilization. *After* fertilization, there is continuity of subsequent development, even if the locus of the embryo alters with implantation (or birth). Any honest biologist must be impressed by these facts, and must be inclined, at least on first glance, to the view that a human life begins at fertilization. Even Dr. Robert Edwards has apparently stumbled over this truth, perhaps inadvertently, in the remark about Louise Brown attributed to him in an article by Peter Gwynne in *Science Digest*: "The last time I saw *her, she* was just eight cells in a test-tube. *She* was beautiful *then*, and she's still beautiful *now!*"[3]

But granting that a human life begins at fertilization, and comes-to-be via a continuous process thereafter, surely—one might say—the blastocyst itself is hardly a human being. I myself would agree that a blastocyst is not, in a *full* sense, a human being—or what the current fashion calls, rather arbitrarily and without clear definition, a person. It does not look like a human being nor can it do very much of what human beings do. Yet, at the same time, I must acknowledge that the human blastocyst is 1) human in origin and 2) *potentially* a mature human being, if all goes well. This too is beyond dispute; indeed it is precisely because of its peculiarly human potentialities that people propose to study *it* rather than the embryos of other mammals. The human blastocyst, even the human blastocyst *in vitro*, is not humanly nothing: it possesses a power to become what everyone will agree is a human being.

Here it may be objected that the blastocyst *in vitro* has today no such power, because there is now no way *in vitro* to bring the blastocyst to that much later fetal stage at which it might survive on its own. There are no published reports of culture of human embryos past the blastocyst stage (though this has been reported for mice). The *in vitro* blastocyst, like the 12-week-old aborted fetus, is *in this sense* not viable (i.e., it is at a stage of maturation before the stage of possible independent existence). But if we distinguish among the *not*-viable embryos, between the *pre*-viable and the *not-at-all* viable—on the basis that the former, though not yet viable is capable of *becoming* or *being made* viable[4]—we note a crucial difference between the blastocyst and the 12-week abortus. Unlike an aborted fetus, the blastocyst is possibly salvageable, and hence *potentially* viable *if it is transferred to a woman for implantation*. It is not strictly true that the *in vitro* blastocyst is *necessarily* not-viable. Until proven otherwise, by embryo transfer and attempted implantation, we are right to consider the human blastocyst *in vitro* as potentially a human being and, in this respect, not fundamentally different from a blastocyst *in utero*. To put the matter more forcefully, the blastocyst *in vitro* is *more* "viable," in the sense of more salvageable, than aborted fetuses at most later stages, up to say 20 weeks.

This is not to say that such a blastocyst is therefore endowed with a so-called right to life, that failure to implant it is negligent homicide, or that experimental touchings of such blastocysts constitute assault and battery. (I myself tend to reject such claims, and indeed think that the ethical questions are not best posed in terms of "rights.") But the blastocyst is not nothing; it is *at least* potential humanity, and as such it elicits, or ought to elicit, our feelings of awe and respect. In the blastocyst, even in the zygote, we face a mysterious and awesome power, a power governed by an immanent plan that may produce an indisputably and fully human being. It deserves our respect not because it has rights or claims or sentience (which it does not have at this stage), but because of what it is, now *and* prospectively.

Let us test this provisional conclusion by considering intuitively our response to two possible fates of such zygotes, blastocysts, and early embryos. First, should such an embryo die, will we be inclined to mourn its passing? When a woman we know miscarries, we are sad—largely for *her* loss and disappointment, but perhaps also at the premature death of a life that might have been. But we do not mourn the departed fetus, nor do we seek ritually to dispose of the remains. In this respect, we do not treat even the fetus as fully one of us.

On the other hand, we would I suppose recoil even from the thought, let alone the practice—I apologize for forcing it upon the reader—of eating such embryos, should someone discover that they would provide a great delicacy, a "human caviar." The human blastocyst would be protected by our taboo against cannibalism, which insists on the humanness of human flesh and which does not permit us to treat even the flesh of the dead as if it were mere meat. *The human embryo is not mere meat; it is not just stuff; it is not a thing.*[5] Because of its origin and because of its capacity, it commands a higher respect.

How much more respect? As much as for a fully developed human being? My own inclination is to say "probably not," but who can be certain? Indeed, there might be prudential and reasonable grounds for an affirmative answer, partly because the presumption of ignorance ought to err in the direction of never underestimating the basis for respect of human life, partly because so many people feel very strongly that even the blastocyst is protectably human. As a first approximation, I would analogize the early embryo *in vitro* to the early embryo *in utero* (because both are potentially viable and human). On this ground alone, *the most sensible policy is to treat the early embryo as a pre-viable fetus, with constraints imposed on early embryo research at least as great as those on fetal research.*

To some this may seem excessively scrupulous. They will argue for the importance of the absence of distinctive humanoid appearance or the absence of sentience. To be sure, we would feel more restraint in invasive procedures conducted on a five-month-old or even 12-week-old living fetus than on a blastocyst. But this added restraint on inflicting suffering on a "look-alike," feeling creature in no way denies the propriety of a prior restraint, grounded in respect for individuated, living, potential humanity. Before I would be persuaded to treat early embryos differently from later ones, I would insist on the establishment of a reasonably clear, naturally grounded boundary that separates "early" and "late," and which provides the basis for respecting "the early" less than "the late." This burden *must* be accepted by proponents of experimentation with human embryos *in vitro* if a decision to permit creating embryos for such experimentation is to be treated as ethically responsible.

IV

Where does the above analysis lead in thinking about treatment of *in vitro* human embryos? I shall indicate, very briefly, the lines toward a possible policy, though that is not my major intent.

The *in vitro* fertilized embryo has four possible fates: 1) *implantation,* in the hope of producing from it a child; 2) *death,* by active "killing" or disaggregation, or by a "natural" demise; 3) use in *manipulative experimentation*—embryological, genetic, etc.; 4) use in attempts at *perpetuation in vitro* beyond the blastocyst stage, ultimately, perhaps, to viability. I will not now consider this fourth and future possibility, though I would suggest that full laboratory growth of an embryo into a viable human being (i.e., ectogenesis), while perfectly compatible with respect owed to its potential humanity as an individual, may be incompatible with the kind of respect owed to its humanity that is grounded in the bonds of lineage and the nature of parenthood.

On the strength of my analysis of the status of the embryo, and the respect due it, no objection would be raised to implantation. *In vitro* fertilization and embryo transfer to treat infertility, as in the case of Mr. and Mrs. Brown, is perfectly compatible with a respect and reverence for human life, including potential human life. Moreover, no disrespect is intended or practiced by the mere fact that several eggs are removed for fertilization, to increase the chance of success. Were it possible to guarantee successful fertilization and normal growth with a single egg, no more would need to be obtained. Assuming nothing further is done with the unimplanted embryos, there is nothing disrespectful going in. The demise of the unimplanted embryos would be analogous to the loss of numerous embryos wasted in the normal *in vivo* attempts to generate a child. It is estimated that over 50 percent of eggs successfully fertilized during unprotected sexual intercourse fail to implant, or do not remain implanted, in the uterine wall, and are shed soon thereafter, before a diagnosis of pregnancy could be made. Any couple attempting to conceive a child tacitly accepts such embryonic wastage as the perfectly acceptable price to be paid for the birth of a (usually) healthy child. Current procedures to initiate pregnancy with laboratory fertilization thus differ from the natural "procedure" in that what would normally be spread over four or five months *in vivo* is compressed into a single effort, using all at once a four or five months' supply of eggs.[6]

Parenthetically, we should note that the natural occurrence of embryo and fetal loss and wastage does not necessarily or automatically justify all deliberate, humanly caused destruction of fetal life. For example, the natural loss of embryos in early pregnancy cannot in itself be a warrant for deliberately aborting them or for invasively experimenting on them *in vitro*, any more than stillbirths could be a justification for newborn infanticide. There are many things that happen naturally that we ought not to do deliberately. It is curious how the same people who deny the relevance of nature as a guide for evaluating human interventions into human generation, and who deny that the term "unnatural" carries any ethical weight, will themselves appeal to "nature's way" when it suits their purposes.[7] Still, in this present matter, the closeness to natural procreation—the goal is the same, the embryonic loss is unavoidable and not desired, and the amount of loss is similar—leads me to believe that we do no more intentional or unjustified harm in the one case than in the other, and practice no disrespect.

But must we allow *in vitro* unimplanted embryos to die? Why should they not be either transferred for "adoption" into another infertile woman, or else used for investigative purposes, to seek new knowledge, say about gene action? The first option raises questions about the nature of parenthood and lineage to which I will return. But even on first glance, it would seem likely to raise a large objection from the original couple, who were seeking a child of their own and not the dissemination of their "own" biological children for prenatal adoption.

But what about experimentation on such blastocysts and early embryos? Is that compatible with the respect they deserve? This is the hard question. On balance, I would think not. Invasive and manipulative experiments involving such embryos very likely presume that they are things or mere stuff, and deny the fact of their possible viability. Certain observational and non-invasive experiments might be different. But on the whole, I would think that the respect for human embryos for which I have argued—I repeat, not their so-called right to life—would lead one to oppose most potentially interesting and useful experimentation. This is a dilemma, but one which cannot be ducked or defined away. Either we accept certain great restrictions on the permissible uses of human embryos or we deliberately decide

to override—though I hope not deny—the respect due to the embryos.

I am aware that I have pointed toward a seemingly paradoxical
conclusion about the treatment of the unimplanted embryos: Leave
them alone, and do not create embryos for experimentation only. To
let them die "naturally" would be the most respectful course,
grounded on a reverence, generically, for their potential humanity,
and a respect, individually, for their being the seed and offspring of a
particular couple who were themselves seeking only to have a child of
their own. An analysis which stressed a "right to life," rather than respect, would of course lead to different conclusions. Only an analysis
of the status of the embryo which denied both its so-called "rights" *or*
its worthiness of all respect would have no trouble sanctioning its use
in investigative research, donation to other couples, commercial
transactions, and other activities of these sorts.

V

The attempt to generate a child with the aid of *in vitro* fertilization constitutes an experiment upon the prospective child. It thus
raises a most peculiar question for the ethics of human experimentation: Can one ethically choose for a yet hypothetical, unconceived
child-to-be the unknown hazards he must face, obviously without
his consent, and simultaneously choose to give him life in which to
face them? This question has been much debated, as it points to a serious and immediate ethical concern: the hazards of manipulating the
embryo as it bears on the health of the child-to-be.

Everyone agrees that human-embryo transfer for the sake of
generation should not be performed until prior laboratory research in
animals has provided a sound basis for estimating the likely risks to
any human beings who will be born as a result of this transfer and
gestation. Argument centers on whether a sufficiently sound basis for
estimating the likely risks to humans *can be* provided by animal experiments, and, if so, whether adequate experimentation has been
done, and what level of risk is acceptable.

There is, it seems to me, good reason for insisting that risk of incidence and likely extent of possible harm be very, very low—lower,
say, than in therapeutic experimentation in children or adults. But I
do not think that the risk of harm must be positively excluded (and it
certainly cannot be). It would suffice if those risks were equivalent to,
or less than, the risks to the child from normal procreation. To insist
on more rigorous standards, especially when we permit known carriers of genetic disease to reproduce, would seem a denial of equal
treatment to infertile couples contemplating *in vitro* assistance. More-

over, it is to give undue weight to the importance of bodily harm over against risks of poor nurture and rearing after birth. Wouldn't the couple's great eagerness for the child count, in the promise of increased parental affection, toward offsetting even a slightly higher but unknown risk of mental retardation?

Finally, to insist on extra-scrupulosity regarding risks in laboratory-assisted reproduction is to attach too much of one's concern to the wrong issue. True, everyone understands about harming children, while very few worry about dehumanization of procreation or problems of lineage. But those are the things that are distinctive about laboratory-assisted reproduction, not the risk of bodily harm to offspring. It should suffice that the risks be comparable to those for ordinary procreation, not greater but no less.

It remains a question whether we now know enough about these risks to go ahead with human-embryo transfer. Here I would defer to the opinions of the cautious experts—for caution is the posture of responsibility toward such prospective children. I would agree with Doctors Luigi Mastroianni, Benjamin Brackett, and Robert Short—all researchers in the field—that the risks for humans have not yet been sufficiently assessed, in large part because the risks in animals have been so poorly assessed (due to the small numbers of such births and to the absence of any *prospective* study to identify and evaluate deviations from the norm).

VI

Many people rejoiced at the birth of Louise Brown. Some were pleased by the technical accomplishment, many were pleased that she was born apparently in good health. But most of us shared the joy of her parents, who after a long, frustrating, and fruitless period, at last had the pleasure and blessing of a child of their own. The desire to have a child of one's own is acknowledged to be a powerful and deep-seated human desire—some have called it "instinctive"—and the satisfaction of this desire, by the relief of infertility, is said to be one major goal of continuing the work with *in vitro* fertilization and embryo transfer. That this is a worthy goal few, if any, would deny.

Yet let us explore what is meant by *"to have a child of one's own."* First, what is meant by *"to have"*? Is the crucial meaning that of gestating and bearing? Or is it "to have" as a possession? Or is it to nourish and to rear, the child being the embodiment of one's activity as teacher and guide? Or is it rather to provide someone who descends and comes after, someone who will replace oneself in the family line or preserve the family tree by new sproutings and branchings?

More significantly, what is meant by *"one's own"*? What sense of one's own is important? A scientist might define "one's own" in terms of carrying one's own genes. Though in some sense correct, this cannot be humanly decisive. For Mr. Brown or for most of us, it would not be a matter of indifference if the sperm used to fertilize the egg were provided by an identical twin brother—whose genes would be, of course, the same as his. Rather, the humanly crucial sense of "one's own," the sense that leads most people to choose their own, rather than to adopt, is captured in such phrases as "my seed," "flesh of my flesh," "sprung from my loins." More accurately, since "one's own" is not the own of one but of *two,* the desire to have a child of "one's own" is *a couple's desire* to embody, out of the conjugal union of their separate bodies, a child who is flesh of their separate flesh made one. This archaic language may sound quaint, but I would argue that this is precisely what is being celebrated by most people who rejoice at the birth of Louise Brown, whether they would articulate it this way or not. Mr. and Mrs. Brown, by the birth of their daughter, fulfill this aspect of their separate sexual natures and of their married life together, they acquire descendants and a new branch of their joined family tree, and the child Louise is given solid and unambiguous roots from which she has sprung and by which she will be nourished.

If this were to be the *only* use made of embryo transfer, and if providing *in this sense* "a child of one's own" were indeed the sole reason for the clinical use of the techniques, there could be no objection. Yet there will almost certainly be other uses, involving third parties, to satisfy the desire "to have" a child of "one's own" in different senses of "to have" and "one's own." I am not merely speculating about future possibilities. With the technology to effect human *in vitro* fertilization and embryo transfer comes the *immediate* possibility of egg donation (egg from donor, sperm from husband), embryo donation (egg and sperm from outside of the marriage), and foster pregnancy (host surrogate for gestation).

Nearly everyone agrees that these circumstances are morally and perhaps psychologically more complicated than the intra-marital case. Here the meaning of "one's own" is no longer so unambiguous; neither is the meaning of motherhood and the status of pregnancy. On the one hand, it is argued that embryo donation, or "prenatal adoption," would be superior to present adoption, because the woman would have the experience of pregnancy and the child would be born of the "adopting" mother, rendering the maternal tie even more close. On the other hand, the mother-child bond rooted in pregnancy and delivery is held to be of little consequence by those who would endorse the use of surrogate gestational "mothers," say for a woman whose infertility is due to uterine disease rather than ovarian disease or oviduct obstruction. Clearly, the "need" and demand for extra-marital embryo transfer are real and probably large, probably even greater than the intra-marital ones. Already, the Chairman of the Ethics Advisory Board has testified in Congress about the need to define the responsibilities of *the donor* and the recipient "parents." Thus the new techniques will not only serve to ensure and preserve lineage, but will also serve to confound and complicate it. The principle truly at work here is not to provide married couples with a child of *their own,* but to provide anyone who wants one with a child, by whatever possible or convenient means.

"So what?" it will be said. First of all, we already practice and enourage adoption. Second, we have permitted artificial insemination—though we have, after some 40 years of this practice, yet to resolve questions of legitimacy. Third, what with the high rate of divorce and remarriage, identification of "mother," "father," and "child" is already complicated. Fourth, there is a growing rate of illegitimacy and husbandless parentages. Fifth, the use of surrogate mothers for foster pregnancy has already occurred, with the aid of artificial insemination.[8] Finally, our age in its enlightenment is no longer so certain about the virtues of family, lineage, and heterosexuality, or even about the taboos against adultery and incest. Against this background, it will be asked, why all the fuss about some little embryos that stray from the nest?

It is not an easy question to answer. Yet, consider. We practice adoption because there are abandoned children who need a good home. We do not, and would not, encourage people deliberately to generate children for others to adopt; partly we wish to avoid baby markets, partly we think it unfair to the child deliberately to deprive him of his natural ties. Recent years have seen a rise in our concern with roots, against the rootless and increasingly homogeneous background of contemporary American life. Adopted children, in particular, are pressing for information regarding their "real parents," and some states now require that such information be made available (on that typically modern ground of "freedom of information," rather than because of the profound importance of lineage for self-identity). The practice of artificial insemination has yet to be evaluated, the secrecy in which it is practiced being an apparent concession to the dangers of publicity.[9] Indeed, most physicians who practice artificial insemination routinely mix in some semen from the husband, to preserve some doubt about paternity—again, a concession to the importance of lineage and legitimacy. Finally, what about the changing mores of marriage, divorce, single-parent families, and sexual behavior? Do we applaud these changes? Do we want to contribute further to the confusion of thought, identity, and practice?[10]

Properly understood, the largely universal taboos against incest, and also the prohibition against adultery, suggest that clarity about who your parents are, clarity in the lines of generation, clarity about who is whose, are the indispensable foundations of a sound family life, itself the sound foundation of civilized community. Clarity about your origins is crucial for self-identity, itself important for self-respect. It would be, in my view, deplorable public policy further to erode such fundamental beliefs, values, institutions, and practices. This means, concretely, no encouragement of embryo adoption or especially of surrogate pregnancy. While it would be perhaps foolish to try to proscribe or outlaw such praactices, it would not be wise for the Federal government to foster them. The Ethics Advisory Board should carefully consider whether it should and can attempt to restrict the use of embryo transfer to the married couple from whom the embryo derives.

The case of surrogate wombs bears a further comment. While expressing no objection to the practice of foster pregnancy itself, some people object that it will be done for pay, largely because of their fear that poor women will be exploited by such a practice. But if there were nothing wrong with foster pregnancy, what would be wrong with making a living at it? Clearly, this objection harbors a *tacit* understanding that to bear another's child for pay is in some sense a degradation of oneself—in the same sense that prostitution is a degradation *primarily* because it entails the loveless surrender of one's body to serve another's lust, and *only derivatively* because the woman is paid. It is to deny the meaning and worth of one's body, to treat it as a mere incubator, divested of its human meaning. It is also to deny the meaning of the bond among sexuality, love, and procreation. The buying and selling of human flesh and the dehumanized uses of the human body ought not to be encouraged. To be sure, the practice of womb donation could be engaged in for love not money, as it apparently has been in the case in Michigan. A woman could bear her sister's child out of sisterly love. But to the degree that one escapes in this way from the degradation and difficulties of the *sale* of human flesh and bodily services, and the treating of the body as stuff (the problem of cannibalism), one approaches instead the difficulties of incest and near-incest.

VII

Objections have been raised about the deliberate technological intervention into the so-called natural processes of human reproduction. Some would simply oppose such interventions as "unnatural," and therefore wrong. Others are concerned about the consequences of these interventions, and about their ends and limits. Again, I think it important to explore the meaning and possible significance of such interventions, present and projected, especially as they bear on fundamental beliefs, institutions, and practices. To do so requires that we consider likely future developments in the laboratory study of human reproduction. Indeed, I shall argue that we *must* consider such future developments in reaching a decision in the present case.

What can we expect in the way of new modes of reproduction, as an outgrowth of present studies? To be sure, prediction is difficult. One can never know with certainty what will happen, much less how soon. Yet uncertainty is not the same as simple ignorance. Some things, indeed, seem likely. They seem likely because 1) they are thought necessary or desirable, at least by some researchers and their sponsors, 2) they are probably biologically possible and technically feasible, and 3) they will be difficult to prevent or control (especially if no one anticipates their development or sees a need to worry about them). One of the things the citizenry, myself included, would expect from an Ethics Advisory Board and our policy makers generally is that they face up to reasonable projections of future accomplishments, consider whether they are cause for social concern, and see whether or not the principles *now* enunciated and the practices *now* established are adequate to deal with any such concerns.

I project at least the following:

1. The growth of human embryos in the laboratory will be extended beyond the blastocyst stage. Such growth must be deemed desirable under all the arguments advanced for developmental research *up* to the blastocyst stage; research on gene action, chromosome segregation, cellular and organic differentiation, fetus-environment interaction, implantation, etc., cannot answer all its questions with the blastocyst. Such *in vitro* post-blastocyst differentiation has apparently been achieved in the mouse, in culture; the use of other mammals as temporary hosts for human embryos is also a possibility. How far such embryos will eventually be perpetuated is anybody's guess, but full-term ectogenesis cannot be excluded. Neither can the existence of laboratories filled with many living human embryos, growing at various stages of development.

2. Experiments will be undertaken to alter the cellular and genetic composition of these embryos, at first without subsequent transfer to a woman for gestation, perhaps later as a prelude to reproductive efforts. Again, scientific reasons now justifying Dr. Soupart's research already justify further embryonic manipulations, including

formation of hybrids or chimeras (within species and between species); gene, chromosome, and plasmid insertion, excision, or alteration; nuclear transplantation or cloning, etc. The techniques of DNA recombination, coupled with the new skills of handling embryos, make prospects for some precise genetic manipulation much nearer than anyone would have guessed ten years ago. And embryological and cellular research in mammals is making astounding progress. On the cover of a recent issue of *Science* is a picture of a hexaparental mouse, born after reaggregation of an early embryo with cells disaggregated from three separate embryos. (Note: That sober journal calls this a "handmade mouse"—i.e., literally a *manu-factured* mouse—and goes on to say that it was "manufactured by genetic engineering techniques.")[11]

3. Storage and banking of living human embryos (and ova) will be undertaken, perhaps commercially. After all, commercial sperm banks are already well-established and prospering.

Space does not permit me to do more than identify a few kinds of questions that must be considered in relation to such possible coming control over human heredity and reproduction: questions about the wisdom required to engage in such practices; questions about the goals and standards that will guide our interventions; questions about changes in the concepts of being human, including embodiment, gender, love, lineage, identity, parenthood, and sexuality; questions about the responsibility of power over future generations; questions about awe, respect, humility; questions about the kind of society we will have if we follow along our present course.[12]

Though I cannot discuss these questions now, I can and must face a serious objection to considering them at all. Most people would agree that the projected possibilities raise far more serious questions than do simple fertilization of a few embryos, their growth *in vitro* to the blastocyst stage, and their possible transfer to women for gestation. Why burden the present decision with these possibilities? Future "abuses," it is often said, do not disqualify present uses (though these same people also often say that "future benefits justify present questionable uses"). Moreover, there can be no certainty that "A" will lead to "B." This thin-edge-of-the-wedge argument has been open to criticism.

But such criticism misses the point, for two reasons. *First*, critics often misunderstand the wedge argument. The wedge argument is not primarily an argument of prediction, that A *will* lead to B, say on the strength of the empirical analysis of precedent and an appraisal of the likely direction of present research. It is primarily an argument about the *logic* of justification. Do the principles of justification *now* used to justify the current research proposal already justify *in advance* the further developments? Consider some of these principles:

1. It is desirable to learn as much as possible about the processes of fertilization, growth, implantation, and differentiation of human embryos and about human gene expression and its control.

2. It would be desirable to acquire improved techniques for *enhancing* conception and implantation, for *preventing* conception and implantation, for the treatment of genetic and chromosomal abnormalities, etc.

3. In the end, only research using *human* embryos can answer these questions and provide these techniques.

4. There should be no censorship or limitation of scientific inquiry or research.

This logic knows no boundary at the blastocyst stage, or for that matter, at any later stage. For these principles *not* to justify future extensions of current work, some independent additional principles, limiting such justification to particular stages of development, would have to be found. Here, the task is to find such a biologically defensible distinction that could be respected as reasonable and not arbitrary, a difficult—perhaps impossible—task, given the continuity of development after fertilization. The citizenry, myself included, will want to know *precisely* what grounds our policy makers will give for endorsing Soupart's research, and whether their principles have not already sanctioned future developments. If they do give such wedge-opening justifications, let them do so deliberately, candidly, and intentionally.

A better case to illustrate the wedge logic is the principle offered for the embryo-transfer procedures as treatment for infertility. Will we support the use of *in vitro* fertilization and embryo transfer because it provides a "child of *one's own*," in a strict sense of *one's own,* to a married couple? Or will we support the transfer because it is treatment of involuntary infertility, which deserves treatment in or out of marriage, hence endorsing the use of any available technical means (which would produce a healthy and normal child), including surrogate wombs, or even ectogenesis?

Second, logic aside, the opponents of the wedge argument do not counsel well. It would be simply foolish to ignore what might come next, and to fail to make the *best possible* assessment of the implications of present action (or inaction). Let me put the matter very bluntly: the Ethics Advisory Board, in the decision it must now make, may very well be helping to decide whether human beings will eventually be produced in laboratories. I say this not to shock—and I do not mean to beg the question of whether that would be desirable or not. I say this to make sure that they and we face squarely the full import and magnitude of this decision. Once the genies let the babies into the bottle, it may be impossible to get them out again.

VIII

So much, then, for the meaning of initiating and manipulating human embryos in the laboratory. These considerations still make me doubt the wisdom of proceeding with these practices, both in research and in their clinical application, notwithstanding that valuable knowledge might be had by continuing the research and identifiable suffering might be alleviated by using it to circumvent infertility. To doubt the wisdom of going ahead makes one at least a fellow-traveller of the opponents of such research, but it does not, either logically or practically, require that one join them in trying to prevent it, say by legal prohibition. Not every folly can or should be legislated against. Attempts at prohibition here would seem to be both ineffective and dangerous—ineffective because impossible to enforce, dangerous because the costs of such precedent-setting interference with scientific research might be greater than the harm it prevents. To be sure, we already have legal restrictions on experimentation with human subjects, which restrictions are manifestly not incompatible with the progress of medical science. Neither is it true that science cannot survive if it must take some direction from the law. Nor is it the case that all research, because it is research, is or should be absolutely protected. But it does not seem to me that *in vitro* fertilization and embryo transfer deserve, *at least at present,* to be treated as sufficiently dangerous for legislative interference.

But if to doubt the wisdom does not oblige one to seek to outlaw the folly, neither does a decision *to permit* require a decision to *encourage or support.* A researcher's freedom to do *in vitro* fertilization, or a woman's right to have a child with laboratory assistance, in no way implies a public (or even a private) obligation to pay for such research or treatment. A right *against* interference is not an entitlement *for assistance.* The question before the Ethics Advisory Board and the Department of Health, Education, and Welfare is *not* whether to permit such research but whether the Federal government should fund it. This is the policy question that needs to be discussed.

The arguments in favor of Federal support are well known. *First,* the research is seen as continuous with, if not quite an ordinary instance of, the biomedical research, which the Federal government supports handsomely; roughly two-thirds of the money spent on biomedical research in the United States comes from Uncle Sam. Why is this research different from all other research? Its scientific merit has been attested to by the normal peer-review process at NIH. For some, that is a sufficient reason to support it.

Second, there are specific practical fruits expected from the anticipated successes of this new line of research. Besides relief for many cases of infertility, the research promises new birth-control measures based upon improved understanding of the mechanisms of fertilization and implantation, which in turn could lead to techniques for blocking these processes. Also, studies on early embryonic development hold forth the promise of learning how to prevent some congenital malformations and certain highly malignant tumors (e.g., hydatidiform mole) that derive from aberrant fetal tissue.

Third, as he who pays the piper calls the tune, Federal support would make easy the Federal regulation and supervision of this research. For the government to abstain, so the argument runs, is to leave the control of research and clinical application in the hands of profit-hungry, adventurous, insensitive, reckless, or power-hungry private physicians, scientists, or drug companies; or, on the other hand, at the mercy of the vindictive, mindless, and superstitious civic groups that will interfere with this research through state and local legislation. Only through Federal regulation—which, it is said, can only follow with Federal funding—can we have reasonable, enforceable, and uniform guidelines.

Fourth is the chauvinistic argument that the United States should lead the way in this brave new research, especially as it will apparently be going forward in other nations. Indeed, one witness testifying before the Ethics Advisory Board deplored the fact that the first Louise Brown was British and not American, and complained, in effect, that the existing moratorium on Federal support has already created what one might call an *"in vitro* fertilization gap." The pre-eminence of American science and technology, so the argument implies, is the center of our pre-eminence among the nations, a position which will be jeopardized if we hang back out of fear.

Let me respond to these arguments, in reverse order. Conceding the premise of the importance of American science for American prestige and strength, it is far from clear that failure to support *this* research would jeopardize American science. Certainly the use of embryo transfer to overcome infertility, though a vital matter for the couples involved, is hardly a matter of vital national interest—at least not unless and until the majority of American women are similarly infertile. The demands of international competition, admittedly often a necessary evil, should be invoked only for things that really matter; a missile gap and an embryo-transfer gap are chasms apart. In areas not crucial to our own survival, there will be many things we should allow other nations to develop, if that is their wish, without feeling obliged to join them. Moreover, one should not rush into potential folly to avoid being the last to commit it.

The argument about governmental regulation has much to recommend it. But it fails to consider that there are other safeguards against recklessness, at least in the clinical applications, known to the high-minded as the canons of medical ethics and to the cynical as liability for malpractice. Also, Federal regulations attached to Federal funding will not in any case regulate research done with private monies, say by the drug companies. Moreover, there are enough concerned practitioners of these new arts who would have a compelling interest in regulating their own practice, if only to escape the wrath and interference of hostile citizen groups in response to unsavory goings-on. The available evidence does not convince me that a sensible practice of *in vitro* experimentation requires regulation by the Federal government.

In turning to the argument about anticipated technological powers, we face difficult calculations of unpredictable and more-or-less-likely costs and benefits, and the all-important questions of priorities in the allocation of scarce resources. Here it seems useful to consider separately the techniques for generating children and the anticipated techniques for birth control or for preventing developmental anomalies and malignancies.

First, accepting that providing a child of their own to infertile couples is a worthy goal—and it is both insensitive and illogical to cite the population problem as an argument for ignoring the problem of infertility—one can nevertheless question its rank relative to other goals of medical research. One can even wonder—and I have done so in print—whether it is indeed a *medical* goal, or a worthy goal for *medicine,* that is, whether alleviating infertility, especially in this way, is part of the art of *healing.* [13] Just as abortion for genetic defect is a peculiar innovation in medicine (or in preventive medicine) in which a disease is treated by eliminating the patient (or, if you prefer, a disease is prevented by "preventing" the patient), so laboratory-fertilization is a peculiar treatment for oviduct obstruction, in that it requires the creation of a new life to "heal" an existing one. All this simply emphasizes the uniqueness of the reproductive organs, in that their proper function involves other people, and calls attention to the fact that infertility is not a "disease," like heart disease or stroke, even though obstruction of a normally patent tube or vessel is the proximate cause of each.

However this may be, there is a more important objection to this approach to the problem. It represents yet another instance of our thoughtless preference for expensive, high-technology, therapy-oriented approaches to disease and dysfunctions. What about spending this money on discovering the causes of infertility? What about the prevention of tubal obstruction? We complain about rising medical costs, but we insist on the most spectacular and the most technological—and thereby the most costly—remedies.

The truth is that we do know a little about the causes of tubal obstruction—though much less than we should or could. For instance, it is estimated that at least one-third of such cases are the aftermath of pelvic-inflammatory disease, caused by that uninvited venereal guest, gonococcus. Leaving aside any question about whether it makes sense for a Federally-funded baby to be the wage of aphrodisiac indiscretion,[14] one can only look with wonder at a society that will have "petri-dish babies"[15] before it has found a vaccine against gonorrhea.

True, there are other causes of blocked oviducts, and blocked oviducts are not the only cause of female infertility. True, it is not logically necessary to choose between prevention and cure. But *practically* speaking, with money for research as limited as it is, research funds targeted for the relief of infertility should certainly go first to epidemiological and preventive measures—especially where the costs in the high-technology cure are likely to be great.

What about these costs? I have already explored some of the nonfinancial costs, in discussing the meaning of this research for our images of humanness. Let us, for now, consider only the financial costs. How expensive was Louise Brown? We do not know, partly because Drs. Edwards and Steptoe have yet to publish their results, indicating how many failures preceded their success, how many procedures for egg removal and for fetal monitoring were performed on Mrs. Brown, and so on. One must add in the costs of monitoring the baby's development to check on her "normality" and, should it come, the costs of governmental regulation. A conservative estimate might place the costs of a successful pregnancy of this kind at between five and ten thousand dollars. If we use the conservative figure of 500,000 for estimating the number of infertile women *with blocked oviducts* in the United States whose *only* hope of having children lies in *in vitro* fertilization,[16] we reach a conservative estimated cost of $2.5 to $5 billion. Is it really even fiscally wise for the Federal government to start down this road?

Clearly not, if it is also understood that the costs of providing the service, rendered possible by a successful technology, will also be borne by the taxpayers. Nearly everyone now agrees that the kidney-machine legislation, obliging the Federal government to pay about

$25,000–$30,000 per patient per year for kidney dialysis for anyone in need (cost to the taxpayers in 1978 was nearly $1 billion), is an impossible precedent—notwithstanding that individual lives have been prolonged as a result. But once the technique of *in vitro* fertilization and embryo transfer is developed and available, how should the baby-making be paid for? Should it be covered under medical insurance? If a National Health Insurance program is enacted, will and should these services be included? (Those who argue that they are part of medicine will have a hard time saying no.) Failure to do so will make this procedure available only to the well-to-do, on a fee-for-service basis. Would that be a fair alternative? Perhaps; but it is unlikely to be tolerated. Indeed, the principle of equality—equal access to equal levels of medical care—is the leading principle in the pressure for medical reform. One can be certain that efforts will be forthcoming to make this procedure available equally to all, independent of ability to pay, under Medicaid or National Health Insurance or in some other way. (I have recently learned that a Boston-based group concerned with infertility has obtained private funding to pay for artificial insemination for women on welfare!!)

Much as I sympathize with the plight of infertile couples, I do not believe that they are entitled to the provision of a child at the public expense, especially at this cost, especially by a procedure that also involves so many moral difficulties. Given the many vexing dilemmas that will surely be spawned by laboratory-assisted reproduction, the Federal government should not be misled by compassion to embark on this imprudent course.

In considering the Federal funding of such research for its other anticipated technological benefits, independent of its clinical use in baby-making, we face a more difficult matter. In brief, as is the case with all basic research, one simply cannot predict what kinds of techniques and uses this research will yield. But here, also, I think good sense would at present say that before one undertakes *human in vitro* fertilization to seek new methods of birth control—e.g., by developing antibodies to the human egg that would physically interfere with its fertilization—one should make adequate attempts to do this in animals. One simply can't get large-enough numbers of human eggs to do this pioneering research well—at least not without subjecting countless women to additional risks not for their immediate benefit. Why not test this conceit first in the mouse or rabbit? Only if the results were very promising—and judged also to be relatively safe in practice—should one consider trying such things in humans. Likewise, the developmental research can and should be first carried out in animals, especially in primates. Though *in vitro* fertilization has yet to be achieved in monkeys, embryo transfer of *in vivo* fertilized eggs has been accomplished, thus permitting the relevant research to proceed. Purely *on scientific grounds,* the Federal government ought not *now* to be investing funds in this research for its promised technological benefits—benefits which, in the absence of pilot studies in animals, must be regarded as mere wishful thoughts in the imaginings of scientists.

There remains the first justification, research for the sake of knowledge: knowledge about cell cleavage, cell-cell and cell-environment interactions, and cell differentiation; knowledge of gene action and of gene regulation; knowledge of the effects and mechanisms of action of various chemical and physical agents on growth and development; knowledge of the basic processes of fertilization and implantation. This is all knowledge worth having, and though much can be learned using animal sources—and these sources have barely begun to be sufficiently exploited—the investigation of these matters in man would, sooner or later, require the use of human-embryonic material. Here, again, there are questions of research priority about which there is room for disagreement, among scientists and laymen alike. But these questions of research priority, while not irrelevant to the decision at hand, are not the questions that the Ethics Advisory Board was constituted to answer.

It was constituted to consider whether such research is consistent with the ethical standards of our community. The question turns in large part on the status of the early embryo. If, as I have argued, the early embryo is deserving of respect because of what it is, now and potentially, it is difficult to justify submitting it to invasive experiments, and especially difficult to justify *creating it solely* for the purpose of experimentation. But even if this argument fails to sway the Board, another one should. For their decision, I remind you, is not whether *in vitro* fertilization should be permitted in the United States, but whether *our* tax dollars should encourage and foster it. One cannot, therefore, ignore the deeply held convictions of a sizeable portion of our population—it may even be a majority on this issue—that regards the human embryo as protectable humanity, not to be experimented upon except for its own benefit. Never mind if these beliefs have a religious foundation—as if that should ever be a reason for dismissing them! The presence, sincerity, and depth of these beliefs, and the grave importance of their subject, is what must concern us. The holders of these beliefs have been very much alienated by the numerous court decisions and legislative enactments regarding abortion and research on fetuses. Many who, by and large, share their opinions about the humanity of prenatal life have with heavy heart gone along with the liberalization of abortion, out of deference to the wishes, desires, interests, or putative rights of pregnant women. But will they go along here with what they can only regard as gratuitous and willful assaults on human life, or at least on potential and salvageable human life, and on human dignity? We can ill afford to alienate them further, and it would be unstatesmanlike, to say the least, to do so, especially in a matter so little important to the national health and one so full of potential dangers.

Technological progress can be but one measure of our national health. Far more important is the affection and esteem in which our citizenry holds its laws and institutions. No amount of relieved infertility is worth the further disaffection and civil contention that the lifting of the moratorium on Federal funding is likely to produce. People opposed to abortion and people grudgingly willing to permit women to obtain elective abortion, at their own expense, will not tolerate having their tax money spent on scientific research requiring what they regard as at best cruelty, at worst murder. A prudent Ethics Advisory Board and a prudent and wise Secretary of Health, Education, and Welfare should take this matter most seriously, and refuse to lift the moratorium—at least until they are persuaded that public opinion will overwhelmingly support them. Imprudence in this matter may be the worst sin of all.

An Afterword

This has been for me a long and difficult exposition. Many of the arguments are hard to make. It is hard to get confident people to face unpleasant prospects. It is hard to get many people to take seriously such "soft" matters as lineage, identity, respect, and self-respect when they are in tension with such "hard" matters as a cure for infertility or new methods of contraception. It is hard to talk about the meaning of sexuality and embodiment in a culture that treats sex increasingly as sport and that has trivialized the significance of gender, marriage, and procreation. It is hard to oppose Federal funding of baby-making in a society which increasingly demands that the Federal government supply all demands, and which—contrary to so much evidence of waste, incompetence, and corruption—continues to believe that only Uncle Sam can do it. And, finally, it is hard to speak about restraint in a culture that seems to venerate very little above man's own attempt to master all. Here, I am afraid, is the biggest question and the one we perhaps can no longer ask or deal with: the question about the reasonableness of the desire to become masters and possessors of nature, human nature included.

Here we approach the deepest meaning of *in vitro* fertilization.

Those who have likened it to artificial insemination are only partly correct. With *in vitro* fertilization, the human embryo emerges for the first time from the natural darkness and privacy of its own mother's womb, where it is hidden away in mystery, into the bright light and utter publicity of the scientist's laboratory, where it will be treated with unswerving rationality, before the clever and shameless eye of the mind and beneath the obedient and equally clever touch of the hand. What does it mean to hold the beginning of human life before your eyes, in your hands—even for 5 days (for the meaning does not depend on duration)? Perhaps the meaning is contained in the following story:

Long ago there was a man of great intellect and great courage. He was a remarkable man, a giant, able to answer questions that no other human being could answer, willing boldly to face any challenge or problem. He was a confident man, a masterful man. He saved his city from disaster and ruled it as a father rules his children, revered by all. But something was wrong in his city. A plague had fallen on generation; infertility afflicted plants, animals, and human beings. The man confidently promised to uncover the cause of the plague and to cure the infertility. Resolutely, dauntlessly, he put his sharp mind to work to solve the problem, to bring the dark things to light. No secrets, no reticences, a full public inquiry. He raged against the representatives of caution, moderation, prudence, and piety, who urged him to curtail his inquiry; he accused them of trying to usurp his rightfully earned power, of trying to replace human and masterful control with submissive reverence. The story ends in tragedy: He solved the problem but, in making visible and public the dark and intimate details of his origins, he ruined his life, and that of his family. In the end, too late, he learns about the price of presumption, of overconfidence, of the overweening desire to master and control one's fate. In symbolic rejection of his desire to look into everything, he punishes his eyes with self-inflicted blindness.

Sophocles seems to suggest that such a man is always in principle—albeit unwittingly—a patricide, a regicide, and a practitioner of incest. We men of modern science may have something to learn from our forebear, Oedipus. It appears that Oedipus, being the kind of man an Oedipus is (the chorus calls him a paradigm of man), had no choice but to learn through suffering. Is it really true that we too have no other choice?

NOTES

1. In the British procedures, several eggs are taken from each woman and fertilized, to increase the chance of success, but only one embryo is transferred for implan-

tation. In Dr. Soupart's proposed experiments, as the embryos will be produced only for the purpose of research and not for transfer, all of them will be discarded or destroyed.

2. A perhaps justifiable exception would be the case of a universal plague on childbirth, say because of some epidemic that fatally attacks all fetuses *in utero* at age 5 months. Faced with the prospect of the end of the race, might we not condone the deliberate institution of pregnancies to provide fetuses for research, in the hope of finding a diagnosis and remedy for this catastrophic blight?

3. Peter Gwynne, "Was the Birth of Louise Brown Only a Happy Accident?" *Science Digest,* October 1978, (emphasis added).

4. For the supporting analysis of the concept of "viability," see my article, "Determining Death and Viability in Fetuses and Abortuses," prepared for the National Commission for the Protection of Human Subjects of Biomedical and Behavioral Research, published in *Appendix: Research on the Fetus,* U.S. Department of Health, Education, and Welfare, HEW Publ. No. (OS) 76-128, 1975.

5. Some people have suggested that the embryo be regarded like a vital organ, salvaged from a newly dead corpse, usable for transplantation or research, and that its donation by egg and sperm donors be governed by the Uniform Anatomical Gift Act, which legitimates pre-mortem consent for organ donation upon death. But though this acknowledges that embryos are not things, it is mistaken in treating embryos as mere organs, thereby overlooking that they are early stages of a *complete, whole* human being. The Uniform Anatomical Gift Act does not apply to, nor should it be stretched to cover, donations of gonads, gametes (male sperm or female eggs), or—especially—zygotes and embryos.

6. There is a good chance that the problem of surplus embryos may be avoidable, for purely technical reasons. Some researchers believe that the uterine receptivity to the transferred embryo might be reduced during the particular menstrual cycle in which the ova are obtained, because of the effects of the hormones given to induce superovulation. They propose that the harvested *eggs* be frozen, and then defrosted one at a time each month for fertilization, culture, and transfer, until pregnancy is achieved. By refusing to fertilize all the eggs at once—i.e., not placing all one's eggs in one uterine cycle—there will not be surplus *embryos,* but at most only surplus eggs. This change in the procedure would make the demise of unimplanted embryos *exactly* analogous to the "natural" embryonic loss in ordinary reproduction.

7. The literature on intervention in reproduction is both confused and confusing on the crucial matter of the meanings of "nature" or "the natural," and their significance for the ethical issues. It may be as much a mistake to claim that "the natural" has *no* moral force as to suggest that the natural way is best, because natural. Though shallow and slippery thought about nature, and its relation to "good," is a likely source of these confusions, the nature of nature may itself be elusive, making it difficult for even careful thought to capture what is natural.

8. An unmarried woman in Dearborn, Michigan, offered to bear a child for her married friend, infertile because of a hysterectomy. She was impregnated by artificial insemination using semen produced by her friend's husband, his wife performing the injection. The threesome lived together all during the pregnancy. The child was delivered at birth by the biological-and-gestational-mother to the wife-and-rearing-mother. The first (pregnancy) mother reports no feelings of attachment to the child she carried and bore. Everyone is reportedly delighted with the event. The trio has publicized its accomplishment and is reported to be considering selling rights to the story for a TV show, a book, and a movie. Their attorney has been swamped with letters requesting similar surrogate "mothers." (*American Medical News,* July 28, 1978, pp. 11–12.)

9. There are today numerous suits pending, throughout the United States, because of artificial insemination with donor semen (AID). Following divorce, the ex-husbands are refusing child support for AID children, claiming, minimally, no paternity, or maximally that the child was the fruit of an adulterous "union." In fact, a few states still treat AID as adultery. The importance of anonymity is revealed in the following bizarre case. A woman wanted to have a child, but abhorred the thought of marriage or of sexual relations with men. She learned a do-it-yourself technique of artificial insemination, and persuaded a male acquaintance to donate his semen. Now some 10 years after this virgin birth, the case has gone to court. The semen donor is suing for visitation privileges, to see his son.

10. To those who point out that the bond between sexuality and procreation has already been effectively and permanently cleaved by "the pill," and that this is therefore an idle worry in the case of *in vitro* fertilization, it must be said that the pill provides only sex without babies. Now the other shoe drops; babies without sex.

11. *Science, 202:5,* October 6, 1978.

12. Some of these questions are addressed, albeit too briefly and polemically, in the latter part of my 1972 "Making Babies" article, to which the reader is referred. It has been pointed out to me by an astute colleague that the tone of the present article is less passionate and more accommodating than the first, which change he regards as an ironic demonstration of the inexorable way in which we get used to, and accept, our technological nightmares. I myself share his concern. I cannot decide whether the decline of my passion is to be welcomed; that is, whether it is due to greater understanding bred of more thought and experience, or to greater callousness and the contempt of familiarity bred from *too much* thought and experience. It does seem to me now that many of the fundamental beliefs and institutions that might be challenged by laboratory growth of human embryos and by laboratory-assisted reproduction are already severely challenged in perhaps more potent and important ways. Here, too, we see the creeping effect of the aggregated powers of modernity and the corrosive power of the familiar. Adaptiveness is our glory and our curse: as Raskolnikov put it, "Man gets used to everything, the beast!"

13. See "Making Babies—the New Biology and the 'Old' Morality," pp. 19–20. See also my "Regarding the End of Medicine and the Pursuit of Health," *The Public Interest,* Number 40, Summer 1975, especially pp. 11–18, and 33–35.

14. Consider the following contributions of Federally-supported programs to rationalizing our sexual and reproductive practices. First, we have Federally-supported programs of sex education in elementary schools, so that the children will know what can happen to them (and what they can make happen). Next, in high school, Uncle Sam provides for teen-age contraception, to prevent the consequences of unavoidable sexual activity. Freed of a major deterrent to unrestricted sexual activity, our teen-agers indulge, but not without consequences: They get gonorrhea, which some of them will have treated, again at the taxpayers' expense through Medicaid. But for some the treatment comes too late to prevent scarring and oviduct obstruction: Federally-supported *in vitro* fertilization research and services come to the rescue, to overcome their infertility. Uncle Sam will, of course, also provide Aid to Dependent Children, if the mother is or goes on welfare.

15. There has been much objection, largely from the scientific community, to the phrase "test-tube baby." More than one commentator has deplored the exploitation of its "flesh-creeping" connotations. They point out that a flat petridish is used, not a test-tube—as if that mattered—and that the embryo spends but a few days in the dish. But they don't ask why the term "test-tube baby" remains the popular designation, and whether it does not embody more of the deeper truth than a more accurate, laboratory appellation. If the decisive difference is between "in the womb" or "in the lab,"

the popular designation conveys it. (See 'Afterword', below.) And it is right on target, and puts us on notice, if the justification for the present laboratory procedures tacitly also *justifies* future extensions, including full ectogenesis—say, if that were the only way a womb-less woman could have a child of her own, without renting a human womb from a surrogate bearer.

16. This figure is calculated from estimates that between 10 and 15 percent of all couples are involuntarily infertile, and that in more than half of these cases the cause is in the female. Blocked oviducts account for perhaps 20 percent of the causes of female infertility. Perhaps 50 percent of these women might be helped to have a child by means of reconstructive surgery on the oviducts; the remainder could conceive *only* with the aid of laboratory fertilization and embryo transfer. These estimates do not include additional candidates with uterine disease (who could "conceive" only by embryo transfer to surrogate-gestators), nor those with ovarian dysfunction who would need egg donation as well, nor that growing population of women who have had tubal ligations and who could later turn to *in vitro* fertilization. It is also worth noting that not all the infertile couples are childless; indeed, a surpassing number are seeking to enlarge an existing family.

27 External Human Fertilization: An Evaluation of Policy

CLIFFORD GROBSTEIN
MICHAEL FLOWER
JOHN MENDELOFF

This article summarizes many of the practices being developed internationally with respect to new birth technologies. The authors describe and evaluate several of these practices, especially in light of their clinical success. Also provided are estimates concerning cost and projections for the demand and supply of such services. On the basis of these data, various policies as well as social, ethical and legal questions are discussed.

Clifford Grobstein is Professor of Biological Sciences and Public Policy. Michael Flowers is an Assistant Research Biologist. John Menideloff is an Assistant Professor of Political Science. All teach at the University of California, San Diego

The first child resulting from fertilization of a human egg outside the body of its mother was born in England on 25 July 1978 (*1, 2*). An assessment of the clinical technology of in vitro fertilization (IVF) thus covers a 5-year period, although related laboratory studies had been under way much earlier (*3*).

Our objective is to offer an early appraisal of a procedure that has engendered significant controversy, both with respect to the procedure itself and to what can be viewed as an opening wedge to broader intervention in human reproduction, heredity, and development (*4*). A series of potential public policy questions can be envisioned that may strain the capability of existing decision mechanisms.

Since the initial clinical success in England, diffusion of the technology has occurred from the pioneer centers in England and Australia to the United States, Europe, and elsewhere (*5*). The diffusion is likely to continue during the next 5 years, as judged by the demand of sterile couples and the heightened efficacies reported by established centers (6, 7). In this article, we will address some of the derivative issues, indicate directions of current policy formation, and touch on the mechanisms being employed for policy decision. Some longer range options and appropriate oversight for such possible developments are also considered.

MOTIVATION, EFFICACY, AND SAFETY

In vitro fertilization falls within the realm of traditional medical motivation—to remove a limitation on normal healthy life. The specific initial objective was to overcome female sterility produced by absence or blockage of the fallopian tubes or oviducts, a condition estimated to occur in some 500,000 American women (8, p. 37). Since the oviducts are normal passageways for egg transport from ovary to uterus, as well as for sperm transport from the vagina and uterus to the egg, fertilization cannot occur without technological intervention. Surgical interventions have been practiced with some success, but there is a significant residue of cases in which surgery is unsuccessful (9).

The rationale for IVF and related procedures is to circumvent the block in the oviduct by (i) capturing the mature egg by laparoscopy just before it would be discharged from its follicle (ovulation), (ii) transferring it to a compatible external medium in which it can be exposed to sperm, (iii) allowing fertilization and early development to occur in the controlled environment of an incubator, and (iv) returning the egg to the natural internal environment beyond the oviductal blockage by inserting it through the cervix into the uterine cavity. The technology is theoretically as simple and direct as the motivation. Both the technology and the motivation, however, become more complicated as theory is turned into practice (10).

The intent of IVF is to provide a baby to an otherwise sterile couple. How well does the procedure accomplish its objective? Available published data (Table 1) (11), though still limited, indicate that efficacy has been significantly improving. For example, the first two births reported by Steptoe, Edwards, and Purdy (12) resulted from a series of 109 embryo transfers (the number of laparoscopies was not reported). This is a success rate (births per embryo transfer) just below 2 percent. The same clinical group (10, p. 414) more recently reported a series of cases involving 330 laparoscopies that resulted in 195 embryo transfers yielding 46 pregnancies. At the time of the report two babies had been delivered, and there were 29 stable pregnancies—an anticipated success rate of about 9 percent (births per laparoscopy). Other groups (Table 1) have reported similar rising success rates with increas-

Table 1. Summary of results from reporting IVF clinics. Successive entries for the same group represent more recent clinical series. Abbreviation: N.R., not reported.

Clinic	Laparo-scopies	Em-bryo trans-fers*	Preg-nancies	Efficacy (%)		Ref-erence
				Preg-nancies/laparo-scopy	Preg-nancies/embryo transfer	
Kershaw's Hospital, Oldham, England	N.R.	77	3		4	(10)
	65	32	4	6	13	(10)
Bourn Hall, Cambridge, England	330	195	46	14	24	(10)
Queen Victoria Medical Centre, Melbourne, Australia	112		16	14		(31)
	252	218	27	11	12	(7)
	90	70	25	28	36	(56)
Royal Women's Hospital, Melbourne, Australia	392	191	8	2	4	(10)
	N.R.	102	14		14	(47)
Eastern Virginia Medical School, Norfolk	40	9	0	0	0	(6)
	31	12	2	6	17	(6)
	24	19	5	21	26	(6)
	79	63	14	18	22	(52)
University of Kiel, Kiel, West Germany	185	19	2	1	11	(10, 53)
Hôpital Antoine Becléré, Clamart, France	139	24	5	4	21	(10)
Hôpital de Sévres, Sévres, France	77	5	2	3	40	(10)
University of Southern California School of Medicine, Los Angeles	28	14	2	7	14	(54)
	16	11	3	18	27	(54)
University of Vienna Medical School, Vienna, Austria	65	19	4	6	21	(10)
University of Göteborg, Göteborg, Sweden	58	3	0	0	0	(10)
University of Adelaide, Adelaide, South Australia	54	27	1	2	4	(55)
Royal North Shore Hospital, Sydney, Australia	N.R.	N.R.	1			(23)
Total	2037	1110	184	8†	16.5	

*One or more embryos per embryo transfer. †Based on the 166 pregnancies achieved after 2037 reported laparoscopies.

483

ing experience (7, 13). The clinical groups with greatest experience (Cambridge, England; Norfolk, Virginia; and two centers in Melbourne, Australia) have now formally reported series of cases with success rates for pregnancies per laparoscopy approaching 20 percent (6, 7).

Major technical modifications have also improved efficacy. For example, hormonally controlled cycles yield multiple instead of single mature eggs (14), incubation before fertilization permits full maturation of externalized eggs (15, 16), and transfer of more than one egg to the uterus increases the pregnancy rate (6, 15). Rates of success of egg recovery, of fertilization, and of achievement of early embryonic cleavage are each reported to be around 90 percent (6, 17, 18). The success of embryo transfer, however, is much lower (6, 7). For example, Table 1 shows a composite total of 1110 embryo transfers leading to 184 pregnancies—a success rate of nearly 17 percent. In contrast, estimates of success in the natural process suggest that roughly 45 percent of fertilized ova achieve implantation (19). Thus the success of embryo transfer in IVF is only about 40 percent that of the comparable phase in the natural process.

Among initial concerns about IVF (20) was the possibility of harm either to the potential offspring or to the mother. For the mother there are two identifiable risks—from the surgical procedures themselves or from the establishment of an ectopic pregnancy (outside of the uterus). Results to date diminish concern about surgical risk. Among more than 2000 laparoscopies for egg recovery, only a single event potentially affecting health or safety has been reported (21). This is a risk well within that of laparoscopy used for other purposes.

Published reports to date show two out of 184 IVF pregnancies that were ectopic (22–24). Although the number of IVF pregnancies is still low, the reported rate of ectopic pregnancy is within the range (0.3 to 3 percent) for the natural process (25). It also is below the recorded rate for pregnancies achieved following tuboplasty to overcome more complex forms of oviductal blockage (26).

Two concerns have been expressed about risk to the embryo—excessive death of early embryos and induced congenital abnormality in those born. It is clear that while the wastage rate is high in the normal process (27) it is even higher in the technology-assisted process. Estimates of the added deaths in the case of IVF must include both the high number of embryos lost during development of the technology and the lower number at its current level of efficacy. Evaluation of the excess of IVF deaths is complicated not only by the hotly debated issue of the status of the early human embryo but by the unresolved question of the percentage of the embryos that would have died anyway because of genetic or other defects. For the moment, it must be assumed that IVF has involved, and continues to involve, some un-quantifiable cost in a higher rate of early embryonic death.

In the matter of induced congenital abnormality, there are likewise no certain conclusions. The number of IVF conceptions and births is as yet insufficient to detect statistically a small increment of abnormality above the natural rate (28). Several abnormalities of IVF embryos have been reported (10, pp. 343–349); neither in number nor kind do they suggest that they were induced by the IVF procedure. Among approximately 125 IVF births (19), there has been only one abnormality reported (29), a cardiac malformation corrected by surgery. However, the earliest IVF children born are only approaching 5 years of age and subtle effects, such as neural defects impairing intelligence, might not yet be apparent. To summarize, there is no dramatic positive evidence reported for IVF-mediated damage to the more than 100 children estimated to have been born to date. Furthermore, whatever the risk to either mother or offspring, it has not proved high enough to deter either the professionals or prospective subjects who are using the procedure in increasing numbers. In fact in March 1982 the board of directors of the American Fertility Society stated that under appropriate specified cicumstances "in vitro fertilization must now be recognized as the acceptable treatment for achieving pregnancy for couples [in which the wife has] absent or irreparably damaged fallopian tubes" (30).

Feasible Extensions of the Basic IVF Procedure

When successful, IVF provides a child to a sterile couple. A number of possible variants of the basic procedure have been outlined (4), all well within technical capability but with quite different motivations and ethical, legal, and social consequences. These fall into several categories.

1) *Male infertility.* Several clinical groups are testing IVF involving male oligospermia—semen with low sperm count, low sperm motility, or other abnormality associated with infertility—and some success has been reported (18, 31, 32). The objective in this case is the same as that of the basic procedure—to provide a child to a sterile couple. New questions might be raised if the wife were fertile and IVF were performed on her to overcome a deficiency of her husband.

2) *Nonspousal sources of gametes (third party).* Biologically it would be expected that egg and sperm from any two fertile members of the human species could be combined to yield an embryo. If the embryo is returned to the uterus of a married donor, use of sperm other than from her husband (if he is also sterile) is equivalent to artificial

insemination by a donor (AID), a procedure that currently is countenanced but not encouraged in the United States. However, IVF also makes possible the converse procedure; that is, the egg might come from a female donor outside the marriage, and the husband might supply the sperm. The egg might be returned for gestation within the hormonally prepared uterus of the otherwise sterile wife. A rationale for such a procedure would be provided by a woman whose ovaries have been removed, but who has a normal uterus. The result of either IVF process, as in AID, would be a child genetically related to only one parent.

3) *Embryo transfer to a uterus other than that of the sterile donor.* The capability for embryo transfer to the hormonally prepared uterus of a nondonor of the egg makes possible several variants with different biological and social relations. The recipient might be a surrogate gestator who agrees to return the child to its genetic parents at birth. There is precedent for such surrogacy, by AID, to compensate for male sterility. The surrogacy option might also be applied simply to suit the convenience of the donor of an egg who did not want pregnancy but did want a child (analogous to wet-nursing). In another variation the recipient might be a woman who wants a child but without insemination, natural or artificial (*33*). In yet another variation, IVF might be used to yield a desired genetic combination without personal interaction, by combining egg and sperm from appropriate donors and transferring the embryo to a third party for gestation. This procedure would separate genetic selection completely from spouse selection and provide a technical base for human breeding programs.

There are few indications that efforts are being made to realize the options outlined above other than an interest [and an early report (*34*) from Melbourne (Queen Victoria Medical Centre)] in transferring "surplus" embryos from one treated couple to another sterile couple (embryo adoption).

4) *Freezing of embryos for storage.* This procedure is being performed by the Monash University Center in Melbourne, where a limited number of embryos have been frozen and viable ones transferred to a receptive uterus (*31*). A first success was reported as a 14-week pregnancy in early May 1983 (*35*). Freezing becomes an option because hormonal stimulation before laparoscopy yields multiple eggs that can be recovered in a single operation. This is advantageous because transfer of more than one embryo gives a higher pregnancy rate (*6, 15*), but also a higher twinning rate than normal, and because embryos not used in a first transfer attempt can be, if frozen and stored, used in a second transfer attempt without repetition of egg recovery.

However, if stored for longer periods, the embryos might constitute an embryo bank. It might, for example, be judged desirable to store embryos early in a marriage (not necessarily involving infertility) for use at some later times. This would provide the ultimate in family planning, as well as possibly allowing later childbearing without added risk of genetic defect (for example, Down syndrome). Success in identifying sex type in cattle embryos has been reported (36), and selection of sex of human offspring may not be far behind. Finally, embryo banks also make possible embryo adoption, if the genetic parents are willing to release the frozen embryos for transfer to other sterile couples or to any woman unable to bear her own child by the natural process.

A number of these extensions of the IVF process lie within the medical model—to correct disability limiting life or health, however these terms may be defined. Others, such as delayed embryo transfer for convenience, clearly go beyond the usual medical sphere. Also, in some of the extensions, such as embryo freezing, there may be added uncertainties as to safety and efficacy. Other species than the human appear to differ in their capability to withstand freezing (37), and there is little reliable information on possible sublethal damage that might become manifest subsequently in offspring.

Nonetheless, it is clear that all the extensions outlined above are within the present technical orbit—that is, if attempted, they are likely to yield some degree of success. In that sense they constitute a set of technological options ready for consideration for developmental trial. The set is not exhaustive since it does not include the possible application of several significant manipulations carried out successfully on mouse embryos at stages comparable to human embryos before transfer; an example is the insertion and expression of genes (38). Nor does the set include the possible development externally of human embryos to stages beyond those needed for transfer to the uterus. Such technical options would have to be undertaken, if at all, under rationales entirely different from those of the original medical impulse toward IVF. Nevertheless, the more direct IVF extensions seem already profound enough in ethical, legal, and social implication to warrant careful policy consideration. The process has begun in Australia and England, but in the United States there has been a hiatus since the report of the Ethics Advisory Board to the secretary of the Department of Health, Education and Welfare in 1979 (8). Several policy issues are discussed in the following sections.

COST AND ITS ALLOCATION

Information about prices charged to patients enrolled in IVF programs is relatively easy to obtain, but determination of the full actual costs of the services is more difficult. The analysis below is based on data from the clinic at the Eastern Virginia Medical School in Norfolk, the first IVF program in the United States. The prices do not appear to differ substantially from those reported at other IVF centers, both here and abroad.

The basic charges to patients at Norfolk are $1650 for a preliminary screening procedure to establish feasibility of subsequent egg recovery, of which $400 is a professional fee and $1000 a hospital expense (Table 2). Charges for a subsequent attempt at egg recovery and embryo transfer, including hospitalization, are $3100—that is, a total of almost $5000 for a single complete treatment, whether or not successful. Excluded are such nonmedical costs as travel, lodgings, time lost from a job, and so on.

From the basic charges and information on home states of Norfolk patients, estimates of actual costs to patients can be made (Table 2). A typical total cost to the patient for an initial treatment (screening plus laparoscopy plus embryo transfer) is about $7500, with each additional

Table 2. Cost estimates for the IVF procedure at Eastern Virginia Medical College, Norfolk. Transportation costs represent two round-trip tickets (husband and wife) from Chicago to Norfolk, the average travel distance for Norfolk patients. Lodging costs represent $30 per night plus $15 per day per person. The screening procedure requires 2 days each for husband and wife; the actual IVF procedure, egg recovery through embryo transfer, and monitoring for signs of pregnancy entails as many as 20 days for the wife and 2 days for the husband. On the basis of occupations of a sample of Norfolk couples, it is estimated that income is lost at a rate of $350 per week for the husband and $210 per week for working wives (approximately two-thirds of the wives are employed). The screening procedure entails the loss of 2 days wages for both husband and wife, while the remaining steps result in the loss of 2 days wages for the husband and as many as 15 days wages for working wives. If vacation or sick leave covers all lost wages for the screening visit and half the loss for the actual IVF procedure, total costs would be reduced by nearly $500. Deductibility of medical expenses from taxable income will also reduce the cost to the couple.

Cost category	Cost of IVF (dollars)	
	Screening	Actual procedure
IVF program		
Administrative charge	100	
Andrology survey	150	
Laboratory		
General		850
Early pregnancy		500
Pergonal		250
Professional fee	400	1000
Hospital deposit	1000	1000
Transportation	500	500
Lodging	120	930
Lost wages	195	560
Total	2465	5590

attempt (omitting screening) costing about $5000. At current levels of efficacy, estimated from overall published data at roughly 10 percent for a given laparoscopy (Table 1), something of the order of $38,000 would be required to ensure a roughly 50 percent chance of a live birth for a particular patient (34). For each child born, aggregate costs are about $50,000, borne by both the successful and unsuccessful couples. It is not unreasonable to anticipate that the overall efficacy could double (6, 7), thereby providing a significant economic saving, as well as reducing discomfort and inconvenience for subjects. By rough estimate, such improved efficacy would also make IVF economically advantageous in comparison with more complicated types of tubal surgery (5).

DEMAND AND SUPPLY OF SERVICES

As more IVF centers are established in the United States (40), it seems important to develop an estimate of the likely demand for and supply of services. Data on infertility from the 1976 National Survey of Family Growth (NSFG) (41) show that about 380,000 married women between 15 and 44, who have had both of their fallopian tubes removed or tied, say that they would like to become pregnant. Adjustments for husband-wife concurrence and for reduced fertility in women over 35 lower the figure for actual candidates to roughly 150,000. In addition, both clinical (42) and survey data (41) indicate that about 850,000 other women have sufficient tubal damage to make pregnancy difficult, if not impossible. If 40 percent of these want children (a reasonable estimate based on the NSFG data), there are another 340,000 potential couples for IVF. If 15 percent of these achieve pregnancy without IVF, 290,000 candidates remain, and together with the 150,000 women without functional fallopian tubes, this constitutes a total pool of 440,000 potential couples for IVF. On the basis of a 12-year period of candidacy for IVF (for a woman between 22 and 34 years of age) and the assumption that each couple would seek only one child, there would be 36,000 candidates annually for IVF because of tubal problems alone.

Rough estimates suggest that if IVF were to be used for idiopathic infertility, oligospermia, and embryo transfers to nondonors the number of candidates might double, to 70,000 patients per year (41, 42). Because a pool of candidates has accumulated, the number seeking IVF is greater now than it will be when this pool is reduced. The percentage of actual candidates is, of course, subject to a number of factors, including insurance coverage, distance to a center, other treatment alternatives, and perceptions of IVF success rate. Because it is not possible to set precise values for any of these variables, we had to choose figures judged to be reasonable (43). For example, if 50 percent choose to attempt IVF the resultant estimated demand clearly is far greater than existing supply—defined as the capacity to deliver services by centers already initiated (see below).

In projecting the possible supply of providers, the first factor to consider is the attitude of specialists dealing with infertility, since establishment of an IVF clinic generally will begin with motivated physicians. Desire to improve treatment effectiveness, to increase income, to enhance prestige and opportunities for productive research are all possible motivations for physicians. Given the technical nature of the procedure, linkage between a clinician and a reproductive biologist is a strong advantage, if not a necessity. Required proficiencies for a team include (i) general medical, (ii) surgical including use of anesthesia, (iii) special skills with laparoscopy, endocrinological monitoring and embryo culture, and (iv) specialized nursing and technical support. In addition, access must be ensured to surgical suites on a priority if not dedicated basis. All of this points to advantages in associating IVF, as it is currently practiced, with large hospitals, particularly those connected with academic medical centers. Many early centers conform to this pattern. In addition, the practice of IVF in settings devoted to infertility will allow its advantages to be objectively evaluated and compared with other treatment.

What number of centers may be required and what criteria need be applied to ensure optimum care? Although it is too early to give definite answers, it is not too early to pose the questions. Our estimates of demand, rough though they are, suggest that with availability of insurance 35,000 patients per year could seek treatment in the United States. The most mature IVF centers have between 200 and 400 patients per year; thus, about 100 centers could handle the estimated demand. Today there may be 10 to 20 established centers in this country, with an equal number in planning stages. Therefore the character of the potential expansion can still be carefully considered so as to yield optimum services economically and therapeutically. No attempts along these lines appear to have been made.

If centers are designed to handle several hundred patients per year, experience at the two Melbourne centers indicates that a team of about 25 persons is required at each center (31, 44). But does the success of a center depend on such a large team and volume of patients? If it does, then the procedure might be carried out in academic medical centers alone (currently there are more than 100). This would have certain advantages initially—quality control, ease of continued research, and relation to other relevant medical expertise. It would also have disadvantages—exclusion of non-academic practitioners, inhibition to miniaturization of the procedure, and excessive emphasis in residency training with possible overproduction of practitioners.

Were the procedure not limited to large centers and large volumes of patients, what then would be the optimum size and distribution of centers in terms of quality and economic considerations? What need is there for setting minimum standards for practitioners and groups? While accessibility of services (and hence certain costs) would be improved if centers were diversified in size and character to fit local circumstances, the problems of quality control would be considerably increased.

Current Status of Relevant Policy

The report of the Ethics Advisory Board (*8*, pp. 13–15) of the Department of Health, Education and Welfare (now Health and Human Services) provides a brief history of the beginnings of federal consideration of IVF. By August 1975 the department had issued regulations that included the following:

> No application or proposal (for research) involving human *in vitro* fertilization may be funded by the Department or any component thereof until the application or proposal has been received by the [Ethics Advisory Board] and the Board has rendered advice as to its acceptability from an ethical standpoint.

There has been no further formal federal policy statement relating to IVF since 1975. Moreover, the advisory board was dissolved shortly after releasing its report in 1979. Accordingly, there is a de facto moratorium on federal support of IVF-related research but no other formulated governmental policy affecting the private sector either with respect to IVF research or practice.

Despite unofficial status, the recommendations of the Ethics Advisory Board are noteworthy since they suggest the kind of policy issues that are raised by IVF. The board's chief conclusions were (*8*, p. 100):

1) The human embryo is entitled to profound respect; but this does not necessarily encompass the full legal and moral rights attributed to persons.

2) The department should consider supporting animal experimentation relevant to IVF.

3) Research on human IVF is ethically acceptable, providing: regulations governing research with human subjects are complied with; the purpose of the research relates primarily to safety and efficacy of

IVF; resulting embryos are not carried in the laboratory beyond implantation stages; the public is advised if risks of producing abnormal offspring through IVF exceed the normal; and all embryos transferred to the uterus are derived from married couples.

4) Proposed research on IVF-derived embryos for purposes other than relief of infertility should be referred for specific Board consideration.

5) The National Institute for Child Health and Human Development should take positive steps to collect national and international data on all aspects of IVF.

6) The Secretary should provide leadership to develop a model law on the legal status of IVF offspring.

The demise of the Ethics Advisory Board came shortly after the creation of the President's Commission for the Study of Ethical Problems in Medicine and Biomedical and Behavioral Research early in 1980. When asked by Senators Edward Kennedy and Orrin Hatch to comment on the six recommendations, the new commission responded that it was satisfied with the adequacy and thoroughness of the study, that the conclusions seemed well-supported, and that the commission might itself take up additional issues. However, at the time of its own termination of authority, in March 1983, the commission had not done so (45, p. 46).

No state has formulated policy specifically addressed to IVF. When planning began to establish the first IVF center in the United States at Norfolk, local groups opposed to IVF sought to block the effort. They were unsuccessful in getting any inhibitory action at either the local or state level. In Massachusetts a law (46) governing fetal research has been interpreted as possibly preventing IVF. A legislative effort to clarify the law to exclude IVF from possible proscription failed, and establishment of an IVF center in the state has been delayed by concern about prosecution under the fetal research law. In Tennessee, New York, Texas, and California, however, IVF centers have been established without challenge.

The practice of IVF primarily is spreading in the private sector and has apparently proceeded in ways that conform to the Ethics Advisory Board recommendations. This is not, however, the case abroad. In both Great Britain and Australia extensions of the basic procedure have been discussed and in certain instances, initiated. These developments have stimulated policy-making in each country that may be of interest in the United States.

Two independent centers in Melbourne, Australia, have put the city in the forefront of IVF practice in terms of numbers of patients treated and of births. Establishment of the centers was accompanied by considerable public discussion and controversy, eventually culminating in May 1982 in the formation, at the initiation of the attorney-general and minister of health of the State of Victoria, of a committee of citizens to consider the social, ethical and legal issues arising from in vitro fertilization. In part, the committee was formed in reaction to the policy of freezing extra embryos at one of the Melbourne centers and of the announced intention to make such embryos available, with the consent of the genetic parents, to sterile nondonor couples.

This citizen committee issued an interim report in September 1982 that contained a list of recommendations (47):

1) A campaign of public education on the nature, causes, and treatment of infertility should be initiated.

2) "Legislation to authorize hospitals as centers in which IVF programs may be conducted" should be enacted.

3) Evidence of 12 mnths or more of attempts to achieve pregnancy through "all other medical procedures" be required for admission to an IVF program.

4) IVF be limited to married couples, with all embryos returned to the donor.

5) Couples seeking IVF receive appropriate counseling.

The committee postponed making recommendations on freeze-thawing of embryos and their transfer to nondonors because disagreements among the members could not be resolved.

Meanwhile, the Australian National Health and Medical Research Council in September 1982 issued, on behalf of the federal government, revised ethical guidelines for the research that it supports. The council stated (48) that IVF "can be a justifiable means of treating infertility" with the approval of institutional ethics committees and within an "accepted family relationship." Although it is assumed that the procedure would normally involve sperm and eggs from married partners, the guidelines allow for egg donation by another woman (AID analogue) and sanction research on embryonic stages prior to implantation so long as the donors give consent.

In England the course has been a little different. The clinical success of the pioneer efforts of Edwards and Steptoe was greeted in 1978 by great publicity and excitement. Although reservations of several kinds were expressed and no public support had been specifically provided, there was sufficient public acceptance to allow an enlarged and better designed center to be established later in Cambridge. Other centers have since been established by other groups (10). However, statements by Edwards to the press and in a scientific paper (49) about advantages to be gained by embryo-freezing and by the experimental use of embryos to improve and extend IVF led to renewed controversy.

Prior to these events four study committees had been established to address concerns about IVF and possible research on human embryos. Two were created by medical professional groups (50), one by a private science and technology group, and one by the national government. The governmental report is expected in 1984.

In November 1982 the British Medical Research Council set out guiding principles for IVF (51); these are directed to its grantees but are likely to have implications beyond. The council sanctioned IVF research that is clinically relevant and involves no transfer of experimentally modified embryos for continued development in vivo. Informed consent from donors whose embryos may be manipulated is required. Surplus embryos from a therapeutic procedure may be used for experiments under the preceding stipulations. In addition, no surplus embryos may be cultured beyond the implantation stage and none may be stored (frozen) for unspecified research use. Experimentation on animal models is encouraged, and interspecific fertilization between human and nonhuman gametes is permitted as an aid to infertility studies, but no fertilized eggs thus produced may be carried beyond early cleavage.

In sum, it appears that as to efficacy, safety, and demand, the practice of IVF is moving toward or has already achieved established status as one therapeutic modality for human sterility. In Australia and Great Britain policy governing its use is actively being formulated; in several other countries, including the United States, application and development of the technique is proceeding solely on the initiative of health professionals and prospective patients. With few exceptions (none that we are aware of in the United States) the procedure is being applied only to married couples. Extensions beyond this, especially freezing of embryos and transfers involving third parties, are the subject of current study in Australia, England, and possibly other countries.

The Policy Horizon

Each of the possible extensions of IVF use noted earlier (4, 49) poses a somewhat different set of ethical, social, and political issues, and each therefore may constitute a different public policy problem. Moreover, the technical status of the several options varies, giving different estimated times at which each extension may become feasible. Thus, embryo freezing and storage is imminent technically whereas safe and successful genetic intervention in embryos, if it ever will be desirable, is technically some distance into the future. The policy problem is how to cope effectively with a series of sequential challenges to current practices and the resultant stresses on the mechanisms of policy formulation.

The problem is not too different from and indeed overlaps that recently considered by the President's Commission for the Study of Ethical Problems (45), which pointed to a number of anticipated impacts of rapidly growing knowledge of molecular genetics: production of drugs and biologics, cancer diagnosis and therapy, genetic screening and diagnosis, and the curing of genetic disorders. With respect to the last, the commission distinguished between genetic intervention in somatic and germinal cells, the latter case being possible by intervention in embryos (referred to as "embryo therapy"), and noted the uncertainties about both the feasibility and desirability of such therapy.

In surveying the range of possible applications of molecular genetics the commission called attention to the breadth and variety of concerns that are raised, more than enough to defy "a simple arithmetical calculation" (45, p. 51) (for example, cost-benefit or risk-benefit analysis). After spelling out the multiplicity of concerns, the commission turned to protecting the future. It suggested that suitable oversight is required by "an evaluation process that is continuing rather than sporadic," allowing "the review body to develop coherent standards and orderly procedures, while making provisions for unexpected development . . ." (45, p. 82). Moreover, the commission envisions a requirement for "a process that is broad-based rather than primarily expert" because the issues will not yield to technical considerations alone and because the experts are likely to have a conflict of interest as "researchers or even as entrepreneurs" (45, p. 82). An oversight mechanism is called for that is primarily educational both for the public and the scientific community, that can exert leadership within the federal government, that is sensitive to public attitudes, that is scientifically well informed and that can exercise oversight without conflict of responsibility for "sponsorship."

Since oversight increasingly seems to be needed for the entire range of potential interventions in human reproduction, a continuing forum at the national level for study and deliberation on such interventions in both heredity and development should be helpful. In whatever form the forum emerges it certainly should update the 1979 report of the Ethics Advisory Board (8) regarding IVF. Moreover, since IVF overlaps and raises issues comparable to those involved in human genetic intervention, a single forum might deal effectively with both. The forum, as the presidential commission report (45) notes, could have several alternate organizational forms. The essential step seems to be to initiate the process, modifying it later as necessary to fit the course of events.

REFERENCES AND NOTES

1. P. C. Steptoe and R. G. Edwards, *Lancet* **1978-II**, 336 (1978).

2. R. G. Edwards, P. C. Steptoe, J. M. Purdy, *Br. J. Obstet. Gynaecol.* **87**, 737 (1980).

3. P. C. Steptoe and R. G. Edwards, *Lancet* **1970-I**, 683 (1970); _____, J. M. Purdy, *Nature (London)* **229**, 132 (1971); A. Lopata *et al., Fertil. Steril.* **25**, 1030 (1974).

4. C. Grobstein, *From Chance To Purpose* (Addison-Wesley, Reading, Mass., 1981).

5. C. Wood and A. Westmore, *Test-Tube Conception* (Hill of Content, Melbourne, 1983), p. 124.

6. H. W. Jones *et al., Fertil. Steril.* **38**, 14 (1982).

7. A. Trounson, *Clin. Reprod. Fertil.* **1**, 56 (1982).

8. Ethics Advisory Board, *Report and Conclusions: HEW Support of Research Involving Human In Vitro Fertilization and Embryo Transfer* (Government Printing Office, Washington, D.C. 1979).

9. Population Information Program, *Pop. Rep. Ser. C* **8**, 97 (1980); G. Betz, T. Engle, L. L. Penney, *Fertil. Steril.* **34**, 534 (1980); J. G. Lauritsen *et al., ibid.* **37**, 68 (1982).

10. R. G. Edwards and J. M. Purdy, Eds, *Human Conception In Vitro* (Academic Press, New York, 1982).

11. Data in Table 1 are complete through February 1983. Changes since then give larger totals but do not significantly alter the efficacy pattern described.

12. P. C. Steptoe, R. G. Edwards, J. M. Purdy, *Br. J. Obstet. Gynaecol.* **87**, 757 (1980).

13. I. Johnston *et al.*, personal communication.

14. A. O. Trounson *et al., Science* **212**, 681 (1981).

15. A. O. Trounson *et al., J. Reprod. Fertil.* **64**, 285 (1982).

16. H. W. Jones *et al., ibid.* **38**, 14 (1982)

17. P. Renou *et al., ibid.* **35**, 409 (1981); C. Wood *et al., Br. J. Obstet. Gynaecol* **88**, 756 (1981).

18. R. G. Edwards, *Nature (London)* **293**, 253 (1981).

19. J. D. Biggers, paper presented at the symposium on "In Vitro Fertilization and Embryo Transfer," Carmel, Calif., October 1982.

20. P. Ramsey, *J. Am. Med. Assoc.* **220**, 1346 (1972); L. R. Kass, *Public Interest* **26**, 18 (1972); L. Walters, *Hastings Cent. Rep.* **9**, 23 (August 1979).

21. L. Mettler, in (*10*), p. 119.

22. P. C. Steptoe and R. G. Edwards, *Lancet* **1976-I**, 880 (1976).

23. D. H. Smith *et al.*, *Fertil. Steril.* **38**, 105 (1982).

24. An additional seven ectopic pregnancies have been reported recently among 76 pregnancies not included in Table 1 [Committee to Consider the Social, Ethical, and Legal Issues Arising from In Vitro Fertilization, Interim Report to the Attorney General, State of Victoria, Australia (April 1983)]. The resulting overall ectopic pregnancy rate (3.4 percent) is not significantly greater than normal.

25. D. A. Edelman, *Int. Plann. Parent. Fed. Med. Bull.* *14*(3), 1 (1980).

26. R. M. L. Winston, *Fertil. Steril.* **34**, 521 (1980).

27. F. E. French and J. M. Bierman, *Public Health Rep.* **77**, 835 (1962); C. J. Roberts and C. R. Lowe, *Lancet* **1975-I**, 498 (1975); J. G. Boue and A. Boue, *Curr. Top. Pathol* **62**, 193 (1976).

28. J. J. Schlesselman, *Am. J. Obstet. Gynecol.* **135**, 135 (1979).

29. C. Wood *et al.*, *Fertil. Steril.* **38**, 22 (1982).

30. American Fertility Society, *Fertil. News* **16** (1982), insert.

31. A. O. Trounson and C. Wood, *Clinics Obstet. Gynecol.* **8**, 681 (1981).

32. H. W. Jones, personal communication.

33. E. Mehren, *Los Angeles Times* (6 February 1983), IV-1.

34. A. Trounson *et al.*, *Br. Med. J.* **286**, 835 (1983).

35. A. Trounson, personal communication; *Los Angeles Times* (4 May 1983); I-4. The pregnancy resulted in a miscarriage at 6 months.

36. D. Shapley, *Nature (London)* **301**, 101 (1983).

37. K. Elliott and J. Whelan, Eds., *The Freezing of Mammalian Embryos* (Elsevier/North-Holland, New York, 1977).

38. J. W. Gordon *et al.*, *Proc. Natl. Acad. Sci. U.S.A.* **77**, 7380 (1980); E. F. Wagner, T. A. Stewart, B. Mintz, *ibid.* **78**, 5016 (1981); F. Constantini and E. Lacy, *Nature (London)* **294**, 92 (1981); J. W. Gordon and F. H. Ruddle, *Science* **214**, 1244 (1981); T. E. Wagner *et al.*, *Proc. Natl. Acad. Sci. U.S.A.* **78**, 6376 (1981); R. L. Brinster *et al.*, *Cell* **27**, 233 (1981); T. A. Stewart, E. F. Wgner, B. Mintz, *Science* **217**, 1046 (1982); R. D. Palmiter *et al.*, *Nature (London)* **300**, 611 (1982).

39. Only after seven attempts is the probability greater than half that a particular couple will have a child $(P = 1 - 0.9^7$.

40. There was only one clinic (Norfolk) operating in 1980. Two more began operation in 1981 and, at present, available information suggests that as many as 20 centers are operational with between 10 and 20 more in early planning stages.

41. National Center for Health Statistics, *Vital and Health Statistics, National Center for Health Statistics* **55**, (1980).

42. Z. S. Jones and K. Pourmond, *Fertil. Steril.* **13**, 398 (1962); A. Raymont *et al., Int. J. Fertil.* **14**, 141 (1969); J. Dor *et al., Fertil. Steril.* **28**, 718 (1977); K. P. Katayma *et al., Am. J. Obstet. Gynecol.* **135**, 207 (1979); M. Roland, *J. Reprod. Med.* **25**, 41 (1980); R. F. Harrison, *Int. J. Fertil.* **25**, 81 (1980).

43. C. Grobstein, M. Flower, J. Mendeloff, in preparation.

44. A. Trounson, personal communication.

45. President's Commission for the Study of Ethical Problems in Medicine and Biomedical and Behavioral Research, *Splicing Life* (Government Printing Office, Washington, D.C., 1982). This report was in part a response to inquiry from three major religious groups. It noted that "gene therapy could also be applied to embryos in conjunction with in vitro fertilization techniques."

46. Mass. Ann. Laws, Ch. 112, §112J(a) IV (Michie/Law Co-op Cum. Supp. 1978); D. M. Flannery *et al., Geo. Law J.* **67**, 1295 (1979).

47. Committee to Consider the Social, Ethical, and Legal Issues Arising from In Vitro Fertilization, Interim Report to the Attorney General, State of Victoria, Australia (September 1982), p. 27.

48. Australian National Health and Medical Research Council, *Monash Univ. Bioethics News* **2**, 25 (1982), supplementary note 4.

49. R. G. Edwards, in (*10*), p. 371.

50. British Medical Association, *Br. Med. J.* **286**, 1594 (1983); Royal College of Obstetricians and Gynaecologists, *ibid.* 1519.

51. British Medical Research Council, *ibid.* **285**, 1480 (1982).

52. H. W. Jones, A. A. Acosta, J. E. Garcia, B. A. Sandow, L. Veeck, *Fertil. Steril.* **39**, 241 (1983).

53. L. Mettler *et al., ibid.* **38**, 30 (1982).

54. R. P. Marrs *et al., ibid.,* p. 270.

55. J. F. P. Kerin *et al., Lancet* **1981-II** 726 (1981).

56. A. Trounson, personal communication.

57. Supported by NSF grant PRA-8020679.

Genetic Engineering
and Genetic Policy/Further Reading

Berger, Brigitte. "A New Interpretation of the I.Q. Controversy" *The Public Interest.* 50 (Winter, 1978), 29–44.

Caplan, Arthur, Editor, *The Sociobiology Debate.* New York: Harper and Row, 1978.

Gaylin, Willard. "The Frankenstein Factor." *New England Journal of Medicine* 297 (September 22, 1977), 665–67.

Goodfield, June. *Playing God: Genetic Engineering and The Manipulation of Life.* New York: Random House, 1977.

Grobstein, Clifford. "External Human Fertilization." *Scientific American* 240 (June, 1979), 57–67.

Hilton, Bruce, et al., Editors. *Ethical Issues in Human Genetics.* New York: Plenum Publishing Corporation, 1973.

Mertens, Thomas R. *Human Genetics: Readings on The Implications of Genetic Engineering.* New York: John Wiley and Sons, 1975.

Ramsey, Paul. "Fabricated Man: The Ethics of Genetic Control." New Haven: Yale University Press, 1970.

Reilly, Philip. *Genetics, Law and Social Policy.* Cambridge: Harvard University Press, 1977.

Wade, Nicholas. *The Ultimate Experiment.* New York: Walker & Co., 1977.

PART SEVEN

THE ALLOCATION OF SCARCE RESOURCES

Gene Outka
Aaron Wildavsky
Willard Gaylin
H. Tristram Engelhardt
Lester C. Thurow

28 Social Justice and Equal Access to Health Care

GENE OUTKA, PH.D.

The problem of the allocation of scarce resources is one of the most common but also most difficult problems in medical ethics as well as in other areas of ethical concern. A variety of means of distribution have been proposed. The article by Outka provides a good introduction to this particular problem by considering a variety of formulations of means of distribution based on different concepts of social justice. Although Outka focuses on a particular problem and argues for a particular resolution of that problem, the article formulates a social and institutional way of thinking about this particular issue. As such it provides a framework for helping us evaluate several significant orientations towards a resolution of the issue.

Dr. Gene Outka, Ph.D., teaches in the Department of Religious Studies at Yale University

I want to consider the following question. Is it possible to understand and to justify morally a societal goal which increasing numbers of people, including Americans, accept as normative? The goal is: the assurance of comprehensive health services for every person irrespective of income or geographic location. Indeed, the goal now has almost the status of a platitude. Currently in the United States politicians in various camps give it at least verbal endorsement (see, e.g., Nixon, 1972:1; Kennedy, 1972:234-252). I do not propose to examine the possible sociological determinants in this emergent consensus. I hope to show that whatever these determinants are, one may offer a plausible case in defense of the goal on reasonable grounds. To demonstrate why appeals to the goal get so successfully under our skins, I shall have recourse to a set of conceptions of social justice. Some of the standard conceptions, found in a number of writings on justice, will do (these writings include Bedau, 1971; Hospers, 1961: 416-468; Lucas, 1972; Perelman, 1963; Rescher, 1966; Ryan, 1916; Vlastos, 1962). By reflecting on them it seems to me a prima facie case can be established, namely, that every person in the entire resident population should have equal access to health care delivery.

The case is prima facie only. I wish to set aside as far as possible a related question which comes readily enough to mind. In the world of "suboptimal alternatives," with the constraints for example which impinge on the government as it makes decisions about resource allocation, what is one to say? What criteria should be employed? Paul Ramsey, in *The Patient as Person* (1970:240), thinks that the large question of how to choose between medical and other societal priorities is "almost, if not altogether, incorrigible to moral reasoning." Whether it is or not is a matter which must be ignored for the present. One may simply observe in passing that choices are unavoidable nonetheless, as Ramsey acknowledges, even where the government allows them to be made by default, so that in some instances they are determined largely by which private pressure groups prove to be dominant. In any event, there is virtue in taking up one complicated question at a time and we need to get the thrust of the case for equal access before us. It is enough to observe now that Americans attach an obviously high priority to organized health care. National health expenditures for the fiscal year 1972 were $83.4 billion (Hicks, 1973:52). Even if such an enormous sum is not entirely adequate, we may still ask: how are we to justify spending whatever we do in accordance as far as possible with the goal of equal access? The answer I propose involves distinguishing various conceptions of social justice and trying to show which of these apply or fail to apply to health care considerations. Only toward the end of the paper will some institutional implications be given more than passing attention, and then in a strictly programmatic way.

Another sort of query should be noted as we begin. What stake does someone in religious ethics have in this discussion? For the reasonable case envisaged is offered after all in the public forum. If the issue is how to justify morally the societal goal which seems so obvious to so many, whether or not they are religious believers, does the religious ethicist then simply participate qua citizen? Here I think we should be wary of simplifying formulae. Why for example should a Jew or a Christian not welcome wide support for a societal goal which he or she can affirm and reaffirm, or reflect only on instances where such support is not forthcoming? If a number of ethical schemes, both religious and humanist, converge in their acceptance of the goal of equal access to health care, so be it. Secularists can join forces with believers, at least at some levels or points, without implying there must be unanimity on every moral issue. Yet it also seems too simple if one claims to wear only the citizen's hat when making the case in question. At least I should admit that a commitment to the basic normative principle which in Christian writings is often called *agape* may influence the account to follow in ways large and small (see Outka, 1972). For example, someone with such a commitment will quite naturally take a special interest in appeals to the generic characteristics all persons share rather than the idiosyncratic attainments which distinguish persons from one another, and in the playing down of desert considerations. As I shall try to show, such appeals are centrally relevant to the case for equal access. And they are nicely in line with the normative pressures agapeic considerations typically exert.

One issue of theoretical importance in religious ethics also emerges in connection with this last point. The approach in this paper may throw a little indirect light on the traditional question, especially prominent in Christian ethics, of how love and justice are related. To distinguish different conceptions of social justice will put us in a better position, I think, to recognize that often it is ambiguous to ask about *"the* relation." There may be different relations to different conceptions. For the conceptions themselves may sometimes produce discordant indications, or turn out to be incommensurable, or reflect, when different ones are seized upon, rival moral points of view. I shall note several of these relations as we proceed.

Which then among the standard conceptions of social justice appear to be particularly relevant or irrelevant? Let us consider the following five:

I.   To each according to his merit or desert.
II. To each according to his societal contribution.
III. To each according to his contribution in satisfying whatever is freely desired by others in the open marketplace of supply and demand.
IV. To each according to his needs.
V.   Similar treatment for similar cases.

In general I shall argue that the first three of these are less relevant because of certain distinctive features which health crises possess. I shall focus on crises here not because I think preventive care is unimportant (the opposite is true), but because the crisis situation shows most clearly the special significance we attach to medical treatment as an institutionalized activity or social practice, and the basic purpose we suppose it to have.

I

To each according to his merit or desert. Meritarian conceptions, above all perhaps, are grading ones: advantages are allocated in accordance with amounts of energy expended or kinds of results achieved. What is judged is particular conduct which distinguishes persons from one another and not only the fact that all the parties are human beings. Sometimes a competitive aspect looms large.

In certain contexts it is illuminating to distinguish between efforts and achievements. In the case of efforts one characteristically focuses on the individual: rewards are based on the pains one takes. Some have supposed, for example, that entry into the kingdom of heaven is linked more directly to energy displayed and fidelity shown than to successful results attained.

To assess achievements is to weigh actual performance and productive contributions. The academic prize is awarded to the student with the highest grade-point average, regardless of the amount of midnight oil he or she burned in preparing for the examinations. Sometimes we may exclaim, "it's just not fair," when person X writes a brilliant paper with little effort while we are forced to devote more time with less impressive results. But then our complaint may be directed against differences in innate ability and talent which no expenditure of effort altogether removes.

After the difference between effort and achievement, and related distinctions, have been acknowledged, what should be stressed I think is the general importance of meritarian or desert criteria in the thinking of most people about justice. These criteria may serve to illuminate a number of disputes about the justice of various practices and institutional arrangements in our society. It may help to explain, for instance, the resentment among the working class against the welfare system. However wrongheaded or self-deceptive the resentment often is, particularly when directed toward those who want to work but for various reasons beyond their control cannot, at its better moments it involves in effect an appeal to desert considerations. "Something for nothing" is repudiated as unjust; benefits should be proportional (or at least related) to costs; those who can make an effort should do so, whatever the degree of their training or significance of their contribution to society; and so on. So, too, persons deserve to have what they have labored for; unless they infringe on the works of others their efforts and achievements are justly theirs.

Occasionally the appeal to desert extends to a wholesale rejection of other considerations as grounds for just claims. The most conspicuous target is need. Consider this statement by Ayn Rand.

A morality that holds *need* as a claim, holds emptiness—

nonexistence—as its standard of value; it rewards an absence, a defect: weakness, inability, incompetence, suffering, disease, disaster, the lack, the fault, the flaw—the *zero*.

Who provides the account to pay these claims? Those who are cursed for being non-zeros, each to the extent of his distance from that ideal. Since all values are the product of virtues, the degree of your virtue is used as the measure of your penalty; the degree of your faults is used as the measure of your gain. Your code declares that the rational man must sacrifice himself to the irrational, the independent man to parasites, the honest man to the dishonest, the man of justice to the unjust, the productive man to thieving loafers, the man of integrity to compromising knaves, the man of self-esteem to sniveling neurotics. Do you wonder at the meanness of soul in those you see around you? The man who achieves these virtues will not accept your moral code; the man who accepts your moral code will not achieve these virtues. (1957:958)

I have noted elsewhere (1972:89-90, 165-167) that *agape*, while it characteristically plays down, need not formally disallow attention to considerations falling under merit or desert; for in the case of merit as well as need it may be possible, the quotation above notwithstanding, to reason solely from egalitarian premises. A major reason such attention is warranted concerns what was called there the differential exercise of an equal liberty. That is, one may fittingly revere another's moral capacities and thus the efforts he makes as well as the ends he seeks. Such reverence may lead one to weigh expenditure of energy and specific achievements. I would simply hold now (1) that the idea of justice is not exhaustively characterized by the notion of desert, even if one agrees that the latter plays an important role; and (2) that the notion of desert is especially ill-suited to play an important role in the determination of policies which should govern a system of health care.

Why is it so ill-suited? Here we encounter some of the distinctive features which it seems to me health crises possess. Let me put it in this way. Health crises seem non-meritarian because they occur so often for reasons beyond our control or power to predict. They frequently fall without discrimination on the (according-to-merit) just and unjust, i.e., the virtuous and the wicked, the industrious and the slothful alike.

While we may believe that virtues and vices cannot depend upon natural contingencies, we are bound to admit, it seems, that many health crises do. It makes sense therefore to say that we are equal in being randomly susceptible to these crises. Even those who ascribe a prominent role to desert acknowledge that justice has also properly to do with pleas of "But I could not help it" (Lucas, 1972:321). One seeks to distinguish such cases from those acknowledged to be praiseworthy or blameworthy. Then it seems unfair as well as unkind to discriminate among those who suffer health crises on the basis of their personal deserts. For it would be odd to maintain that a newborn child deserves his hemophilia or the tumor afflicting her spine.

These considerations help to explain why the following rough distinction is often made. Bernard Williams, for example, in his discussion of "equality in unequal circumstances," identifies two different sorts of inequality, inequality of merit and inequality of need, and two corresponding goods, those earned by effort and those demanded by need (1971:126-137). Medical treatment in the event of illness is located under the umbrella of need. He concludes: "Leaving aside preventive medicine, the proper ground of distribution of medical care is ill health: this is a necessary truth" (1971:127). An irrational state of affairs is held to obtain if those whose needs are the same are treated unequally, when needs are the ground of the treatment. One might put the point this way. When people are equal in the relevant respects—in this case when their needs are the same and occur in a context of random, undeserved susceptibility—that by itself is a good reason for treating them equally (see also Nagel, 1973:354).

In many societies, however, a second necessary condition for the receipt of medical treatment exists de facto: the possession of money. This is not the place to consider the general question of when inequalities in wealth may be regarded as just. It is enough to note that one can plausibly appeal to all of the conceptions of justice we are embarked in sorting out. A person may be thought to be entitled to a higher income when he works more, contributes more, risks more, and not simply when he needs more. We may think it fair that the industrious should have more money than the slothful and the surgeon more than the tobacconist. The difficulty comes in the misfit between the reasons for differential incomes and the reasons for receiving medical treatment. The former may include a pluralistic set of claims in which different notions of justice must be meshed. The latter are more monistically focused on needs, and the other notions not accorded a similar relevance. Yet money may nonetheless remain as a causally necessary condition for receiving medical treatment. It may be the power to secure what one needs. The senses in which health crises are distinctive may then be insufficiently determinative for the policies which govern the actual availability of treatment. The nearly automatic links between income, prestige, and the receipt of comparatively higher quality medical treatment should then be subjected to critical scrutiny. For unequal treatment of the rich ill and the poor ill is unjust if, again, needs rather than differential income constitute the ground of such treatment.

Suppose one agrees that it is important to recognize the misfit between the reasons for differential incomes and the reasons for receiving medical treatment, and that therefore income as such should not govern the actual availability of treatment. One may still ask whether the case so far relies excessively on "pure" instances where desert considerations are admittedly out of place. That there are such pure instances, tumors afflicting the spine, hemophilia, and so on, is not denied. Yet it is an exaggeration if we go on and regard all health crises as utterly unconnected with desert. Note for example that Williams leaves aside preventive medicine. And if in a cool hour we examine the statistics, we find that a vast number of deaths occur each year due to causes not always beyond our control, e.g., automobile accidents, drugs, alcohol, tobacco, obesity, and so on. In some final reckoning it seems that many persons (though crucially, not all) have an effect on, and arguably a responsibility for, their own medical needs. Consider the following bidders for emergency care: (1) a person with a heart attack who is seriously overweight; (2) a football hero who has suffered a concussion; (3) a man with lung cancer who has smoked cigarettes for forty years; (4) a 60 year old man who has always taken excellent care of himself and is suddenly stricken with leukemia; (5) a three year old girl who has swallowed poison left out carelessly by her parents; (6) a 14 year old boy who has been beaten without provocation by a gang and suffers brain damage and recurrent attacks of uncontrollable terror; (7) a college student who has slashed his wrists (and not for the first time) from a psychological need for attention; (8) a woman raised in the ghetto who is found unconscious due to an overdose of heroin.

These cases help to show why the whole subject of medical treatment is so crucial and so perplexing. They attest to some melancholy elements in human experience. People suffer in varying ratios the effects of their natural and undeserved vulnerabilities, the irresponsibility and brutality of others, and their own desires and weaknesses. In some final reckoning then desert considerations seem not irrelevant to many health crises. The practical applicability of this admission, however, in the instance of health care delivery, appears limited. We may agree that it underscores the importance of preventive health care by stressing the influence we sometimes have over our medical needs. But if we try to foster such care by increasing the penalties for neglect, we normally confine ourselves to calculations about incentives. At the risk of being denounced in some quarters as censorious and puritannical, perhaps we should for example levy far higher taxes on alcohol and tobacco and pump the dollars directly into health care programs rather than (say) into highway building. Yet these steps would by no means lead necessarily to a demand that we correlate in some strict way a demonstrated effort to be temperate with the receipt of privileged medical treatment as a reward. Would it be feasible to allocate the additional tax monies to the man with leukemia before the overweight man suffering a heart attack on the ground of a difference in desert? At the point of emergency care at least, it seems impracticable for the doctor to discriminate between these cases, to make meritarian judgments at the point of catastrophe. And the number of persons who are in need of medical treatment for reasons utterly beyond their control remains a datum with tenacious relevance. There are those who suffer the ravages of a tornado, are handicapped by a genetic defect, beaten without provocation, etc. A commitment to the basic purpose of medical care and to the institutions for achieving it involves the recognition of this persistent state of affairs.

II

To each according to his societal contribution. This conception gives moral primacy to notions such as the public interest, the common good, the welfare of the community, or the greatest good of the greatest number. Here one judges the social consequences of particular conduct. The formula can be construed in at least two ways (Rescher, 1966:79-80). It may refer to the interest of the social group considered collectively, where the group has some independent life all its own. The group's welfare is the decisive criterion for determining what constitutes any member's proper share. Or the common good may refer only to an aggregation of distinct individuals and considered distributively.

Either version accords such a primacy to what is socially advantageous as to be unacceptable not only to defenders of need, but also, it would seem, of desert. For the criteria of effort and achievement are often conceived along rather individualistic lines. The pains an agent takes or the results he brings about deserve recompense, whether or not the public interest is directly served. No automatic harmony then is necessarily assumed between his just share as individually earned and his proper share from the vantage point of the common good. Moreover, the test of social advantage *simpliciter* obviously threatens the agapeic concern with some minimal consideration due each person which is never to be disregarded for the sake of long-range social benefits. No one should be considered as *merely* a means or instrument.

The relevance of the canon of social productiveness to health crises may accordingly also be challenged. Indeed, such crises may cut against it in that they occur more frequently to those whose comparative contribution to the general welfare is less, e.g., the aged, the disabled, children.

Consider for example Paul Ramsey's persuasive critique of social and economic criteria for the allocation of a single scarce medical resource. He begins by recounting the imponderables which faced the widely-discussed "public committee" at the Swedish Hospital in Seattle when it deliberated in the early 1960's. The sparse resource in this case was the kidney machine. The committee was charged with the responsibility of selecting among patients suffering chronic renal failure those who were to receive dialysis. Its criteria were broadly social and economic. Considerations weighed included age, sex, marital status, number of dependents, income, net worth, educational background, occupation, past performance and future potential. The application of such criteria proved to be exceedingly problematic. Should someone with six children always have priority over an artist or composer? Were those who arranged matters so that their families would not burden society to be penalized in effect for being provident? And so on. Two critics of the committee found "a disturbing picture of the bourgeoisie sparing the bourgeoisie" and observed that "the Pacific Northwest is no place for a Henry David Thoreau with bad kidneys" (quoted in Ramsey, 1970:248).

The mistake, Ramsey believes, is to introduce criteria of social worthiness in the first place. In those situations of choice where not all can be saved and yet all need not die, "the equal right of every human being to live, and not relative personal or social worth, should be the ruling principle" (1970:256). The principle leads to a criterion of "random choice among equals" expressed by a lottery scheme or a practice of "first-come, first-served." Several reasons stand behind Ramsey's defense of the criterion of random choice. First, a religious belief in the equality of persons before God leads intelligibly to a refusal to choose between those who are dying in any way other than random patient selection. Otherwise their equal value as human beings is threatened. Second, a moral primacy is ascribed to survival over other (perhaps superior) interests persons may have, in that it is the condition of everything else. ". . . Life is a value incommensurate with all others, and so not negotiable by bartering one man's worth against another's" (1970:256). Third, the entire enterprise of estimating a person's social worth is viewed with final skepticism. ". . . We have no way of knowing how really and truly to estimate a man's societal worth or his worth to others or to himself in unfocused social

situations in the ordinary lives of men in their communities"
(1970:256). This statement, incidentally, appears to allow something
other than randomness in *focused* social situations; when, say, a President or Prime Minister and the owner of the local bar rush for the last
place in the bomb shelter, and the knowledge of the former can save
many lives. In any event, I have been concerned with a restricted
point to which Ramsey's discussion brings illustrative support. The
canon of social productiveness is notoriously difficult to apply as a
workable criterion for distributing medical services to those who need
them.

One may go further. A system of health care delivery which
treats people on the basis of the medical care required may often go
against (at least narrowly conceived) calculations of societal advantage. For example, the health care needs of people tend to rise during
that period of their lives, signaled by retirement, when their incomes
and social productivity are declining. More generally:

> Some 40 to 50 per cent of the American people—the aged,
> children, the dependent poor, and those with some significant
> chronic disability are in categories requiring relatively large
> amounts of medical care but with inadequate resources to pur-
> chase such care. (Somers, 1971a:20)

If one agrees, for whatever reasons, with the agapeic judgment
that each person should be regarded as irreducibly valuable, then one
cannot succumb to a social productiveness criterion of human worth.
Interests are to be equally considered even when people have ceased to
be, or are not yet, or perhaps never will be, public assets.

III

*To each according to his contribution in satisfying whatever is
freely desired by others in the open marketplace of supply and demand.* Here we have a test which, though similar to the preceding one,
concentrates on what is desired de facto by certain segments of the
community rather than the community as a whole, and on the relative
scarcity of the service rendered. It is tantamount to the canon of supply and demand as espoused by various laissez-faire theoreticians (cf.
Rescher, 1966:80-81). Rewards should be given to those who by virtue of special skill, prescience, risk-taking, and the like discern what is
desired and are able to take the requisite steps to bring satisfaction. A
surgeon, it may be argued, contributes more than a nurse because of
the greater training and skill required, burdens borne, and effective
care provided, and should be compensated accordingly. So too per-

haps, a star quarterback on a pro-football team should be remunerated even more highly because of the rare athletic prowess needed, hazards involved, and widespread demand to watch him play.

This formula does not then call for the weighing of the value of various contributions, and tends to conflate needs and wants under a notion of desires. It also assumes that a prominent part is assigned to consumer free-choice. The consumer should be at liberty to express his preferences, and to select from a variety of competing goods and services. Those who resist many changes currently proposed in the organization and financing of health care delivery in the U.S.A.—such as national health insurance—often do so by appealing to some variant of this formula.

Yet it seems health crises are often of overriding importance when they occur. They appear therefore not satisfactorily accommodated to the context of a free marketplace where consumers may freely choose among alternative goods and services.

To clarify what is at stake in the above contention, let us examine an opposing case. Robert M. Sade, M.D., published an article in *The New England Journal of Medicine* entitled "Medical Care as a Right: A Refutation" (1971). He attacks programs of national health insurance in the name of a person's right to select one's own values, determine how they may be realized, and dispose of them if one chooses without coercion from other men. The values in question are construed as economic ones in the context of supply and demand. So we read:

> In a free society, man exercises his right to sustain his own life by producing economic values in the form of goods and services that he is, or should be, free to exchange with other men who are similarly free to trade with him or not. The economic values produced, however, are not given as gifts by nature, but exist only by virtue of the thought and effort of individual men. Goods and services are thus owned as a consequence of the right to sustain life by one's own physical and mental effort. (1971:1289)

Sade compares the situation of the physician to that of the baker. The one who produces a loaf of bread should as owner have the power to dispose of his own product. It is immoral simply to expropriate the bread without the baker's permission. Similarly, "medical care is neither a right nor a privilege: it is a service that is provided by doctors and others to people who wish to purchase it" (1971:1289). Any coercive regulation of professional practices by the society at large is held to be analogous to taking the bread from the baker without his consent. Such regulation violates the freedom of the physician over his own services and will lead inevitably to provider-apathy.

The analogy surely misleads. To assume that doctors autonomously produce goods and services in a fashion closely akin to a baker is grossly oversimplified. The baker may himself rely on the agricultural produce of others, yet there is a crucial difference in the degree of dependence. Modern physicians depend on the achievements of medical technology and the entire scientific base underlying it, all of which is made possible by a host of persons whose salaries are often notably less. Moreover, the amount of taxpayer support for medical research and education is too enormous to make any such unqualified case for provider-autonomy plausible.

However conceptually clouded Sade's article may be, its stress on a free exchange of goods and services reflects one historically influential rationale for much American medical practice. And he applies it not only to physicians but also to patients or "consumers."

> The question is whether the decision of how to allocate the consumer's dollar should belong to the consumer or to the state. It has already been shown that the choice of how a doctor's services should be rendered belongs only to the doctor: in the same way the choice of whether to buy a doctor's service rather than some other commodity or service belongs to the consumer as a logical consequence of the right to his own life. (1971:1291)

This account is misguided, I think, because it ignores the overriding importance which is so often attached to health crises. When lumps appear on someone's neck, it usually makes little sense to talk of choosing whether to buy a doctor's service rather than a color television set. References to just trade-offs suddenly seem out of place. No compensation suffices, since the penalties may differ so much.

There is even a further restriction on consumer choice. One's knowledge in these circumstances is comparatively so limited. The physician makes most of the decisions: about diagnosis, treatment, hospitalization, number of return visits, and so on. In brief:

> The consumer knows very little about the medical services he is buying—probably less than about any other service he purchases. . . . While [he] can still play a role in policing the market, that role is much more limited in the field of health care than in almost any other area of private economic activity. (Schultze, 1972:214-215)

For much of the way, then, an appeal to supply and demand and consumer choice is not quite fitting. It neglects the issue of the value of various contributions. And it fails to allow for the recognition that medical treatments may be overridingly desired. In contexts of catastrophe at any rate, when life itself is threatened, most persons (other than those who are apathetic or seek to escape from the terrifying prospects) cannot take medical care to be merely one option among others.

IV

To each according to his needs. The concept of needs is sometimes taken to apply to an entire range of interests which concern a person's "psycho-physical existence" (Outka, 1972:esp. 264-265). On this wide usage, to attribute a need to someone is to say that the person lacks what is thought to conduce to his or her "welfare"—understood in both a physiological sense (e.g., for food, drink, shelter, and health) and a psychological one (e.g., for continuous human affection and support).

Yet even in the case of such a wide usage, what the person lacks is typically assumed to be basic. Attention is restricted to recurrent considerations rather than to every possible individual whim or frivolous pursuit. So one is not surprised to meet with the contention that a preferable rendering of this formula would be: "to each according to his essential needs" (Perelman, 1963:22). This contention seems to me well taken. It implies, for one thing, that basic needs are distinguishable from felt needs or wants. For the latter may encompass expressions of personal preference unrelated to considerations of survival or subsistence, and sometimes artificially generated by circumstances of rising affluence in the society at large.

Essential needs are also typically assumed to be given rather than acquired. They are not constituted by any action for which the person is responsible by virtue of his or her distinctively greater effort. It is almost as if the designation "innocent" may be linked illuminatingly to need, as retribution, punishment, and so on, are to desert, and in complex ways, to freedom. Thus essential needs are likewise distinguishable from deserts. Where needs are unequal, one thinks of them as fortuitously distributed; as part, perhaps, of a kind of "natural lottery" (see Rawls, 1971:e.g., 104). So very often the advantages of health and the burdens of illness, for example, strike one as arbitrary effects of the lottery. It seems wrong to say that a newborn child deserves as a reward all of his faculties when he has done nothing in particular which distinguishes him from another newborn who comes into the world deprived of one or more of them. Similarly, though crudely, many religious believers do not look on natural events as personal deserts. They are not inclined to pronounce sentences such as, "That evil person with incurable cancer got what he deserved." They are disposed instead to search for some distinction between what they may call the conditions of finitude on the one hand and sin and moral evil on the other. If the distinction is "ultimately" invalid, in this life it seems inscrutably so. Here and now it may be usefully drawn. Inequalities in the need for medical treatment are taken, it appears, to reflect the conditions of finitude more than anything else.

One can even go on to argue that among our basic or essential needs, the case of medical treatment is conspicuous in the following sense. While food and shelter are not matters about which we are at liberty to please ourselves, they are at least predictable. We can plan, for instance, to store up food and fuel for the winter. It may be held that responsibility increases along with the power to predict. If so, then many health crises seem peculiarly random and uncontrollable. Cancer, given the present state of knowledge at any rate, is a contingent disaster, whereas hunger is a steady threat. Who will need serious medical care, and when, is then perhaps a classic example of uncertainty.

Finally, and more theoretically, it is often observed that a need-conception of justice comes closest to charity or *agape* (e.g., Perelman, 1963:23). I think there are indeed crucial overlaps (see Outka, 1972:91-92, 309-312). To cite several of them: the equal consideration *agape* enjoins has to do in the first instance with those generic endowments which people share, the characteristics of a person qua human existent. Needs, as we have seen, likewise concern those things essential to the life and welfare of men considered simply as men (see also Honoré, 1968). They are not based on particular conduct alone, on those idiosyncratic attainments which contribute to someone's being such-and-such a kind of person. Yet a certain sort of inequality is recognized, for needs differ in divergent circumstances and so treatments must if benefits are to be equalized. *Agape* too allows for a distinction between equal consideration and identical treatment. The aim of equalizing benefits is implied by the injunction to consider the interests of each party equally. This may require differential treatments of differing interests.

Overlaps such as these will doubtless strike some as so extensive that it may be asked whether *agape* and a need-conception of justice are virtually equivalent. I think not. One contrast was pointed out before. The differential treatment enjoined by *agape* is more complex and goes deeper. In the case of *agape*, attention may be appropriately given to varying *efforts* as well as to unequal *needs*. More generally one may say that agapeic considerations extend to all of the psychological nuances and contextual details of individual persons and their circumstances. Imaginative concern is enjoined for concrete human beings: for what someone is uniquely, for what he or she—as a matter of personal history and distinctive identity—wants, feels, thinks, celebrates, and endures. The attempt to establish and enhance mutual affection between individual persons is taken likewise to be fitting. Conceptions of social justice, including "to each according to his essential needs," tend to be more restrictive; they call attention to considerations which obtain for a number of persons, to impersonally specified criteria for assessing collective policies and practices. *Agape* involves more, even if one supposes never less.

Other differences could be noted. What is important now however is the recognition that, in matters of health care in particular, *agape* and a need-conception of justice are conjoined in a number of relevant respects. At least this is so for those who think that, again, justice has properly to do with pleas of "But I could not help it." It seeks to distinguish such cases from those acknowledged to be praiseworthy or blameworthy. The formula "to each according to his needs" is one cogent way of identifying the moral relevance of these pleas. To ignore them may be thought to be unfair as well as unkind when they arise from the deprivation of some essential need. The move to confine the notion of justice wholly to desert considerations is thereby resisted as well. Hence we may say that sometimes "questions of social justice arise just because people are unequal in ways they can do very little to change and . . . only by attending to these inequalities can one be said to be giving their interests equal consideration" (Benn, 1971:164).

V

Similar treatment for similar cases. This conception is perhaps the most familiar of all. Certainly it is the most formal and inclusive one. It is frequently taken as an elementary appeal to consistency and linked to the universalizability test. One should not make an arbitrary exception on one's own behalf, but rather should apply impartially whatever standards one accepts. The conception can be fruitfully applied to health care questions and I shall assume its relevance. Yet as literally interpreted, it is necessary but not sufficient. For rightly or not, it is often held to be as compatible with no positive treatment whatever as with active promotion of other people's interests, as long as all are equally and impartially included. Its exponents sometimes assume such active promotion without demonstrating clearly how this is built into the conception itself. Moreover, it may obscure a distinction which we have seen agapists and others make: between equal consideration and identical treatment. Needs may differ and so treatments must, if benefits are to be equalized.

I have placed this conception at the end of the list partly because it moves us, despite its formality, toward practice. Let me suggest briefly how it does so. Suppose first of all one agrees with the case so far offered. Suppose, that is, it has been shown convincingly that a need-conception of justice applies with greater relevance than the earlier three when one reflects about the basic purpose of medical care. To treat one class of people differently from another because of income or geographic location should therefore be ruled out, because such reasons are irrelevant. (The irrelevance is conceptual, rather than always, unfortunately, causal.) In short, all persons should have equal access, "as needed, without financial, geographic, or other barriers, to the whole spectrum of health services" (Somers and Somers, 1972a:122).

Suppose however, secondly, that the goal of equal access collides on some occasions with the realities of finite medical resources and needs which prove to be insatiable. That such collisions occur in fact it would be idle to deny. And it is here that the practical bearing of the formula of similar treatment for similar cases should be noticed. Let us recall Williams' conclusion: "the proper ground of distribution of medical care is ill health: this is a necessary truth." While I agree with the essentials of his argument—for all the reasons above—I would prefer, for practical purposes, a slightly more modest formulation. Illness is the proper ground for the *receipt* of medical care. However, the *distribution* of medical care in less-than-optimal circumstances requires us to face the collisions. I would argue that in such circumstances the formula of similar treatment for similar cases may be construed so as to guide actual choices in the way most compatible with the goal of equal access. The formula's allowance of no positive treatment whatever may justify exclusion of entire classes of cases from a priority list. Yet it forbids doing so for irrelevant or arbitrary reasons. So (1) if we accept the case for equal access, but (2) if we simply cannot, physically cannot, treat all who are in need, it seems more just to discriminate by virtue of categories of illness, for example, rather than between the rich ill and poor ill. All persons with a certain rare, noncommunicable disease would not receive priority, let us say, where the costs were inordinate, the prospects for rehabilitation remote, and for the sake of equalized benefits to many more. Or with Ramsey we may urge a policy of random patient selection when one must decide between claimants for a medical treatment unavailable to all. Or we may acknowledge that any notion of "comprehensive benefits" to which persons should have equal access is subject to practical restrictions which will vary from society to society depending on resources at a given time. Even in a country as affluent as the United States there will surely always be items excluded, e.g., perhaps over-the-counter drugs, some teenage orthodontia, cosmetic surgery, and the like (Somers and Somers, 1972b:182). Here too the formula of similar treatment for similar cases may serve to modify the application of a need-conception of justice in order to address the insatiability-problem and limit frivolous use. In all of the foregoing instances of restriction, however, the relevant feature remains the illness, discomfort, etc. itself. The goal of equal access then retains its prima facie authoritativeness. It is imperfectly realized rather than disregarded.

VI

These latter comments lead on to the question of institutional implications. I cannot aim here of course for the specificity rightly sought by policy-makers. My endeavor has been conceptual elucidation. While the ethicist needs to be apprised about the facts, he or she does not, qua ethicist, don the mantle of the policy-expert. In any case, only rarely does anyone do both things equally well. Yet cross-fertilization is extremely desirable. For experts should not be isolated from the wider assumptions their recommendations may reflect. I shall merely list some of the topics which would have to be discussed at length if we were to get clear about the implications. Examples will be limited to the current situation in the United States.

Anyone who accepts the case for equal access will naturally be concerned about de facto disparities in the availability of medical treatment. Let us consider two relevant indictments of current American practice. They appear in the writings not only of those who attack indiscriminately a system seen to be governed only by the appetite for profit and power, but also of those who denounce in less sweeping terms and espouse more cautiously reformist positions. The first shortcoming has to do with the maldistribution of supply. Per capita ratios of physicians to populations served vary, sometimes notoriously, between affluent suburbs and rural and inner city areas. This problem is exacerbated by the distressing data concerning the greater health needs of the poor. Chronic disease, frequency and duration of hospitalization, psychiatric disorders, infant death rates, etc.—these occur in significantly larger proportions to lower income members of American society (Appel, 1970; Hubbard, 1970). A further complication is that "the distribution of health insurance coverage is badly skewed. Practically all the rich have insurance. But among the poor, about two-thirds have none. As a result, among people aged 25 to 64 who die, some 45 to 50 per cent have neither hospital nor surgical coverage" (Somers, 1971a:46). This last point connects with a second shortcoming frequently cited. Even those who are otherwise economically independent may be shattered by the high cost of a "catastrophic illness" (see some eloquent examples in Kennedy, 1972).

Proposals for institutional reforms designed to overcome such disparities are bound to be taken seriously by any defender of equal access. What he or she will be disposed to press for, of course, is the removal of any double standard or "two class" system of care. The viable procedures for bringing this about are not obvious, and comparisons with certain other societies (for relevant alternative models) are drawn now with perhaps less confidence (see Anderson, 1973). One set of commonly discussed proposals includes (1) incentive subsidies to physicians, hospitals, and medical centers to provide services in regions of poverty (to overcome in part the unwillingness—to which no unique culpability need be ascribed—of many providers and their spouses to work and live in grim surroundings); (2) licensure controls to avoid comparatively excessive concentrations of physicians in regions of affluence; (3) a period of time (say, two years) in an underserved area as a requirement for licensing; (4) redistribution facilities which allow for population shifts.

A second set of proposals is linked with health insurance itself. While I cannot venture into the intricacies of medical economics or comment on the various bills for national health insurance presently inundating Congress, it may be instructive to take brief note of one proposal in which, once more, the defender of equal access is bound to take an interest (even if he or she finally rejects it on certain practical grounds). The precise details of the proposal are unimportant for our purposes (for one much-discussed version, see Feldstein, 1971). Consider this crude sketch. Each citizen is (in effect) issued a card by the government. Whenever "legitimate" medical expenses (however determined for a given society) exceed, say, 10 per cent of his or her annual taxable income, the card may be presented so that additional costs incurred will be paid for out of general tax revenues. The reasons urged on behalf of this sort of arrangement include the following. In the case of medical care there is warrant for proportionately equalizing what is spent from anyone's total taxable income. This warrant reflects the conditions, discussed earlier, of the natural lottery. Insofar as the advantages of health and the burdens of illness are random and undeserved, we may find it in our common interest to share risks. A fixed percentage of income attests to the misfit, also mentioned previously, between the reasons for differential total income and the reasons for receiving medical treatment. If money remains a causally necessary condition for receiving medical treatment, then a way must be found to place it in the hands of those who need it. The card is one such means. It is designed effectively to equalize purchasing power. In this way it seems to accord nicely with the goal of equal access. On the other side, the requirement of initial out-of-pocket expenses—sufficiently large in comparison to average family expenditures on health care—is designed to discourage frivolous use and foster awareness that medical care is a benefit not to be simply taken as a matter of course. It also safeguards against an excessively large tax burden while providing universal protection against the often disastrous costs of serious illness. Whether 10 per cent is too great a chunk for the very poor to pay, and whether by itself the proposal will feed price inflation and neglect of preventive medicine are questions which would have to be answered.

Another kind of possible institutional reform will also greatly interest the defender of equal access. This has to do with the "design of health care systems" or "care settings." The prevalent setting in American society has always been "fee-for-service." It is left up to each person to obtain the requisite care and to pay for it as he or she goes along. Because costs for medical treatment have accelerated at such an alarming rate, and because the sheer diffusion of energy and effort so characteristic of American medical practice leaves more and more people dissatisfied, alternatives to fee-for-service have been considered of late with unprecedented seriousness. The alternative care setting most widely discussed is prepaid practice, and specifically the "health maintenance organization" (HMO). Here one finds "an organized system of care which accepts the responsibility to provide or otherwise assure comprehensive care to a defined population for a fixed periodic payment per person or per family . . ." (Somers, 1972b:v). The best-known HMO is the Kaiser-Permanente Medical Care Program (see also Garfield, 1971). Does the HMO serve to realize the goal of equal access more fully? One line of argument in its favor is this. It is plausible to think that equal access will be fostered by the more economical care setting. HMO's are held to be less costly per capita in at least two respects: hospitalization rates are much below the national average; and less often noted, physician manpower is as well. To be sure, one should be sensitive to the corruptions in each type of setting. While fee-for-service has resulted in a suspiciously high number of surgeries (twice as many per capita in the United States as in Great Britain), the HMO physician may more frequently permit the patient's needs to be overridden by the organization's pressure to economize. It may also be more difficult in an HMO setting to provide for close personal relations between a particular physician and a particular patient (something commended, of course, on all sides). After such corruptions are allowed for, the data seem encouraging to such an extent that a defender of equal access will certainly support the repeal of any law which limits the development of prepaid practice, to approve of "front-aid" subsidies for HMO's to increase their number overall and achieve a more equitable distribution throughout the country, and so on. At a minimum, each care setting should be available in every region. If we assume a common freedom to choose between them, each may help to guard against the peculiar temptations to which the other is exposed.

To assess in any serious way proposals for institutional reform such as the above is beyond the scope of this paper. We would eventually be led, for example, into the question of whether it is consistent for the rich to pay more than the poor for the same treatment when, again, needs rather than income constitute the ground of the treatment (Ward, 1973), and from there into the tangled subject of the "ethics of redistribution" in general (see, e.g., Benn and Peters, 1965:155-178; de Jouvenal, 1952). Other complex issues deserve to be considered as well, e.g., the criteria for allocation of limited resources,[2] and how conceptions of justice apply to the providers of health care.[3]

Those committed to self-conscious moral and religious reflection about subjects in medicine have concentrated, perhaps unduly, on issues about care of individual patients (as death approaches, for instance). These issues plainly warrant the most careful consideration. One would like to see in addition, however, more attention paid to social questions in medical ethics. To attend to them is not necessarily to leave behind all of the matters which reach deeply into the human condition. Any detailed case for institutional reforms, for example, will be enriched if the proponent asks soberly whether certain conflicts and certain perplexities allow for more than partial improvements and provisional resolutions. Can public and private interests ever be made fully to coincide by legislative and administrative means? Will the commitment of a physician to an individual patient and the commitment of the legislator to the "common good" ever be harmonized in every case? Our anxiety may be too intractable. Our fear of illness and of dying may be so pronounced and immediate that we will seize the nearly automatic connections between privilege, wealth, and power if we can. We will do everything possible to have our kidney machines even if the charts make it clear that many more would benefit from mandatory immunization at a fraction of the cost. And our capacity for taking in rival points of view may be too limited. Once we have witnessed tangible suffering, we cannot just return with ease to public policies aimed at statistical patients. Those who believe that justice is the pre-eminent virtue of institutions and that a case can be convincingly made on behalf of justice for equal access to health care would do well to ponder such conflicts and perplexities. Our reforms might then seem, to ourselves and to others, less abstract and jargon-filled in formulation and less sanguine and piecemeal in substance. They would reflect a greater awareness of what we have to confront.

NOTES

1. Much of the research for this paper was done during the Fall Term, 1972-73, when I was on leave in Washington, D.C. I am very grateful for the two appointments which made this leave possible: as Service Fellow, Office of Special Projects, Health Services and Mental Health Administration, Department of Health, Education, and Welfare; and as Visiting Scholar, Kennedy Center for Bioethics, Georgetown University.

2. The issue of priorities is at least threefold: (1) between improved medical care and other social needs, e.g., to restrain auto accidents and pollution; (2) between different sorts of medical treatments for different illnesses, e.g., prevention vs. crisis intervention and exotic treatments; (3) between persons all of whom need a single scarce resource and not all can have it, e.g., Ramsey's discussion of how to decide among those who are to receive dialysis. Moreover, (1) can be subdivided between (a) improved medical care and other social needs which affect health directly, e.g., drug addiction, auto accidents, and pollution; (b) improved medical care and other social needs which serve the overall aim of community-survival, e.g., a common defense. In the case of (2), one would like to see far more careful discussion of some general criteria which might be employed, e.g., numbers affected, degree of contagion, prospects for rehabilitation, and so on.

3. What sorts of appeals to justice might be cogently made to warrant, for instance, the differentially high income physicians receive? Here are three possibilities: (1) the greater skill and responsibility involved should be rewarded proportionately, i.e., one should attend to considerations of *desert*; (2) there should be *compensation* for the money invested for education and facilities in order to restore circumstances of approximate equality (this argument, while a common one in medical circles, would need to consider that medical education is received in part at public expense and that the modern physician is the highest paid professional in the country); (3) the difference should benefit the least advantaged more than an alternative arrangement where disparities are less. We prefer a society where the medical profession flourishes and everyone has a longer life expectancy to one where everyone is poverty-stricken with a shorter life expectancy ("splendidly equalized destitution"). Yet how are we to ascertain the minimum degree of differential income required for the least advantaged members of the society to be better off?

Discussions of "justice and the interests of providers" are, I think, badly needed. Physicians in the United States have suffered a decline in prestige for various reasons, e.g., the way many used Medicare to support and increase their own incomes. Yet one should endeavor to assess their interests fairly. A concern for professional autonomy is clearly important, though one may ask whether adequate attention has been paid to the distinction between the imposition of cost-controls from outside and interference with professional medical judgments. One may affirm the former, it seems, and still reject—energetically—the latter.

REFERENCES

Anderson, Odin
1973   Health Care: Can There Be Equity? The United States, Sweden and England. New York: Wiley.
Appel, James Z.
1970   "Health care delivery." Pp. 141-166 in Boisfeuillet Jones (ed.), The Health of Americans. Englewood Cliffs, N.J.: Prentice-Hall, Inc.
Bedau, Hugo A.
1971   "Radical egalitarianism." Pp. 168-180 in Hugo A. Bedau (ed.), Justice and Equality. Englewood Cliffs, N.J.: Prentice-Hall, Inc.
Benn, Stanley I.
1971   "Egalitarianism and the equal consideration of interests." Pp. 152-167 in Hugo A. Bedau (ed.), Justice and Equality. Englewood Cliffs, N.J.: Prentice-Hall, Inc.
Benn, Stanley I. and Richard S. Peters.
1965   The Principles of Political Thought. New York: The Free Press.
de Jouvenel, Bertrand
1952   The Ethics of Redistribution. Cambridge: University Press.
Feldstein, Martin S.
1971   "A new approach to national health insurance." The Public Interest 23 (Spring):93-105.
Garfield, Sidney R.
1971   "Prevention of dissipation of health services resources." American Journal of Public Health 61:1499-1506.
Hicks, Nancy
1973   "Nation's doctors move to police medical care." Pp. 1, 52 in New York Times, Sunday, October 28.
Honoré, A.M.
1968   "Social justice." Pp. 61-94 in Robert S. Summers (ed.), Essays in Legal Philosophy. Oxford: Basil Blackwell.
Hospers, John
1961   Human Conduct. New York: Harcourt, Brace and World, Inc.
Hubbard, William N.
1970   "Health knowledge." Pp. 93-120 in Boisfeuillet Jones (Ed.), The Health of Americans. Englewood Cliffs, N.J.: Prentice-Hall, Inc.
Kennedy, Edward M.
1972   In Critical Condition: The Crisis in America's Health Care. New York: Simon and Schuster.
Lucas, J. R.
1972   "Justice." Philosophy 47, No. 181 (July):229-248.
Nagel, Thomas
1973   "Equal treatment and compensatory discrimination." Philosophy and Public Affairs 2, No. 4 (Summer):348-363.
Nixon, Richard M.
1972   "President's message on health care system." Document No. 92-261 (March 2). House of Representatives, Washington, D.C.
Outka, Gene
1972   Agape: An Ethical Analysis. New Haven and London: Yale University Press
Perelman, Ch.
1963   The Idea of Justice and the Problem of Argument. Trans. John Petrie. London: Routledge and Kegan Paul.
Ramsey, Paul
1970   The Patient as Person. New Haven and London: Yale University Press.
Rand, Ayn
1957   Atlas Shrugged. New York: Signet.

Rawls, John
1971   *A Theory of Justice.* Cambridge, Mass.: Harvard University Press.
Rescher, Nicholas
1966   *Distributive Justice.* Indianapolis: The Bobbs-Merrill Company, Inc.
Ryan, John A.
1916   *Distributive Justice.* New York: The Macmillan Company.
Sade, Robert M.
1971   "Medical care as a right: a refutation." *The New England Journal of Medicine* 285 (December): 1288-1292.
Schultze, Charles L., Edward R. Fried, Alice M. Rivlin and Nancy H. Teeters
1972   *Setting National Priorities: The 1973 Budget.* Washington, D.C.: The Brookings Institution.
Somers, Anne R.
1971a *Health Care in Transition: Directions for the Future.* Chicago: Hospital Research and Educational Trust.
1971b (ed.), *The Kaiser-Permanente Medical Care Program.* New York: The Commonwealth Fund.
Somers, Anne R. and Herman M. Somers
1972a "The organization and financing of health care: issues and directions for the future." *American Journal of Orthopsychiatry* 42 (January), 119-136.
1972b "Major issues in national health insurance." *Milbank Memorial Fund Quarterly* 50, No. 2, Part 1 (April):177-210.
Vlastos, Gregory
1962   "Justice and equality." Pp. 31-72 in Richard B. Brandt (ed.), *Social Justice.* Englewood Cliffs, N.J.: Prentice-Hall, Inc.
Ward, Andrew
1973   "The idea of equality reconsidered." *Philosophy* 48 (January):85-90.
Williams, Bernard A.O.
1971   "The idea of equality." Pp. 116-137 in Hugo A. Bedau (ed.), *Justice and Equality.* Englewood Cliffs, N.J.: Prentice-Hall, Inc.

29 Doing Better and Feeling Worse: The Political Pathology of Health Policy

AARON WILDAVSKY

This entertaining but extremely provocative article provides an analysis of a number of slogans that have characterized most discussions on health policy as well as pro and con arguments for a national health insurance system. Wildavsky also analyzes a number of financial and programmatic issues related to the development of health policy and evaluates their outcomes.

Aaron Wildavsky is Dean of the Graduate School of Public Policy at the University of California, Berkeley

According to the great equation, Medical Care equals Health. But the Great Equation is wrong. More available medical care does not equal better health. The best estimates are that the medical system (doctors, drugs, hospitals) offers about 10 per cent of the usual indices for measuring health whether you live at all (infant mortality), how well you live (days lost due to sickness), how long you live (adult mortality). The remaining 90 per cent are determined by factors over which doctors have little or no control, from individual life style (smoking, exercise, worry), to social conditions (income, eating habits, physiological inheritance), to the physical environment (air and water quality). Most of the bad things that happen to people are at present beyond the reach of medicine.

Everyone knows that doctors do help. They can mend broken bones, stop infections with drugs, operate successfully on swollen appendices. Inoculations, internal infections, and external repairs are other good reasons for keeping doctors, drugs, and hospitals around. More of the same, however, is counterproductive. Nobody needs unnecessary operations; and excessive use of drugs can create dependence or allergic reactions or merely enrich the nation's urine.

More money alone, then, cannot cure old complaints. In the absence of medical knowledge gained through new research, or of administrative knowledge to convert common practice into best practice, current medicine has gone as far as it can. It will not burn brighter if more money is poured on it. No one is saying that medicine is good for nothing, only that it is not good for everything. Thus the marginal value of one—or one billion—dollars spent on medical care will be close to zero in improving health. And, for purposes of public policy, it is not the bulk of present medical expenditures, which do have value, but the proposed future spending, which is of dubious value, that should be our main concern.

When people are polled, they are liable, depending on what they are asked, to say that they are getting good care but that there is a crisis in the medical-care system. Three-quarters to four-fifths of the population, depending on the survey, are satisfied with their doctors and the care they give; but one-third to two-thirds think the system that produces these results is in bad shape. Opinions about the family doctor, of course, are formed from personal experience. "The system," on the other hand, is an abstract entity—and here people may well imitate the attitudes of those interested and vocal elites who insist the system is in crisis. People do, however, have specific complaints related to their class position. The rich don't like waiting, the poor don't like high prices, and those in the middle don't like both. Everyone would like easier access to a private physician in time of need. As we shall see, the widespread belief that doctors are good but the system is bad has a plausible explanation. That's the trouble: everyone behaves reasonably; it is only the systemic effects of all this reasonable behavior that are unreasonable.

If most people are healthier today than people like themselves have ever been, and if access to medical care now is more evenly distributed among rich and poor, why is there said to be a crisis in medical care that requires massive change? If the bulk of the population is satisfied with the care it is getting, why is there so much pressure in government for change? Why, in brief, are we doing better but feeling worse? Let us try to create a theory of the political pathology of health policy.

PARADOXES, PRINCIPLES, AXIOMS, IDENTITIES, AND LAWS

The fallacy of the Great Equation is based on the Paradox of Time: past successes lead to future failures. As life expectancy increases and as formerly disabling diseases are conquered, medicine is faced with an older population whose disabilities are more difficult to defeat. The cost of cure is higher, both because the easier ills have already been dealt with and because the patients to be treated are older. Each increment of knowledge is harder won; each improvement in health is more expensive. Thus time converts one decade's achievements into the next decade's dilemmas. Yesterday's victims of tuberculosis are today's geriatric cases. The Paradox of Time is that success lies in the past and (possibly) the future, but never the present.

The Great Equation is rescued by the *Principle of Goal Displacement*, which states that any objective that cannot be attained will be replaced by one that can be approximated. Every program needs an opportunity to be successful; if it cannot succeed in terms of its ostensible goals, its sponsors may shift to goals whose achievement they can control. The process subtly becomes the purpose. And that is exactly what has happened as "health" has become equivalent to "equal access to" medicine.

When government goes into public housing, it actually provides apartments; when it goes into health, all it can provide is medicine. But medicine is far from health. So what the government can do then is try to equalize access to medicine, whether or not that access is related to improved health. If the question is, "Does health increase with government expenditure on medicine?," the answer is likely to be "No." Just alter the question—"Has access to medicine been improved by government programs?"—and the answer is most certainly, with a little qualification, "Yes."

By "access," of course, we mean quantity, not quality, of care. Access, moreover, can be measured, and progress toward an equal number of visits to doctors can be reported. But better access is not the same as better health. Something has to be done about the distressing stickiness of health rates, which fail to keep up with access. After all, if medical care does not equal health, access to medical care is irrelevant to health—unless, of course, health is not the real goal but merely a cover for something more fundamental, which might be called "mental health" (reverently), or "shamanism" (irreverently), or "caring" (most accurately).

Any doctor will tell you, say sophisticates, that most patients are not sick, at least physically, and that the best medicine for them is reassurance. Tranquilizers, painkillers, and aspirin would seem to be the functional equivalents, for these are the drugs most often prescribed. Wait a minute, says the medical sociologist (the student not merely of medicine's manifest, but also of its latent, functions), pain is just as real when it's mental as when it's physical. If people want to know somebody loves them, if today they prefer doctors of medicine to doctors of theology, they are entitled to get what they want.

Once "caring" has been substituted for (or made equivalent to) "doctoring," access immediately becomes a better measure of attainment. The number of times a person sees a doctor is probably a better measure of the number of times he has been reassured than of his well-being or a decline in his disease. So what looks like a single goal substitution (access to medicine in place of better health) is actually a double displacement: caring instead of health, and access instead of caring.

This double displacement is fraught with consequences. Determining how much medical care is sufficient is difficult enough; determining how much "caring" is, is virtually impossible. The treatment of physical ills is partially subjective; the treatment of mental ills is almost entirely subjective. If a person is in pain, he alone can judge how much it hurts. How much caring he needs depends upon how much he wants. In the old days he took his tension chiefly to the private sector, and there he got as much attention as he could pay for. But now with government subsidy of medicine looming so large, the question of how much caring he should get inevitably becomes public.

By what standard should this public question be decided? One objective criterion—equality of access—inevitably stands out among the rest. For if we don't quite know what caring is or how much of it there should be, we can always say that at least it should be equally distributed. Medicaid has just about equalized the number of doctor visits per year between the poor and the rich. In fact, the upper class is showing a decrease in visits, and the life expectancy of richer males is going down somewhat. Presumably, no one is suggesting remedial action in favor of rich men. Equality, not health, is the issue.

Equality

One can always assert that even if the results of medical treatment are illusory, the poor are entitled to their share. This looks like a powerful argument, but it neglects the *Axiom of Inequality*. That axiom states that every move to increase equality in one dimension necessarily decreases it in another. Consider space. The United States has unequal rates of development. Different geographic areas vary considerably in such matters as income, custom, and expectation. Establishing a uniform national policy disregards these differences; allowing local variation means that some areas are more unequal than others. Think of time. People not only have unequal incomes, they also differ in the amount of time they are prepared to devote to medical care. In equalizing the effects of money on medical care—by removing money as a consideration—care is likely to be allocated by the distribution of available time. To the extent that the pursuit of money takes time, people with a monetary advantage will have a temporal disadvantage. You can't have it both ways, as the Axiom of Allocation makes abundantly clear.

"No system of care in the world," says David Mechanic, summing up the *Axiom of Allocation,* "is willing to provide as much care as people will use, and all such systems develop mechanisims that ration . . . services." Just as there is no free lunch, so there is *no free medicine.* Rationing can be done by time (waiting lists, lines), by distance (people farther from facilities use them less than those who are closer), by complexity (forms, repeated visits, communications difficulties), by space (limiting the number of hospital beds and available doctors), or by any or all of these methods in combination. But why do people want more medical service than any system is willing to provide? The answer has to do with uncertainty.

If medicine is only partially and imperfectly related to health, it follows that doctor and patient both will often be uncertain as to what is wrong or what to do about it. Otherwise—if medicine were perfectly related to health—either there would be no health problem or it would be a very different one. Health rates would be on one side and health resources on the other; costs and benefits could be neatly compared. But they can't, because we often don't know how to produce the desired benefits. Uncertainty exists because medicine is a quasi-science—more science than, say, political science; less science than physics. How the participants in the medical system resolve their uncertainties matters a great deal.

The *Medical Uncertainty Principle* states that there is always one more thing that might be done—another consultation, a new drug, a different treatment. Uncertainty is resolved by doing more: the patient asks for more, the doctor orders more. The patient's simple rule for resolving uncertainty is to seek care up to the level of his insurance. If everyone uses all the care he can, total costs will rise; but the individual has so little control over the total that he does not appreciate the connection between his individual choice and the collective result. A corresponding phenomenon occurs among doctors. They can resolve uncertainty by prescribing up to the level of the patient's insurance, a rule reinforced by the high cost of malpractice. Patients bringing suit do not consider the relationship between their own success and higher medical costs for everyone. The patient is anxious, the doctor insecure; this combination is unbeatable until the irresistible force meets the immovable object—the Medical Identity.

The *Medical Identity* states that use is limited by availability. Only so much can be gotten out of so much. Thus, if medical uncertainty suggests that existing services will be used, Identity reminds us to add the words "up to the available supply." That supply is primarily doctors, who advise on the kind of care to provide and the number of hospital beds to maintain. But patients, considering only their own desires in time of need, want to maximize supply, a phenomenon that follows inexorably from the *Principle of Perspective*.

That principle states that social conditions and individual feelings are not the same thing. A happy social statistic may obscure a sad personal situation. A statistical equilibrium may hide a family crisis. Morbidity and mortality, in tabulating aggregate rates of disease and death, describe you and me but do not touch us. We do not think of ourselves as "rates." Our chances may be better or worse than the aggregate. To say that doctors are not wholly (or even largely) successful in alleviating certain symptoms is not to say that they don't help some people and that one of those people won't be me. Taking the chance that it will be me often seems to make sense, even if there is reason to believe that most people can't be helped and that some may actually be harmed. Most people, told that the same funds spent on other purposes may increase social benefits, will put their personal needs first. This is why expenditures on medical care are always larger than any estimate of the social benefit received. Now we can understand, by combining into one law the previous principles and Medical Identity, why costs rise so far and so fast.

The *Law of Medical Money* states that medical costs rise to equal the sum of all private insurance and government subsidy. This occurs because no one knows how much medical care ought to cost. The patient is not sure he is getting all he should, and the doctor does not want to be faulted for doing less than he might. Consider the triangular relationship between doctor, patient, and hospital. With private insurance, the doctor can use the hospital resources that are covered by the insurance while holding down his patient's own expenditures. With public subsidies, the doctor may charge his highest usual fee, abandon charitable work, and ignore the financial benefits of eliminating defaults on payments. His income rises. His patient doesn't have to pay, and his hospital expands. The patient, if he is covered by a government program or private insurance (as about 90 per cent are) finds that his out-of-pocket expenses have remained the same. His insurance costs more, but either it comes out of his paycheck, looking like a fixed expense, or it is taken off his income tax as a deduction. Hospitals work on a cost-plus basis. They offer the latest and the best, thus pleasing both doctor and patient. They pay their help better; or, rather, they get others to pay their help. It's on the house—or at least on the insurance.

Perhaps our triangle ought to be a square: maybe we should include insurance companies. Why are they left out of almost all discussions of this sort? Why don't they play a cost-cutting role in medical care as they do in other industries? After all, the less the outlay, the more income for the company. Here the simplest explanation seems the best: insurance companies make no difference because they are no different from the rest of the healty-care industry. The largest, Blue Cross *and* Blue Shield, are run by the hospital establishment on behalf of doctors. After all, hospitals do not so much have patients as they have doctors who have patients. Doctors run hospitals, not the other way around. Insurance companies not willing to play this game have left the field.

What process ultimately limits medical costs? If the Law of Medical Money predicts that costs will increase to the level of available funds, then that level must be limited to keep costs down. Insurance may stop increasing when out-of-pocket payments exceed the growth in the standard of living; at that point individuals may not be willing to buy more. Subsidy may hold steady when government wants to spend more on other things or when it wants to keep its total tax take down. Costs will be limited when either individuals or governments reduce the amount they put into medicine.

No doubt the Law of Medical Money is crude, even rude. No doubt it ignores individual instances of self-sacrifice. But it has the virtue of being a powerful and parsimonious predictor. Costs have risen (and are continuing to rise) to the level of insurance and subsidy.

WHY THERE IS A CRISIS

If more than three-quarters of the population are satisfied with their medical care, why is there a crisis? Surveys on this subject are inadequate, but invariably they reveal two things: (one) the vast majority are satisfied, but (two) they wish medical care didn't cost so much and they would like to be assured of contact with their doctor. So far as the people are concerned, then, the basic problems are cost and access. Why, to begin at the end, aren't doctors where patients want them to be?

To talk about physicians being maldistributed is to turn the truth upside down: it is the potential patients who are maldistributed. For doctors to be in the wrong place, they would have to be where people aren't, and yet they are accused of sticking to the main population centers. If distant places with little crowding and less pollution, far away from the curses of civilization, attracted the same people who advocate their virtues, doctors would live there, too. Obviously, they prefer the amenities of metropolitan areas. Are they wrong to live where they want to live? Or are the rural and remote wrong to demand that others come where they are?

Doctors can be offered a government subsidy—more money, better facilities—on the grounds that it is a national policy for medical care to be available wherever citizens choose to live. Virtually all students in medical schools are heavily subsidized, so it would not be entirely unjust to demand that they serve several years in places not of their own choosing. The reason such policies do not work well—from Russia to the "Ruritanias" of this world—is that people who are forced to live in places they don't like make endless efforts to escape.

Because the distribution of physicians is determined by rational choice—doctors locate where their psychic as well as economic income is highest—there is no need for special laws to explain what happens. But the political pathology of health policy—the more the government spends on medicine, the less credit it gets—does require explanation.

The syndrome of "the more, the less" has to be looked at as it developed over time. First we passed Medicare for the elderly and Medicaid for the poor. The idea was to get more people into the mainstream of good medical care. Following the Law of Medical Money, however, the immediate effect was to increase costs, not merely for the poor and elderly but for all the groups in between. You can't simply add the costs of the new coverage to the costs of the old; you have to multiply them both by higher figures up to the limits of the joint coverage. This is where the *Axiom of Inequality* takes over. The wealthier aged, who can afford to pay, receive not merely the same benefits as the aged poor, but even more, because they are better able to negotiate the system. Class tells. Inequalities are immediately created within the same category. Worse still is the "notch effect" under Medicaid, through which those just above the eligibles in income may be worse off than those below. Whatever the cutoff point, there must always be a "near poor" who are made more unequal. And so is everybody else who pays twice, first in taxes to support care for others and again in increased costs for themselves. Moreover, with increased utilization of medicine, the system becomes crowded; medical care is not only more costly but harder to get. So there we have the Paradox of Time—as things get better, they get worse.

The politics of medical care becomes a minus-sum game in which every institutional player leaves the table poorer than when he sat down. In the beginning, the number of new patients grows arithmetically while costs rise geometrically. The immediate crisis is cost. Medicaid throws state and federal budgets out of whack. The talk is all about chiselers, profiteers, and reductions. Forms and obstacles multiply. The Medical Identity is put in place. Uncle Sam becomes Uncle Scrooge. One would hardly gather that billions more are actually being spent on medicine for the poor. But the federal government is not the only participant who is doing better and feeling worse.

Unequal levels of development within states pit one location against another. A level of benefits adequate for New York City would result in coverage of half or more of the population in upstate areas as well as nearly all of Alaska's Eskimos and Arizona's Indians. The rich pay more; the poor get hassled. Patients are urged to take more of their medicine only to discover they are targets of restrictive practices. They are expected to pay deductibles before seeing a doctor and to contribute a co-payment (part of the cost) afterward. Black doctors are criticized if their practice consists predominantly of white patients, but they are held up to scorn if they increase their income by treating large numbers of the poor and aged in the ghettos. Doctors are urged to provide more patients with better medicine, and then they are criticized for making more money. The *Principle of Perspective* leads each patient to want the best for himself disregarding the social cost; and, at the same time, doctors are criticized for giving high-cost care to people who want it. The same holds true for hospitals: keeping wages down is exploitation of workers; raising them is taking advantage of insurance. Vast financial incentives are offered to encourage the establishment of nursing homes to serve the aged, and the operators are then condemned for taking advantage of the opportunity.

Does anyone win? Just try to abolish Medicare and Medicaid. Crimes against the poor and aged would be the least of the accusations. Few argue that the country would be better off without these programs than with them. Yet, as the programs operate, the smoke they generate is so dense that their supporters are hard to find.

By now it should be clear how growing proportions of people in need of medicine can be getting it in the midst of what is universally decried as a crisis in health care. Governments face phenomenal increases in cost. Administrators alternately fear charges of incompetence for failing to restrain real financial abuse and charges of niggardliness toward the needy. Patients are worried about higher costs, especially as serious or prolonged illnesses threaten them with financial catastrophe. That proportionally few people suffer this way does not decrease the concern, because it *can* happen to anyone. Doctors fear federal control, because efforts to lower costs lead to more stringent regulations. The proliferation of forms makes them feel like bureaucrats; the profusion of review committees threatens to keep them permanently on trial. New complaints increase faster than old ones can be remedied. Specialists in public health sing their ancient songs—you are what you eat, as old as you feel, as good as the air you breathe—with more conviction and less effect. True but trite: what can be done isn't worth doing; what is worth doing can't be done. The watchwords are malaise, stasis, crisis.

If money is a barrier to medicine, the system is discriminatory. If money is no barrier, the system gets overcrowded. If everyone is insured, costs rise to the level of the insurance. If many remain underinsured, their income drops to the level of whatever medical disaster befalls them. Inability to break out of this bind has made the politics of health policy pathological.

POLITICAL PATHOLOGY

Health policy began with a laudable effort to help people by resolving the polarized conflict between supporters of universal, national health insurance ("socialized" medicine) and the proponents of private medicine. Neither side believed a word uttered by the other. The issue was sidestepped by successfully implementing medical care for the aged under Social Security. Agreement that the aged needed help was easier to achieve than consensus on any overall medical system. The obvious defect was that the poor, who needed financial help the most, were left out unless they were also old and covered by Social Security. The next move, therefore, was Medicaid for the poor, at least for those reached by state programs.

Even if one still believed that medicine equaled health, it became impossible to ignore the evidence that availability of medical services was not the same as their delivery and use. Seeing a doctor was not the same as actually doing what he prescribed. It is hard to alleviate stress in the doctor's office when the patient goes back to the same stress at home and on the street.

"Health delivery" became the catchword. At times it almost seemed as if the welcome wagon was supposed to roll up to the door and deliver health, wrapped in a neat package. One approach brought services to the poor through neighborhood health centers. The idea was that local control would increase sensitivity to the patients' needs. But experience showed that this "sensitivity" had its price. Local "needs" encompassed a wider range of services, including employment. The costs per patient-visit for seeing a doctor or social worker were three to four times those for seeing a private practitioner. Achieving local control meant control by inside laymen rather than outside professionals, a condition doctors were loath to accept. Innovation both in medical practice and in power relationships proved a greater burden than distant federal sponsors could bear, so they tried to co-opt the medical powers by getting them to sponsor health centers. The price was paid in higher costs and lower local control. Amid universal complaints, programs were maintained where feasible, phased out where necessary, and forgotten where possible.

By now the elite participants have exceeded their thresholds of pain: government can't make good on its promises to deliver services;

administrators are blamed for everything from malpractice by doctors to overcharges by hospitals; doctors find their professional prerogatives invaded by local activists from below and by state and federal bureaucrats from above. From the left come charges that the system is biased against the poor because local residents are unable to obtain, or maintain, control of medical facilities, and because the rates by which health is measured are worse for them than for the better off. Loss of health is tied to lack of power. From the right come charges that the system penalizes the professional and the productive: excessive governmental intervention leads to lower medical standards and higher costs of bureaucracy, so that costs go up while health does not.

As neighborhood health centers (NHCs) phased out, the new favorites, the health-maintenance organizations (HMOs), phased in. If the idea behind the NHCs was to bring services to the people, the idea behind the HMOs is to bring the people to the services. If a rationale for NHCs was to exert lay control over doctors, the rationale for HMOs is to exert medical control over costs. The concept is ancient. Doctors gather together in a group facility. Individuals or groups, such as unions and universities, join the HMO at a fixed rate for specified services. Through efficiencies in the division of labor and through features such as bonuses to doctors for less utilization, downward control is exerted on costs.

Since the basic method of cutting costs is to reduce the supply of hospital beds and physician services (the Medical Identity), HMOs work by making people wait. Since physicians are on salary, they must be given a quota of patients or a cost objective against which to judge their efforts. Both incentives may have adverse effects on patients. HMO patients complain about the difficulty of building up a personal relationship with a doctor who can be seen quickly when the need arises. Establishing such a relationship requires communication skills most likely to be found among the middle class. The patient's ability to shop around for different opinions is minimized, unless he is willing to pay extra by going outside the system. Doctors are motivated to engage in preventive practices, though evidence on the efficacy of these practices is hard to come by. They are also motivated to engage in bureaucratic routines to minimize the patients' demands on their time; and they may divert patients to various specialties or ask them to return, so as to fit them into each physician's assigned quota. In a word, HMOs are a mixed bag, with no one quite sure yet what the trade-off is between efficiency and effectiveness. Turning the Great Equation into an Identity—where Health = Health Maintenance Organization—does, however, solve a lot of problems by definition.

HMOs may be hailed by some as an answer to the problem of medical information. How is the patient-consumer to know whether he is getting proper care at reasonable cost? If it were possible to rate HMOs, and if they were in competition, people might find it easier to choose among them than among myriads of private doctors. Instead of being required to know whether all those tests and special consultations were necessary, or how much an operation should cost, the patients (or better still, their sponsoring organizations) might compare records of each HMO's ability to judge. Our measures of medical quality and cost, however, are still primitive. Treatment standards are notoriously subjective. Health rates are so tenuously connected to medicine that they are bound to be similar among similar populations so long as everyone has even limited access to care.

If health is only minimally related to care, less expertise may be about as good as more professional training. If by "care" many or most people mean simply a sympathetic listener as much as, or more than, they mean a highly trained, cold diagnostician, cheaper help may be as good as, or even better than, expensive assistance. Enter the nurse-practitioner or the medical corpsman or the old Russian *feldsher*—medical assistants trained to deal with emergencies, make simple diagnoses, and refer more complicated problems to medical doctors. They cost less, and they actually make home visits. The main disadvantage is their apparent challenge to the prestige of doctors, but it could work the other way around: doctors might be elevated because they deal with more complicated matters. But the success of the medical assistant might nonetheless raise questions about the mystique of medical doctors. In response the doctors might deny that anyone else can really know what is going on and what needs to be done, and they might then use assistants as additions to (but not substitutes for) their services. That would mean another input into the medical system and therefore an additional cost. The politics of medicine is just as much about the power of doctors as it is about the authority of politicians.

Now we see again, but from a different angle, why the medical system seems in crisis although most people are satisfied with the care they are receiving. At any one time, most people are reasonably healthy. When they do need help, they can get it. The quality of care is generally impressive; or whatever ails them goes away of its own accord. But these comments apply only to the mass of patients. The elite participants—doctors, administrators, politicians—are all frustrated. Anything they turn to rebounds against them. Damned if they do and cursed if they don't, it is not surprising that they feel that any future position is bound to be less uncomfortable than the one they hold today. Things can always get worse, of course, but it is not easy for them to see that.

GOVERNMENTAL LEGITIMACY: CURING THE SICKNESS OF HEALTH

Why should government pay billions for health and get back not even token tribute? If government is going to be accused of abusing the poor, neglecting the middle classes, and milking the rich; if it is to be condemned for bureaucratizing the patient and coercing the doctor, it can manage all that without spending billions. Slanders and calumnies are easier to bear when they are cost-free. Spending more for worse treatment is as bad a policy for government as it would be for any of us. The only defendant without counsel is the government. What should it do?

The Axiom of Inequality cannot be changed; it is built into the nature of things. What government can do is to choose the kinds of inequalities with which it is prepared to live. Increasing the waiting time of the rich, for instance—that is, having them wait as long as everybody else—may not seem outrageous. Decreasing subsidies in New York City and increasing them in Jacksonville may seem a reasonable price to pay for national uniformity. From the standpoint of government, however, the political problem is not to achieve equal treatment but to get support, at least from those it intends to benefit. Government needs gratitude, not ingrates.

The Principle of Goal Displacement, through the double-displacement effect, succeeds only in substituting access to care for health; it by no means guarantees that people will value the access they get. Equal access to care will not necessarily be equated with the best care available or with all that patients believe they require. Government's task is to resolve the Paradox of Time so that, as things get better, people will see themselves as better off.

Proposals for governmental support of medical care have ranged from modest subsidies to private insurance (the AMA's Medicredit) to public control of the medical industry on the British model. The latter has never had much support in this country, because of widespread opposition to socializing doctors by turning them into de facto government employees. The former has lost whatever support it once had as respect for the AMA has declined, its internal unity has diminished, and its congressional supporters have nearly vanished. Private insurance seems as much the problem as the solution.

The two most prominent proposals would resolve the political problems of medical care in contrasting ways, but substantively they are similar. Both the Comprehensive Health Insurance Plan (CHIP), introduced in the last days of the Nixon administration, and the Kennedy-Mills proposal would involve billions of dollars in additional expenditures. Estimates put each of them at $42 billion to start, less substantial existing expenditures—but then no estimates in this field have ever come remotely close to reality. Both proposals would provide health insurance for virtually everyone and would cover almost everything (including catastrophic and long-term illness) except for prolonged mental illness and nursing-home care. Both include a string of deductibles and co-insurance mechanisms, with CHIP so complex as almost to defy description. Both seek to hold down costs by giving individuals a financial incentive to limit use. Neither provides incentives for the medical community to contain costs, other than the importunings of insurance companies and state governments (CHIP) or the federal government (Kennedy-Mills), which have not been noticeably effective in the past.

CHIP would be financed largely through employer-employee contributions, with employees making a per capita payment; Kennedy-Mills substitutes a more (though by no means entirely) progressive proportionate tax. CHIP mandates insurance and gives a choice of private plans supervised through state agencies. Kennedy-Mills works largely through a special fund collected and administered by the federal government. The basic difference between them is that more of the cost of Kennedy-Mills shows up in the federal budget, while most of the cost of CHIP, as its acronym suggests, is diffused through the private sector.

The most likely consequence of both proposals would be a vast inflation of costs without a corresponding increase in services. Since medical manpower and facilities could not increase proportionately with demand, prices would rise. It would be Medicaid all over again, only worse because so many new things would be attempted and so many old things expanded. Almost before the ink dried on the legislation, efforts would be under way to delay this provision, lessen the cost of that one, introduce rationing in nonmonetary ways, find more forms for doctors and patients to fill out, and on and on. Cries of systemic crisis would be replaced by prophecies of systemic failure. But enough. My purpose is not to predict the medical consequences of these proposals but to analyze their political rationale.

Based on the political premise that some form of national health insurance was inevitable, CHIP sought to limit the government's liability. By joining the opposition, the Nixon administration hoped to control the apparatus so as to lessen its impact on the federal budget and bureaucracy. If people were determined to have something that wasn't going to help them, the government could at least see to it that the totals did not swamp its budget or overload its administration.

The costs of failure would be spread around among the states, the various insurance companies, and innumerable individual and group medical practices. Just as revenue sharing was designed to channel demands to state and local governments, instead of the national government (here's a little money and lot of trouble, and don't bother me!) so CHIP was devised to diffuse responsibility.

What the Republican administration did not foresee was that the rapid breakdown of the existing medical system would inevitably lead to demands for a federal takeover. When a company goes bankrupt, it is usually returned, not to its owners, but to its creditors. This insight belongs to the sponsors of the Kennedy-Mills bill. They seized on the Nixon plan to advance one that would load additional clients, services, and billions onto the shoulders of government. Wouldn't this proposal be too expensive and cumbersome? The worse the better, politically! For then the stage would be set for a national health service.

Under the Kennedy-Griffith (now Kennedy-Corman) proposal, which was the senator's original preference, every person in the United States would, without personal payment, be covered for a wide variety of services, thus replacing all public programs and private insurance with an all-inclusive federal system. Every public and personal medical expense would be transferred to the federal government, paid for half by additional payroll taxes and higher taxes on unearned income and half from general revenues. Obviously, as the sole direct payer, the federal government would have control over costs, but, by the same token, it would have to make all the decisions on how much of what service would be provided to which people in what way for how long.

The difference between Kennedy-Mills and the Kennedy-Corman Health Society Act (HSA) is that the latter would work directly on the Law of Medical Money by limiting the financial resources flowing into the medical system. Whatever the federal government allocated would be all that could be spent, except for the sums spent by those people choosing to pay extra to go outside the system. To put HSA in proper perspective, it is useful to contrast it with another proposal, one that would also limit supply but from a different direction. Senators Long and Ribicoff proposed to deal with the costs of catastrophic illness by setting individual-expenditure limits beyond which costs would be paid by the government. But Long-Ribicoff did not relate individual payments to income. For our comparison, therefore, it is more helpful to concentrate on Martin Feldstein's proposal for an income-graded program in which each person pays medical costs up to a specified proportion of his income, after which the government picks up the remaining (defined as catastrophic) expenses. Medicare and Medicaid are replaced, as all benefits are related to income. The poor pay less, the rich pay more, but everyone is protected against the costs of catastrophe. Although the catastrophic portion would rise in cost, especially for long-term disability, it would represent a relatively small proportion of medical expenditures. Total costs would be determined by overall financial inputs, which would be limited by the willingness of people to pay instead of inflated by using up their insurance or subsidy.

At first glance it might appear strange for national health insurance (whether through private intermediaries or direct government operation) to be conceived of as a method for limiting costs; but experience in practice, as well as deduction from theory, bears out that conception. The usual complaint in Britain, for example, is that the National Health Service is being starved for funds: hospital construction has been virtually nil; the number of doctors per capita has hardly increased; long queues persist for hospitalization in all but emergency cases. Why? Because health care accounts for a sizable proportion of both government expenditure and gross national product and must compete with family allowances, housing, transportation, and all the rest. While there are pressures to increase medical expenditures, they are counterbalanced by demands from other sectors. In times of extreme financial stringency, all too frequent as government expenditure approaches half of the GNP, it is not likely that priority will go to medicine.

So much for current trends. In the future, the nation will probably move toward (and vacillate between) three generic types of health care policies: (1) a mixed public and private system like the one we have now, only bigger; (2) total coverage through a national health service; and (3) income-graded catastrophic health insurance. It will be convenient to refer to these approaches as "mixed," "total," and "income."

The total and income approaches have weaknesses. The income-catastrophic approach might encourage a "sky's the limit" attitude toward large expenditures; the other side of the coin is that resources would flow to those chronically and/or extremely ill people who most need help. The total approach would strain the national budget, putting medical needs at the mercy of other concerns, such as tax increases; on the other hand, making medicine more political might have the advantage of providing more informed judgment on its relative priority. The two approaches, however, are more interesting for their different strengths than for their weaknesses.

The income approach would magnify individual choice until the level of catastrophic cost is reached. Holding ability to pay relatively constant, each person would be able to decide how much (in terms of what money can buy) he is willing to give up to purchase medical services. There would be no need to regulate the medical industry as to cost and service: supply and demand would determine the price. Paperwork would be minimized. So would bureaucracy. Under- or over-utilization could be dealt with by raising or lowering the percentage limits at each level of income, rather than by dealing with tens of thousands of doctors, hospitals, pharmacies, and the like. The total approach, by contrast, could promise a kind of collective rationality in the sense that the government would make a more direct determination of how much the nation wanted to spend on health versus other desired expenditures.

How might we choose between an essentially administrative and a primarily market-oriented mechanism? Each is as political as the other, but they come to their politics in different ways. An income approach would be simpler to administer and easier to abandon. If it didn't work, more ambitious programs could readily be subsidized. A total approach could promise more, because no one under existing programs would be worse off (except taxpayers), and everyone with insufficient coverage would come under its comprehensive umbrella. The backers of totality fear that the income approach would preempt the health field for years to come. The proponents of income grading fear that, once a comprehensive program is begun, there will be no getting out of it—too many people would lose benefits they already have, and the medical system would have unalterably changed its character. The choice (not only now but in the future) really has to be made on fundamental grounds of a modified-market versus an almost entirely administrative approach. Which proposal would be not only proper for the people but good for the government?

MARKET VERSUS ADMINISTRATIVE MECHANISMS

At the outset, I should state my conviction that doing either one consistently would be better than mixing them up. Both methods would give government a better chance to know what it is doing and to get credit for what it does. Expenditures on the medical system, whether too high or too low for some tastes, would be subject to overall control instead of sudden and unpredictable increases. Patients would have a system they could understand and would therefore be able to hold government accountable for how it was working. Under one system they would know that care was comprehensive, crediting government with the program and criticizing it for quality and cost. Under the other, they would know they were being encouraged to exercise discretion, but within boundaries guaranteeing them protection against catastrophe. Under the present system, they can't figure out what's going on (who can?); or why their coverage is inadequate; or why, if there is no effective government control, there are so many governmental forms. Mixed approaches will only exacerbate these unfortunate tendencies, multiplying ambiguities about deductibles and co-payment amid startling increases in cost. If we want our future to be better than our past, then let us look more closely at the bureaucratic and market models for medical care.

What do we know about medical care in a bureaucratic setting? Distressingly little. But there may be just enough collected from studies of HMOs and of systems in other countries, especially Britain, to provide a few clues. Doctors in HMOs work fewer hours than do doctors in private practice. This is not surprising. One of the attractions of HMOs for doctors is the limit on the hours they can be put on call. Market physicians respond to increases in patient load by increasing the hours they see patients; physicians working in a bureaucratic context respond by spending less time with patients. Two consequences of a public system are immediately apparent: more doctors will be needed, and less time will be spent listening and examining. Patients' demands for more time with the doctor will be met by repeated visits rather than longer ones. But will doctors be distributed more equally over the nation? The evidence suggests not. Britain has failed to achieve this goal in the quarter-century since the National Health Service began. The reason is that not only economic but also political allocations are subject to biases, one of which, incidentally, is called majority rule. The same forces that gather doctors in certain areas are reflected in the political power necessary to supply funds to keep them there.

Surely the ratio of specialists to general practitioners could be better controlled by central direction than by centrifugal market forces. Agreed. But a price is paid that should be recognized. The much higher proportion of general practitioners in Britain is achieved through a class bias that values "consultants" (their "specialists") more highly than ordinary doctors. (Consultants are called "Mister," as if to emphasize their individual excellence, while general practitioners are given the collective title of "Doctor.") The much higher proportion of specialists in America may stem in part from a desire to maintain equality among doctors—a nice illustration of the Axiom of Inequality. One result of the British custom is to lower the quality of general practice; another is to deny general practitioners access to hospitals. They lose control of their patients at the portal, leaving them without the comfort they may need in a stressful time and subjecting them to a bewildering maze of specialists and subspecialists, separated by custom and procedure, none of whom may be in charge of the whole person.

Would a bureaucratic system based on fixed charges and predetermined salaries place more emphasis on cheaper prevention than on more expensive maintenance, or on outpatient rather than hospital service? Possibly. (No one knows for sure whether preventive medicine actually works.) Doctors, in any event, do not cease to be doctors once they start operating in a bureaucratic setting. Cure, to doctors, is intrinsically more interesting than prevention; it is also something they know they can attempt, whereas they cannot enforce measures such as "no smoking." If it were true, moreover, that providing ample opportunities to see doctors outside the hospital would reduce the need to use hospitals, then providing outpatient services should hold down costs. The little evidence available, however, suggests otherwise. A natural experiment for this purpose takes place when patients have generous coverage for both in- and out-patient medical services. Visits to the doctor go up, but so does utilization of hospitals. More frequent visits generate awareness of more things wrong, for which more hospitalization is indicated. The way to limit hospital costs, if that is the objective, is to limit access to hospitals by reducing the number of available beds.

The great advantage of a comprehensive health service is that it keeps expenditures in line with other objectives. The Principle of Perspective works both ways: if an individual is not an aggregate, neither is an aggregate an individual. Left to our own devices, at near zero cost, you and I use as much as we and ours need. At the governmental level, however, it is not a question of personal needs and desires but of collective choice among different levels of taxation and expenditure. Hence, it should not be surprising that our collective choice would be less than the sum total of our individual preferences.

The usual complaint about the market method is money. Poor people are kept out of the medical system by not having enough. No one disputes this. And whatever evidence exists also suggests that the use of deductibles and co-payment exerts a disproportionate effect in deterring the poor from acquiring medical care. Therefore, to preserve as much of the market as possible, the response is to provide the poor with additional funds they can use for any purpose they desire, including (but not limited to) medical care. This immediately raises the issue of services in kind versus payment in cash. Enabling the poor to receive medical services without financial cost to themselves means they cannot choose alternative expenditures. A negative way of looking at this is to say that it reveals distrust of the poor: presumably, the poor are not able to make rational decisions for themselves, so the government must decide for them. A positive approach is to say that health is so important that society has an interest in assuring that the poor receive access to care. I almost said, "whether they want it or not," but, the argument continues, the choice of seeking or not seeking health care is neither easy nor simple: the poor—because they are poor, because money means more to them, because they have so many other vital needs—are under great temptation to sacrifice future health to present concerns. The alleged short-sighted psychology of the poor requires that they be protected against themselves.

The problem is not with the intellectually insubstantial (though politically potent) arguments that medical care is a right and that money should have nothing to do with medicine. The Axiom of Allocation assures us that medical care must be allocated in some way, and that, if it is not done at the bottom through individual income, it will be done at the top through national income. If medicine is a right, so is education, housing, food, employment (without which other rights can no longer be enjoyed), and so on, until we are led to the same old problems of resource allocation. The real question is whether care will be allocated by governmental mechanisms, in which one-man-one-vote is the ideal, or by the distribution of income, in which one-dollar-one-preference is the ideal, modified to assist the poor.

The problem for market men is not to demonstrate resource scarcity but to show that one of the essential conditions of buying and selling really is operating. I refer to consumer information about the cost and quality of care. The same problems crop up in many other areas involving technical advice: without knowing as much as the lawyer, builder, garage mechanic, or television repair man, how can the consumer determine whether the advice is good and the work performed properly and at reasonable cost?

The image in the literature is amateur patient versus professional doctor: the patient is not sure what is wrong, who the best doctor is, and how much the treatment should cost. Worse still, doctors deliberately withhold information by making it unethical to advertise prices or criticize peers. Should the doctor be less than competent or more than usually inclined to run up a bill, there is little the patient can do.

There are elements of reality in this picture, as all of us will recognize, but it is exaggerated. People can and do ask others about their experiences with various doctors; mothers endlessly compare pediatricians, for example. The abuses with which we are concerned are more likely to occur when patients lack a stable relationship with at least one doctor, and when there is no community whose opinions the doctor values and the patient learns to consult.

Nevertheless, it is obvious that patient-consumers do lack full information about the medical services they are buying. So, in fact, do doctors lack full knowledge of the services they are selling. How, then, might the imperfect medical market be improved? Would some alternative provision of medical services ensure better information?

Since all costs would be paid by taxpayers, government would have an incentive to keep the expenditures on a national health service in proportion to the expenditures for other vital activities. The very feature that has so far made a national health service politically unpalatable—it would take over about $50 billion of now private expenditures, thus requiring a massive tax increase—would immediately make the government financially responsible. Under a total governmental program, central authorities would have to determine how much should be spent and how these funds should be allocated to regional authorities. Basing the formula on numbers would put remote places at a disadvantage; basing it on area would put populous places at a disadvantage. How would regional authorities decide how much money to put toward hospital beds versus outpatient clinics, versus drugs, versus long-term care? There are few objective criteria. Would teams of medical specialists make the decisions? Professional boundaries would cause problems. Would administrators? Lack of medical expertise would cause problems. Administrative committees would have to decide who receives how much treatment, given the limited resources available from the central authority. Would their collective judgment be better or worse than that of individuals negotiating with doctors and hospitals? No one knows. But something can be said about the trade-off between quality and cost.

Suppose the question is: Under which type of system are costs likely to be highest per capita? The answer is: first, mixed public and private; second, mostly private; third, mostly public. Costs are greater under a mixed system because potential quality is valued over real cost: it pays each individual to use up his insurance and subsidy, because the quality-cost ratio is set high. Under the mostly private system, the individual has an incentive to keep his costs down. Under the largely public one, the government has an incentive to keep its costs within bounds. Because each individual regards his personal worth more than his social value, however, a series of individual payments will add up to something more than the payments determined by the very same people's collective judgment. At the margins, then, the economic market, preferring quality over cost, would produce somewhat larger expenditures than would the political arena.

Who would value a public medical system? Those who want government to exert maximum control over at least cost. The term "cost" here may be used in two ways—financial and political. Government does more, is able to allocate more resources, and has more of a chance of getting support for what it does. People who are more concerned with equality than with quality of care—though, of course, they want both—also should prefer public financing. It assures reasonably equal access, and it also places medical care in the context of other public needs. Doctors who value independence and patients who value responsiveness would be less in favor of a public system.

Who would prefer a private system, providing the effects of income were mitigated? People who want less governmental direction and more personal control over costs. These include doctors who want less governmental control, patients who want more choice, and politicians who want more leeway in resource allocation and less blame for bureaucratizing medicine.

I would prefer the income approach, because it is readily reversible; it means less bureaucracy and more choice. The total approach, however, could be infused with choice: Under the rubric of a single national health service, there could be three to six competitive and alternative programs, each organized on a different basis. There could be HMOs, foundation plans (under which individual doctors contract with a central service), and other variants. Patients could use any of these programs, all of which would be competing for their favor. The total sum to be spent each year would be fixed at the federal level, and each service would be paid its proportionate share according to the number and type of patients it had enrolled. Thus, we could mitigate the worst features of a bureaucratic system while maintaining its strengths.

Thought and Action

Let us summarize. Basically there are two sites for relating cost to quality—that is, for disciplining needs, which may be infinite, by controlling resources, which are limited. One is at the level of the individual; the other, at the level of the collectivity. By comparing his individual desires with his personal resources, through the private market, the individual internalizes an informal cost-effectiveness analysis. Since incomes differ, the break-even point differs among individuals. And if incomes were made more equal, individuals would still differ in the degree to which they choose medical care over other goods and services. These other valued objects would compete with medicine, leading some individuals to choose lower levels of medicine and thus reducing the inputs into (and cost of) the system. This creative tension can also be had at the collective level. There it is a tension between some public services, such as medicine, and others, such as welfare, and a tension between the resources left in private hands and those devoted to the public sector. The fatal defect of the mixed system, a defect that undermines the worth of its otherwise valuable pluralism, is that it does not impose sufficient discipline either at the individual or at the collective level. The individual need not face his full costs, and the government need not carry the full burden.

My purpose in writing this essay has not been to assess current political feasibility but to determine longer-lasting political virtue. The proposals I believe to be the worst for sustaining the legitimacy of government are at present the most popular. Proposals that deserve the most serious attention are ignored. The falsely assumed excessive cost of total care and the falsely believed inequality of the income approach have removed them from serious consideration. Perhaps this is the way it has to be. But I believe there is still time to change our ways of thinking about medical care. Medicine is by no means the only field where how we think affects what we believe, where what we believe is the key to how we feel, and where how we feel determines how we act.

If politicians did not believe that better health would emerge from greater effort, could they justify pouring billions more into the medical system? It could be argued that belief in medicine—doctor as witchdoctor—is so deeply ingrained that no evidence to the contrary would be accepted. Maybe. But this argument does not reach the question of what politicians would do if they believed otherwise.

Suppose the people were told that additional increments devoted to medicine would not improve their collective health but would give them more opportunity to express their individual feelings to doctors. How much more would they pay for this "caring"? Would it be as much as $10 billion? Would it be that high if the program contained no guarantee—and none do—that doctors would care more or be more available?

In any event, after the mixed approach fails, as it surely will, this country will be faced with the same alternatives—putting together the pieces administratively through a national health service, or dismantling what exists in favor of a modified market mechanism. But this is all too neat.

It could be, of course, that the future will find the worst is really the best. The three systems I have separated for analytical convenience—private, public, and mixed—may in practice refuse to reveal their pristine purity. What life has joined together no abstraction may be able to put asunder. A national health service, for instance, might quickly lose its putatively public character as numerous individuals opt for private care. In Scandinavian countries, even those in the professional strata who are convinced supporters of public medicine often prefer to use private doctors. They pay out to jump queues, so as to be treated when they wish, and to have private hospital rooms to carry on business or just to receive extra attention. By paying twice, once through taxes and once through fees for services, they raise the total cost of medicine to society. Would not a public system that was 20 or 30 per cent private be, in reality, mixed?

Consider an income-graded catastrophic system. It would, to begin with, have to pay all costs for those below the poverty line. As time passed, political pressure might increase the proportion of the population subsidized to 25 or 30 per cent. As costs increased, administrative action might be undertaken to limit coverage of expensive long-term illness. How different, then, would this presumably private system be from the mixed system it was designed to replace?

The present as future may be replaced by the future as future only to be superseded by the future as past. First the mixed system (the present as future) will be intensified by pouring billions into it (à la Kennedy-Mills). When that fails, an income-graded catastrophic plan or a national health service (the future as future) will be tried. Efforts to make the former system wholly private will be unfeasible, because public sentiment is against rationing medical care solely by money. Efforts to make the latter system wholly public will fail, because forbidding private fees for service will appear to citizens as an intolerable restraint on their liberty. Then we can expect the future as past. By the next century, we may have learned that a mixed system is bad in every respect except one—it mirrors our ambivalence. Whether we will grow up by learning to live with faults we do not wish to do without is a subject for a seer, not a social scientist.

Health policy is pathological because we are neurotic and insist on making our government psychotic. Our neurosis consists in knowing what is required for good health (Mother was right: Eat a good breakfast! Sleep eight hours a day! Don't drink! Don't smoke! Keep clean! *And* don't worry!) but not being willing to do it. Government's ambivalence consists in paying coming and going: once for telling people how to be healthy and once for paying their bills when they disregard this advice. Psychosis appears when government persists in repeating this self-defeating play. Maybe twenty-first-century man will come to cherish his absurdities.*

* I wish to thank Eli Ginzberg, Osler Peterson, Jack Fein, Lee Friedman, William Niskanen, Marc Pauley, Otto Davis, and Merlin DuVal for their helpful comments on various drafts of this paper. Responsibility for the final version, however, is mine.

BIBLIOGRAPHY

Eugene Feingold, *Medicare: Policy and Politics, A Case Study and Policy Analysis* (San Francisco, 1966).

Martin S. Feldstein, *The Rising Cost of Hospital Care* (a publication of the National Center for Health Services Research and Development, Information Resources Press, Washington, D.C., 1971).

Elliot Friedson, *Doctoring Together* (New York, 1976).

Victor R. Fuchs, ed., *Essays in the Economics of Health and Medical Care* (National Bureau of Economic Research, New York, 1972).

Eli Ginzberg, "Preventive Health: No Easy Answers," *The Sight-Saving Review*, Winter, 1973–74, pp. 187–93.

Edward Hughes, et al., "Utilization of Surgical Manpower in a Prepaid Group Practice," *The New England Journal of Medicine*, October 10, 1974, pp. 759–63.

Herbert E. Klarman, "Application of Cost-Benefit Analysis to the Health Services and the Special Case of Technologic Innovation," *International Journal of Health Services*, 4:2 (1974), pp. 325–52.

Theodore R. Marmor, "Can the U.S. Learn from Canada?," in S. Andreopoulos, ed., *National Health Insurance: Can We Learn from Canada?* (New York, 1975).

Thomas McKeown, *Medicine in Modern Society* (London, 1965).

David Mechanic, *The Growth of Bureaucratic Medicine: An Inquiry into the Dynamics of Patient Behavior and the Organization of Medical Care* (New York, 1976).

Osler Peterson, M.D., "Is Medical Care Worth the Price?," *Bulletin of the American Academy of Arts and Sciences*, 29:1 (October, 1975), pp. 17–23.

Robert Stevens and Rosemary Stevens, *Welfare Medicine in America: A Case Study of Medicaid* (New York, 1974).

Alan Williams, "Measuring the Effectiveness of Health Care Systems," *British Journal of Preventive and Social Medicine*, 28:3 (August, 1974), pp. 196–202.

Warren Winkelstein, Jr., "Epidemiological Considerations Underlying the Allocation of Health and Disease Care Resources," *International Journal of Epidemiology*, 1:1 (1972), pp. 69–74.

30 *Harvesting the Dead*

WILLARD GAYLIN, M.D.

Scarcity of organs and tissue is the most obvious major problem in transplantation. Gaylin suggests a not-too-fanciful solution: declaring people with a flat EEG to be dead and then maintaining them on respirators for the purposes of experimentation, transplantation, training of the physicians, and the production of needed hormones and antibodies. Such a solution has many obvious benefits and few major costs, except as Gaylin suggests, those costs on a level which may eventuate our paying more than we had ever imagined. The technology for such a procedure is with us now; serious ethical analysis of such use of the legally dead yet breathing corpses has not yet been made.

Dr. Willard Gaylin, M.D., is the President of the Institute of Society, Ethics, and the Life Sciences

Nothing in life is simple anymore, not even the leaving of it. At one time there was no medical need for the physician to consider the concept of death; the fact of death was sufficient. The difference between life and death was an infinite chasm breached in an infinitesimal moment. Life and death were ultimate, self-evident opposites.

Redefining Death

With the advent of new techniques in medicine, those opposites have begun to converge. We are now capable of maintaining visceral functions without any semblance of the higher functions that define a person. We are, therefore, faced with the task of deciding whether that which we have kept alive is still a human being, or, to put it another way, whether that human being that we are maintaining should be considered "alive."

Until now we have avoided the problems of definition and reached the solutions in silence and secret. When the life sustained was unrewarding—by the standards of the physician in charge—it was discontinued. Over the years, physicians have practiced euthanasia on an ad hoc, casual, and perhaps irresponsible basis. They have withheld antibiotics or other simple treatments when it was felt that a life did not warrant sustaining, or pulled the plug on the respirator when they were convinced that what was being sustained no longer warranted the definition of life. Some of these acts are illegal and, if one wished to prosecute, could constitute a form of manslaughter, even though it is unlikely that any jury would convict. We prefer to handle all problems connected with death by denying their existence. But death and its dilemmas persist.

New urgencies for recognition of the problem arise from two conditions: the continuing march of technology, making the sustaining of vital processes possible for longer periods of time; and the increasing use of parts of the newly dead to sustain life for the truly living. The problem is well on its way to being resolved by what must have seemed a relatively simple and ingenious method. As it turned out, the difficult issues of euthanasia could be evaded by redefining death.

In an earlier time, death was defined as the cessation of breathing. Any movie buff recalls at least one scene in which a mirror is held to the mouth of a dying man. The lack of fogging indicated that indeed he was dead. The spirit of man resided in his *spiritus* (breath). With increased knowledge of human physiology and the potential for reviving a nonbreathing man, the circulation, the pulsating heart, became the focus of the definition of life. This is the tradition with which most of us have been raised.

There is of course a relationship between circulation and respiration, and the linkage, not irrelevantly, is the brain. All body parts require the nourishment, including oxygen, carried by the circulating blood. Lack of blood supply leads to the death of an organ; the higher functions of the brain are particularly vulnerable. But if there is no respiration, there is no adequate exchange of oxygen, and this essential ingredient of the blood is no longer available for distribution. If a part of the heart loses its vascular supply, we may lose that part and still survive. If a part of the brain is deprived of oxygen, we may, depending on its location, lose it and survive. But here we pay a special price, for the functions lost are those we identify with the self, the soul, or humanness, i.e., memory, knowledge, feeling, thinking, perceiving, sensing, knowing, learning, and loving.

Most people are prepared to say that when all of the brain is destroyed the "person" no longer exists; with all due respect for the complexities of the mind/brain debate, the "person" (and personhood) is generally associated with the functioning part of the head—the brain. The higher functions of the brain that have been described are placed, for the most part, in the cortex. The brain stem (in many ways more closely allied to the spinal cord) controls primarily visceral functions. When the total brain is damaged, death in all forms will ensue because the lower brain centers that control the circulation and respiration are destroyed. With the development of modern respirators, however, it is possible to artificially maintain respiration and with it, often, the circulation with which it is linked. It is this situation that has allowed for the redefinition of death—a redefinition that is being precipitously embraced by both scientific and theological groups.

The movement toward redefining death received considerable impetus with the publication of a report sponsored by the Ad Hoc Committee of the Harvard Medical School in 1968. The committee offered an alternative definition of death based on the functioning of the brain. Its criteria stated that if an individual is unreceptive and unresponsive, i.e., in a state of irreversible coma; if he has no movements or breathing when the mechanical respirator is turned off; if he demonstrates no reflexes; and if he has a flat electroencephalogram for at least twenty-four hours, indicating no electrical brain activity (assuming that he has not been subjected to hypothermia or central nervous system depressants), he may then be declared dead.

What was originally offered as an optional definition of death is, however, progressively becoming *the* definition of death. In most states there is no specific legislation defining death;[1] the ultimate responsibility here is assumed to reside in the general medical community. Recently, however, there has been a series of legal cases which seem to be establishing brain death as a judicial standard. In California in May of this year an ingenious lawyer, John Cruikshank, offered as a defense of his client, Andrew D. Lyons, who had shot a man in the head, the argument that the cause of death was not the bullet but the removal of his heart by a transplant surgeon, Dr. Norman Shumway. Cruikshank's argument notwithstanding, the jury found his client guilty of voluntary manslaughter. In the course of that trial, Dr. Shumway said: "The brain in the 1970s and in the light of modern day medical technology is the sine qua non—the criterion for death. I'm saying anyone whose brain is dead is dead. It is the one determinant that would be universally applicable, because the brain is the one organ that can't be transplanted."

This new definition, independent of the desire for transplant, now permits the physician to "pull the plug" without even committing an act of passive euthanasia. The patient will first be defined as dead; pulling the plug will merely be the harmless act of halting useless treatment on a cadaver. But while the new definition of death avoids one complex problem, euthanasia, it may create others equally difficult which have never been fully defined or visualized. For if it grants the right to pull the plug, it also implicitly grants the privilege *not* to pull the plug, and the potential and meaning of this has not at all been adequately examined.

These cadavers would have the legal status of the dead with none of the qualities one now associates with death. They would be warm, respiring, pulsating, evacuating, and excreting bodies requiring nursing, dietary, and general grooming attention—*and could probably be maintained so for a period of years.* If we chose to, we could, with the technology already at hand, legally avail ourselves of these new cadavers to serve science and mankind in dramatically useful ways. The autopsy, that most respectable of medical traditions, that last gift of the dying person to the living future, could be extended in principle beyond our current recognition. To save lives and relieve suffering—traditional motives for violating tradition—we could develop hospitals (an inappropriate word because it suggests the presence of living human beings), banks, or farms of cadavers which require feeding and maintenance, in order to be harvested. To the uninitiated the "new cadavers" in their rows of respirators would seem indistinguishable from comatose patients now residing in wards of chronic neurological hospitals.

Precedents

The idea of wholesale and systematic salvage of useful body parts may seem startling, but it is not without precedent. It is simply magnified by the technology of modern medicine. Within the confines of one individual, we have always felt free to transfer body parts to places where they are needed more urgently, felt free to reorder the priorities of the naturally endowed structure. We will borrow skin from the less visible parts of the body to salvage a face. If a muscle is paralyzed, we will often substitute a muscle that subserves a less crucial function. This was common surgery at the time that paralytic polio was more prevalent.

It soon becomes apparent, however, that there is a limitation to this procedure. The person in want does not always have a second-best substitute. He may then be forced to borrow from a person with a surplus. The prototype, of course, is blood donation. Blood may be seen as a regeneratable organ, and we have a long-standing tradition of blood donation. What may be more important, and perhaps dangerous, we have established the precedent in blood of commercialization—not only are we free to borrow, we are forced to buy and, indeed, in our country at least, permitted to sell. Similarly, we allow the buying or selling of sperm for artificial insemination. It is most likely that in the near future we will allow the buying and selling of ripened ova so that a sterile woman may conceive her baby if she has a functioning uterus. Of course, once *in vitro* fertilization becomes a reality (an imminent possibility), we may even permit the rental of womb space for gestation for a woman who does manufacture her own ova but has no uterus.

Getting closer to our current problem, there is the relatively long-standing tradition of banking body parts (arteries, eyes, skin) for short periods of time for future transplants. Controversy has arisen with recent progress in the transplanting of major organs. Kidney transplants from a near relative or distant donor are becoming more common. As heart transplants become more successful, the issue will certainly be heightened, for while the heart may have been reduced by the new definition of death to merely another organ, it will always have a core position in the popular thinking about life and death. It has the capacity to generate the passion that transforms medical decisions into political issues.

The ability to use organs from cadavers has been severely limited in the past by the reluctance of heirs to donate the body of an individual for distribution. One might well have willed one's body for scientific purposes, but such legacies had no legal standing. Until recently, the individual lost control over his body once he died. This has been changed by the Uniform Anatomical Gift Act. This model piece of legislation, adopted by all fifty states in an incredibly short period of time, grants anyone over eighteen (twenty-one in some states) the right to donate en masse all "necessary organs and tissues" simply by filling out and mailing a small card.

Beyond the postmortem, there has been a longer-range use of human bodies that is accepted procedure—the exploitation of cadavers as teaching material in medical schools. This is a long step removed from the rationale of the transplant—a dramatic gift of life from the dying to the near-dead; while it is true that medical education will inevitably save lives, the clear and immediate purpose of the donation is to facilitate training.

It is not unnatural for a person facing death to want his usefulness to extend beyond his mortality; the same biases and values that influence our life persist in our leaving of it. It has been reported that the Harvard Medical School has no difficulty in receiving as many donations of cadavers as they need, while Tufts and Boston Universities are usually in short supply. In Boston, evidently, the cachet of getting into Harvard extends even to the dissecting table.

The way is now clear for an ever-increasing pool of usable body parts, but the current practice minimizes efficiency and maximizes waste. Only a short period exists between the time of death of the patient and the time of death of his major parts.

Uses of the Neomort

In the ensuing discussion, the word *cadaver* will retain its usual meaning, as opposed to the new cadaver, which will be referred to as a *neomort*. The "ward" or "hospital" in which it is maintained will be called a *bioemporium* (purists may prefer *bioemporion*).

Whatever is possible with the old embalmed cadaver is extended to an incredible degree with the neomort. What follows, therefore, is not a definitive list but merely the briefest of suggestions as to the spectrum of possibilities.

TRAINING: Uneasy medical students could practice routine physical examinations—auscultation, percussion of the chest, examination of the retina, rectal and vaginal examinations, et cetera—indeed, everything except neurological examinations, since the neomort by definition has no functioning central nervous system.

Both the student and his patient could be spared the pain, fumbling, and embarrassment of the "first time."

Interns also could practice standard and more difficult diagnostic procedures, from spinal taps to pneumoencephalography and the making of arteriograms, and residents could practice almost all of their surgical skills—in other words, most of the procedures that are now normally taught with the indigent in wards of major city hospitals could be taught with neomorts. Further, students could practice more exotic procedures often not available in a typical residency—eye operations, skin grafts, plastic facial surgery, amputation of useless limbs, coronary surgery, etc.; they could also practice the actual removal of organs, whether they be kidneys, testicles, or what have you, for delivery to the transplant teams.

TESTING: The neomort could be used for much of the testing of drugs and surgical procedures that we now normally perform on prisoners, mentally retarded children, and volunteers. The efficacy of a drug as well as its toxicity could be determined beyond limits we might not have dared approach when we were concerned about permanent damage to the testing vehicle, a living person. For example, operations for increased vascularization of the heart could be tested to determine whether they truly do reduce the incidence of future heart attacks before we perform them on patients. Experimental procedures that proved useless or harmful could be avoided; those that succeed could be available years before they might otherwise have been. Similarly, we could avoid the massive delays that keep some drugs from the marketplace while the dying clamor for them.

Neomorts would give us access to other forms of testing that are inconceivable with the living human being. We might test diagnostic instruments such as sophisticated electrocardiography by selectively damaging various parts of the heart to see how or whether the instrument could detect the damage.

EXPERIMENTATION: Every new medical procedure demands a leap of faith. It is often referred to as an "act of courage," which seems to me an inappropriate terminology now that organized medicine rarely uses itself as the experimental body. Whenever a surgeon attempts a procedure for the first time, he is at best generalizing from experimentation with lower animals. Now we can protect the patient from too large a leap by using the neomort as an experimental bridge.

Obvious forms of experimentation would be cures for illnesses which would first be induced in the neomort. We could test antidotes by injecting poison, induce cancer or virus infections to validate and compare developing therapies.

Because they have an active hematopoietic system, neomorts would be particularly valuable for studying diseases of the blood. Many of the examples that I draw from that field were offered to me by Dr. John F. Bertles, a hematologist at St. Luke's Hospital Center in New York. One which interests him is the utilization of marrow transplants. Few human-to-human marrow transplants have been successful, since the kind of immunosuppression techniques that require research could most safely be performed on neomorts. Even such research as the recent experimentation at Willowbrook—where mentally retarded children were infected with hepatitis virus (which was not yet culturable outside of the human body) in an attempt to find a cure for this pernicious disease—could be done without risking the health of the subjects.

BANKING: While certain essential blood antigens are readily storable (e.g., red cells can now be preserved in a frozen state), others are not, and there is increasing need for potential means of storage. Research on storage of platelets to be used in transfusion requires human recipients, and the data are only slowly and tediously gathered at great expense. Use of neomorts would permit intensive testing of platelet survival and probably would lead to a rapid development of a better storage technique. The same would be true for white cells.

As has been suggested, there is great wastage in the present system of using kidney donors from cadavers. Major organs are difficult to store. A population of neomorts maintained with body parts computerized and catalogued for compatibility would yield a much more efficient system. Just as we now have blood banks, we could have banks for all the major organs that may someday be transplantable—lungs, kidney, heart, ovaries. Beyond the obvious storage uses of the neomort, there are others not previously thought of because there was no adequate storage facility. Dr. Marc Lappé of the Hastings Center has suggested that a neomort whose own immunity system had first been severely repressed might be an ideal "culture" for growing and storing our lymphoid components. When we are threatened by malignancy or viral disease, we can go to the "bank" and withdraw our stored white cells to help defend us.

HARVESTING: Obviously, a sizable population of neomorts will provide a steady supply of blood, since they can be drained periodically. When we consider the cost-benefit analysis of this system, we would have to evaluate it in the same way as the lumber industry evaluates sawdust—a product which in itself is not commercially feasible but which supplies a profitable dividend as a waste from a more useful harvest.

The blood would be a simultaneous source of platelets, leukocytes, and red cells. By attaching a neomort to an IBM cell separator, we could isolate cell types at relatively low cost. The neomort could also be tested for the presence of hepatitis in a way that would be impossible with commercial donors. Hepatitis as a transfusion scourge would be virtually eliminated.

Beyond the blood are rarer harvests. Neomorts offer a great potential source of bone marrow for transplant procedures, and I am assured that a bioemporium of modest size could be assembled to fit most transplantation antigen requirements. And skin would, of course, be harvested—similarly bone, corneas, cartilage, and so on.

MANUFACTURING: In addition to supplying components of the human body, some of which will be continually regenerated, the neomort can also serve as a manufacturing unit. Hormones are one obvious product, but there are others. By the injection of toxins, we have a source of antitoxin that does not have the complication of coming from another animal form. Antibodies for most of the major diseases can be manufactured merely by injecting the neomort with the viral or bacterial offenders.

Perhaps the most encouraging extension of the manufacturing process emerges from the new cancer research, in which immunology is coming to the fore. With certain blood cancers, great hope attaches to the use of antibodies. To take just one example, it is conceivable that leukemia could be generated in individual neomorts—not just to provide for *in vivo* (so to speak) testing of antileukemic modes of therapy but also to generate antibody immunity responses which could then be used in the living.

Cost-Benefit Analysis

If seen only as the harvesting of products, the entire feasibility of such research would depend on intelligent cost-benefit analysis. Although certain products would not warrant the expense of maintaining a community of neomorts, the enormous expense of other products, such as red cells with unusual antigens, would certainly warrant it. Then, of course, the equation is shifted. As soon as one economically sound reason is found for the maintenance of the community, all of the other ingredients become gratuitous by-products, a familiar problem in manufacturing. There is no current research to indicate the maintenance cost of a bioemporium or even the potential duration of an average neomort. Since we do not at this point encourage sustaining life in the brain-dead, we do not know the limits to which it could be extended. This is the kind of technology, however, in which we have previously been quite successful.

Meantime, a further refinement of death might be proposed. At present we use total brain function to define brain death. The source of electroencephalogram activity is not known and cannot be used to distinguish between the activity of higher and lower brain centers. If, however, we are prepared to separate the concept of "aliveness" from "personhood" in the adult, as we have in the fetus, a good argument can be made that death should be defined not as cessation of total brain function but merely as cessation of cortical function. New tests may soon determine when cortical function is dead. With this proposed extension, one could then maintain neomorts without even the complication and expense of respirators. The entire population of decorticates residing in chronic hospitals and now classified among the incurably ill could be redefined as dead.

But even if we maintain the more rigid limitations of total brain death it would seem that a reasonable population could be maintained if the purposes warranted it. It is difficult to assess how many new neomorts would be available each year to satisfy the demand. There are roughly 2 million deaths a year in the United States. The most likely sources of intact bodies with destroyed brains would be accidents (about 113,000 per year), suicides (around 24,000 per year), homicides (18,000), and cerebrovascular accidents (some 210,000 per year). Obviously, in each of these categories a great many of the individuals would be useless—their bodies either shattered or scattered beyond value or repair.

And yet, after all the benefits are outlined, with the lifesaving potential clear, the humanitarian purposes obvious, the technology ready, the motives pure, and the material costs justified—how are we to reconcile our emotions? Where in this debit-credit ledger of limbs and livers and kidneys and costs are we to weigh and enter the repugnance generated by the entire philanthropic endeavor?

Cost-benefit analysis is always least satisfactory when the costs must be measured in one realm and the benefits in another. The analysis is particularly skewed when the benefits are specific, material, apparent, and immediate, and the price to be paid is general, spiritual, abstract, and of the future. It is that which induces people to abandon freedom for security, pride for comfort, dignity for dollars.

William May, in a perceptive article,[2] defended the careful distinctions that have traditionally been drawn between the newly dead and the long dead. "While the body retains its recognizable form, even in death, it commands a certain respect. No longer a human presence, it still reminds us of that presence which once was utterly inseparable from it." But those distinctions become obscured when, years later, a neomort will retain the appearance of the newly dead, indeed, more the appearance of that which was formerly described as living.

Philosophers tend to be particularly sensitive to the abstract needs of civilized man; it is they who have often been the guardians of values whose abandonment produces pains that are real, if not always quantifiable. Hans Jonas, in his *Philosophical Essays*, anticipated some of the possibilities outlined here, and defended what he felt to be the sanctity of the human body and the unknowability of the borderline between life and death when he insisted that "Nothing less than the maximum definition of death will do—brain death plus heart death plus any other indication that may be pertinent—before final violence is allowed to be done." And even then Jonas was only contemplating *temporary* maintenance of life for the collection of organs.

The argument can be made on both sides. The unquestionable benefits to be gained are the promise of cures for leukemia and other diseases, the reduction of suffering, and the maintenance of life. The proponents of this view will be mobilized with a force that may seem irresistible.

They will interpret our revulsion at the thought of a bioemporium as a bias of our education and experience, just as earlier societies were probably revolted by the startling notion of abdominal surgery, which we now take for granted. The proponents will argue that the revulsion, not the technology, is inappropriate.

Still there will be those, like May, who will defend that revulsion as a quintessentially human factor whose removal would diminish us all, and extract a price we cannot anticipate in ways yet unknown and times not yet determined. May feels that there is "a tinge of the inhuman in the humanitarianism of those who believe that the perception of social need easily overrides all other considerations and reduces the acts of implementation to the everyday, routine, and casual."

This is the kind of weighing of values for which the computer offers little help. Is the revulsion to the new technology simply the fear and horror of the ignorant in the face of the new, or is it one of those components of humanness that barely sustain us at the limited level of civility and decency that now exists, and whose removal is one more step in erasing the distinction between man and the lesser creatures—beyond that, the distinction between man and matter?

Sustaining life is an urgent argument for any measure, but not if that measure destroys those very qualities that make life worth sustaining.

[1] Kansas and Maryland have recently legislated approval for a brain definition of death.

[2] "Attitudes Toward the Newly Dead," *The Hastings Center Studies*, volume 1, number 1, 1973.

31 *Allocating Scarce Medical Resources and the Availability of Organ Transplantation: Some Moral Presuppositions*

H. Tristram Engelhardt

Engelhardt argues that some ethical dilemmas have a staying problem because of their complexity, morally and conceptually. The organ transplantation debates raise profound issues of public policy, the allocation of medical and financial resources, problems of procurement and distribution, and the right to health care. Engelhardt further focuses the ethical dilemmas by relating the transplantation dilemmas to circumstances of life which are unfortunate and fair and unfortunate and unfair. The article provides a careful ethical analysis of the profound dilemmas at the heart of the organ transplantation debates.

H. Tristram Engelhardt is at the Center for Ethics, Baylor College of Medicine in Houston, Texas.

THE PROBLEM

Some controversies have a staying power because they spring from unavoidable moral and conceptual puzzles. The debates concerning transplantation are a good example. To begin with, they are not a single controversy. Rather, they are examples of the scientific debates with heavy political and ethical overlays that characterize a large area of public-policy discussions.[1]

The determination of whether or not heart or liver transplantation is an experimental or nonexperimental procedure for which it is reasonable and necessary to provide reimbursement is not simply a determination on the basis of facts regarding survival rates or the frequency with which the procedure is employed. Nor is it a purely moral issue.[2]

It is an issue similar to that raised regarding the amount of pollutants that ought to be considered safe in the work place. The question cannot be answered simply in terms of scientific data, unless one presumes that there will be a sudden inflection in the curve expressing the relationship of decreasing parts per billion of the pollutant and the incidence of disease or death, after which very low concentrations do not contribute at all to an excess incidence of disability or death. If one assumes that there is always some increase in death and disability due to the pollutant, one is not looking for an absolutely safe level but rather a level at which the costs in lives and health do not outbalance the costs in jobs and societal vexation that most more stringent criteria would involve. Such is not a purely factual judgment but requires a balancing of values. Determinations of whether a pollutant is safe at a particular level, of whether a procedure is reasonable and necessary, of whether a drug is safe, of whether heart and liver transplantations should be regarded as nonexperimental procedures are not simply factual determinations. In the background of those determinations is a set of moral judgments regarding equity, decency, and fairness, cost–benefit trade-offs, individual rights, and the limits of state authority.

Since such debates are structured by the intertwining of scientific, ethical, and political issues, participants appeal to different sets of data and rules of inference, which leads to a number of opportunities for confusion. The questions that cluster around the issue of providing for the transplantation of organs have this distracting heterogeneity. There are a number of questions with heavy factual components, such as, "Is the provision of liver transplants an efficient use of health-care resources?" and "Will the cost of care in the absence of a transplant approximate the costs involved in the transplant?" To answer such questions, one will need to continue to acquire data concerning the long-term survival rates of those receiving transplants.[3-8] There are, as well, questions with major moral and political components, which give public-policy direction to the factual issues. "Does liver or heart transplantation offer a proper way of using our resources, given other available areas of investment?" "Is there moral authority to use state force to redistribute financial resources so as to provide transplantations for all who would benefit from the procedure?" "How ought one fairly to resolve controversies in this area when there is important moral disagreement?"

These serious questions have been engaged in a context marked by passion, pathos, and publicity. George Deukmejian, governor of California, ordered the state to pay for liver transplantation for Koren Crosland, and over $265,000 was raised through contributions from friends and strangers to support the liver transplantation of Amy Hardin of Cahokia, Illinois.[9] Charles and Marilyn Fiske's testimony to the Subcommittee on Investigations and Oversight of the House Committee on Science and Technology provided an example of how fortuitous publicity can lead to treatment[10]—in this case, to their daughter Jamie's receiving payment through Blue Cross of Massachusetts by agreement on October 1, 1982,[11] along with contingency authorization for coverage for liver-transplantation expenses through the Commonwealth of Massachusetts on October 29, 1982.[12] The proclamation by President Reagan of a National Organ Donation Awareness Week, which ran from April 22 through 28, further underscored the public nature of the issues raised.[13] In short, several serious and difficult moral and political dilemmas have been confronted under the spotlight of media coverage and political pressures.[14-17] What is needed is an examination of the moral and conceptual assumptions that shape the debate, so that one can have a sense of where reasonable answers can be sought.

Why Debates about Allocating Resources Go On and On

The debates concerning the allocation of resources to the provision of expensive, life-saving treatment such as transplantation have recurred repeatedly over the past two decades and show no promise of abating.[18-21] To understand why that is the case, one must recall the nature of the social and moral context within which such debates are carried on. Peaceable, secular, pluralist societies are by definition ones that renounce the use of force to impose a particular ideology or view of the good life, though they include numerous communities with particular, often divergent, views of the ways in which men and women should live and use their resources. Such peaceable, secular societies require at a minimum a commitment to the resolution of disputes in ways that are not fundamentally based on force.[22] There will thus be greater clarity regarding how peaceably to discuss the allocation of resources for transplantation than there will be regarding the importance of the allocation of resources itself.[23] The latter requires a more concrete view of what is important to pursue through the use of our resources than can be decisively established in general secular terms. As a consequence, it is clearer that the public has a right to determine particular expenditures of common resources than that any particular use of resources, as for the provision of transplantation, should be embraced.

This is a recurring situation in large-scale, secular, pluralist states. The state as such provides a relatively neutral bureaucracy that transcends the particular ideological and religious commitments of the communities it embraces, so that its state-funded health-care service (or its postal service) should not be a Catholic, Jewish, or even Judeo-Christian service. This ideal of a neutral bureaucracy is obviously never reached. However, the aspiration to this goal defines peaceable, secular, pluralist societies and distinguishes them from the political vision that we inherited from Aristotle and which has guided us and misguided us over the past two millennia. Aristotle took as his ethical and political ideal the city-state with no more than 100,000 citizens, who could then know each other, know well whom they should elect, and create a public consensus.[24,25] It is ironic that Aristotle fashioned this image as he participated in the fashioning of the first large-scale Greek state.

We do not approach the problems of the proper allocations of scarce resources within the context of a city-state, with a relatively clear consensus of the ways in which scarce resources ought to be used. Since the Reformation and the Renaissance, the hope for a common consensus has dwindled, and with good cause. In addition, the Enlightenment failed to provide a fully satisfactory secular surrogate. It failed to offer clearly convincing moral arguments that would have established a particular view of the good life and of the ways in which resources ought to be invested. One is left only with a general commitment to peaceable negotiation as the cardinal moral canon of large-scale peaceable, secular, pluralist states.[26]

As a result, understandings about the proper use of scarce resources tend to occur on two levels in such societies. They occur within particular religious bodies, political and ideological communities, and interest groups, including insurance groups. They take place as well within the more procedurally oriented vehicles and structures that hold particular communities within a state. The more one addresses issues such as the allocation of scarce resources in the context of a general secular, pluralist society, the more one will be pressed to create an answer in some procedurally fair fashion, rather than hope to discover a proper pattern for the distribution of resources to meet medical needs. However, our past has left us with the haunting and misguided hope that the answer can be discovered.

There are difficulties as well that stem from a tension within morality itself: a conflict between respecting freedom and pursuing the good. Morality as an alternative to force as the basis for the resolution of disputes focuses on the mutual respect of persons. This element of morality, which is autonomy-directed, can be summarized in the maxim, Do not do unto others what they would not have done unto themselves. In the context of secular pluralist ethics, this element has priority, in that it can more clearly be specified and justified. As a result, it sets limits to the moral authority of others to act and thus conflicts with that dimension of morality that focuses on beneficence, on achieving the good for others. This second element of morality may be summarized in the maxim, Do to others their good. The difficulty is that the achievement of the good will requires the cooperation of others who may claim a right to be respected in their nonparticipation. It will require as well deciding what goods are to be achieved and how they are to be ranked. One might think here of the conflict between investing communal resources in liver and heart transplantations and providing adequate general medical care to the indigent and near indigent. The more one respects freedom, the more difficult it will be for a society to pursue a common view of the good. Members will protest that societal programs restrict their freedom of choice, either through restricting access to programs or through taxing away their disposable income.

The problem of determining whether and to what extent resources should be invested in transplantation is thus considerable. The debate must be carried on in a context in which the moral guidelines are more procedural than supplied with content. Moreover, the debate will be characterized by conflicting views of what is proper to do, as well as by difficulties in showing that there is state authority to force the participation of unwilling citizens. Within these vexing constraints societies approach the problem of allocating scarce medical resources and in particular of determining the amount of resources to be diverted to transplantation. This can be seen as a choice among possible societal insurance mechanisms. As with the difficulty of determining a safe level of pollutants, the answer with respect to the correct level of insurance will be as much created as discovered.

INSURANCE AGAINST THE NATURAL AND SOCIAL LOTTERIES

Individuals are at a disadvantage or an advantage as a result of the outcomes of two major sets of forces than can be termed the natural and social lotteries.[27,28] By the natural lottery I mean those forces of nature that lead some persons to be healthy and others to be ill and disabled through no intention or design of their own or of others. Those who win the natural lottery do not need transplantations. They live long and healthy lives and die peacefully. By the social lottery I mean the various interventions, compacts, and activities of persons that, with luck, lead to making some rich and others poor. The natural lottery surely influences the social lottery. However, the natural lottery need not conclusively determine one's social and economic power, prestige, and advantage. Thus, those who lose at the natural lottery and who are in need of heart and liver transplantation may still have won at the social lottery by having either inherited or earned sufficient funds to pay for a transplantation. Or they may have such a social advantage because their case receives sufficient publicity so that others contribute to help shoulder the costs of care.

An interest in social insurance mechanisms directed against losses at the natural and social lotteries is usually understood as an element of beneficence-directed justice. The goal is to provide the amount of coverage that is due to all persons. The problem in such societal insurance programs is to determine what coverage is due. Insofar as societies provide all citizens with a minimal protection against losses at the natural and the social lotteries, they give a concrete understanding of what is due through public funds. At issue here is whether coverage must include transplantation for those who cannot pay.

However, there are moral as well as financial limits to a society's protection of its members against such losses. First and foremost, those limits derive from the duty to respect individual choices and to recognize the limits of plausible state authority in a secular, pluralist society. If claims by society to the ownership of the resources and services of persons have limits, then there will always be private property that individuals will have at their disposal to trade for the services of others, which will create a second tier of health care for the affluent. Which is to say, the more it appears reasonable that property is owned neither totally societally nor only privately, and insofar as one recognizes limits on society's right to constrain its members, two tiers of health-care services will by right exist: those provided as a part of the minimal social guarantee to all and those provided in addition through the funds of those with an advantage in the social lottery who are interested in investing those resources in health care.

In providing a particular set of protections against losses at the social and natural lotteries, societies draw one of the most important societal distinctions—namely, between outcomes that will be socially recognized as unfortunate and unfair and those that will not be socially recognized as unfair, no matter how unfortunate they may be. The Department of Health and Human Services, for instance, in not recognizing heart transplantation as a nonexperimental procedure, removed the provision of such treatment from the social insurance policy. The plight of persons without private funds for heart transplantation, should they need heart transplantation, would be recognized as unfortunate but not unfair.[29-31] Similarly, proposals to recognize liver transplantation for children and adults as nonexperimental are proposals to alter the socially recognized boundary between losses at the natural and social lotteries that will be understood to be unfortunate and unfair and those that will simply be lamented as unfortunate but not seen as entitling the suffering person to a claim against societal resources.[32]

The need to draw this painful line between unfortunate and unfair outcomes exists in great measure because the concerns for beneficence do not exhaust ethics. Ethics is concerned as well with respecting the freedom of individuals. Rendering to each his or her due also involves allowing individuals the freedom to determine the use of their private energies and resources. In addition, since secular pluralist arguments for the authority of peaceable states most clearly establish those societies as means for individuals peaceably to negotiate the disposition of their communally owned resources, difficulties may arise in the allocation of scarce resources to health care in general and to transplantation in particular. Societies may decide to allocate the communal resources that would have been available for liver and heart transplantation to national defense or the building of art museums and the expansion of the national park system. The general moral requirement to respect individual choice and procedurally fair societal decisions will mean that there will be a general secular, moral right for individuals to dispose of private resources, and for societies to dispose of communal resources, in ways that will be wrong from a number of moral perspectives. As a result, the line between outcomes that will count as unfortunate and those that will count as unfair will often be at variance with the moral beliefs and aspirations of particular ideological and moral communities encompassed by any large-scale secular society.

Just as one must create a standard of safety for pollutants in the work place by negotiations beween management and labor and through discussions in public forums one will also need to create a particular policy for social insurance to cover losses at the natural and social lotteries. This will mean that one will not be able to discover that any particular investment in providing health care for those who cannot pay is morally obligatory. One will not be able to show that societies such as that of the United Kingdom, which do not provide America's level of access to renal dialysis for end-stage renal disease, have made a moral mistake.[33,34] Moral criticism will succeed best in examining the openness of such decisions to public discussion and control.

It is difficulties such as these that led the President's Commission for the Study of Ethical Problems in Medicine and Biomedical and Behavioral Research to construe equity in health care neither as equality in health care nor as access to whatever would benefit patients or meet their needs. The goal of equality in health care runs aground on both conceptual and moral difficulties. There is the difficulty of understanding whether equality would embrace equal amounts of health care or equal amounts of funds for health care. Since individual health needs differ widely, such interpretations of equality are fruitless. Attempting to understand equality as providing health care only from a predetermined list of services to which all would have access conflicts with the personal liberty to use private resources in the acquisition of additonal care not on the list. Construing equity as providing all with any health care that would benefit them would threaten inordinately to divert resources to health care. It would conflict as well with choices to invest resources in alternative areas. Substituting "need" for "benefit" leads to similar difficulties unless one can discover, among other things, a notion of need that would not include the need to have one's life extended, albeit at considerable cost.

The commission, as a result, construed equity in health care as the provision of an "adequate level of health care." The commission defined adequate care as "enough care to achieve sufficient welfare, opportunity, information, and evidence of interpersonal concern to facilitate a reasonably full and satisfying life."[35] However, this definition runs aground on the case of children needing liver transplants and other such expensive health-care interventions required to secure any chance of achieving "a reasonably full and satisfying life." There is a tension in the commission's report between an acknowledgment that a great proportion of one's meaning of "adequate health care" must be created and a view that the lineaments of that meaning can be discovered. Thus, the commission states that "[i]n a democracy, the appropriate values to be assigned to the consequences of policies must ultimately be determined by people expressing their values through social and political processes, as well as in the marketplace."[36] On the other hand, the commission states that "adequacy does require that everyone receive care that meets standards of sound medical practice."[37] The latter statement may suggest that one could discover what would constitute sound medical practice. In addition, an appeal to a notion of "excessive burdens" will not straightforwardly determine the amount of care due to individuals, since a notion of "excessiveness" requires choosing a particular hierarchy of costs and benefits.[38] Neither will an appeal to excessive burdens determine the amount of the tax burden that others should bear,[39] since there will be morally determined upper limits to taxation set by that element of property that is not communal. People, insofar as they have private property in that sense, have the secular moral right, no matter how unfeeling and uncharitable such actions may appear to others, not to aid those with excessive burdens, even if the financial burdens of those who could be taxed would not be excessive.

Rather, it would appear, following other suggestions from the commission, that "adequate care" will need to be defined by considering, among other things, professional judgments of physicians, average current use, lists of services that health-maintenance organizations and others take to be a part of decent care, as well as more general perceptions of fairness.[40] Such factors influence what is accepted generally in a society as a decent minimal or adequate level of health care. As reports considering the effects of introducing expensive new technology suggest, there is a danger that treatments may be accepted as part of "sound medical practice" before the full financial and social consequences of that acceptance are clearly understood. Much of the caution that has surrounded the development of liver and heart transplantation has been engendered by the experience with renal dialysis, which was introduced with overly optimistic judgments regarding the future costs that would be involved.

Even if, as I have argued, the concrete character of "rights to health care" is more created as an element of societal insurance programs than discovered and if the creation is properly the result of the free choice of citizens, professional and scientific bodies will need to aid in the assessment of the likely balance of costs and benefits to be embraced with the acceptance of any new form of treatment as standard treatment, such as heart and liver transplantation. A premature acceptance may lead to cost pressures on services that people will see under mature consideration to be more important. At that point it may be very difficult to withdraw the label of "standard treatment" from a technologic approach that subsequent experience shows to be too costly, given competing opportunities for the investment of resources. On the other hand, new technologic developments may offer benefits worth the cost they will entail, such as the replacement by computerized tomography of pneumoencephalography. But in any event, there is no reason to suppose that there is something intrinsically wrong with spending more than 10.5 per cent of the gross national product on health care.

Is Transplantation Special?

All investments in expensive life-saving treatment raise a question of prudence: Could the funds have been better applied elsewhere? Will the investment in expensive life-saving treatment secure an equal if not greater decrease in morbidity and mortality than an investment in improving the health care of the millions who lack health-care insurance or have only marginal coverage? If the same funds were invested in prenatal health care or the treatment of hypertension, would they secure a greater extension of life and diminution of morbidity for more people? When planning for the rational use of communal funds, it is sensible to seek to maximize access and contribution to the greatest number of people as a reasonable test of what it means to use communal resources for the common good. However, not everything done out of the common purse need be cost effective. It is unclear how one could determine the cost effectiveness of symphony orchestras or art museums. Societies have a proclivity to save the lives of identifiable individuals while failing to come to the aid of unidentified, statistical lives that could have been saved with the same or fewer resources. Any decision to provide expensive life-saving treatment out of communal funds must at least frankly acknowledge when it is not a cost-effective choice but instead a choice made because of special sympathies for those who are suffering or because of special fears that are engendered by particular diseases.

The moral framework of secular, pluralist societies in which rights to health care are more created than discovered will allow such choices as morally acceptable, even if they are less than prudent uses of resources. It will also be morally acceptable for a society, if it pursues expensive life-saving treatment, to exclude persons who through their own choices increase the cost of care. One might think here of the question whether active alcoholics should be provided with liver transplants. There is no invidious discrimination against persons in setting a limit to coverage or in precluding coverage if the costs are increased through free choice. However, societies may decide to provide care even when the costs are incurred by free decision.

Though none of the foregoing is unique to transplantation, the issue of transplantation has the peculiarity of involving the problem not only of the allocation of monetary resources and of services but of that of organs as well. In a criticism of John Rawls' *Theory of Justice,* which theory attempts to provide a justification for a patterned distribution of resources that would redound to the benefit of the least-well-off class, Robert Nozick tests his readers' intuitions by asking whether societal rights to distribute resources would include the right to distribute organs as well.[41] He probably chose this as a test case because our bodies offer primordial examples of private property. The example is also forceful, given the traditional Western reluctance, often expressed in religious regulations, to use corpses for dissection. There is a cultural reluctance to consider parts of the body as objects for the use of persons. No less a figure than Immanuel Kant argued for a position that would appear to preclude the sale or gift of a body part to another.[42] This view of Kant's, one should note, is very close to the traditional Roman Catholic notion that one has a duty to God regarding one's self not to alter one's body except to preserve health.[43]

The concern to have a sufficient supply of organs for transplantation has expressed itself in recent political proposals and counterproposals regarding the rights of individuals to sell their organs, the provision of federal funds for the support of organ procurement, the study of the medical and legal issues that procurement may raise, and even the taking of organs from cadavers by society with the presumption of consent unless individuals have indicated the contrary.[44-49] It will be easier to show that persons have a right to determine what ought to be done with their bodies, even to the point of making donor consent decisive independently of the wishes of the family, than to show that society may presume consent. A clarification of policy, to make donor decisions definitive, would be in accord with the original intentions of the Uniform Act of Donation of Organs and would ease access to needed organs. It would not impose on people the burden of having to announce to others that they do not want their organs used for transplantation. The more one presumes that organs are not societal property, the more difficult it is to justify shifting the burden to individuals to show that they do not want their organs used. If sufficient numbers of organs are not available, it will be unfortunate, but from the point of view of general secular morality, not unfair. Free individuals will have valued other goals (e.g., having an intact body for burial) more highly than the support of transplantation. One will have encountered again one of the recurring limitations on establishing and effecting a general consensus regarding the ways in which society ought to respond to the unfortunate deliverances of nature.

LIVING WITH THE UNFORTUNATE, WHICH IS NOT UNFAIR

Proposals for the general support of transplantation are thus restricted by various elements of the human condition. There is not simply a limitation due to finite resources, making it impossible to do all that is conceivably possible for all who might marginally benefit. There are restrictions as well that are due to the free decisions of both individuals and societies. Individuals will often decide in ways unsympathetic to transplantation programs that would involve the use of their private resources, including their organs. Insofar as one takes seriously respect for persons, one must live with the restrictions that result from numerous free choices. One may endeavor to educate, entice, and persuade people to participate. However, free societies are characterized by the commitment to live with the tragedies that result from the decisions of free individuals not to participate in the beneficent endeavors of others. There are then also the restrictions due to the inability to give a plausible account of state authority that would allow the imposition of a concrete view of the good life. Secular, pluralist societies are more neutral moral frameworks for negotiation and creation of ways to use their common resources than modes for discovering the proper purpose for those resources. If societies freely decide to give a low priority to transplantation and invest instead in generally improving health care for the indigent in the hope of doing greater good, there will be an important sense in which they have acted within their right, even if from particular moral perspectives that may seem wrongheaded.

These reflections on the human condition suggest that we will need in the future to learn to live with the fact that some may receive expensive life-saving treatment while others do not, because some have the luck of access to the media, the attention of a political leader, or sufficient funds to purchase care in their own right. The differences in need, both medical and financial, must be recognized as unfortunate. They are properly the objects of charitable response. However, it must be understood that though unfortunate circumstances are always grounds for praiseworthy charity, they do not always provide grounds, by that fact, for redrawing the line between the circumstances we will count as unfortunate but not unfair and those we will count as unfortunate and unfair. To live with circumstances we must acknowledge as unfortunate but not unfair is the destiny of finite men and women who have neither the financial nor moral resources of gods and goddesses. We must also recognize the role of these important conceptual and moral issues in the fashioning of what will count as reasonable and necessary care, safe and efficacious procedures, nonexperimental treatment, or standard medical care. Though we are not gods and goddesses, we do participate in creating the fabric of these "facts."

REFERENCES

1. Engelhardt HT Jr. Caplan AL, eds. Scientific controversies. London: Cambridge University Press. (in press).

2. Newman H. Medicare program: solicitation of hospitals and medical centers to participate in a study of heart transplants. Fed Regist. January 22, 1981; 46:7072–5.

3. Copeland JG, Mammana RB, Fuller JK, Campbell DW, McAleer MJ. Salier JA. Heart transplantation: four years' experience with conventional immunosuppression. JAMA 1984; 251:1563–6.

4. DeVries WC, Anderson JL, Joyce LD, et al. Clinical use of the total artifical heart. N Engl J Med 1984; 310:273–8.

5. Dummer JS, Hardy A, Poorsattar A, Ho M. Early infections in kidney, heart, and liver transplant recipients on cyclosporine. Transplantation 1983; 36:259–67.

6. Shunzaburo I, Byers WS, Starzl TE. Current status of hepatic transplantation. Semin Liver Dis 1983; 3:173–80.

7. Starzl TE, Iwatsuki S, Van Thiel DH, et al. Evolution of liver transplantation. Hepatology 1982; 2:614–36.

8. Van Thiel DH, Schade RR, Starzl TE, et al. Liver transplantation in adults. Hepatology 1982; 2:637–40.

9. Wessel D. Transplants increase, and so do disputes over who pays bills. Wall Street Journal. April 12, 1984; 73:1, 12.

10. Spirito TH. Letter of October 29, 1982. In: Organ transplants: hearings before the subcommittee on investigations and oversight. 98th Congress, 1st Session. Washington, D.C.: Government Printing Office, 1983:226.

11. Litos PA. Letter of October 1, 1982. In: Organ transplants: hearings before the subcommittee on investigations and oversight. 98th Congress, 1st Session. Washington, D.C.: Government Printing Office, 1983:227.

12. Fiske C, Fiske M. Statements of Charles and Marilyn Fiske, and daughter Jamie, liver transplant patient. In: Organ transplants: hearings before the subcommittee on investigations and oversight. 98th Congress, 1st Session. Washington, D.C.: Government Printing Office, 1983:212–8. [see 4].

13. Gunby P. Organ transplant improvements, demands draw increasing attention. JAMA 1984; 251:1521–3, 1527.

14. *Idem.* Media-abetted liver transplants raise questions of 'equity and decency.' JAMA 1983; 249:1973–4, 1980–2.

15. Iglehart JK. Transplantation: the problem of limited resources. N Engl J Med 1983; 309:123–8.

16. *Idem.* The politics of transplantation. N. Engl J Med 1984; 310:864–8.

17. Strauss MJ. The political history of the artificial heart. N Engl J Med 1984; 310:332–6.

18. Ad Hoc Task Force on Cardiac Replacement. Cardiac replacement: medical ethical psychological and economic implications. Washington D.C.: Government Printing Office, 1969.

19. Artificial Heart Assessment Panel. The totally implantable artificial heart. Bethesda, Md.: National Institutes of Health, 1973. (DHEW publication no. (NIH)74–191).

20. Leaf A. The MGH trustees say no to heart transplants. N Engl J Med 1980; 302:1087–8.

21. Barnes BA, Dunphy ME, Koff RS, et al. Final report of the task force on liver transplantation in Massachusetts. Boston: Blue Cross and Blue Shield, 1983.

22. Engelhardt HT Jr. Bioethics in pluralist societies. Perspect Biol Med 1982; 26:64–78.

23. *Idem.* The physician-patient relationship in a secular, pluralist society. In: Shelp EE, ed. The clinical encounter. Dordrecht, Holland: D Reidel, 1983: 253–66.

24. Aristotle. Nicomachaean ethics. ix 10. 1170b.

25. *Idem.* Politics. vii 4.1326b.

26. Engelhardt HT. Bioethics: an introduction and critique. New York: Oxford University Press. (in press).

27. Rawls J. A theory of justice. Cambridge, Mass.: Belknap Press, 1971.

28. Nozick R. Anarchy, state, and utopia. New York: Basic Books, 1974.

29. Newman H. Exclusion of heart transplantation procedures from Medicare coverage. Fed Regist 1980; 45:52296.

30. Knox RA. Heart transplants; to pay or not to pay. Science 1980; 209:570–2,574–5.

31. Evans RW, Anderson A, Perry B. The national heart transplantation study: an overview. Heart Transplant 1982; 2(1):85–7.

32. Consensus Conference. Liver transplantation. JAMA 1983; 250:2961–4.

33. Who shall be dialysed? Lancet 1983; 1:717.

34. Aaron HJ, Schwartz WB. The painful prescription: rationing hospital care. Washington, D.C.: Brookings Institute, 1984.

35. President's Commission for the Study of Ethical Problems in Medicine and Biomedical and Behavioral Research. Securing access to health care. Vol. 1. Washington, D.C.: Government Printing Office, 1983:20.

36. President's Commission, [35] p. 37.

37. President's Commission, [35] p. 37.

38. President's Commission, [35] p. 42–3.

39. President's Commission, [35] p. 43–6.

40. President's Commission, [35] p. 37–47.

41. Nozick R. Anarchy, state and utopia. New York: Basic Books, 1974:206–7.

42. Kant I. Kants werke: akademie textausgabe. Vol. 6. Berlin: Walter de Gruyter, 1968:423.

43. Kelly G. Medico-moral problems. St. Louis: Catholic Hospital Association, 1958:245–52.

44. Caplan AL. Organ transplants: the costs of success. Hastings Cent Rep 1983; 13(6):23–32.

45. Kolata G. Organ shortage clouds new transplant era. Science 1983; 221:32–3.

46. Overcast TD, Evans RW, Bowen LE, Hoe MM, Livak CL. Problems in the identification of potential organ donors: misconceptions and fallacies associated with donor cards. JAMA 1984; 251:1559–62.

47. Prottas JM. Encouraging altruism: public attitudes and the marketing of organ donation. Milbank Mem Fund Q 1983; 61:278–306.

48. U.S. Congress, House. To amend the public health service act to authorize financial assistance for organ procurement organizations, and for other purposes. By: Gore A. 98th Congress, 1st Session. H. Rept. 4080. 1983.

49. U.S. Congress, Senate. To provide for the establishment of a task force on organ procurement and transplantation and an organ procurement and transplantation registry, and for other purposes. By: Hatch O. 98th Congress, 1st Session. S. Rept. 2048, 1983.

32 *Medicine Versus Economics*

LESTER C. THUROW

An underdeveloped area of biomedical ethics is the cost of health care. While much has been written about the allocation of resources, few articles take a hard look at the economic issues. The value of this article is that, while it provides economic data related to the cost of health care, the author also examines the policy and value implications of economic decisions. Thurow is anxious to avoid an unequal health care system, and recognizes that substantial changes in the practice of medicine and social expectations will be necessary to effect this.

Lester C. Thurow is at the Sloan School of Management of the Massachusetts Institute of Technology

Discussions of the economics of health care usually start with the observation that health care spending has risen from 5 to 11 per cent of the gross national product over the past two decades. Despite spending more of its gross national product on health care than any other country, the United States is 15th in male life expectancy, 7th in female life expectancy, and 13th in infant mortality.[1,2] Although these are generally relevant facts if one is thinking about health care as a social problem, such conditions have long existed and are not the source of today's acute pressures to change the American health care system. Those pressures flow from a narrower set of budgetary issues. Basically, each of the institutions that pays today's health care bills wants to get out from under that obligation.

The federal government has a budget deficit of $200 billion plus. It spends more than $100 billion on health care.[3] If it is to reduce its budget deficit by cutting expenditures, it must cut health care spending. The federal government used to view health care as a social problem. Today it views it almost solely as a budget-deficit problem. The shift in perspectives is important. Social problems can be left to fester; budget-deficit problems require more immediate solution.

To cut its own spending, the federal government is reducing grants-in-aid to state and local governments. This places state and local governments in a position in which they must raise taxes or cut expenditures simply to maintain their present financial positions. Since state and local governments spend more than $60 billion on health care, cuts in health care spending stand front and center in the federally induced budget-balancing exercises confronting state and local governments.[3]

Since governments provide health care primarily to the elderly and the poor, government deficit-reduction measures systematically dismantle the existing system of paying for health care for these groups. This immediately raises the question of what, if anything, is going to be put in its place.

Although government has been the principal force pushing for cost containment in the past decade, private corporations are going to assume that role in the next decade. American business faces rapidly mounting foreign competition. In 1984 imports exceeded exports by $123 billion. Health insurance has become a big cost of doing business. Health care costs add $600 to the price of a car at the Chrysler Corporation,[4] but this is probably an extreme case. With foreign competition, American industry can no longer pass its health care costs along to the consumer in the form of higher prices. American industry is losing its markets at current prices and must reduce costs and prices if it is not to be run out of business.

As a result, higher health care costs today mean lower profits. Corporate health care spending is approaching $100 billion and, within the foreseeable future, will surpass total after-tax corporate profits. Business magazines have started to publish articles on how corporations can and must shake costs out of their health care systems.[5] Cutting health care costs is going to be a central business objective in the next five years. Whereas government cost-containment measures focus attention on the elderly and the poor, corporate cost containment focuses attention on the health care systems for the middle class.

Cost containment has become a central objective because of both what has been happening to costs and what seems to be happening to medical technology. Modern technology has made almost everyone a candidate for a "catastrophic" illness.[6] That is to say, modern technology makes it likely that everyone will die of an illness that requires immense amounts of money, except those lucky enough to die quietly in their sleep. In any given year, 70 per cent of Medicare's money goes for 9 per cent of those covered, but most of us will be in that 9 per cent at some point before we die.[7]

Given medicine's potential ability to spend almost unlimited amounts of money on almost everyone before reaching the traditional "do no harm" stopping point for giving up, all the major payers want to reduce their role in the health care system sharply. They need to hold costs down, but just as important, they do not want to be in the position of having to say that such-and-such a treatment cannot be given to Patient X because it costs too much.

From the perspective of those who pay, the problem is clear. Under the current system, costs are out of control. They must be brought under control. The source of the problem is equally clear. When a retrospective fee-for-service, insured-reimbursement system is used, no one has an interest in cost containment. For doctors, patients, hospitals, and insurance companies the system is essentially a pass-through system. The payer (government or corporation) bears the burden yet has no say about how much is to be spent.

From the perspective of those who pay, the solution is also clear. The current system must be replaced by one in which the people involved have a direct interest in cost containment. To achieve this, the system must shift away from retrospective fees for service to prospective, so-much-per-patient payments. With prospective payments the payers can limit their total costs, yet do not get involved in making decisions about which treatments should be given to which patients. The payer decides how much money can be spent, and the medical community must decide how that money is allocated among patients.

The details will differ and evolve, but the Medicare diagnostic-related group (DRG) system is the ripple that will build into the wave of the future. Today's DRG system pays providers on the basis of the diagnostic categories into which patients fall. Tomorrow's systems will pay providers a fixed fee to take care of a group of potential patients regardless of their individual diagnoses. I would predict that corporations, not governments, will take the lead in this effort. Once the idea becomes legitimate for middle-class workers, the government will extend it to the poor and elderly.

Such a system meets the needs of the payers, but it also conforms to the currently popular idea that the health care system should become more of a market system. No one is ever willing to come right out and say so, but the long-run aim is to return the system to the point at which a large fraction of health care costs once again comes directly out of individual pockets. The goal is to make the patient the main cost container.

This is why the government is raising deductibles in its health insurance systems and proposing to tax both health insurance contributions and health insurance benefits.[8] Larger deductibles force the individual patient to become a cost container by virtue of the fact that a substantial up-front fraction of the total costs has to come out of his or her own funds. Private health insurance must be taxed to discourage its use, since those who purchase private health insurance to cover the gap created by the higher government deductibles vitiate the whole purpose of the higher deductibles. For those who buy private health insurance, there is once again no direct patient incentive for cost containment. Ideally, the government would like to prohibit the purchase of private health care insurance to cover what the government does not cover, but since this is not politically possible, taxing health insurance is the next best option.

In its efforts to raise deductibles and force the patient to become the cost container, government is going to be emulated by corporations. They, too, would like to move to much higher deductibles so that the patient becomes the chief cost container in their systems.

There is no question that DRG systems can work if the sole question is cost containment. They are in fact working.[9] The combination of higher deductibles and the DRG system has sharply reduced admisssions and the average length of stay for Medicare patients. If the limit were per person rather than per disease, even more drastic reductions could have been achieved.

The problems spring from the inequities in health care services that will result. About 12 per cent of the population is not now insured.[10] Few of the uninsured are rich, yet they are not dying in the streets. Somewhere in the system their costs are being covered. Overtly (by having insurance systems contribute to a pool to pay for the costs of the uninsured) or covertly (by charging paying patients more than their costs and using the extra funds to subsidize those not insured), funds are being extracted from the current system to pay for the uninsured. In a prospective, so-much-per-patient system, this is not going to be possible. The insured are going to need all of their own insurance funds plus some of their own personal funds to cover their own costs. There is going to be no slack in the system to cover those not directly covered.

This immediately raises two questions: Who is going to be the residual provider for those not covered elsewhere? and At what level of quality is that residual care to be set? Is it to be a level of care equal to that of the rest of the population, or something less—a basic-necessities, no-frills, no-heroic-measures type of health care?

Clearly, it is not going to be equal care. A prospective-payment system does not stop those with money from buying health care over and above that provided by governments and corporations. There will be a market for those able and willing to pay for more health care. But markets exist to distribute goods and services in accordance with the distribution of income. Since the top 20 per cent of the population has 11 times as much income as the bottom 20 per cent, any market system will end up providing at least 11 times as much health care to the top 20 per cent as to the bottom 20 per cent.[11] And if health care is what economists call a "superior" good (i.e., people are willing to spend a larger fraction of their income on it as their income goes up), as it probably is, the gap could be much larger than 11 to 1.

The most likely outcome is a segregated, three-tiered health care system. There will be a set of government health care providers who will provide the minimal level of health care for the poor and the elderly. Government will pay health care providers a fixed annual fee to cover a certain population. The level of health care will be determined by the per capita grant that the government is willing to pay. Health care providers will have to decide whether they wish to work in this segment of the health care market and to bid for such government contracts or whether they want to compete in one of the other two tiers.

No one knows how low the minimal cost and quality might be. If, for example, their political willingness to cut back on government food programs for the poor is any indication, Americans may be willing to tolerate a minimal level of health care that is much lower than some of us thought politically possible. Although I will confess to being an egalitarian when it comes to health care, it is possible that most Americans do not share my values. What makes me doubt this, however, is the fact that I know of few Americans who would be willing to see themselves given care noticeably worse than that being given to others. And if they aren't willing to see themselves cared for in the minimal health care system, then they aren't being politically honest when they prescribe it for others.

The quality of the second tier will be established by private corporations and will depend on the level of health care that they are willing to provide for their employees. The system will be similar in form to that of the governmental first tier (corporations will sign fixed-price contracts with health care providers to cover their workers for some fixed period), but the prospective per capita payment is apt to be substantially higher than that provided by the government's health care system.

The third tier will be a free-market, individual health care system. This will be the market in which people can buy health care in excess of that provided by their employers or the government. The only limit on treatment will be the amount of money that people are willing to spend on themselves or their family.

Basically, each market will set buyer (payer) against seller (provider). In the government and corporate markets, the buyer is apt to be dominant. Buyers dominate sellers in most capitalistic markets, and they are almost certain to do so in an industry with enormous excessive productive capacity. In 1984 the average hospital occupancy rate was only 67 percent.[10] There will be a lot of very hungry bidders for those government and corporate contracts.

In the third market, health care providers may have their traditional dominance. Insured people will be dealing with their own lives and health and may well be willing to allow profit levels well in excess of those that can be earned in the first two tiers. Certainly—taking the profit margins for cars as an example—General Motors can earn much fatter profit margins selling Cadillacs than it can earn selling Chevrolets. On the basis of this marketing fact of life, one would predict that most health care providers will try to compete in the third tier. The profits and incomes will be fatter. Those who fail to make it in the third tier will be forced to compete in the other two tiers.

Although what I have sketched out is what I think is likely to happen, as one who believes in an egalitarian distribution of health care I don't find it a very attractive prospect. Is there any alternative? Maybe.

That "maybe" proceeds from the fact that there are sharp differences from region to region in the use of many of the expensive treatments now proliferating so rapidly, with no observable differences in outcomes (life expectancy, morbidity, or days missed from work because of illness).[12] At one time, observers had a crude explanation for such differences. If a region had a lot of surgeons, it would do a lot of surgery. But this crude explanation does not seem to be accurate.

Different practice styles, based on the local concept of what constitutes good medical practice, seem to prevail from region to region. If one could convert all American doctors to the practice style of the group of competent doctors that uses each medical technique the least, it would be possible to effect enormous savings without having to employ the unequal three-tiered health care system toward which we are now moving.

In doing so, it would be possible to preserve the real improvements in access to health care that have been made over the past 20 years. The current system does not provide equal health care for everyone, but it certainly provides care that is more equal than that of 25 years ago.

But let no one underestimate the changes that would be required within the community of physicians. Their practice style would have to shift from one based on the motto "Do no harm" to one based on the precept "Employ a treatment only when you are sure that it will make a noticeable improvement." Instead of optimistically using new procedures that "just might" work when old procedures don't, doctors would not employ new procedures until they could be proved to work well. Experimental procedures would not become commonplace overnight. Heroic measures would not be employed unless there was a high probability that they would work.

Let me descibe a mental experiment—what the Germans call a *gedanken* experiment—that illustrates the changes that must come about in medical thinking. At the moment, the medical community knows that if it prescribes a marginally effective but inexpensive treatment, substantial costs will be incurred, but they will be met by the taking of small amounts of money from many people. Doctors can reassure themselves that the amounts will be so small that no one will notice.

Suppose that the payment system were to work differently. Instead of taking the necessary money from many people, the doctor had to choose the person who would have to give up all of his or her income to pay for the treatment prescribed. In 1984 the average American full-time worker earned just about $20,000.[13] Imagine that every time doctors prescribed a treatment costing $20,000, they would also have to pick a particular American worker and effectively tell that worker that he or she had been sentenced to one year of slavery to pay the medical bills of the patient receiving treatment. If that were the way the system worked, would you as the physician be willing to say that the benefits of a given treatment were so great it was worth sentencing another human being to one year of slavery to pay for them? If the answer is yes, the treatment should be given. If no, the treatment should not be given. Effectively, this is the choice that we as a society are now making. Every $20,000 treatment requires the collection of $20,000 worth of income from someone, but at the level at which medical decisions are actually made, we don't see the choice in this light.

The time for change is here. Can the medical community systematically change its practice styles to encourage the least costly alternatives? I don't know. That is a question for the medical community itself to answer.

Similar attitudinal changes will be required within the larger society. Americans will have to realize that the best medical care is not the care that employs every experimental technique known to humankind. Americans will have to learn that doctors should not be sued for not incurring every possible expenditure in hopeless situations, and if they do sue, the courts will have to realize that a failure to spend is not in itself evidence of bad medical practice.

If neither the medical community nor the larger society is willing to make such changes, then the current health care system is going to be very different 10 years from now.

REFERENCES

1. Reinhardt UE. Hard choices in health care: a matter of ethics. In: Health care: how to improve it: alternatives for the 1980s. No. 7. Center for National Policy, p. 21.

2. Marmor TR, Dunham A. The politics of health policy reform: problems, origins, alternatives, and a possible prescription. In: Health care: how to improve it: alternatives for the 1980s. No. 17. Center for National Policy, p. 33.

3. U.S. Department of Commerce. Survey of current business. Washington, D.C.: U.S. Department of Commerce. 1984:54.

4. The soaring cost of health care: national issues forum. Domestic Policy Association, Public Agenda Foundation, 1984:6.

5. Chapman FS. Deciding who pays to save lives. Fortune. May 27, 1985:59.

6. Bernstein BJ. The misguided quest for the artificial heart. Technology Review. Nov/Dec 1984:3.

7. Davis K. Access to health care: a matter of fairness. In: Health care: how to improve it: alternatives for the 1980s. No. 17. Center for National Health Policy, p. 47.

8. Rosenbaum DE. Tax urged on health premiums. New York Times. May 3, 1985:D1.

9. Sullivan R. Decline in hospital use tied to new U.S. policies. New York Times. April 16, 1985:1.

10. Updated report on access to health care for the American people. Princeton, N.J.: Robert Wood Johnson Foundation, 1983. (Special report no. 1).

11. Money income of households, families, and persons in the United States: 1983. Series P-60. No. 146. Washington, D.C.: Bureau of the Census, p. 18.

12. Bunker JP. When doctors disagree. New York Review of Books. April 25, 1985:7.

13. Survey of current business. Washington, D.C.: United States Department of Commerce, March 1985:7.

The Allocation
of Scarce Resources/Further Reading

Fox, Renee and Swazey, Judith P. *The Courage to Fail: A Social View of Organ Transplant and Dialysis.* Chicago: University of Chicago Press, 1974.

Fost, Norman. "Children as Renal Donors." *New England Journal of Medicine* 296 (February 17, 1977), 363–67.

Jonson, A. R. "The Totally Implantable Artificial Heart." *Hastings Center Report* 3 (November, 1973), 1–4.

Katz, J. and Capron, Alexander Morgan. *Catastrophic Diseases: Who Decides What? A Psychological and Legal Analysis of the Problems Posed by Hemodialysis and Organ Transplantation.* New York: Russell Sage Foundation, 1975.

Rettig, Richard A. "The Policy Debate on Patient Care Financing for Victims of End-Stage Renal Disease." *Law and Contemporary Problems* 40 (Autumn, 1976), 196–230.

Robertson, John A. "Organ Donations by Incompetents and the Substituted Judgement Doctrine." *Columbia Law Review* 76 (January, 1976), 48–78.

"The Sale of Human Body Parts" *Michigan Law Review* 72 (May, 1974), 1182–1264.

Shapiro, Michael H. "Who Merits Merit? Problems in Distributive Justice and Utility Posed by the New Biology." *Southern California Law Review* 49 (November, 1974), 318–70.

Simmons, Roberta G. et al., *Gift of Life: The Social and Psychological Impact of Organ Transplantation.* New York: John Wiley and Sons, 1977.

Titmuss, Richard. *The Gift Relationship: From Human Blood to Social Policy.* New York: Pantheon Books, 1971. (Penguin Paperback, 1973.)

Instruction on Respect for Human Life in Its Origin and on the Dignity of Procreation; Replies to Certain Questions of the Day

CONGREGATION FOR THE DOCTRINE OF THE FAITH

Foreword

The Congregation for the Doctrine of the Faith has been approached by various Episcopal Conferences or individual Bishops, by theologians, doctors and scientists, concerning biomedical techniques which make it possible to intervene in the initial phase of the life of a human being and in the very processes of procreation and their conformity with the principles of Catholic morality. The present Instruction, which is the result of wide consultation and in particular of a careful evaluation of the declarations made by Episcopates, does not intend to repeat all the Church's teaching on the dignity of human life as it originates and on procreation, but to offer, in the light of the previous teaching of the Magisterium, some specific replies to the main questions being asked in this regard.

The exposition is arranged as follows: an introduction will recall the fundamental principles, of an anthropological and moral character, which are necessary for a proper evaluation of the problems and for working out replies to those questions; the first part will have as its subject respect for the human being from the first moment of his or her existence; the second part will deal with the moral questions raised by technical interventions on human procreation; the third part will offer some orientations on the relationships between moral law and civil law *in terms of the respect due to human embryos and foetuses* and as regards the legitimacy of techniques of artificial procreation.*

INTRODUCTION: 1. BIOMEDICAL RESEARCH AND THE TEACHING OF THE CHURCH

The gift of life which God the Creator and Father has entrusted to man calls him to appreciate the inestimable value of what he has been given and to take responsibility for it: this fundamental principle must be placed at the centre of one's reflection in order to clarify and solve the moral problems raised by artificial interventions on life as it originates and on the processes of procreation.

Thanks to the progress of the biological and medical sciences, man has at his disposal ever more effective therapeutic resources; but he can also acquire new powers, with unforeseeable consequences, over human life at its very beginning and in its first stages. Various procedures now make it possible to intervene not only in order to assist but also to dominate the processes of procreation. These techniques can enable man to "take in hand his own destiny", but they also expose him "to the temptation to go beyond the limits of a reasonable dominion over nature".[1] They might constitute progress in the service of man, but they also involve serious risks. Many people are therefore expressing an urgent appeal that in interventions on procreation the values and rights of the human person be safeguarded. Requests for clarification and guidance are coming not only from the faithful but also from those who recognize the Church as "an expert in humanity"[2] with a mission to serve the "civilization of love"[3] and of life.

The Church's Magisterium does not intervene on the basis of a particular competence in the area of the experimental sciences; but having taken account of the data of research and technology, it intends to put forward, by virtue of its evangelical mission and apostolic duty, the moral teaching corresponding to the dignity of the person and to his or her integral vocation. It intends to do so by expounding the criteria of moral judgment as regards the applications of scientific research and technology, especially in relation to human life and its beginnings. These criteria are the respect, defence and promotion of man, his "primary and fundamental right" to life,[4] his dignity as a

---

* The terms "zygote", "pre-embryo", "embryo" and "foetus" can indicate in the vocabulary of biology successive stages of the development of a human being. The present Instruction makes free use of these terms, attributing to them an identical ethical relevance, in order to designate the result (whether visible or not) of human generation, from the first moment of its existence until birth. The reason for this usage is clarified by the text (cf I, 1).

person who is endowed with a spiritual soul and with moral responsibility,[5] and who is called to beatific communion with God.

The Church's intervention in this field is inspired also by the love which she owes to man, helping him to recognize and respect his rights and duties. This love draws from the fount of Christ's love: as she contemplates the mystery of the Incarnate Word, the Church also comes to understand the "mystery of man";[6] by proclaiming the Gospel of salvation, she reveals to man his dignity and invites him to discover fully the truth of his own being. Thus the Church once more puts forward the divine law in order to accomplish the work of truth and liberation.

For it is out of goodness—in order to indicate the path of life—that God gives human beings his commandments and the grace to observe them: and it is likewise out of goodness—in order to help them persevere along the same path—that God always offers to everyone his forgiveness. Christ has compassion on our weaknesses: he is our Creator and Redeemer. May his spirit open men's hearts to the gift of God's peace and to an understanding of his precepts.

2. SCIENCE AND TECHNOLOGY
AT THE SERVICE OF THE HUMAN PERSON

God created man in his own image and likeness: "male and female he created them" (*Gen* 1:27), entrusting to them the task of "having dominion over the earth" (*Gen* 1:28). Basic scientific research and applied research constitute a significant expression of this dominion of man over creation. Science and technology are valuable resources for man when placed at his service and when they promote his integral development for the benefit of all; but they cannot of themselves show the meaning of existence and of human progress. Being ordered to man, who initiates and develops them, they draw from the person and his moral values the indication of their purpose and the awareness of their limits.

It would on the one hand be illusory to claim that scientific research and its applications are morally neutral; on the other hand one cannot derive criteria for guidance from mere technical efficiency, from research's possible usefulness to some at the expense of others, or, worse still, from prevailing ideologies. Thus science and technology require, for their own intrinsic meaning, an unconditional respect for the fundamental criteria of the moral law: that is to say, they must be at the service of the human person, of his inalienable rights and his true and integral good according to the design and will of God.[7]

The rapid development of technological discoveries gives greater urgency to this need to respect the criteria just mentioned: science without conscience can only lead to man's ruin. "Our era needs such wisdom more than bygone ages if the discoveries made by man are to be further humanized. For the future of the world stands in peril unless wiser people are forthcoming".[8]

3. Anthropology and Procedures in the Biomedical Field

Which moral criteria must be applied in order to clarify the problems posed today in the field of biomedicine? The answer to this question presupposes a proper idea of the nature of the human person in his bodily dimension.

For it is only in keeping with his true nature that the human person can achieve self-realization as a "unified totality";[9] and this nature is at the same time corporal and spiritual. By virtue of its substantial union with a spiritual soul, the human body cannot be considered as a mere complex of tissues, organs and functions, nor can it be evaluated in the same way as the body of animals; rather it is a constitutive part of the person who manifests and expresses himself through it.

The natural moral law expresses and lays down the purposes, rights and duties which are based upon the bodily and spiritual nature of the human person. Therefore this law cannot be thought of as simply a set of norms on the biological level; rather it must be defined as the rational order whereby man is called by the Creator to direct and regulate his life and actions and in particular to make use of his own body.[10]

A first consequence can be deduced from these principles: an intervention on the human body affects not only the tissues, the organs and their functions but also involves the person himself on different levels. It involves, therefore, perhaps in an implicit but none-theless real way, a moral significance and responsibility. Pope John Paul II forcefully reaffirmed this to the World Medical Association when he said: "Each human person, in his absolutely unique singular-ity, is constituted not only by his spirit, but by his body as well. Thus, in the body and through the body, one touches the person himself in his concrete reality. To respect the dignity of man consequently amounts to safeguarding this identity of the man 'corpore et anima unus', as the Second Vatican Council says (*Gaudium et Spes*, 14, par. 1). It is on the basis of this anthropological vision that one is to find the fundamental criteria for decision-making in the case of procedures which are not strictly therapeutic, as, for example, those aimed at the improvement of the human biological condition".[11]

Applied biology and medicine work together for the integral good of human life when they come to the aid of a person stricken by illness and infirmity and when they respect his or her dignity as a creature of God. No biologist or doctor can reasonably claim, by virtue of his scientific competence, to be able to decide on people's origin and destiny. This norm must be applied in a particular way in the field of sexuality and procreation, in which man and woman actualize the fundamental values of love and life.

God, who is love and life, has inscribed in man and woman the vocation to share in a special way in his mystery of personal communion and in his work as Creator and Father.[12] For this reason marriage possesses specific goods and values in its union and in procreation which cannot be likened to those existing in lower forms of life. Such values and meanings are of the personal order and determine from the moral point of view the meaning and limits of artificial interventions on procreation and on the origin of human life. These interventions are not to be rejected on the grounds that they are artificial. As such, they bear witness to the possibilities of the art of medicine. But they must be given a moral evaluation in reference to the dignity of the human person, who is called to realize his vocation from God to the gift of love and the gift of life.

4. FUNDAMENTAL CRITERIA FOR A MORAL JUDGMENT

The fundamental values connected with the techniques of artificial human procreation are two: the life of the human being called into existence and the special nature of the transmission of human life in marriage. The moral judgment on such methods of artificial procreation must therefore be formulated in reference to these values.

Physical life, with which the course of human life in the world begins, certainly does not itself contain the whole of a person's value, nor does it represent the supreme good of man who is called to eternal life. However it does constitute in a certain way the "fundamental" value of life, precisely because upon this physical life all the other values of the person are based and developed.[13] The inviolability of the innocent human being's right to life "from the moment of conception until death"[14] is a sign and requirement of the very inviolability of the person to whom the Creator has given the gift of life.

By comparison with the transmission of other forms of life in the universe, the transmission of human life has a special character of its own, which derives from the special nature of the human person. "The transmission of human life is entrusted by nature to a personal and conscious act and as such is subject to the all-holy laws of God:

immutable and inviolable laws which must be recognized and observed. For this reason one cannot use means and follow methods which could be licit in the transmission of the life of plants and animals".[15]

Advances in technology have now made it possible to procreate apart from sexual relations through the meeting *in vitro* of the germ-cells previously taken from the man and the woman. But what is technically possible is not for that very reason morally admissible. Rational reflection on the fundamental values of life and of human procreation is therefore indispensable for formulating a moral evaluation of such technological interventions on a human being from the first stages of his development.

5. Teachings of the Magisterium

On its part, the Magisterium of the Church offers to human reason in this field too the light of Revelation: the doctrine concerning man taught by the Magisterium contains many elements which throw light on the problems being faced here.

From the moment of conception, the life of every human being is to be respected in an absolute way because man is the only creature on earth that God has "wished for himself"[16] and the spiritual soul of each man is "immediately created" by God;[17] his whole being bears the image of the Creator. Human life is sacred because from its beginning it involves "the creative action of God"[18] and it remains forever in a special relationship with the Creator, who is its sole end.[19] God alone is the Lord of life from its beginning until its end: no one can, in any circumstance, claim for himself the right to destroy directly an innocent human being.[20]

Human procreation requires on the part of the spouses responsible collaboration with the fruitful love of God;[21] the gift of human life must be actualized in marriage through the specific and exclusive acts of husband and wife, in accordance with the laws inscribed in their persons and in their union.[22]

* * *

I.
Respect for Human Embryos

Careful reflection on this teaching of the Magisterium and on the evidence of reason, as mentioned above, enables us to respond to the numerous moral problems posed by technical interventions upon the human being in the first phases of his life and upon the processes of his conception.

1. WHAT RESPECT IS DUE TO THE HUMAN EMBRYO, TAKING INTO ACCOUNT HIS
   NATURE AND IDENTITY?

*The human being must be respected—as a person—from the very
first instant of his existence.*

The implementation of procedures of artificial fertilization has
made possible various interventions upon embryos and human foetuses. The aims pursued are of various kinds: diagnostic and therapeutic, scientific and commercial. From all of this, serious problems arise.
Can one speak of a right to experimentation upon human embryos for
the purpose of scientific research? What norms or laws should be
worked out with regard to this matter? The response to these problems
presupposes a detailed reflection on the nature and specific identity—
the word "status" is used—of the human embryo itself.

At the Second Vatican Council, the Church for her part presented
once again to modern man her constant and certain doctrine according
to which: "Life once conceived, must be protected with the utmost
care; abortion and infanticide are abominable crimes"[23] More recently,
the *Charter of the Rights of the Family*, published by the Holy See,
confirmed that "Human life must be absolutely respected and protected from the moment of conception."[24]

This Congregation is aware of the current debates concerning the
beginning of human life, concerning the individuality of the human
being and concerning the identity of the human person. The Congregation recalls the teachings found in the *Declaration on Procured Abortion*: "From the time that the ovum is fertilized, a new life is begun
which is neither that of the father nor of the mother; it is rather the life
of a new human being with his own growth. It would never be made
human if it were not human already. To this perpetual evidence . . .
modern genetic science brings valuable confirmation. It has demonstrated that, from the first instant, the programme is fixed as to what
this living being will be: a man, this individual-man with his characteristic aspects already well determined. Right from fertilization is begun
the adventure of a human life, and each of its great capacities requires
time . . . to find its place and to be in a position to act".[25] This teaching
remains valid and is further confirmed, if confirmation were needed,
by recent findings of human biological science which recognize that in
the zygote* resulting from fertilization the biological identity of a new
human individual is already constituted.

---

* The zygote is the cell produced when the nuclei of the two gametes have fused.

Certainly no experimental datum can be in itself sufficient to bring us to the recognition of a spiritual soul; nevertheless, the conclusions of science regarding the human embryo provide a valuable indication for discerning by the use of reason a personal presence at the moment of this first appearance of a human life: how could a human individual not be a human person? The Magisterium has not expressly committed itself to an affirmation of a philosophical nature, but it constantly reaffirms the moral condemnation of any kind of procured abortion. This teaching has not been changed and is unchangeable.[26]

Thus the fruit of human generation, from the first moment of its existence, that is to say from the moment the zygote has formed, demands the unconditional respect that is morally due to the human being in his bodily and spiritual totality. The human being is to be respected and treated as a person from the moment of conception; and therefore from that same moment his rights as a person must be recognized, among which in the first place is the inviolable right of every innocent human being to life.

This doctrinal reminder provides the fundamental criterion for the solution of the various problems posed by the development of the biomedical sciences in this field: since the embryo must be treated as a person, it must also be defended in its integrity, tended and cared for, to the extent possible, in the same way as any other human being as far as medical assistance is concerned.

2. IS PRENATAL DIAGNOSIS MORALLY LICIT?

If prenatal diagnosis respects the life and integrity of the embryo and the human foetus and is directed towards its safeguarding or healing as an individual, then the answer is affirmative.

For prenatal diagnosis makes it possible to know the condition of the embryo and of the foetus when still in the mother's womb. It permits, or makes it possible to anticipate earlier and more effectively, certain therapeutic, medical or surgical procedures.

Such diagnosis is permissible, with the consent of the parents after they have been adequately informed, if the methods employed safeguard the life and integrity of the embryo and the mother, without subjecting them to disproportionate risks.[27] But this diagnosis is gravely opposed to the moral law when it is done with the thought of possibly inducing an abortion depending upon the results: a diagnosis which shows the existence of a malformation or a hereditary illness must not be the equivalent of a death-sentence. Thus a woman would be committing a gravely illicit act if she were to request such a diagnosis with the deliberate intention of having an abortion should the results confirm the existence of a malformation or abnormality. The spouse or relatives or anyone else would similarly be acting in a manner contrary to the moral law if they were to counsel or impose such a diagnostic procedure on the expectant mother with the same intention of possibly proceeding to an abortion. So too the specialist would be guilty of illicit collaboration if, in conducting the diagnosis and in communicating its results, he were deliberately to contribute to establishing or favouring a link between prenatal diagnosis and abortion.

In conclusion, any directive or programme of the civil and health authorities or of scientific organizations which in any way were to favour a link between prenatal diagnosis and abortion, or which were to go as far as directly to induce expectant mothers to submit to prenatal diagnosis planned for the purpose of eliminating foetuses which are affected by malformations or which are carriers of heredi-tary illness, is to be condemmed as a violation of the unborn child's right to life and as an abuse of the prior rights and duties of the spouses.

3. ARE THERAPEUTIC PROCEDURES CARRIED OUT ON THE HUMAN EMBRYO LICIT?

As with all medical interventions on patients, *one must uphold as licit procedures carried out on the human embryo which respect the life and integrity of the embryo and do not involve disproportionate risks for it but are directed towards its healing, the improvement of its condition of health, or its individual survival.*

Whatever the type of medical, surgical or other therapy, the free and informed consent of the parents is required, according to the deontological rules followed in the case of children. The application of this moral principle may call for delicate and particular precautions in the case of embryonic or foetal life.

The legitimacy and criteria of such procedures have been clearly stated by Pope John Paul II: "A strictly therapeutic intervention whose explicit objective is the healing of various maladies such as those stemming from chromosomal defects will, in principle, be considered desirable, provided it is directed to the true promotion of the personal well-being of the individual without doing harm to his integrity or worsening his conditions of life. Such an intervention would indeed fall within the logic of the Christian moral tradition."[28]

4. HOW IS ONE TO EVALUATE MORALLY RESEARCH AND EXPERIMENTATION* ON HUMAN EMBRYOS AND FOETUSES?

Medical research must refrain from operations on live embryos, unless there is a moral certainty of not causing harm to the life or integrity of the unborn child and the mother, and on condition that the parents have given their free and informed consent to the procedure. It follows that all research, even when limited to the simple observation of the embryo, would become illicit were it to involve risk to the embryo's physical integrity or life by reason of the methods used or the effects induced.

As regards experimentation, and presupposing the general distinction between experimentation for purposes which are not directly therapeutic and experimentation which is clearly therapeutic for the subject himself, in the case in point one must also distinguish between experimentation carried out on embryos which are still alive and experimentation carried out on embryos which are dead. *If the embryos are living, whether viable or not, they must be respected just like any other human person; experimentation on embryos which is not directly therapeutic is illicit.*[29]

No objective, even though noble in itself, such as a foreseeable advantage to science, to other human beings or to society, can in any way justify experimentation on living human embryos or foetuses, whether viable or not, either inside or outside the mother's womb. The informed consent ordinarily required for clinical experimentation on adults cannot be granted by the parents, who may not freely dispose of the physical integrity or life of the unborn child. Moreover, experimentation on embryos and foetuses always involves risk, and indeed in most cases it involves the certain expectation of harm to their physical integrity or even their death.

To use human embryos or foetuses as the object or instrument of

---

* Since the terms "research" and "experimentation" are often used equivalently and ambiguously, it is deemed necessary to specify the exact meaning given them in this document.

1) By *research* is meant any inductive-deductive process which aims at promoting the systematic observation of a given phenomenon in the human field or at verifying a hypothesis arising from previous observations.

2) By *experimentation* is meant any research in which the human being (in the various stages of his existence: embryo, foetus, child or adult) represents the object through which or upon which one intends to verify the effect, at present unknown or not sufficiently known, of a given treatment (e.g. pharmacological, teratogenic, surgical, etc.).

experimentation constitutes a crime against their dignity as human beings having a right to the same respect that is due to the child already born and to every human person.

The *Charter of the Rights of the Family* published by the Holy See affirms: "Respect for the dignity of the human being excludes all experimental manipulation or exploitation of the human embryo."[30] The practice of keeping alive human embryos *in vivo* or *in vitro* for experimental or commercial purposes is totally opposed to human dignity.

In the case of experimentation that is clearly therapeutic, namely, when it is a matter of experimental forms of therapy used for the benefit of the embryo itself in a final attempt to save its life, and in the absence of other reliable forms of therapy, recourse to drugs or procedures not yet fully tested can be licit.[31]

The corpses of human embryos and foetuses, whether they have been deliberately aborted or not, must be respected just as the remains of other human beings. In particular, they cannot be subjected to mutilation or to autopsies if their death has not yet been verified and without the consent of the parents or of the mother. Furthermore, the moral requirements must be safeguarded that there be no complicity in deliberate abortion and that the risk of scandal be avoided. Also, in the case of dead foetuses, as for the corpses of adult persons, all commercial trafficking must be considered illicit and should be prohibited.

5. HOW IS ONE TO EVALUATE MORALLY THE USE FOR RESEARCH PURPOSES OF EMBRYOS OBTAINED BY FERTILIZATION 'IN VITRO'?

Human embryos obtained *in vitro* are human beings and subjects with rights: their dignity and right to life must be respected from the first moment of their existence. *It is immoral to produce human embryos destined to be exploited as disposable "biological material".*

In the usual practice of *in vitro* fertilization, not all of the embryos are transferred to the woman's body; some are destroyed. Just as the Church condemns induced abortion, so she also forbids acts against the life of these human beings. *It is a duty to condemn the particular gravity of the voluntary destruction of human embryos obtained 'in vitro' for the sole purpose of research, either by means of artificial insemination or by means of "twin fission".* By acting in this way the researcher usurps the place of God; and, even though he may be unaware of this, he sets himself up as the master of the destiny of others inasmuch as he arbitrarily chooses whom he will allow to live and whom he will send to death and kills defenceless human beings.

Methods of observation or experimentation which damage or impose grave and disproportionate risks upon embryos obtained *in vitro* are morally illicit for the same reasons. Every human being is to be respected for himself, and cannot be reduced in worth to a pure and simple instrument for the advantage of others. *It is therefore not in conformity with the moral law deliberately to expose to death human embryos obtained 'in vitro'.* In consequence of the fact that they have been produced *in vitro*, those embryos which are not transferred into the body of the mother and are called "spare" are exposed to an absurd fate, with no possibility of their being offered safe means of survival which can be licitly pursued.

6. WHAT JUDGMENT SHOULD BE MADE ON OTHER PROCEDURES OF MANIPULATING EMBRYOS CONNECTED WITH THE "TECHNIQUES OF HUMAN REPRODUCTION"?

Techniques of fertilization *in vitro* can open the way to other forms of biological and genetic manipulation of human embryos, such as attempts or plans for fertilization between human and animal gametes and the gestation of human embryos in the uterus of animals, or the hypothesis or project of constructing artificial uteruses for the human embryo. *These procedures are contrary to the human dignity proper to the embryo, and at the same time they are contrary to the right of every person to be conceived and to be born within marriage and from marriage.*[32] *Also, attempts or hypotheses for obtaining a human being without any connection with sexuality through "twin fission", cloning or parthenogenesis are to be considered contrary to the moral law, since they are in opposition to the dignity both of human procreation and of the conjugal union.*

The freezing of embryos, even when carried out in order to preserve the life of an embryo—cryopreservation—*constitutes an offence against the respect due to human beings* by exposing them to grave risks of death or harm to their physical integrity and depriving them, at least temporarily, of maternal shelter and gestation, thus placing them in a situation in which further offences and manipulation are possible.

Certain attempts to influence chromosomic or genetic inheritance are not therapeutic but are aimed at producing human beings selected according to sex or other predetermined qualities. These manipulations are contrary to the personal dignity of the human being and his or her integrity and identity. Therefore in no way can they be justified on the grounds of possible beneficial consequences for future humanity.[33] Every person must be respected for himself: in this consists the dignity and right of every human being from his or her beginning.

II.

INTERVENTIONS UPON HUMAN PROCREATION

By "artificial procreation" or "artificial fertilization" are understood here the different technical procedures directed towards obtaining a human conception in a manner other than the sexual union of man and woman. This Instruction deals with fertilization of an ovum in a test-tube (*in vitro* fertilization) and artificial insemination through transfer into the woman's genital tracts of previously collected sperm.

A preliminary point for the moral evaluation of such technical procedures is constituted by the consideration of the circumstances and consequences which those procedures involve in relation to the respect due the human embryo. Development of the practice of *in vitro* fertilization has required innumerable fertilizations and destructions of human embryos. Even today, the usual practice presupposes a hyperovulation on the part of the woman: a number of ova are withdrawn, fertilized and then cultivated *in vitro* for some days. Usually not all are transferred into the genital tracts of the woman; some embryos, generally called "spare", are destroyed or frozen. On occasion, some of the implanted embryos are sacrificed for various eugenic, economic or psychological reasons. Such deliberate destruction of human beings or their utilization for different purposes to the detriment of their integrity and life is contrary to the doctrine on procured abortion already recalled.

The connection between *in vitro* fertilization and the voluntary destruction of human embryos occurs too often. This is significant: through these procedures, with apparently contrary purposes, life and death are subjected to the decision of man, who thus sets himself up as the giver of life and death by decree. This dynamic of violence and domination may remain unnoticed by those very individuals who, in wishing to utilize this procedure, become subject to it themselves. The facts recorded and the cold logic which links them must be taken into consideration for a moral judgment on IVF and ET (*in vitro* fertilization and embryo transfer): the abortion-mentality which has made this procedure possible thus leads, whether one wants it or not, to man's domination over the life and death of his fellow human beings and can lead to a system of radical eugenics.

Nevertheless, such abuses do not exempt one from a further and thorough ethical study of the techniques of artificial procreation considered in themselves, abstracting as far as possible from the destruction of embryos produced *in vitro*.

The present Instruction will therefore take into consideration in the first place the problems posed by heterologous artificial fertilization (II, 1-3),* and subsequently those linked with homologous artificial fertilization (II, 4-6).**

Before formulating an ethical judgment on each of these procedures, the principles and values which determine the moral evaluation of each of them will be considered.

A

Heterologous Artificial Fertilization

1. Why must human procreation take place in marriage?

Every human being is always to be accepted as a gift and blessing of God. However, from the moral point of view a truly responsible procreation vis-à-vis the unborn child must be the fruit of marriage.

For human procreation has specific characteristics by virture of the personal dignity of the parents and of the children: the procreation of a new person, whereby the man and the woman collaborate with the power of the Creator, must be the fruit and the sign of the mutual self-giving of the spouses, of their love and of their fidelity.[34] *The fidelity of the spouses in the unity of marriage involves reciprocal respect of their right to become a father and a mother only through each other.*

The child has the right to be conceived, carried in the womb, brought into the world and brought up within marriage: it is through the secure and recognized relationship to his own parents that the child can discover his own identity and achieve his own proper human development.

---

* By the term *heterologous artificial fertilization* or *procreation,* the Instruction means techniques used to obtain a human conception artificially by the use of gametes coming from at least one donor other than the spouses who are joined in marriage. Such techniques can be of two types:

a) *Heterologous IVF and ET:* the technique used to obtain a human conception through the meeting *in vitro* of gametes taken from at least one donor other than the two spouses joined in marriage.

b) *Heterologous artificial insemination:* the technique used to obtain a human conception through the transfer into the genital tracts of the woman of the sperm previously collected from a donor other than the husband.

** By *artificial homologous fertilization or procreation,* the Instruction means the technique used to obtain a human conception using the gametes of the two spouses joined in marriage. Homologous artificial fertilization can be carried out by two different methods:

a) *Homologous IVF and ET:* the technique used to obtain a human conception through the meeting *in vitro* of the gametes of the spouses joined in marriage.

b) *Homologous artificial insemination:* the technique used to obtain a human conception through the transfer into the genital tracts of a married woman of the sperm previously collected from her husband.

The parents find in their child a confirmation and completion of their reciprocal self-giving: the child is the living image of their love, the permanent sign of their conjugal union, the living and indissoluble concrete expression of their paternity and maternity.[35]

By reason of the vocation and social responsibilities of the person, the good of the children and of the parents contributes to the good of civil society; the vitality and stability of society require that children come into the world within a family and that the family be firmly based on marriage.

The tradition of the Church and anthropological reflection recognize in marriage and in its indissoluble unity the only setting worthy of truly responsible procreation.

2. DOES HETEROLOGOUS ARTIFICIAL FERTILIZATION CONFORM TO THE DIGNITY OF THE COUPLE AND TO THE TRUTH OF MARRIAGE?

Through IVF and ET and heterologous artificial insemination, human conception is achieved through the fusion of gametes of at least one donor other than the spouses who are united in marriage. *Heterologous artificial fertilization is contrary to the unity of marriage, to the dignity of the spouses, to the vocation proper to parents, and to the child's right to be conceived and brought into the world in marriage and from marriage.*[36]

Respect for the unity of marriage and for conjugal fidelity demands that the child be conceived in marriage; the bond existing between husband and wife accords the spouses, in an objective and inalienable manner, the exclusive right to become father and mother solely through each other.[37] Recourse to the gametes of a third person, in order to have sperm or ovum available, constitutes a violation of the reciprocal commitment of the spouses and a grave lack in regard to that essential property of marriage which is its unity.

Heterologous artificial fertilization violates the rights of the child; it deprives him of his filial relationship with his parental origins and can hinder the maturing of his personal identity. Furthermore, it offends the common vocation of the spouses who are called to fatherhood and motherhood: it objectively deprives conjugal fruitfulness of its unity and integrity; it brings about and manifests a rupture between genetic parenthood, gestational parenthood and responsibility for upbringing. Such damage to the personal relationships within the family has repercussions on civil society: what threatens the unity and stability of the family is a source of dissension, disorder and injustice in the whole of social life.

These reasons lead to a negative moral judgment concerning heterolo-

gous artificial fertilization: consequently fertilization of a married woman with the sperm of a donor different from her husband and fertilization with the husband's sperm of an ovum not coming from his wife are morally illicit. Futhermore, the artificial fertilization of a woman who is unmarried or a widow, whoever the donor may be, cannot be morally justified.

The desire to have a child and the love between spouses who long to obviate a sterility which cannot be overcome in any other way constitute understandable motivations; but subjectively good intentions do not render heterologous artificial fertilization conformable to the objective and inalienable properties of marriage or respectful of the rights of the child and of the spouses.

3. IS "SURROGATE"* MOTHERHOOD MORALLY LICIT?

No, for the same reasons which lead one to reject heterologous artificial fertilization: for it is contrary to the unity of marriage and to the dignity of the procreation of the human person.

Surrogate motherhood represents an objective failure to meet the obligations of maternal love, of conjugal fidelity and of responsible motherhood; it offends the dignity and the right of the child to be conceived, carried in the womb, brought into the world and brought up by his own parents; it sets up, to the detriment of families, a division between the physical, psychological and moral elements which constitute those families.

B

HOMOLOGOUS ARTIFICIAL FERTILIZATION

Since heterologous artificial fertilization has been declared unacceptable, the question arises of how to evaluate morally the process of homologous artificial fertilization: IVF and ET and artificial insemination between husband and wife. First a question of principle must be clarified.

* By "surrogate mother" the Instruction means:

a) the woman who carries in pregnancy an embryo implanted in her uterus and who is genetically a stranger to the embryo because it has been obtained through the union of the gametes of "donors". She carries the pregnancy with a pledge to surrender the baby once it is born to the party who commissioned or made the agreement for the pregnancy.

b) the woman who carries in pregnancy an embryo to whose procreation she has contributed the donation of her own ovum, fertilized through insemination with the sperm of a man other than her husband. She carries the pregnancy with a pledge to surrender the child once it is born to the party who commissioned or made the agreement for the pregnancy.

4. WHAT CONNECTION IS REQUIRED FROM THE MORAL POINT OF VIEW BETWEEN
PROCREATION AND THE CONJUGAL ACT?

a) The Church's teaching on marriage and human procreation
affirms the "inseparable connection, willed by God and unable to be
broken by man on his own initiative, between the two meanings of the
conjugal act: the unitive meaning and the procreative meaning. Indeed,
by its intimate structure, the conjugal act, while most closely uniting
husband and wife, capacitates them for the generation of new lives,
according to laws inscribed in the very being of man and of woman".[38]
This principle, which is based upon the nature of marriage and the
intimate connection of the goods of marriage, has well-known consequences on the level of responsible fatherhood and motherhood. "By
safeguarding both these essential aspects, the unitive and the procreative, the conjugal act preserves in its fullness the sense of true mutual
love and its ordination towards man's exalted vocation to
parenthood".[39]

The same doctrine concerning the link between the meanings of
the conjugal act and between the goods of marriage throws light on the
moral problem of homologous artificial fertilization, since "it is never
permitted to separate these different aspects to such a degree as positively to exclude either the procreative intention or the conjugal
relation".[40]

Contraception deliberately deprives the conjugal act of its openness to procreation and in this way brings about a voluntary dissociation of the ends of marriage. Homologous artificial fertilization, in
seeking a procreation which is not the fruit of a specific act of conjugal
union, objectively effects an analogous separation between the goods
and the meanings of marriage.

Thus, *fertilization is licitly sought when it is the result of a
"conjugal act which is per se suitable for the generation of children to
which marriage is ordered by its nature and by which the spouses become
one flesh".[41] But from the moral point of view procreation is deprived of its
proper perfection when it is not desired as the fruit of the conjugal act, that
is to say of the specific act of the spouses' union.*

b) The moral value of the intimate link between the goods of
marriage and between the meanings of the conjugal act is based upon
the unity of the human being, a unity involving body and spiritual
soul.[42] Spouses mutually express their personal love in the "language
of the body", which clearly involves both "spousal meanings" and
parental ones.[43] The conjugal act by which the couple mutually express
their self-gift at the same time expresses openness to the gift of life. It
is an act that is inseparably corporal and spiritual. It is in their bodies

and through their bodies that the spouses consummate their marriage and are able to become father and mother. In order to respect the language of their bodies and their natural generosity, the conjugal union must take place with respect for its openness to procreation; and the procreation of a person must be the fruit and the result of married love. The origin of the human being thus follows from a procreation that is "linked to the union, not only biological but also spiritual, of the parents, made one by the bond of marriage".[44] Fertilization achieved outside the bodies of the couple remains by this very fact deprived of the meanings and the values which are expressed in the language of the body and in the union of human persons.

c) Only respect for the link between the meanings of the conjugal act and respect for the unity of the human being make possible procreation in conformity with the dignity of the person. In his unique and irrepeatable origin, the child must be respected and recognized as equal in personal dignity to those who give him life. The human person must be accepted in his parents' act of union and love; the generation of a child must therefore be the fruit of that mutual giving[45] which is realized in the conjugal act wherein the spouses cooperate as servants and not as masters in the work of the Creator who is Love. [46]

In reality, the origin of a human person is the result of an act of giving. The one conceived must be the fruit of his parents' love. He cannot be desired or conceived as the product of an intervention of medical or biological techniques; that would be equivalent to reducing him to an object of scientific technology. No one may subject the coming of a child into the world to conditions of technical efficiency which are to be evaluated according to standards of control and dominion.

The moral relevance of the link between the meanings of the conjugal act and between the goods of marriage, as well as the unity of the human being and the dignity of his origin, demand that the procreation of a human person be brought about as the fruit of the conjugal act specific to the love between spouses. The link between procreation and the conjugal act is thus shown to be of great importance on the anthropological and moral planes, and it throws light on the positions of the Magisterium with regard to homologous artificial fertilization.

5. IS HOMOLOGOUS 'IN VITRO' FERTILIZATION MORALLY LICIT?

The answer to this question is strictly dependent on the principles just mentioned. Certainly one cannot ignore the legitimate aspirations of sterile couples. For some, recourse to homologous IVF and ET appears to be the only way of fulfilling their sincere desire for a child.

The question is asked whether the totality of conjugal life in such situations is not sufficient to ensure the dignity proper to human procreation. It is acknowledged that IVF and ET certainly cannot supply for the absence of sexual relations[47] and cannot be preferred to the specific acts of conjugal union, given the risks involved for the child and the difficulties of the procedure. But it is asked whether, when there is no other way of overcoming the sterility which is a source of suffering, homologous *in vitro* fertilization may not constitute an aid, if not a form of therapy, whereby its moral licitness could be admitted.

The desire for a child—or at the very least an openness to the transmission of life—is a necessary prerequisite from the moral point of view for responsible human procreation. But this good intention is not sufficient for making a positive moral evaluation of *in vitro* fertilization between spouses. The process of IVF and ET must be judged in itself and cannot borrow its definitive moral quality from the totality of conjugal life of which it becomes part nor from the conjugal acts which may precede or follow it. [48]

It has already been recalled that, in the circumstances in which it is regularly practised, IVF and ET involves the destruction of human beings, which is something contrary to the doctrine on the illicitness of abortion previously mentioned.[49] But even in a situation in which every precaution was taken to avoid the death of human embryos, homologous IVF and ET dissociates from the conjugal act the actions which are directed to human fertilization. For this reason the very nature of homologous IVF and ET also must be taken into account, even abstracting from the link with procured abortion.

Homologous IVF and ET is brought about outside the bodies of the couple through actions of third parties whose competence and technical activity determine the success of the procedure. Such fertilization entrusts the life and identity of the embryo into the power of doctors and biologists and establishes the domination of technology over the origin and destiny of the human person. Such a relationship of domination is in itself contrary to the dignity and equality that must be common to parents and children.

Conception *in vitro* is the result of the technical action which presides over fertilization. *Such fertilization is neither in fact achieved nor positively willed as the expression and fruit of a specific act of the conjugal union. In homologous IVF and ET, therefore, even if it is considered in the context of 'de facto' existing sexual relations, the generation of the human person is objectively deprived of its proper perfection: namely, that of being the result and fruit of a conjugal act* in which the spouses can become "cooperators with God for giving life to a new person".[50]

These reasons enable us to understand why the act of conjugal love is considered in the teaching of the Church as the only setting worthy of human procreation. For the same reasons the so-called "simple case", i.e. a homologous IVF and ET procedure that is free of any compromise with the abortive practice of destroying embryos and with masturbation, remains a technique which is morally illicit because it deprives human procreation of the dignity which is proper and connatural to it.

Certainly, homologous IVF and ET fertilization is not marked by all that ethical negativity found in extra-conjugal procreation; the family and marriage continue to constitute the setting for the birth and the upbringing of the children. Nevertheless, in conformity with the traditional doctrine relating to the goods of marriage and the dignity of the person, *the Church remains opposed from the moral point of view to homologous 'in vitro' fertilization. Such fertilization is in itself illicit and in opposition to the dignity of procreation and of the conjugal union, even when everything is done to avoid the death of the human embryo.*

Although the manner in which human conception is achieved with IVF and ET cannot be approved, every child which comes into the world must in any case be accepted as a living gift of the divine Goodness and must be brought up with love.

6. HOW IS HOMOLOGOUS ARTIFICIAL INSEMINATION TO BE EVALUATED FROM THE MORAL POINT OF VIEW?

Homologous artificial insemination within marriage cannot be admitted except for those cases in which the technical means is not a substitute for the conjugal act but serves to facilitate and to help so that the act attains its natural purpose.

The teaching of the Magisterium on this point has already been stated.[51] This teaching is not just an expression of particular historical circumstances but is based on the Church's doctrine concerning the connection between the conjugal union and procreation and on a consideration of the personal nature of the conjugal act and of human procreation. "In its natural structure, the conjugal act is a personal action, a simultaneous and immediate cooperation on the part of the husband and wife, which by the very nature of the agents and the proper nature of the act is the expression of the mutual gift which, according to the words of Scripture, brings about union 'in one flesh' ".[52] Thus moral conscience "does not necessarily proscribe the use of certain artificial means destined solely either to the facilitating of the natural act or to ensuring that the natural act normally performed achieves its proper end".[53] If the technical means facilitates the conjugal act or helps it to reach its natural objectives, it can be morally acceptable. If, on the other hand, the procedure were to replace the conjugal act, it is morally illicit.

Artificial insemination as a substitute for the conjugal act is prohibited by reason of the voluntarily achieved dissociation of the two meanings of the conjugal act. Masturbation, through which the sperm is normally obtained, is another sign of this dissociation: even when it is done for the purpose of procreation, the act remains deprived of its unitive meaning: "It lacks the sexual relationship called for by the moral order, namely the relationship which realizes 'the full sense of mutual self-giving and human procreation in the context of true love' ".[54]

7. WHAT MORAL CRITERION CAN BE PROPOSED WITH REGARD TO MEDICAL INTERVENTION IN HUMAN PROCREATION?

The medical act must be evaluated not only with reference to its technical dimension but also and above all in relation to its goal which is the good of persons and their bodily and psychological health. The moral criteria for medical intervention in procreation are deduced from the dignity of human persons, of their sexuality and of their origin.

Medicine which seeks to be ordered to the integral good of the person must respect the specifically human values of sexuality.[55] *The doctor is at the service of persons and of human procreation. He does not have the authority to dispose of them or to decide their fate.* A medical intervention respects the dignity of persons when it seeks to assist the conjugal act either in order to facilitate its performance or in order to enable it to achieve its objective once it has been normally performed".[56]

On the other hand, it sometimes happens that a medical procedure technologically replaces the conjugal act in order to obtain a procreation which is neither its result nor its fruit. In this case the medical act is not, as it should be, at the service of conjugal union but rather appropriates to itself the procreative function and thus contradicts the dignity and the inalienable rights of the spouses and of the child to be born.

The humanization of medicine, which is insisted upon today by everyone, requires respect for the integral dignity of the human person first of all in the act and at the moment in which the spouses transmit life to a new person. It is only logical therefore to address an urgent appeal to Catholic doctors and scientists that they bear exemplary witness to the respect due to the human embryo and to the dignity of procreation. The medical and nursing staff of Catholic hospitals and clinics are in a special way urged to do justice to the moral obligations which they have assumed, frequently also, as part of their contract. Those who are in charge of Catholic hospitals and clinics and who are often Religious will take special care to safeguard and promote a diligent observance of the moral norms recalled in the present Instruction.

8. THE SUFFERING CAUSED BY INFERTILITY IN MARRIAGE

The suffering of spouses who cannot have children or who are afraid of bringing a handicapped child into the world is a suffering that everyone must understand and properly evaluate.

On the part of the spouses, the desire for a child is natural: it expresses the vocation to fatherhood and motherhood inscribed in conjugal love. This desire can be even stronger if the couple is affected by sterility which appears incurable. Nevertheless, marriage does not confer upon the spouses the right to have a child, but only the right to perform those natural acts which are *per se* ordered to procreation.[57]

A true and proper right to a child would be contrary to the child's dignity and nature. The child is not an object to which one has a right, nor can he be considered as an object of ownership: rather, a child is a gift, "the supreme gift" [58] *and the most gratuitous gift of marriage, and is a living testimony of the mutual giving of his parents. For this reason, the child has the right, as already mentioned, to be the fruit of the specific act of the conjugal love of his parents; and he also has the right to be respected as a person from the moment of his conception.*

Nevertheless, whatever its cause or prognosis, sterility is certainly a difficult trial. The community of believers is called to shed light upon and support the suffering of those who are unable to fulfill their legitimate aspiration to motherhood and fatherhood. Spouses who find themselves in this sad situation are called to find in it an opportunity for sharing in a particular way in the Lord's Cross, the source of spiritual fruitfulness. Sterile couples must not forget that "even when procreation is not possible, conjugal life does not for this reason lose its value. Physical sterility in fact can be for spouses the occasion for other important services to the life of the human person, for example, adoption, various forms of educational work, and assistance to other families and to poor or handicapped children".[59]

Many researchers are engaged in the fight against sterility. While fully safeguarding the dignity of human procreation, some have achieved results which previously seemed unattainable. Scientists therefore are to be encouraged to continue their research with the aim of preventing the causes of sterility and of being able to remedy them so that sterile couples will be able to procreate in full respect for their own personal dignity and that of the child to be born.

III.

MORAL AND CIVIL LAW

THE VALUES AND MORAL OBLIGATIONS
THAT CIVIL LEGISLATION
MUST RESPECT AND SANCTION IN THIS MATTER

The inviolable right to life of every innocent human individual and the rights of the family and of the institution of marriage constitute fundamental moral values, because they concern the natural condition and integral vocation of the human person; at the same time they are constitutive elements of civil society and its order.

For this reason the new technological possibilities which have opened up in the field of biomedicine require the intervention of the political authorities and of the legislator, since an uncontrolled application of such techniques could lead to unforeseeable and damaging consequences for civil society. Recourse to the conscience of each individual and to the self-regulation of researchers cannot be sufficient for ensuring respect for personal rights and public order. If the legislator responsible for the common good were not watchful, he could be deprived of his prerogatives by researchers claiming to govern humanity in the name of the biological discoveries and the alleged "improvement" processes which they would draw from those discoveries. "Eugenism" and forms of discrimination between human beings could come to be legitimized: this would constitute an act of violence and a serious offense to the equality, dignity and fundamental rights of the human person.

The intervention of the public authority must be inspired by the rational principles which regulate the relationships between civil law and moral law. The task of the civil law is to ensure the common good of people through the recognition of and the defence of fundamental rights and through the promotion of peace and of public morality.[60] In no sphere of life can the civil law take the place of conscience or dictate norms concerning things which are outside its competence. It must sometimes tolerate, for the sake of public order, things which it cannot forbid without a greater evil resulting. However, the inalienable rights of the person must be recognized and respected by civil society and the political authority. These human rights depend neither on single individuals nor on parents; nor do they represent a concession made by society and the State: they pertain to human nature and are inherent in the person by virtue of the creative act from which the person took his or her origin.

Among such fundamental rights one should mention in this regard: *a*) every human being's right to life and physical integrity from the moment of conception until death; *b*) the rights of the family and of marriage as an institution and, in this area, the child's right to be conceived, brought into the world and brought up by his parents. To each of these two themes it is necessary here to give some further consideration.

In various States certain laws have authorized the direct suppression of innocents: the moment a positive law deprives a category of human beings of the protection which civil legislation must accord them, the State is denying the equality of all before the law. When the State does not place its power at the service of the rights of each citizen, and in particular of the more vulnerable, the very foundations of a State based on law are undermined. The political authority consequently cannot give approval to the calling of human beings into existence through procedures which would expose them to those very grave risks noted previously. The possible recognition by positive law and the political authorities of techniques of artificial transmission of life and the experimentation connected with it would widen the breach already opened by the legalization of abortion.

As a consequence of the respect and protection which must be ensured for the unborn child from the moment of his conception, the law must provide appropriate penal sanctions for every deliberate violation of the child's rights. The law cannot tolerate—indeed it must expressly forbid—that human beings, even at the embryonic stage, should be treated as objects of experimentation, be mutilated or destroyed with the excuse that they are superfluous or incapable of developing normally.

The political authority is bound to guarantee to the institution of the family, upon which society is based, the juridical protection to which it has a right. From the very fact that it is at the service of people, the political authority must also be at the service of the family. Civil law cannot grant approval to techniques of artificial procreation which, for the benefit of third parties (doctors, biologists, economic or governmental powers), take away what is a right inherent in the relationship between spouses; and therefore civil law cannot legalize the donation of gametes between persons who are not legitimately united in marriage.

Legislation must also prohibit, by virtue of the support which is due to the family, embryo banks, *post mortem* insemination and "surrogate motherhood".

It is part of the duty of the public authority to ensure that the civil law is regulated according to the fundamental norms of the moral law in matters concerning human rights, human life and the institution of the family. Politicians must commit themselves, through their interventions upon public opinion, to securing in society the widest possible consensus on such essential points and to consolidating this consensus wherever it risks being weakened or is in danger of collapse.

In many countries, the legalization of abortion and juridical tolerance of unmarried couples makes it more difficult to secure respect for the fundamental rights recalled by this Instruction. It is to be hoped that States will not become responsible for aggravating these socially damaging situations of injustice. It is rather to be hoped that nations and States will realize all the cultural, ideological and political implications connected with the techniques of artificial procreation and will find the wisdom and courage necessary for issuing laws which are more just and more respectful of human life and the institution of the family.

The civil legislation of many states confers an undue legitimation upon certain practices in the eyes of many today; it is seen to be incapable of guaranteeing that morality which is in conformity with the natural exigencies of the human person and with the "unwritten laws" etched by the Creator upon the human heart. All men of good will must commit themselves, particularly within their professional field and in the exercise of their civil rights, to ensuring the reform of morally unacceptable civil laws and the correction of illicit practices. In addition, "conscientious objection" vis-à-vis such laws must be supported and recognized. A movement of passive resistance to the legitimation of practices contrary to human life and dignity is beginning to make an ever sharper impression upon the moral conscience of many, especially among specialists in the biomedical sciences.

Conclusion

The spread of technologies of intervention in the processes of human procreation raises very serious moral problems in relation to the respect due to the human being from the moment of conception, to the dignity of the person, of his or her sexuality, and of the transmission of life.

With this Instruction the Congregation for the Doctrine of the Faith, in fulfilling its responsibility to promote and defend the Church's teaching in so serious a matter, addresses a new and heartfelt invitation to all those who, by reason of their role and their commitment, can exercise a positive influence and ensure that, in the family and in society, due respect is accorded to life and love. It addresses this invitation to those responsible for the formation of consciences and of public opinion, to scientists and medical professionals, to jurists and politicians. It hopes that all will understand the incompatibility between recognition of the dignity of the human person and contempt for life and love, between faith in the living God and the claim to decide arbitrarily the origin and fate of a human being.

In particular, the Congregation for the Doctrine of the Faith addresses an invitation with confidence and encouragement to theologians, and above all to moralists, that they study more deeply and make ever more accessible to the faithful the contents of the teaching of the Church's Magisterium in the light of a valid anthropology in the matter of sexuality and marriage and in the context of the necessary interdisciplinary approach. Thus they will make it possible to understand ever more clearly the reasons for and the validity of this teaching. By defending man against the excesses of his own power, the Church of God reminds him of the reasons for his true nobility; only in this way can the possibility of living and loving with that dignity and liberty which derive from respect for the truth be ensured for the men and women of tomorrow. The precise indications which are offered in the present Instruction therefore are not meant to halt the effort of reflection but rather to give it a renewed impulse in unrenounceable fidelity to the teaching of the Church.

In the light of the truth about the gift of human life and in the light of the moral principles which flow from that truth, everyone is invited to act in the area of responsibility proper to each and, like the good Samaritan, to recognize as a neighbour even the littlest among the children of men (Cf. *Lk* 10:29-37). Here Christ's words find a new and particular echo: "What you do to one of the least of my brethren, you do unto me" (*Mt* 25:40).

NOTES

1. POPE JOHN PAUL II, *Discourse to those taking part in the 81st Congress of the Italian Society of Internal Medicine and the 82nd Congress of the Italian Society of General Surgery*, 27 October 1980: *AAS* 72 (1980) 1126.

2. POPE PAUL VI, *Discourse to the General Assembly of the United Nations Organization*, 4 October 1965: *AAS* 57 (1965) 878; Encyclical *Populorum Progressio*, 13: *AAS* 59 (1967) 263.

3. POPE PAUL VI, *Homily during the Mass closing the Holy Year*, 25 December 1975: *AAS* 68 (1976) 145; POPE JOHN PAUL II, Encyclical *Dives in Misericordia*, 30: *AAS* 72 (1980) 1224.

4. Pope John Paul II, *Discourse to those taking part in the 35th General Assembly of the World Medical Association*, 29 October 1983: *AAS* 76 (1984) 390.

5. Cf. Declaration *Dignitatis Humanae*, 2.

6. Pastoral Constitution *Gaudium et Spes*, 22; Pope John Paul II, Encyclical *Redemptor Hominis*, 8: *AAS* 71 (1979) 270-272.

7. Cf. Pastoral Constitution *Gaudium et Spes*, 35.

8. Pastoral Constitution *Gaudium et Spes*, 15; cf. also Pope Paul VI, Encyclical *Populorum Progressio*, 20: *AAS* 59 (1967) 267; Pope John Paul II, Encyclical *Redemptor Hominis*, 15: *AAS* 71 (1979) 286-289; Apostolic Exhortation *Familiaris Consortio*, 8: *AAS* 74 (1982) 89.

9. Pope John Paul II, Apostolic Exhortation *Familiaris Consortio*, 11: *AAS* 74 (1982) 92.

10. Cf. Pope Paul VI, Encyclical *Humanae Vitae*, 10: *AAS* 60 (1968) 487-488.

11. Pope John Paul II, *Discourse to the members of the 35th General Assembly of the World Medical Association*, 29 October 1983: *AAS* 76 (1984) 393.

12. Cf. Pope John Paul II, Apostolic Exhortation *Familiaris Consortio*, 11: *AAS* 74 (1982) 91-92; cf. also Pastoral Constitution *Gaudium et Spes*, 50.

13. Sacred Congregation for the Doctrine of the Faith, *Declaration on Procured Abortion*, 9, *AAS* 66 (1974) 736-737.

14. Pope John Paul II, *Discourse to those taking part in the 35th General Assembly of the World Medical Association*, 29 October 1983: *AAS* 76 (1984) 390.

15. Pope John XXIII, Encyclical *Mater et Magistra*, III: *AAS* 53 (1961) 447.

16. Pastoral Constitution *Gaudium et Spes*, 24.

17. Cf. Pope Pius XII, Encyclical *Humani Generis: AAS* 42 (1950) 575; Pope Paul VI. *Professio Fidei: AAS* 60 (1968) 436.

18. Pope John XXIII, Encyclical *Mater et Magistra*, III: *AAS* 53 (1961) 447; cf. Pope John Paul II, *Discourse to priests participating in a seminar on "Responsible Procreation"*, 17 September 1983, *Insegnamenti di Giovanni Paolo II*, VI, 2 (1983) 562: "At the origin of each human person there is a creative act of God: no man comes into existence by chance; he is always the result of the creative love of God".

19. Cf. Pastoral Constitution *Gaudium et Spes*, 24.

20. Cf. Pope Pius XII, *Discourse to the Saint Luke Medical-Biological Union*, 12 November 1944: *Discorsi e Radiomessagi* VI (1944-1945) 191-192.

21. Cf. Pastoral Constitution *Gaudium et Spes*, 50.

22. Cf. Pastoral Constitution *Gaudium et Spes,* 51: "When it is a question of harmonizing married love with the responsible transmission of life, the moral character of one's behaviour does not depend only on the good intention and the evaluation of the motives: the objective criteria must be used, criteria drawn from the nature of the human person and human acts, criteria which respect the total meaning of mutual self-giving and human procreation in the context of true love".

23. Pastoral Constitution *Gaudium et Spes,* 51.

24. Holy See, *Charter of the Rights of the Family,* 4: *L'Osservatore Romano,* 25 November 1983.

25. Sacred Congregation for the Doctrine of the Faith, *Declaration on Procured Abortion,* 12-13: *AAS* 66 (1974) 738.

26. Cf. Pope Paul VI, *Discourse to participants in the Twenty-third National Congress of Italian Catholic Jurists,* 9 December 1972: *AAS* 64 (1972) 777.

27. The obligation to avoid disproportionate risks involves an authentic respect for human beings and the uprightness of therapeutic intentions. It implies that the doctor "above all ... must carefully evaluate the possible negative consequences which the necessary use of a particular exploratory technique may have upon the unborn child and avoid recourse to diagnostic procedures which do not offer sufficient guarantees of their honest purpose and substantial harmlessness. And if, as often happens in human choices, a degree of risk must be undertaken, he will take care to assure that it is justified by a truly urgent need for the diagnosis and by the importance of the results that can be achieved by it for the benefit of the unborn child himself" (Pope John Paul II, *Discourse to Participants in the Pro-Life Movement Congress,* 3 December 1982: *Insegnamenti di Giovanni Paolo II,* V, 3 [1982] 1512). This clarification concerning "proportionate risk" is also to be kept in mind in the following sections of the present Instruction, whenever this term appears.

28. Pope John Paul II, *Discourse to the Participants in the 35th General Assembly of the World Medical Association,* 29 October 1983: *AAS* 76 (1984) 392.

29. Cf. Pope John Paul II, *Address to a Meeting of the Pontifical Academy of Sciences,* 23 October 1982: *AAS* (1983) 37: "I condemn, in the most explicit and formal way, experimental manipulations of the human embryo, since the human being, from conception to death, cannot be exploited for any purpose whatsoever".

30. Holy See, *Charter of the Rights of the Family,* 4b: *L'Osservatore Romano,* 25 November 1983.

31. Cf. Pope John Paul II, *Address to the Participants in the Convention of the Pro-Life Movement,* December 1982: *Insegnamenti di Giovanni Paolo II,* V, 3 (1982) 1511: "Any form of experimentation on the foetus that may damage its integrity or worsen its condition is unacceptable, except in the case of a final effort to save it from death". Sacred Congregation for the Doctrine of the Faith, *Declaration on Euthanasia,* 4: *AAS* 72 (1980) 550: "In the absence of other sufficient remedies, it is permitted, with the patient's consent, to have recourse to the means provided by the most advanced medical techniques, even if these means are still at the experimental stage and are not without a certain risk".

32. No one, before coming into existence, can claim a subjective right to begin to exist; nevertheless, it is legitimate to affirm the right of the child to have a fully human origin through conception in conformity with the personal nature of the human being. Life is a gift that must be bestowed in a manner worthy both of the subject receiving it and of the subjects transmitting it. This statement is to be borne in mind also for what will be explained concerning artificial human procreation.

33. Cf. Pope John Paul II, *Discourse to those taking part in the 35th General Assembly of the World Medical Association,* 29 October 1983: *AAS* 76 (1984) 391.

34. Cf. Pastoral Constitution on the Church in the Modern World, *Gaudium et Spes,* 50.

35. Cf. Pope John Paul II, Apostolic Exhortation *Familiaris Consortio,* 14: *AAS* 74 (1982) 96.

36. Cf. Pope Pius XII, *Discourse to those taking part in the 4th International Congress of Catholic Doctors,* 29 September 1949: *AAS* 41 (1949) 559. According to the plan of the Creator, "A man leaves his father and his mother and cleaves to his wife, and they become one flesh" (*Gen* 2:24). The unity of marriage, bound to the order of creation, is a truth accessible to natural reason. The Church's Tradition and Magisterium frequently make reference to the Book of Genesis, both directly and through the passages of the New Testament that refer to it: *Mt* 19:4-6; *Mk* 10:5-8; *Eph* 5:31. Cf. Athenagoras, *Legatio pro christianis, 33: PG* 6,965-967; St Chrysostom, *In Matthaeum homiliae,* LXII, 19, 1: *PG* 58 597; St Leo the Great, *Epist. ad Rusticum, 4: PL* 54, 1204; Innocent III, Epist. *Gaudemus in Domino: DS* 778; Council of Lyons II, *IV Session: DS* 860; Council of Trent, XXIV *Session: DS* 1798. 1802; Pope Leo XIII, Encyclical *Arcanum Divinae Sapientiae: ASS* 12 (1879/80) 388-391; Pope Pius XI, Encyclical *Casti Connubii: AAS* 22 (1930) 546-547; Second Vatican Council, *Gaudium et Spes,* 48; Pope John Paul II, Apostolic Exhortation *Familiaris Consortio,* 19: *AAS* 74 (1982) 101-102; *Code of Canon Law,* Can. 1056.

37. CF. Pope Pius XII, *Discourse to those taking part in the 4th International Congress of Catholic Doctors,* 29 September 1949: *AAS* 41 (1949) 560: *Discourse to those taking part in the Congress of the Italian Catholic Union of Midwives,* 29 October 1951: *AAS* 43 (1951) 850; *Code of Canon Law,* Can. 1134.

38. Pope Paul VI, Encyclical Letter *Humanae Vitae,* 12: *AAS* 60 (1968) 488-489.

39. *Loc. cit, ibid.,* 489.

40. Pope Pius XII, *Discourse to those taking part in the Second Naples World Congress on Fertility and Human Sterility,* 19 May 1956: *AAS* 48 (1956) 470.

41. *Code of Canon Law,* Can. 1061. According to this Canon, the conjugal act is that by which the marriage is consummated if the couple "have performed (it) between themselves in a human manner".

42. Cf. Pastoral Constitution *Gaudium et Spes,* 14.

43. Cf. POPE JOHN PAUL II, *General Audience on 16 January 1980: Insegnamenti di Giovanni Paolo II,* III, 1 (1980) 148-152.

44. POPE JOHN PAUL II, *Discourse to those taking part in the 35th General Assembly of the World Medical Association,* 29 October 1983: *AAS* 76 (1984) 393.

45. Cf. Pastoral Constitution *Gaudium et Spes,* 51.

46. Cf. Pastoral Constitution *Gaudium et Spes,* 50.

47. Cf. POPE PIUS XII, *Discourse to those taking part in the 4th International Congress of Catholic Doctors,* 29 September 1949: *AAS* 41 (1949) 560: "It would be erroneous ... to think that the possibility of resorting to this means (artificial fertilization) might render valid a marriage between persons unable to contract it because of the *impedimentum impotentiae''.*

48. A similar question was dealt with by POPE PAUL VI, Encyclical *Humanae Vitae,* 14: *AAS* 60 (1968) 490-491.

49. Cf. *supra:* I, 1 ff.

50. POPE PAUL II, Apostolic Exhortation *Familiaris Consortio,* 14: *AAS* 74 (1982) 96.

51. Cf. *Response of the Holy Office,* 17 March 1897: *DS* 3323; POPE PIUS XII, *Discourse to those taking part in the 4th International Congress of Catholic Doctors,* 29 September 1949: *AAS* 41 (1949) 560; *Discourse to the Italian Catholic Union of Midwives,* 29 October 1951: *AAS* 43 (1951) 850; *Discourse to those taking part in the Second Naples World Congress on Fertility and Human Sterility,* 19 May 1956: *AAS* 48 (1956) 471-473; *Discourse to those taking part in the 7th International Congress of the International Society of Haematology,* 12 September 1958: *AAS* 50 (1958) 733; POPE JOHN XXIII, Encyclical *Mater et Magistra,* III: *AAS* 53 (1961) 447.

52. POPE PIUS XII, *Discourse to the Italian Catholic Union of Midwives,* 29 October 1951: *AAS* 43 (1951) 850.

53. POPE PIUS XII, *Discourse to those taking part in the 4th International Congress of Catholic Doctors,* 29 September 1949: *AAS* 41 (1949) 560.

54. SACRED CONGREGATION FOR THE DOCTRINE OF THE FAITH, *Declaration on Certain Questions Concerning Sexual Ethics,* 9: *AAS* 68 (1976) 86, which quotes the Pastoral Constitution *Gaudium et Spes,* 51. Cf. *Decree of the Holy Office,* 2 August 1929: *AAS* 21 (1929) 490; POPE PIUS XII, *Discourse to those taking part in the 26th Congress of the Italian Society of Urology,* 8 October 1953: *AAS* 45 (1953) 678.

55. Cf. POPE JOHN XXIII, Encyclical *Mater et Magistra,* III: *AAS* 53 (1961) 447.

56. Cf. POPE PIUS XII, *Discourse to those taking part in the 4th International Congress of Catholic Doctors,* 29 September 1949: *AAS* 41 (1949), 560.

57. Cf. POPE PIUS XII, *Discourse to those taking part in the Second Naples World Congress on Fertility and Human Sterility,* 19 May 1956: *AAS* 48 (1956) 471-473.

58. Pastoral Constitution *Gaudium et Spes*, 50.

59. Pope John Paul II, Apostolic Exhortation *Familiaris Consortio*, 14: *AAS* 74 (1982) 97.

60. Cf. Declaration *Dignitatis Humanae*, 7.